*Study Guide for*

# Fundamentals of Nursing

## The Art and Science of Person-Centered Care

*Study Guide for*

# Fundamentals of Nursing

## The Art and Science of Person-Centered Care

**Ninth Edition**

**Marilee LeBon, BA**
Editor/Writer
Brigantine, New Jersey

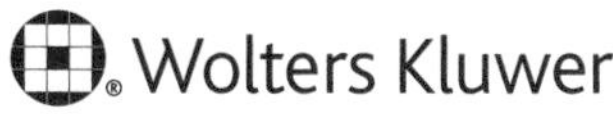

Philadelphia • Baltimore • New York • London
Buenos Aires • Hong Kong • Sydney • Tokyo

*Vice President and Publisher:* Julie K. Stegman
*Director of Product Development:* Jennifer K. Forestieri
*Acquisitions Editor:* Natasha McIntyre
*Development Editor:* Kelly Horvath
*Editorial Coordinators:* Emily Buccieri, Lindsay Ries
*Marketing Manager:* Brittany Clements
*Production Project Manager:* Linda Van Pelt
*Design Coordinator:* Holly McLaughlin
*Manufacturing Coordinator:* Karin Duffield
*Prepress Vendor:* Aptara, Inc.

9th edition



Printed in the United States

ISBN: 9781496382542



LWW.com

# Preface

Marilee LeBon, in close consultation with the authors of the ninth edition of *Fundamentals of Nursing: The Art and Science of Person-Centered Care*, has carefully developed this Study Guide. We recognize that beginning students in nursing must learn an enormous amount of information and skills in a short period of time. The Study Guide is structured to help you integrate the knowledge you have gained and begin to apply it to the practice of nursing. To help you accomplish this goal, the following types of exercises are provided in each chapter of the Study Guide.

## ASSESSING YOUR UNDERSTANDING

These exercises group similar types of questions together to help you learn the information in a variety of formats. The types of questions included follow the same format in each Study Guide chapter, but not every type of question is used in each chapter. The format includes:

- Identification Questions
- Fill in the Blanks
- Matching Exercises
- Correct the False Statements
- Short Answer

## APPLYING YOUR KNOWLEDGE

These questions challenge you to reflect on the critical thinking and blended skills developed in the classroom and apply them to your own practice of the *art and science of person-centered nursing care.*

- Critical Thinking Questions: these questions offer an exciting and practical means to challenge the assumptions you bring to nursing and to "stretch" your application of new theoretical concepts.
- Reflective Practice: Cultivating QSEN Competencies: these exercises offer opportunities to use your critical thinking ability and knowledge of blended skills to respond to real-life scenarios, similar to those that may occur in your practice.
- Patient Care Studies: these studies in the clinical nursing care chapters provide a unique opportunity for you to "encounter" an actual patient and to use the nursing process to assess and diagnose the patient's nursing needs and brainstorm ways to best meet these needs.

## PRACTICING FOR NCLEX

*Multiple Choice Questions:* Each chapter contains a section of multiple choice questions presented in the NCLEX-RN exam format.
*Alternate-Format Questions:* The alternate-format-style questions for the NCLEX-RN exam include the types of questions described below. Several of these types are provided in each chapter to help you become familiar with this NCLEX format. They are:

- Multiple Response Questions: questions with a detailed stem that require you to select more than one correct answer.
- Prioritization Questions: questions with a detailed stem that require you to place the options provided in the correct order.
- Hot Spot Questions: questions that require you to identify a specific area on an illustration or a graph.
- Chart/Exhibit Questions: multiple choice questions with a detailed stem that require

you to review information in a chart or an exhibit in order to select the correct answer.

## ANSWER KEY

The answers to the Assessing Your Understanding, Reflective Practice, Patient Care Study, and Practicing for NCLEX questions are included in the Answer Key at the back of the book so that you can immediately assess your own learning as you complete each chapter.

The nursing diagnoses used in this book are from T. Heather Herdman and Shigemi Kamitsuru (Eds.), NANDA International, Inc. *Nursing Diagnoses: Definitions and Classification 2018-2020*, Eleventh Edition © 2017 NANDA International, ISBN 978-1-62623-929-6. Used by arrangement with the Thieme Group, Stuttgart/New York. To make safe and effective judgments using NANDA-I nursing diagnoses, it is essential that nurses refer to the definitions and defining characteristics of the diagnoses listed in the Appendix found on thePoint.

The authors and Wolters Kluwer hope you find this Study Guide to be helpful and enjoyable, and we wish you every success as you begin the exciting journey toward becoming a nurse.

# Contents

CHAPTER 1

# Introduction to Nursing

## ASSESSING YOUR UNDERSTANDING

### FILL IN THE BLANKS

1. The ICN, founded in 1899, was the first international organization of professional women.
2. Founded in the late 1800s, the ANA is a professional organization for registered nurses in the United States.
3. The ANA's 2015 Scope & standards of practice defines the activities of nurses that are specific and unique to nursing.
4. nurse Practice acts are laws established in each state in the United States to regulate the practice of nursing.
5. One of the major guidelines for nursing practice, the nursing Process, integrates both the art and science of nursing and allows nurses to implement their roles.

### CORRECT THE FALSE STATEMENTS

***Circle the word "true" or "false" that follows the statement. If you circled "false," change the underlined word or words to make the statement true. Place your answer in the space provided.***

1. Nursing (QSEN) competencies include nurse-centered care, teamwork and collaboration, quality improvement, safety, evidence-based practice, and informatics.
   a. True
   b. False patient-Centered Care
2. The ANA defines continuing education as those professional development experiences designed to enrich the nurse's contribution to health.
   a. True
   b. False ________
3. The legal authority to practice nursing is termed professional standards.
   a. True
   b. False licensure
4. When a nurse completes a diploma, associate degree, or baccalaureate program, he or she becomes licensed as a licensed practical nurse.
   a. True
   b. False RN
5. In early civilizations influenced by the theory of animism, the roles of health care provider and nurse were interchangeable.
   a. True
   b. False distinct & Separate
6. The Doctor of Nursing Practice (DNP) degree is designed for nurses seeking a terminal degree in nursing practice and offers an alternative approach to research-focused doctoral programs.
   a. True
   b. False ________
7. All nursing actions focus on the orders of the health care provider.
   a. True
   b. False the Patient

8. Practical nursing was developed to prepare nurses to give bedside nursing care to patients.
   a. True
   b. False ______

9. When the major goals of health care—promoting, maintaining, or restoring health—can no longer be met, the nurse's duties are terminated.
   a. True
   b. False ______

10. Nursing has evolved through history from a technical service to a knowledge-centered process that allows maximizing of human potential.
    a. True
    b. False ______

## SHORT ANSWER

***Nursing has been defined in many ways, but there are essential elements present in most thoughtful perspectives. Use your own words to expand the following short definitions of nursing.***

1. Nursing is caring. ______

2. Nursing is sharing. ______

3. Nursing is touching. ______

4. Nursing is feeling. ______

5. Nursing is listening. ______

6. Nursing is accepting. ______

7. Nursing is respecting. ______

8. Give an example in which a nurse may incorporate the following broad aims of nursing into a nursing care plan for a patient who is undergoing diagnostic tests for lung cancer and who smokes two packs of cigarettes a day.
   a. Promoting health: ______
   b. Preventing illness: ______
   c. Restoring health: ______
   d. Facilitating coping: ______

9. List the criteria that define the following concepts:
   a. A profession: ______
   b. A discipline: ______

10. The National League for Nursing (NLN) recently identified 10 trends to watch for nursing education (Heller, Oros, & Durneey-Crowley, 2000). Describe how these trends are affecting nursing in transition:
    a. Changing demographics and increasing diversity: ______
    b. Technologic explosion: ______
    c. Globalization of the world's economy and society: ______

**d.** The era of the educated consumer, alternative therapies and genomics, and palliative care: ______________________

______________________

**e.** Shift to population-based care and the increasing complexity of patient care:

______________________

______________________

**f.** The cost of health care and the challenge of managed care: ______________________

______________________

**g.** Impact of health policy and regulation:

______________________

______________________

**h.** The growing need for interdisciplinary education for collaborative practice:

______________________

______________________

**i.** The current nursing shortage and opportunities for life-long learning and workforce development: ______________________

______________________

**j.** Significant advances in nursing science and research: ______________________

______________________

**11.** Give an example of a nursing action that might be performed by a nurse relying on the following four competencies:

**a.** Cognitive skills: ______________________

**b.** Technical skills: ______________________

**c.** Interpersonal skills: ______________________

**d.** Ethical/legal skills: ______________________

**12.** Complete the following table with the correct word or phrase to differentiate among the nursing roles that are listed.

| Title | Education/Preparation | Role Description |
|---|---|---|
| *Example:* Nurse researcher | Advanced degree | Conducts research relevant to practice and education |
| Clinical nurse specialist | | |
| Nurse midwife | | |
| Nurse practitioner | | |
| Nurse anesthetist | | |
| Nurse administrator | | |
| Nurse entrepreneur | | |
| Nurse educator | | |

## APPLYING YOUR KNOWLEDGE

### CRITICAL THINKING QUESTIONS

1. Think of nursing situations in which the nurse involved promoted each of nursing's aims.
   a. Describe an instance of each.
      Promoting health
      Preventing illness
      Restoring health
      Facilitating coping
   b. Describe the factors that might warrant a particular nursing aim in each case.
   c. How would you evaluate whether your nursing aims were successful?
2. Research a historical figure in nursing whom you respect and admire. Write a nursing philosophy that best expresses his or her nursing goals. Then interview a modern-day nurse about his or her nursing philosophy. Note how the two philosophies are similar or different. Form your own nursing philosophy based on your results.

### REFLECTIVE PRACTICE: CULTIVATING QSEN COMPETENCIES

***Use the following expanded scenario from Chapter 1 in your textbook to answer the questions below.***

*Scenario:* Roberto Pecorini is a 38-year-old man diagnosed with metastatic colon cancer. Having undergone radiation treatments and chemotherapy, he is extremely weak and malnourished. He is receiving intravenous fluids via a central venous catheter. He has two pressure injuries on his sacrum, each approximately 2 cm in diameter, requiring wound care. He also has a colostomy that he cannot care for independently. His wife is distraught and tells the nurse that she has two children at home under the age of 5 and is worried about caring for them and her husband at the same time.

1. What basic human needs should the nurse address to provide individualized, holistic care for the Pecorini family?

______________________________

______________________________

______________________________

2. What would be a successful outcome for this patient?

______________________________

______________________________

______________________________

3. What intellectual, technical, interpersonal, and/or ethical/legal competencies are most likely to bring about the desired outcome?

______________________________

______________________________

______________________________

4. What resources might be helpful for the Pecorini family?

______________________________

______________________________

______________________________

## PRACTICING FOR NCLEX

### MULTIPLE CHOICE QUESTIONS

***Circle the letter that corresponds to the best answer for each question.***

1. A nurse practicing in the early Christian period might perform which nursing action characteristic of this era?
   a. Carrying out menial tasks based on the orders of the priest–health care provider
   b. Making organized visits to the sick
   c. Providing physical care and herbal remedies to the mother of a family
   d. Providing nursing care in lieu of serving a jail sentence
2. Florence Nightingale was a nursing pioneer who challenged prejudices against women and elevated the status of all nurses. Which statement describes one of her accomplishments?
   a. She established the fact that nursing is the same as medicine.
   b. She promoted adding nursing education as part of a medical degree.
   c. She established the tenets of the American Red Cross.
   d. She promoted the publication of books about nursing and health care.

3. A nurse educator is discussing the role of nursing based on the American Nurses Association (ANA). Which statement **best** describes this role?
   a. Nursing is a profession dependent upon the medical community as a whole.
   b. It is the role of the health care provider, not the nurse, to assist patients in understanding their health problems.
   c. It is the role of nursing to provide a caring relationship that facilitates health and healing.
   d. The essential components of professional nursing care are strength, endurance, and cure.
4. A nurse is providing care for patients in a long-term care facility. Based on the definitions of nursing in the textbook, what should be the central focus of this care?
   a. The nursing actions provided by the nurse
   b. The patient receiving the care
   c. The nurse as the caregiver
   d. Nursing as a profession
5. A nurse is helping a patient on hospice make an informed decision about his own health and life. Which nursing role has this nurse performed?
   a. Advocate
   b. Counselor
   c. Caregiver
   d. Communicator
6. A person practicing nursing in the 1950s would most likely have been influenced by what trend?
   a. Large numbers of women began to work outside the home, asserting their independence.
   b. Nursing practice was broadened to include practice in a wide variety of health care settings.
   c. Male dominance in the health care profession slowed the progress of professionalism in the nursing practice.
   d. Hospital schools were established to provide more easily controlled and less expensive staff for the hospital.
7. A nurse manager is teaching staff how to use a new piece of hospital equipment. What educational setting would be most appropriate for this process?
   a. Continuing education
   b. Graduate education
   c. In-service education
   d. Undergraduate studies
8. A nurse completes a nursing degree at a local community college in 2 years. This nurse has completed what type of nursing education program?
   a. Diploma in nursing
   b. Associate degree in nursing
   c. Baccalaureate degree in nursing
   d. Graduate education in nursing
9. A nurse identifies a patient's health care needs and devises a care plan to meet those needs. Which guideline is being followed in this case?
   a. Nursing standards
   b. Nursing orders
   c. Nurse practice acts
   d. Nursing process

## ALTERNATE-FORMAT QUESTIONS

### Multiple Response Questions

***Circle the letters that correspond to the best answers for each question.***

1. Which nursing actions demonstrate the aim of nursing to promote health? *(Select all that apply.)*
   a. Increasing student awareness of sexually transmitted diseases by distributing informational pamphlets at a college health center
   b. Performing diagnostic measurements and examinations in an outpatient setting
   c. Serving as a role model of health for patients by maintaining a healthy weight
   d. Helping a person with paraplegia learn how to use a wheelchair
   e. Facilitating decisions about lifestyles that would enhance the well-being of a teenager
   f. Administering an insulin shot to a diabetic patient

2. Which nursing actions demonstrate the aim of nursing to facilitate coping? *(Select all that apply.)*
   a. Teaching a class on the nutritional needs of pregnant women
   b. Changing the bandages of a patient who has undergone heart surgery
   c. Teaching a patient and his/her family how to live with diabetes
   d. Assisting a patient and his/her family to prepare for death
   e. Starting an intravenous line for a malnourished older adult patient
   f. Providing counseling for the family of a teenager with an eating disorder
3. A nurse educator is teaching students the criteria that define nursing as a profession. Which nursing actions are based on these criteria? *(Select all that apply.)*
   a. A nurse accesses a well-defined body of specific and unique knowledge to plan nursing care for patients.
   b. A nurse performs actions based on the standards of performance determined by the medical community.
   c. A nurse follows an established code of ethics when performing actions for hospice patients.
   d. A nurse is committed to using ongoing research when planning nursing care for patients.
   e. A nurse graduate applies for selective membership in the ANA.
   f. A nurse independently chooses nursing interventions for a patient and uses self-regulation to ensure they are performed properly.
4. A nurse applies for membership in a professional nursing organization that is operating in the United States. To which organizations might this nurse apply? *(Select all that apply.)*
   a. ANA
   b. NNO
   c. ICN
   d. AACN
   e. NASN
   f. ANO
5. A newly hired nurse consults the nurse practice act affecting her new facility. What are examples of the realm of authority of a nurse practice act? *(Select all that apply.)*
   a. Defining the legal scope of nursing practice
   b. Enforcing federally regulated nursing legislation
   c. Excluding untrained and unlicensed people from practicing nursing
   d. Enforcing rules and regulations defined by the nurse practice act
   e. Establishing the criteria for the education and licensure of nurses
   f. Defining legal requirements and titles for RNs and LPNs
6. A graduate nurse applies for a nursing license in Pennsylvania. Which actions are examples of the jurisdiction of the licensing board? *(Select all that apply.)*
   a. Allowing graduates of approved schools of nursing to take the NCLEX
   b. Authorizing nurses to practice nursing in any state
   c. Licensing nurses during the lifetime of the holder
   d. Denying licensing due to criminal actions
   e. Protecting nurses from being suspended for professional misconduct
   f. Issuing special licenses to nurses practicing in long-term care facilities

**Prioritization Questions**

1. The role of medicine developed from the precivilization era, through the eras signifying the beginning of civilization, the beginning of the 16th century, the 18th and 19th centuries, and the World War II era to the present. Place the events that defined these eras listed below in the correct chronologic order to follow this timeline.
   a. An explosion of knowledge in medicine and technology occurred.
   b. Focus on religion was replaced by a focus on warfare, exploration, and expansion of knowledge.
   c. Belief in good and evil spirits bringing health or illness existed; medicine men were health care providers.

**d.** Hospital schools were organized; female nurses were under control of male hospital administrators and health care providers; males dominated the health care setting.

**e.** Varied health care settings developed.

**f.** Temples were the centers of medical care; belief that illness is caused by sin and the displeasure of the gods existed; priests were health care providers.

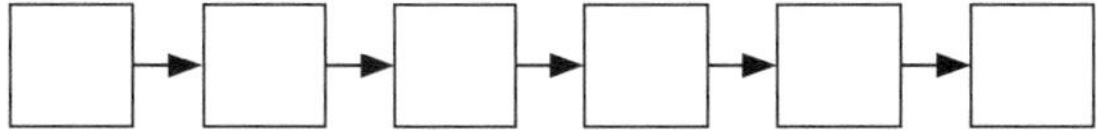

**2.** The role of the nurse developed from the pre-civilization era, through the eras signifying the beginning of civilization, the beginning of the 16th century, the 18th and 19th centuries, and the World War II era to the present. Place the following roles of the nurse listed below in the correct chronologic order to follow this timeline.

**a.** There was a shortage of nurses; criminals were recruited as nurses; nursing was viewed as disreputable.

**b.** Nursing was broadened in all areas and was practiced in a wide variety of settings; nursing was viewed as a profession.

**c.** Nurses were portrayed as mothers, caring for family and delivering physical care and health remedies.

**d.** Nurses were viewed as slaves, carrying out menial tasks based on the orders of the priest.

**e.** Florence Nightingale elevated nursing to a respected occupation and founded modern methods in nursing education.

**f.** Efforts were made to upgrade nursing education, and women were more assertive and independent.

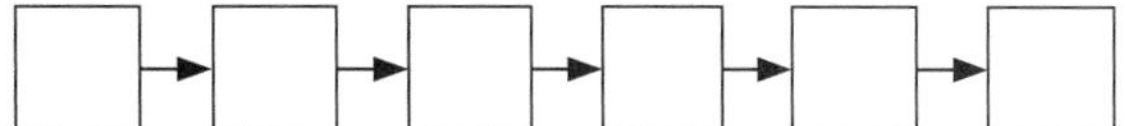

CHAPTER 2

# Theory, Research, and Evidence-Based Practice

## ASSESSING YOUR UNDERSTANDING

### FILL IN THE BLANKS

1. ____________ research involves the concepts of basic and applied research.
2. ____________ are abstract impressions organized into symbols of reality.
3. The ____________ theory describes the process by which living matter adjusts to other living things and to environmental conditions.
4. ____________ is the patient's right to agree knowledgeably, to participate in a study without coercion, or to refuse to participate without jeopardizing the care he or she will receive.
5. ____________ is provided nursing care that is supported by reliable research-based evidence.

### MATCHING EXERCISES

***Match the term in Part A with the correct definition listed in Part B.***

**PART A**

**a.** Adaptation theory
**b.** General systems theory
**c.** Philosophy
**d.** Concept
**e.** Theory
**f.** Process
**g.** Developmental theory
**h.** Nursing theory
**i.** System
**j.** Knowledge system

**PART B**

____ **1.** The action phase of a conceptual framework; a series of actions, changes, or functions that bring about a desired goal

____ **2.** The study of wisdom, fundamental knowledge, and the processes used to develop and construct our perceptions of life

____ **3.** A set of interacting elements, all serving the common purpose of contributing to an overall goal

____ **4.** Differentiates nursing from other disciplines and activities in that it serves the purposes of describing, explaining, predicting, and controlling desired outcomes of nursing care practices

____ **5.** Abstract impressions from the environment organized into symbols of reality; describes objects, properties, and events and the relationships among them

____ **6.** A statement that explains or characterizes an action, occurrence, or event that is based on observed facts but lacks absolute or direct proof

____ 7. Emphasizes relationships between the whole and the parts and describes how parts function and behave

____ 8. Defines a continuously occurring process that effects change and involves interaction and response

____ 9. Outlines human growth as a predictable and orderly process beginning with conception and ending with death

**SHORT ANSWER**

1. Nursing theories are often based on, and influenced by, other broadly applicable processes and theories. Briefly describe the ideas and principles of the following theories that are basic to many nursing concepts.

   a. General systems theory: ____________

   b. Adaptation theory: ____________

   c. Developmental theory: ____________

2. List four basic characteristics of nursing theories:

   a. ____________

   b. ____________

   c. ____________

   d. ____________

3. Explain how the following factors have influenced the nursing profession.

   a. Cultural influences on nursing: ____________

   b. Educational influences on nursing: ____________

   c. Research and publishing in nursing: ____________

   d. Improved communication in nursing: ____________

   e. Improved autonomy of nursing: ____________

4. List four reasons that nursing research develops knowledge according to the National Institute of Nursing Research (NINR):

   a. ____________

   b. ____________

   c. ____________

   d. ____________

5. Which nursing theorist(s) best defines your own personal beliefs about nursing practice and why?

   ____________

## APPLYING YOUR KNOWLEDGE

**CRITICAL THINKING QUESTIONS**

1. Describe how three different theories of nursing would direct the nursing care (identification and management of health/nursing needs) of the family described here: A 15-year-old girl who self-mutilates by cutting is admitted to the psychiatric ward for evaluation. Her family is anxious about her behavior and worried about her prognosis. A teacher who reported the incident is close to the girl and asks to speak to the attending health care provider.

2. Write the theories discussed in this chapter on a piece of paper, along with a brief description of their basic tenets (refer to Table 2-2 in the textbook). Interview your faculty, nurses you know, and classmates and have them rank the theories in order of importance based on their own system of beliefs. Ask the participants to give you an example of their personal philosophy that they would like to incorporate into their nursing practice. Note which theory was most widely respected and determine its value to your own practice.

### REFLECTIVE PRACTICE: CULTIVATING QSEN COMPETENCIES

***Use the following expanded scenario from Chapter 2 in your textbook to answer the questions below.***

*Scenario:* Charlotte Horn, the daughter of a 57-year-old patient being discharged with an order for intermittent nasogastric tube feedings, is being taught how to perform the procedure. During one of the teaching sessions, Charlotte asks several questions: "How will I know the tube is in the right place? Will someone be available if I have a problem inserting the tube? What can I do to keep my mother comfortable with this tube in her?"

1. How might the nurse respond to Ms. Horn's concerns regarding the care of her mother?

_______________________________________

_______________________________________

_______________________________________

2. What would be a successful outcome for this patient?

_______________________________________

_______________________________________

_______________________________________

3. What intellectual, technical, interpersonal, and/or ethical/legal competencies are most likely to bring about the desired outcome?

_______________________________________

_______________________________________

_______________________________________

4. What resources might be helpful for Ms. Horn?

_______________________________________

_______________________________________

_______________________________________

## PRACTICING FOR NCLEX

### MULTIPLE CHOICE QUESTIONS

***Circle the letter that corresponds to the best answer for each question.***

1. A nurse researcher is studying female patients who have survived breast cancer. The nurse asks each patient to describe her experience and then analyzes the data for the meaning of the experience within each person's own reality. This nurse has used what type of qualitative research method?
   a. Phenomenology
   b. Grounded theory
   c. Ethnography
   d. Historical

2. A nurse observes that the past five patients referred from a certain community clinic have been treated for drug and/or alcohol overdose. Based on this information, the nurse assumes that the clinic specializes in the treatment of substance abuse. This is an example of what type of reasoning?
   a. Inductive reasoning
   b. Nursing process
   c. Deductive reasoning
   d. General systems theory

3. A nursing theorist examines a hospital environment by studying each ward and how it works individually and then relating this information to the hospital as a whole working entity. This is an example of the use of what theory?
   a. Adaptation theory
   b. Developmental theory
   c. General systems theory
   d. Psychosocial theory

4. A nursing theorist studies health care systems in communities. Which statement accurately describes a characteristic of these systems?
   a. The system is an entity in itself and cannot communicate with or react to its environment.
   b. Boundaries separate health care systems both from each other and from the environment.
   c. The system is closed in that it does not allow energy, matter, or information to move between it and its boundaries.
   d. The system is independent of its subsystems in that a change in one element does not affect the whole.

5. A nurse who works in a pediatric practice assesses the developmental level of children of various ages to determine their psychosocial development. These assessments are based on the work of:
   a. Erikson
   b. Maslow
   c. Watson
   d. Rogers

6. Nurses on a busy hospital ward plan nursing care for patients. Which nursing action best exemplifies the primary focus of nursing?
   a. The nurse adjusts the environment of the patient to facilitate provision of care.
   b. The nurse concentrates on the health status of a patient.
   c. The nurse focuses on the procedures being performed for patients that day.
   d. The nurse comforts a patient who received bad results from a test.

7. A nurse providing care for patients has a personal philosophy that nursing interventions should be instituted for patients when they demonstrate ineffective adaptive responses. This nurse's philosophy is based on the theory of:
   a. Imogene M. King
   b. Madeleine Leininger
   c. Sister Callista Roy
   d. Jean Watson

8. A nurse caring for patients in a hospital setting focuses on ill patients as the center of all nursing activities performed daily. The nurse also provides care based on helping patients to adapt to the hospital environment. This nurse is following the principles of:
   a. Florence Nightingale
   b. Myra E. Levine
   c. Martha Rogers
   d. Dorothea Orem

## ALTERNATE-FORMAT QUESTIONS

### Multiple Response Questions

***Circle the letters that correspond to the best answers for each question.***

1. A nurse is writing an article for a nursing journal describing a study of the emergency protocols in a hospital emergency department. Which statements accurately describe elements of this process? *(Select all that apply.)*
   a. The abstract summarizes the article and is found at the end of the article.
   b. The introduction reviews the literature and states the purpose of the article.
   c. The method section provides details of how the study was conducted.
   d. The results are often presented in words, charts, tables, or graphs.
   e. The discussion provides details about the subjects, design, and data collection.
   f. The references are listed at the beginning and include articles and books used.

2. A nurse is using the quantitative research process to study the cause of healthcare-associated infections and how to prevent them. Which actions are examples of the components of this process? *(Select all that apply.)*
   a. The nurse collects data from subjects in the study.
   b. The nurse defines the purpose of the study after conclusions have been made.
   c. The nurse formulates a hypothesis and variables in the study.
   d. The nurse uses instruments to determine the variables in the study.
   e. The nurse uses grounded theory to discover the beliefs of the subjects.
   f. The nurse formulates an abstract to state the relationship between the variables.

3. Nurse researchers use both quantitative and qualitative research in their practices. Which actions are examples of the use of qualitative research? *(Select all that apply.)*
   a. The nurse examines nursing issues related to the Native American patient.
   b. The nurse investigates past nursing trends to understand the current profession.
   c. The nurse examines the effect of nursing interventions on patient outcomes.
   d. The nurse examines cause-and-effect relationships between variables in a lab.
   e. The nurse discovers how people describe the effect of illness in their lives.
   f. The nurse explores events in real-life situations to generate new knowledge.
4. A nurse manager is attempting to switch the medical records in an orthopedic office to a computerized format. The nurse asks questions about the accuracy and efficiency of the current record keeping system by using the PICOT format. Which statements illustrate the components of this process?
   a. P: The nurse purchases computers from a computer store.
   b. P: The nurse chooses the population involved (orthopedic patients).
   c. I: The nurse considers interventions to make the plan work.
   d. C: The nurse compares the written records to the computerized records.
   e. O: The nurse determines the occurrence of problems in the systems.
   f. T: The nurse finishes comparing the records and evaluates the outcome.

**Prioritization Question**

1. A nurse researcher is using the steps of the quantitative research process to study the impact of managed care on the U.S. health care system. Place the following steps of this process in the order in which they would be performed.
   a. The nurse defines the purpose of the study.
   b. The nurse develops a plan to find answers to the questions of the study.
   c. The nurse publishes the research in the *American Journal of Nursing.*
   d. The nurse uses statistical procedures to analyze the data found.
   e. The nurse states the research problem.
   f. The nurse reviews the literature already published on the topic.
   g. The nurse formulates a hypothesis and defines the variables in the study.
   h. The nurse selects the group to be studied and specific samples to use for data.
   i. The nurse collects the data using interviews, questionnaires, and examinations.

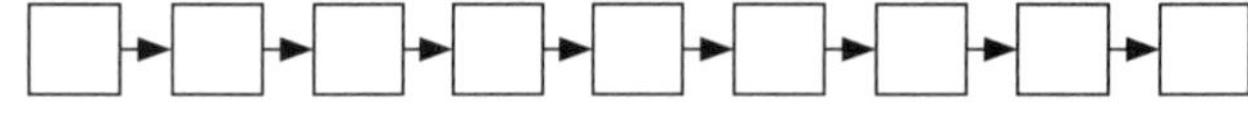

CHAPTER 3

# Health, Wellness, and Health Disparities

## ASSESSING YOUR UNDERSTANDING

### FILL IN THE BLANKS

1. ____________ is a medical term meaning that there is a pathologic change in the structure or function of the body or mind.
2. Arthritis is an example of a(n) ____________ illness.
3. A(n) ____________ illness generally has a rapid onset of symptoms and lasts only a relatively short time.
4. The reappearance of symptoms of a chronic disease in a patient who has been in remission is known as a period of ____________.
5. A landscaper's increased risk for developing skin cancer because of excessive exposure to the sun is considered a(n) ____________ risk factor.

### MATCHING EXERCISES

***Match the risk factors listed in Part A with their appropriate examples listed in Part B. Answers may be used more than once.***

#### PART A

**a.** Age
**b.** Genetic composition
**c.** Physiologic factors
**d.** Health habits
**e.** Lifestyle
**f.** Environment

#### PART B

____ **1.** A mother and her school-aged child are concerned about increasing gang-related violence in their neighborhood.

____ **2.** A teenager who is a new driver is admitted to the emergency room with multiple fractures after wrecking his car.

____ **3.** A woman with multiple sex partners tests positive for HIV.

____ **4.** A woman is worried about breast cancer because it "runs in the family."

____ **5.** An overweight executive presents with high blood pressure.

____ **6.** An alcoholic man develops a liver abscess.

____ **7.** A patient tells you his father died of colon cancer.

____ **8.** A smoker develops a chronic cough.

____ **9.** A toddler presents with a mild concussion following a fall.

____ **10.** A pregnant woman has toxemia in her 5th month.

____ **11.** A 40-year-old man has a father and brother who died of heart attacks at an early age.

____ **12.** An older adult fractures a hip and ankle bone when falling down a flight of stairs in his home.

***Match the model of health and illness listed in Part A with the correct definition in Part B.***

**PART A**

**a.** Agent–host–environment model
**b.** Health belief model
**c.** Health–illness continuum
**d.** High-level wellness model
**e.** Health promotion model

**PART B**

____ **13.** This model views health as a constantly changing state, with high-level wellness and death being on opposite ends of a graduated scale.

____ **14.** Halbert Dunn's model of health is based on a person functioning to maximum potential while maintaining balance and a purposeful direction in the environment.

____ **15.** This model, developed by Leavell and Clark for use in community health, is helpful for examining the causes of disease in a person by looking at and understanding risk factors.

____ **16.** Rosenstock's model of health is based on three components of disease perception: (1) perceived susceptibility to a disease, (2) perceived seriousness of a disease, and (3) perceived benefits of action.

____ **17.** This model, developed by Pender, illustrates the multidimensional nature of people interacting with their environment as they pursue health.

## SHORT ANSWER

**1.** Describe how your own self-concept has been influenced by the following factors:

**a.** Interpersonal interactions: ____________________

____________________

____________________

**b.** Physical and cultural influences: ____________________

____________________

____________________

**c.** Education: ____________________

____________________

____________________

**d.** Illness: ____________________

____________________

____________________

**2.** Compare and contrast the two types of illnesses listed below:

**a.** Acute illness: ____________________

____________________

____________________

**b.** Chronic illness: ____________________

____________________

____________________

**3.** Describe where you personally fit on the health–illness continuum and why:

____________________

____________________

**4.** List two examples of nursing actions that would be performed at each of the following levels of health promotion and illness prevention.

**a.** Primary health promotion: ____________________

____________________

____________________

**b.** Secondary health promotion: ____________________

____________________

____________________

**c.** Tertiary health promotion: ____________________

____________________

____________________

5. Describe Dunn's processes (high-level wellness health model) that are a part of each person's perception of his or her own wellness state and help that person know who and what he or she is.
   a. Being: ____________________
   b. Belonging: ____________________
   c. Becoming: ____________________
   d. Befitting: ____________________

## APPLYING YOUR KNOWLEDGE

### CRITICAL THINKING QUESTIONS

1. Identify and compare the factors affecting the health and illness of the following patients:
   a. A 39-year-old pregnant woman who has been in good health throughout her pregnancy is admitted to the obstetrics unit for vaginal bleeding in her 16th week of pregnancy. Her husband is at her bedside.
   b. A 20-year-old woman in her 23rd week of pregnancy, who is addicted to crack cocaine, is brought to the emergency room by her boyfriend. She is having contractions.
   c. Determine the nurse's role in assisting these patients and their families.
2. Interview two patients: one who has recently experienced an acute illness and one who is chronically ill. Identify the individual health risk factors, basic human needs, and self-concepts of each patient. Explore and compare the different ways acute and chronic illnesses affect patients and their families.

### REFLECTIVE PRACTICE: CULTIVATING QSEN COMPETENCIES

***Use the following expanded scenario from Chapter 3 in your textbook to answer the questions below.***

***Scenario:*** Ruth Jacobi is a 62-year-old woman who was hospitalized after a "mini-stroke." While hospitalized, she was prescribed medication for high blood pressure and was referred to a smoking cessation support group. She has now returned to her pre-event level of functioning and is being prepared for discharge. She says, "I know I have an increased risk for a major stroke, so I want to do everything possible to stay as active and healthy as I can."

1. How might the nurse respond to Ms. Jacobi's stated desire for a higher level of wellness?
2. What would be a successful outcome for this patient?
3. What intellectual, technical, interpersonal, and/or ethical/legal competencies are most likely to bring about the desired outcome?
4. What resources might be helpful for Ms. Jacobi?

## PRACTICING FOR NCLEX

### MULTIPLE CHOICE QUESTIONS

*Circle the letter that corresponds to the best answer for each question.*

1. A nurse is immunizing children against measles. This is an example of what level of preventive care?
   a. Primary
   b. Secondary
   c. Tertiary
2. A nurse refers an HIV-positive patient to a local support group. This is an example of what level of preventive care?
   a. Primary
   b. Secondary
   c. Tertiary
3. A nurse is caring for a patient who has breast cancer. The patient tells the nurse: "I don't know why this happened to me, but I'm ready to move on and do whatever I need to do to get healthy again." This patient is in which stage of acute illness?
   a. Stage 1
   b. Stage 2
   c. Stage 3
   d. Stage 4
4. A nurse is caring for a patient who has COPD, a chronic illness of the lungs. The patient is in remission. Which statement best describes a period of remission in a patient with a chronic illness?
   a. The symptoms of the illness reappear.
   b. The disease is no longer present.
   c. New symptoms occur at this time.
   d. Symptoms are not experienced.
5. A nurse observes that a patient who has pneumonia is in the recovery and rehabilitation stage of the illness. What statement describes the patient response that the nurse would expect at this stage of the illness?
   a. The patient gives up the dependent role.
   b. The patient assumes a dependent role.
   c. The patient seeks medical attention.
   d. The patient recognizes symptoms of illness.
6. Nurses promote the needs of patients as an integral part of each person's human dimension. Which needs are being met when a nurse recommends a senior citizen community center for an older adult who is living alone?
   a. Spiritual needs
   b. Sociocultural needs
   c. Intellectual needs
   d. Emotional needs

### ALTERNATE-FORMAT QUESTIONS

#### Multiple Response Questions

*Circle the letters that correspond to the best answers for each question.*

1. A hospital nurse assesses patients in various stages of illness. Which statements accurately describe patient responses to illness based on Suchman's stages of illness? *(Select all that apply.)*
   a. In stage 1, the person defines himself or herself as being sick, seeks validation of this experience from others, and gives up normal activities.
   b. In stage 2, most people focus on their symptoms and bodily functions.
   c. When help from a health care provider is sought, the person becomes a patient and enters stage 3, assuming a dependent role.
   d. When a patient decides to accept a diagnosis and follow a prescribed treatment plan, he or she is in stage 4, achieving recovery and rehabilitation.
   e. In stage 1, pain is the most significant symptom indicating illness, although other symptoms, such as a rash, fever, bleeding, or cough, may be present.
   f. Most patients complete the final stage of illness behavior in the hospital or a long-term care setting.
2. A nurse provides interventions for patients in a long-term care facility to help them meet their intellectual needs. Which nursing actions promote these needs? *(Select all that apply.)*
   a. A nurse provides patient teaching about foot care to a diabetic patient.
   b. A nurse manager shuts down a cafeteria to investigate cases of food poisoning.

**c.** A nurse refers a patient experiencing dysfunctional grief to a grief counselor.

**d.** A nurse explains to an obese patient the benefits of following a healthy diet.

**e.** A nurse shows residents a video discussing modified activities for older adults.

**f.** A nurse sets up a pet therapy program for the residents.

**3.** The nurse is using Leavell and Clark's Agent–Host–Environment Health Model to help plan nursing interventions for patients in a hospital setting. Which examples of nursing actions to prevent healthcare-associated infections (HAIs) in these patients best illustrate the principles of this model? *(Select all that apply.)*

**a.** The nurse should assess the patients for risk factors for infection when planning nursing care.

**b.** The nurse should assess patients' ability to fight off infection by using a graduated scale with high-level wellness on one end and death on the other.

**c.** The nurse should consider the patients' family history and age when assessing risk factors for infection.

**d.** The nurse should consider patients' past behavior when determining goals for recovery.

**e.** The nurse should assess what the patients believe to be true about themselves and their illnesses when developing a nursing plan to prevent HAIs.

**f.** The nurse should examine environmental stressors in patients' lives to see how they might affect their recovery and ability to ward off infection.

**4.** A nurse is performing health promotion activities for patients at a local health care clinic. Which nursing actions exemplify the focus of secondary preventive care? *(Select all that apply.)*

**a.** Scheduling immunizations for a child

**b.** Teaching parents about child safety in the home

**c.** Performing range-of-motion exercises on a patient

**d.** Screening patients for hypertension

**e.** Scheduling a mammogram for a patient

**f.** Referring a patient to family counseling

### Chart/Exhibit Questions

***Refer to the chart below and identify the type of human dimension(s) represented by the examples listed.***

| Human Dimensions | Basic Human Needs | Examples |
|---|---|---|
| Physical dimension | Physiologic needs | Circulation |
| Environmental dimension | Safety and security needs | Climate |
| Sociocultural dimension | Love and belonging needs | Support systems |
| Emotional | Self-esteem needs | Loneliness dimension |
| Intellectual and spiritual dimension | Self-actualization needs | Values |

**1.** An older adult must live with and control his diabetes. ___________

**2.** Worried about losing his job, a 35-year-old executive exacerbates his ulcer. ___________

**3.** The mother of a toddler must learn how to childproof her house. ___________

**4.** An older woman has a raised toilet seat installed in her bathroom. ___________

**5.** A homeless man does not seek treatment for pneumonia. ___________

**6.** A Catholic woman refuses treatment for cancer and arranges a pilgrimage to a holy site where miraculous cures have been recorded by her religious leaders. ___________

**7.** A 15-year-old pregnant woman must learn how to care for her baby when it is born. ___________

**8.** A woman with rheumatoid arthritis improves her mobility with the use of pain medications. ___________

CHAPTER 4

# Health of the Individual, Family, and Community

## ASSESSING YOUR UNDERSTANDING

### FILL IN THE BLANKS

1. The most essential of all basic human needs is ___________.
2. According to Maslow's hierarchy of basic human needs, physical activity and rest are considered to be ___________ needs.
3. Relatives such as aunts, uncles, and grandparents are part of what is known as the ___________ family.
4. The function of the family that helps a family member meet his or her basic needs by providing emotional comfort and helping to establish and maintain an identity in times of stress is ___________.
5. The number and availability of health care institutions and services would be considered a(n) ___________ risk factor.

### MATCHING EXERCISES

***Match the correct risk factor category listed in Part A with the appropriate example of family risks listed in Part B. Answers may be used more than once.***

**PART A**

**a.** Lifestyle

**b.** Psychosocial

**c.** Developmental

**d.** Environmental

**e.** Biologic

**PART B**

____ **1.** A child with severe birth defects is born into a family.

____ **2.** A teacher reports to a teenage boy's parents that drugs have been found in his locker.

____ **3.** A recently divorced single parent of a 2-year-old must return to work but cannot afford adequate childcare.

____ **4.** Two families are forced to live together in cramped conditions to make ends meet.

____ **5.** Families in a city ghetto area fear walking to school/work because of gang activity on their street.

____ **6.** An older adult living with her son's family cannot tolerate what she feels is inadequate discipline of her grandchildren.

____ **7.** A mother returns home from the hospital with a premature baby for whom she must provide care.

____ **8.** A 13-year-old in her first trimester of pregnancy tells you she didn't think she could become pregnant the first time she had sexual relations.

____ **9.** A family vacationing in Mexico becomes ill after drinking the local water.

____ **10.** An older adult who lives alone cannot afford his prescriptions.

____ **11.** A couple learns that their infant has sickle cell anemia.

____ **12.** A 5-year-old girl accuses her uncle of touching her inappropriately.

____ **13.** A 3-month-old infant fails to thrive because of malnutrition.

____ **14.** A woman whose mother died of breast cancer finds a lump in her breast during her monthly breast examination.

## SHORT ANSWER

**1.** Give an example of the following family functions and explain how each meets the needs of individual family members and society as a whole.

**a.** Physical: ____________________

**b.** Economic: ____________________

**c.** Reproductive: ____________________

**d.** Affective and coping: ____________________

**e.** Socialization: ____________________

**2.** A first-time mother-to-be is taken to the surgical unit for an emergency cesarean birth. Her husband is standing nearby with a look of confusion and apprehension on his face. Give an example of how each of the following basic needs can be met by the nurse in caring for this couple.

**a.** Physiologic needs: ____________________

**b.** Safety and security needs: ____________________

**c.** Love and belonging needs: ____________________

**d.** Self-esteem needs: ____________________

**e.** Self-actualization needs: ____________________

**3.** List three types of families you have dealt with in your life experience. Describe how each family differs from one another. Which families do you feel have been most effective in preparing their members to meet individual, family, and community needs? Explain your choices.

**a.** ____________________

**b.** ____________________

**c.** ____________________

4. List typical questions that should be part of a family assessment.

______________________________________

______________________________________

______________________________________

______________________________________

______________________________________

______________________________________

5. Describe the provisions of the Patient Protection and Affordable Care Act (PPACA), often referred to as the Affordable Care Act.

______________________________________

______________________________________

## APPLYING YOUR KNOWLEDGE

### CRITICAL THINKING QUESTIONS

1. Volunteer some of your time at a local homeless shelter or any other service-oriented organization. Identify the individual immediate and long-term needs of the people served. List each of these needs in order of importance. What can be done to help promote health in these people? Explain how you could attempt to provide the following basic needs for the people served:
   a. Physiologic needs
   b. Safety and security needs
   c. Love and belonging needs
   d. Self-esteem needs
   e. Self-actualization needs
2. Review the lifestyles of some of the characters in your favorite TV dramas. Identify their risk factors and give an example of a character at risk for each of the following:
   a. Lifestyle
   b. Social/psychological
   c. Environmental
   d. Biologic

   Describe an appropriate nursing response for each example noted above.

### REFLECTIVE PRACTICE: CULTIVATING QSEN COMPETENCIES

***Use the following expanded scenario from Chapter 4 in your textbook to answer the questions below.***

***Scenario:*** Samuel Kaplan is an 80-year-old man who walks with a cane after recent knee surgery. His wife, aged 76 years, was diagnosed with Alzheimer's disease 1 year ago. The couple has no family living nearby, but a son lives with his wife and children about 200 miles away. After it is suggested that his wife be admitted to a long-term care facility, Mr. Kaplan breaks into tears and says, "I don't think I can continue to care for my wife at home anymore. But how can I even consider putting her in a nursing home?"

1. What basic human needs should be addressed by the nurse to provide individualized, holistic care for Mr. Kaplan?

______________________________________

______________________________________

______________________________________

2. What would a successful outcome be for this patient?

______________________________________

______________________________________

______________________________________

3. What intellectual, technical, interpersonal, and/or ethical/legal competencies are most likely to bring about the desired outcome?

______________________________________

______________________________________

______________________________________

4. What resources might be helpful for Mr. Kaplan?

______________________________________

______________________________________

______________________________________

______________________________________

## PRACTICING FOR NCLEX

### MULTIPLE CHOICE QUESTIONS

***Circle the letter that corresponds to the best answer for each question.***

1. A nurse is caring for a 78-year-old male patient who has been hospitalized following a stroke. Which nursing action has the highest priority for this patient?
   a. Ensuring that the patient has family and friends visit him
   b. Helping the patient to fill out an advanced directives form
   c. Finding a safe environment for the patient upon discharge
   d. Measuring the patient's I&O during recovery
2. A nurse is working at a community clinic that serves mostly families with young children. What would be a priority intervention for patients in this developmental stage?
   a. Setting up parenting classes
   b. Providing alcohol and drug information
   c. Screening for congenital defects
   d. Providing sex education
3. A nurse is caring for an adolescent who lost a leg in a motor vehicle accident. Which human need would the nurse most likely need to address?
   a. Love and belonging needs
   b. Safety and security needs
   c. Self-actualization needs
   d. Self-esteem needs
4. A home health care nurse who works in a low-income community assesses the risk factors for patients being serviced. What is an example of a community risk factor?
   a. A woman finds out that she is genetically inclined to develop crippling arthritis.
   b. An 80-year-old man is at risk for falls in his home due to clutter in his hallways and stairways.
   c. Children are kept inside the home on a sunny summer day because of lack of recreational opportunities.
   d. A child is born with severe intellectual disability.

### ALTERNATE-FORMAT QUESTIONS

#### Multiple Response Questions

***Circle the letters that correspond to the best answers for each question.***

1. Priority nursing interventions are geared to meeting the physiologic needs of patients. What are examples of physiologic needs according to Maslow's hierarchy of needs? *(Select all that apply.)*
   a. A nurse washes her hands and puts on gloves before inserting a catheter in a patient.
   b. A nurse invites a patient's estranged son to visit him.
   c. A nurse counsels an overweight teenager about proper nutrition.
   d. A nurse administers pain medication to a postoperative patient.
   e. A nurse attains a master's degree in nursing by going to school in the evening.
   f. A home care practitioner requests a quiet environment so her older adult patient can get some rest.
2. Once physiologic needs are met, nurses can concentrate on meeting self-actualization needs of patients. What are examples of self-actualization needs according to Maslow's hierarchy of needs? *(Select all that apply.)*
   a. A nurse attains a master's degree in nursing by going to school in the evening.
   b. A nurse refers a patient's spouse to an Al-Anon group meeting.
   c. A student nurse takes a course in communication to improve her ability to relate to patients.
   d. A nurse raises the side rails on the bed of a patient at risk for falls.
   e. A nurse administers insulin to a patient with diabetes.
   f. A nurse subscribes to several nursing journals to stay abreast of developments in the profession.

3. A nurse is providing family-centered care to patients in a community health care clinic. Which statements about the family unit are accurate? *(Select all that apply.)*
   a. According to Friedman, Bowden, and Jones (2003), the members of a group home would not be considered a family.
   b. The family is a buffer between the needs of individual members and society.
   c. The family should not be concerned with meeting the needs of society.
   d. Duvall (1985) identified critical family developmental tasks and stages in the family life cycle.
   e. The nuclear family is composed of two parents and their children.
   f. A blended family exists when parents adopt a child from another culture.
4. A nurse is caring for a family consisting of three middle-aged adults. Which examples describe developmental tasks of this type of family structure? *(Select all that apply.)*
   a. The family must adjust to the cost of family life.
   b. The family must maintain ties with younger and older generations.
   c. The family must prepare for retirement.
   d. The family must adjust to loss of spouse.
   e. The family must support moral and ethical family values.
   f. The family must cope with loss of energy and privacy.

**Prioritization Question**

1. A nurse is prioritizing care for patients in a hospital setting. Place the following examples of interventions to meet human needs in order from highest-level needs to lower-level needs based on Maslow's hierarchy:
   a. A nurse includes family members in the care of a patient.
   b. A nurse places a No Smoking sign on the door of a patient who is receiving oxygen.
   c. A nurse provides nutrition for a patient through a feeding tube.
   d. A nurse prepares a room for a clerical visit requested by a patient.
   e. A nurse helps a patient focus on her strengths following a diagnosis of breast cancer.

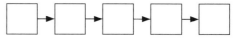

CHAPTER 5

# Cultural Diversity

## ASSESSING YOUR UNDERSTANDING

### FILL IN THE BLANKS

1. Nurses work in a local community clinic within the larger health care system. The clinic is considered a(n) ___________ of the larger cultural group.
2. Hispanics living in a neighborhood of a large city maintain their own language and cultural practices. This sense of identification that a cultural group has collectively, based on the group's common heritage, is known as its ___________.
3. A nurse believes that her patient care practices are better than those of other nurses. This idea that one's own ideas, practices, and beliefs are superior to, or are preferred to, those of others is termed ___________.
4. ___________ occurs when a nurse ignores differences in the cultures of patients and proceeds as though they do not exist.
5. A nurse who practiced nursing in Puerto Rico immigrates to the United States. The psychological feelings this nurse might experience when practicing in this different, strange culture is termed culture ___________.
6. A nurse assumes that all Native American patients use a shaman for healing practices. This is an example of ___________.

### MATCHING EXERCISES

***Match the cultural group listed in Part A with common health problems occurring in these populations listed in Part B. Answers may be used more than once.***

**PART A**

**a.** Native Americans and Alaska Natives
**b.** African Americans
**c.** Asians
**d.** Hispanics
**e.** Whites
**f.** Eastern European Jews

**PART B**

____ **1.** Sickle cell anemia
____ **2.** Cancer of the liver
____ **3.** Breast cancer
____ **4.** Cystic fibrosis
____ **5.** Fetal alcohol syndrome
____ **6.** Obesity
____ **7.** Keloids
____ **8.** Gaucher's disease
____ **9.** Tay–Sachs' disease
____ **10.** Thalassemia

### SHORT ANSWER

1. Describe how you would advise impoverished patients who are not meeting their health care needs due to the following conditions:
   a. Lack of transportation to clinic, hospital, or health care provider's office:
   ______________________________
   ______________________________
   b. Living in overcrowded conditions; absence of running water and adequate sanitation:
   ______________________________
   ______________________________
   c. Lack of health insurance:
   ______________________________
   ______________________________
2. Using the *Transcultural Assessment: Health-Related Beliefs and Practices* located in your textbook, assess the health-related beliefs of a patient of a different culture. How do this patient's beliefs differ from yours? What nursing actions could you take to help this patient express and practice his or her beliefs?
   Patient, culture, and medical condition: ______
   ______________________________
   ______________________________
   Health-related beliefs: ______________
   ______________________________
   ______________________________
   How my beliefs differ: ______________
   ______________________________
   ______________________________
   Nursing actions for patient: ___________
   ______________________________
   ______________________________
3. Explain why the following groups of people are at high risk for living in poverty.
   a. Families headed by single women: ________
   ______________________________
   ______________________________
   b. Older adults: ______________
   ______________________________
   ______________________________
   c. Future generations of those now in poverty:
   ______________________________
   ______________________________
4. List five characteristics often found in people living within the culture of poverty.
   a. ______________________________
   b. ______________________________
   c. ______________________________
   d. ______________________________
   e. ______________________________

## APPLYING YOUR KNOWLEDGE

### CRITICAL THINKING QUESTIONS

1. How would you respond to the individual nursing needs of the following patients?
   a. A Jewish man refuses to let a female nurse perform a nursing history and asks for a male doctor to examine him instead.
   b. A girl, age 13, delivers her first baby. She tells you she had an abortion earlier but is ready for this new baby.
   c. A man who speaks limited English brings his grandfather (who speaks no English) to the emergency room. The grandfather presents with the warning signs of a myocardial infarction.
2. Interview a fellow classmate you have not yet met about his or her cultural background. Ask him or her what cultural practices are important at home as well as how his or her culture might influence his or her beliefs about health care.

### REFLECTIVE PRACTICE: CULTIVATING QSEN COMPETENCIES

***Use the following expanded scenario from Chapter 5 in your textbook to answer the questions below.***

***Scenario:*** Danielle Dorvall, a 45-year-old Haitian woman, has been in the United States for approximately 8 months. She recently had a surgical repair of a fractured femur and is now confined to bed in skeletal traction. When the nurse appears to change Ms. Dorvall's dressings, she asks that a Haitian folk healer from her neighborhood be allowed to come to the hospital to help heal her broken leg.

1. How might the nurse respond to Ms. Dorvall's request for a Haitian folk healer?

_______________________________________

_______________________________________

_______________________________________

2. What would be a successful outcome for this patient?

_______________________________________

_______________________________________

_______________________________________

3. What intellectual, technical, interpersonal, and/or ethical/legal competencies are most likely to bring about the desired outcome?

_______________________________________

_______________________________________

_______________________________________

4. What resources might be helpful for Ms. Dorvall?

_______________________________________

_______________________________________

_______________________________________

## PRACTICING FOR NCLEX

### MULTIPLE CHOICE QUESTIONS

***Circle the letter that corresponds to the best answer for each question.***

1. A nurse working in a free community clinic serving low-income patients researches socioeconomic factors and statistics contributing to the formation of a culture of poverty in the United States. Which statement accurately describes one of these factors?
   a. The U.S. Census Bureau (2014) noted that an estimated 25% of the U.S. population had an income below the poverty threshold.
   b. In 2014, 10% of all children in the United States lived in poverty.
   c. The feminization of poverty tends to decrease the number of people who are living at poverty level.
   d. The socioeconomic status of older adults often differs based on their culture.

2. A nurse is performing nutritional assessments of new residents of a long-term care facility. Which resident would the nurse assess as being at greater risk for having lactose intolerance?
   a. African American male
   b. White female
   c. Native American male
   d. Alaska Native female

3. A nurse specializing in transcultural nursing teaches students that in some cases the culture of poverty is passed from generation to generation. Which population would the nurse designate *least* at risk for this trend?
   a. Families living on public assistance
   b. Families living in inner cities
   c. Families of migrant farm workers
   d. Families living in isolated areas

4. A nurse is caring for an older adult in a long-term care facility. The patient appears disoriented and complains of the "bright lights and constant activity." The nurse appropriately documents what condition in the patient chart?
   a. Culture assimilation
   b. Culture disorientation
   c. Culture blindness
   d. Culture shock

### ALTERNATE-FORMAT QUESTIONS

#### Multiple Response Questions

***Circle the letters that correspond to the best answers for each question.***

1. A nurse is providing care for patients of different cultures in a blended community clinic. Which characteristics of culture should the nurse consider when planning culturally competent care? *(Select all that apply.)*
   a. Culture guides behavior into acceptable ways for people in a specific group.
   b. Culture is not affected by a group's social and physical environment.
   c. Cultural practices and beliefs are constantly evolving and changing over time to satisfy a group's needs.
   d. Culture influences the way people of a group view themselves.
   e. There are differences both within cultures and among cultures.
   f. Subcultures exist within most cultures.

**2.** A nurse is practicing transcultural nursing in a long-term care facility. Which nursing actions reflect the use of culturally respectful care? *(Select all that apply.)*

**a.** The nurse uses open-ended questions when performing cultural assessments on patients.

**b.** The nurse uses past experiences of members of a culture exclusively to solve any cultural issues that may arise.

**c.** The nurse ignores any personal beliefs, values, practices, and family experiences that may cause personal biases that affect the nursing care of culturally diverse patients.

**d.** The nurse uses the techniques of observation and listening to acquire knowledge of the beliefs and values of patients.

**e.** The nurse discourages families from bringing food from home for the patient to help the patient adapt to the food provided by the facility.

**f.** The nurse incorporates the suggestions of a patient's folk medicine practitioner into the care plan.

CHAPTER 6

# Values, Ethics, and Advocacy

## ASSESSING YOUR UNDERSTANDING

### FILL IN THE BLANKS

1. When a young boy is left to explore values on his own with no guidance from his parents, the parents are using a(n) ____________ approach to value transmission.
2. Parents who encourage their children to seek more than one solution to a problem and weigh the consequences of each are practicing the ____________ mode of value transmission.
3. A nurse analyzes personal feelings regarding choices that need to be made when several alternatives for patient care are presented and decides whether these choices are rationally made. This nurse is engaging in the practice of ____________.
4. A nurse who is proud and happy about a decision to obtain further education is involved in the ____________ step of the process of valuing.
5. A nurse ranks personal values along a continuum of importance leading to a personal code of conduct. This organization of values is termed a(n) ____________.
6. A nurse who is committed to protecting the right of a legal minor to refuse medical treatment is practicing patient ____________.

### MATCHING EXERCISES

***Match the term in Part A with the correct definition listed in Part B.***

**PART A**

**a.** Value
**b.** Moral facility
**c.** Advocacy
**d.** Values clarification
**e.** Ethics
**f.** Morals
**g.** Ethical dilemma
**h.** Value system
**i.** Ethical distress

**PART B**

____ **1.** Two (or more) clear moral principles apply, but they support mutually inconsistent courses of action

____ **2.** A process of discovery allowing a person to discover what choices to make when alternatives are presented and to identify whether these choices are rationally made or the result of previous conditioning

____ **3.** A personal belief about worth that acts as a standard to guide one's behavior

____ **4.** Personal or communal standards of right and wrong

____ **5.** Ethical problem in which the person knows the right thing to do, but institutional constraints make it nearly impossible to pursue the right actions

____ **6.** A commitment to developing one's ability to act ethically

____ **7.** A systematic inquiry into the principles of right and wrong conduct, of virtue and vice, and of good and evil, as they relate to conduct

____ **8.** The protection and support of another's rights

***Match the mode of value transmission in Part A with the appropriate example listed in Part B. Answers may be used more than once.***

**PART A**

**a.** Modeling
**b.** Moralizing
**c.** Laissez-faire
**d.** Rewarding and punishing
**e.** Responsible choice

**PART B**

____ **9.** A boy receiving good grades in school is taken to a video arcade to celebrate

____ **10.** A girl is encouraged by her parents to explore all aspects of her own personal code of ethics

____ **11.** A child whose parents smoke decides to give it a try

____ **12.** A boy is left to his own devices when confronted with moral issues

____ **13.** A child is taught by teachers and parents that premarital sex is sinful

____ **14.** A child is encouraged to interact with people of various cultures to explore different values

____ **15.** A boy is sent to his room following an altercation with his sibling

____ **16.** A boy learns to eat a healthy diet by following his parents' example

____ **17.** A boy is allowed to determine his own bedtime

**SHORT ANSWER**

**1.** Describe how you, as a nurse, would help the following patient to define her values and choose a plan of action using the steps listed in your text: A 36-year-old mother of a 10-year-old child with cystic fibrosis works during the day as a cashier and is going to school at night to study nursing. Her husband is a salesman who has constant overnight travel. The child needs more attention than the mother has time to supply, and the mother feels guilty for spending time to better herself. She cannot afford to hire a full-time caretaker for her child.

**a.** Values clarification: ____________________

____________________

**b.** Choosing: ____________________

____________________

**c.** Prizing: ____________________

____________________

**d.** Acting: ____________________

____________________

**2.** Identify four ethical issues confronted by nurses in their daily nursing practice. How would you deal with these issues in your own practice?

**a.** ____________________

____________________

**b.** ____________________

____________________

**c.** ____________________

____________________

**d.** ____________________

____________________

**3.** Briefly describe the five principles of bioethics and give an example of each.

**a.** Autonomy: ____________________

____________________

____________________

**b.** Nonmaleficence: ____________________

____________________

____________________

c. Beneficence: ______________________

d. Justice: ______________________

e. Fidelity: ______________________

4. Describe how you, as a nurse, would act as an advocate for the following patients:
   a. An infant born addicted to crack cocaine whose mother wants to take him home: ______________________
   b. A 12-year-old girl who seeks a pregnancy test at a Planned Parenthood clinic without her parents' knowledge: ______________________
   c. A 15-year-old girl who is anorexic and who refuses to eat anything during her hospital stay: ______________________
   d. A 28-year-old man who contracted AIDS from an infected male partner, and who tells you that the other nurses have been avoiding him: ______________________
   e. A 48-year-old mother with emphysema who refuses to quit smoking: ______________________
   f. A 78-year-old woman in a long-term care facility who is dying of cancer and asks you to help her "end the pain" through assisted suicide: ______________________

5. List the qualities you possess that you feel are most important in developing your own personal code of ethics: ______________________

6. Use the five-step model of ethical decision making listed in your text to resolve the following moral distress: You believe that a homeless patient, diagnosed with high blood pressure, needs a psychological workup. She appears confused and unable to care for herself or manage her medication. She is alternately withdrawn and combative. You suspect she may have early Alzheimer's disease. Your superiors insist she be discharged without further treatment, and you are told there is no room for her on the psychiatric ward.
   a. Assess the situation: ______________________
   b. Diagnose the ethical problem: ______________________
   c. Plan: ______________________
   d. Implement your decision: ______________________
   e. Evaluate your decision: ______________________

7. Give an example of an ethical problem that may occur among the following health care personnel, patients, and institutions.
   a. Nurse/patient: ______________________
   b. Nurse/nurse: ______________________
   c. Nurse/health care provider: ______________________
   d. Nurse/institution: ______________________

## APPLYING YOUR KNOWLEDGE

### CRITICAL THINKING QUESTIONS

1. Describe how you would respond in an ethical manner to the following patient requests:
   a. The anxious father of a 17-year-old gay patient asks you to perform an HIV test on his son without his son's knowledge.
   b. A woman who presents with contusions and marks consistent with domestic abuse tells you that her husband pushed her down the steps. She asks you not to tell anyone. When her husband arrives, he hovers over her in an obsessive and overly protective manner.
2. Describe what you would do in the following situations:
   a. A doctor asks you to falsify a report that he prescribed medicine contraindicated for a patient's condition.
   b. A nurse coworker refuses to bathe an HIV-positive patient.
   c. Due to administrative cutbacks, there are not enough nurses scheduled to cover the critical care unit in which you work.

   Share your responses with a classmate and explore the difference in your responses. What competencies and character traits promote ethical behavior?

### REFLECTIVE PRACTICE: CULTIVATING QSEN COMPETENCIES

***Use the following expanded scenario from Chapter 6 in your textbook to answer the questions below.***

*Scenario:* William Raines, a homeless 68-year-old man diagnosed with schizophrenia, developmental delays, and uncontrolled hypertension, was admitted for control of moderately severe elevation of his blood pressure. A review of his medical record reveals that Mr. Raines, who has no medical insurance, was getting samples of medications for blood pressure treatment from the pharmaceutical representatives at the clinic. A recent policy change stopped this practice approximately 4 weeks ago. Mr. Raines is about to be discharged with several prescriptions for medications, but he refuses to take the prescriptions, saying, "Why take that useless paper? I haven't got any money to buy those pills with, anyway."

1. How might the nurse react to Mr. Raines response to filling his prescriptions?

   ______________________________

   ______________________________

   ______________________________

2. What would be a successful outcome for this patient?

   ______________________________

   ______________________________

   ______________________________

3. What intellectual, technical, interpersonal, and/or ethical/legal competencies are most likely to bring about the desired outcome?

   ______________________________

   ______________________________

   ______________________________

4. What resources might be helpful for Mr. Raines?

   ______________________________

   ______________________________

   ______________________________

## PRACTICING FOR NCLEX

### MULTIPLE CHOICE QUESTIONS

***Circle the letter that corresponds to the best answer for each question.***

1. A nurse who is caring for a new mother realizes that the woman is not prepared to go home with her newborn after a hospital stay of only 24 hours, but hospital policy dictates that the mother be discharged. This nurse may be faced with which moral problem?
   a. Ethical uncertainty
   b. Ethical distress
   c. Ethical dilemma
   d. Ethical dissatisfaction

2. A nurse uses the utilitarian action guiding theory when deciding how to handle the following ethical conflict: A 13-year-old female patient with anorexia refuses to eat food despite slowly starving to death. The parents insist the nurse use a feeding tube to feed her. Which statement is an example of this theory in practice?
   a. The nurse forces food via an eating tube because the end result is good in that it will save the patient's life.
   b. The nurse refuses to force feed the patient because the nurse believes that force feeding a patient who refuses food is wrong even if it is a life-saving measure.
   c. The nurse believes that force feeding a patient could be right or wrong depending on the process used to accomplish the action.
   d. The nurse believes that force feeding a patient violates the principles of autonomy and nonmaleficence.
3. A nurse demonstrates the professional value known as altruism when caring for patients in a long-term care facility. What is an example of a nursing action based on this value?
   a. A nurse consults a patient when planning nursing care to determine priorities.
   b. A nurse researches the culture of a Muslim patient when planning nursing care.
   c. A nurse helps an older adult patient fill out an informed consent form.
   d. A nurse promotes universal access to health care for underserved populations.
4. A nurse cultivates dispositions that enable practicing nursing in a manner in which he or she believes in. This nurse is displaying what essential element of moral facility?
   a. Moral sensibility
   b. Moral responsiveness
   c. Moral capacity
   d. Moral valuing
5. A nurse who provides the information and support that patients and their families need to make the decision that is right for them is practicing what principle of bioethics?
   a. Autonomy
   b. Nonmaleficence
   c. Justice
   d. Fidelity
6. Nurses who value patient advocacy follow what guideline?
   a. They value their loyalty to an employing institution or to a colleague over their commitment to their patient.
   b. They give priority to the good of the individual patient rather than to the good of society in general.
   c. They choose the claims of the patient's well-being over the claims of the patient's autonomy.
   d. They make decisions for patients who are uninformed concerning their rights and opportunities.

## ALTERNATE-FORMAT QUESTIONS

### Multiple Response Questions

***Circle the letters that correspond to the best answers for each question.***

1. A school nurse interviewing parents of a child who is doing poorly in school determines that the parents practice a laissez-faire method of discipline. What are examples of this form of value transmission? *(Select all that apply.)*
   a. A boy says a prayer before meals that he learned from his parents.
   b. A boy is taken for ice cream to celebrate his good report card.
   c. A teenage boy explores religions of friends in hopes of developing his own faith.
   d. A boy is taught how to behave in public by his schoolteacher.
   e. A teenage girl is punished for staying out too late with her friends.
   f. A teenage girl tries alcohol at a party with her friends.

2. Nurses practice the professional value of autonomy when providing nursing care for patients. Which nursing actions best describe the use of this value? *(Select all that apply.)*
   a. A nurse stays later than his or her shift to continue caring for a patient in critical condition.
   b. A nurse researches a new procedure that would benefit his or her patient.
   c. A nurse keeps her promise to call a patient's doctor regarding pain relief.
   d. A nurse reads the Patient Bill of Rights to a visually impaired patient.
   e. A nurse collaborates with other health care team members to ensure the best possible treatment for a patient.
   f. A novice nurse seeks the help of a more experienced nurse to insert a catheter in a patient.
3. Which nursing actions best describe the use of the professional value of altruism? *(Select all that apply.)*
   a. A nurse demonstrates an understanding of the culture of his or her patient.
   b. A nurse becomes a mentor to a student nurse working on her floor.
   c. A nurse is accountable for the care provided to a mentally challenged patient.
   d. A nurse lobbies for universal access to health care.
   e. A nurse respects the right of a Native American to call in a shaman for a consultation.
   f. A nurse protects the privacy of a patient with AIDS.
4. Which nursing actions best describe the use of the professional value of human dignity? *(Select all that apply.)*
   a. A nurse plans nursing care together with his or her patient.
   b. A nurse provides honest information to a patient about his or her illness.
   c. A nurse provides privacy for an older adult patient.
   d. A nurse reports an error made by an incompetent coworker.
   e. A nurse plans individualized nursing care for his or her patients.
   f. A nurse refuses to discuss a patient with a curious friend.
5. A nurse instructor is teaching students about the use of moral facility in nursing practice. Which statements accurately represent the basic principles of ethics? *(Select all that apply.)*
   a. The term "ethics" generally refers to personal or communal standards of right or wrong.
   b. The ability to be ethical begins in childhood and develops gradually.
   c. An action that is legal or customary is ethically right.
   d. Ethics is a systematic inquiry into the principles of right and wrong conduct, of virtue and vice, and of good and evil, as they relate to conduct.
   e. A commitment to developing the ability to act ethically is known as moral facility.
   f. Most nurses are born with a natural ability to behave in an ethically professional way.
6. A nurse seeks to incorporate the principle of bioethics known as nonmaleficence when caring for patients in a long-term care facility. Which nursing actions best exemplify this principle?
   a. The nurse performs regular patient assessments for pressure injuries.
   b. The nurse follows "medication rights" when administering medicine to patients.
   c. The nurse provides information to patients to help them make decisions about treatment options.
   d. The nurse arranges for hospice for a patient who is terminally ill.
   e. The nurse keeps promises to provide diligent care to patients.
   f. The nurse acts fairly when allocating time and resources to patients.

CHAPTER 7

# Legal Dimensions of Nursing Practice

## ASSESSING YOUR UNDERSTANDING

### FILL IN THE BLANKS

1. The *Education for all Handicapped Children Act* passed by the United States federal governing bodies is a form of ____________ law.
2. A state's ____________ protects the public by broadly defining the legal scope of nursing practice.
3. ____________ is a specialized form of credentialing based on laws passed by a state legislature.
4. A nurse called by either attorney to explain to the judge and jury what happened, based on the patient's record, and to offer an opinion about whether the nursing care met acceptable standards is called a(n) ____________.
5. When the nurse participates in establishing, maintaining, and improving health care environments and conditions of employment, he or she is participating in a practice known as ____________.
6. When a nurse documents the fall of an older adult patient, he or she is filing a(n) ____________ report.
7. The Joint Commission defines a(n) ____________ as an unexpected occurrence involving death or serious or psychological injury, or the risk thereof.

### MATCHING EXERCISES

***Match the type of tort listed in Part A with an example of the tort listed in Part B.***

**PART A**

**a.** Assault
**b.** Battery
**c.** Slander
**d.** Liability
**e.** Invasion of privacy
**f.** False imprisonment
**g.** Fraud
**h.** Negligence
**i.** Libel

**PART B**

____ **1.** A nurse seeking a middle-management position in long-term care claims to be certified in gerontologic nursing, which is not the case.

____ **2.** A nurse tapes an interview with a patient without his knowledge.

____ **3.** A nurse threatens to slap an older adult patient who refuses to clean up after herself.

____ **4.** A nurse spreads a rumor that a patient is a compulsive gambler.

____ **5.** A nurse forgets to replace an IV bag that is empty.

____ **6.** A nurse uses restraints on a patient unnecessarily.

____ **7.** A nurse physically attacks a patient who complains that she is not being cared for properly.

____ **8.** A nurse circulates a petition among her coworkers in an attempt to remove a coworker from her unit who has engaged in inappropriate behavior with a patient. This behavior is described at the top of the petition.

***Match the terms listed in Part A with their definitions listed in Part B.***

**PART A**

**a.** Litigation
**b.** Plaintiff
**c.** Defendant
**d.** Crime
**e.** Credentialing
**f.** Felony
**g.** Tort
**h.** Contract
**i.** Testator
**j.** Beneficiary
**k.** Misdemeanor
**l.** Precedent

**PART B**

____ **9.** The person who makes a will

____ **10.** The exchange of promises between two parties

____ **11.** The process of a lawsuit

____ **12.** The case that first sets down the rule by decision

____ **13.** The one being accused in a lawsuit

____ **14.** A wrong against a person or his/her property, considered to be against the public as well

____ **15.** Crimes that are commonly punishable with fines or imprisonment for less than 1 year, or with both, or with parole

____ **16.** The person or government bringing suit against another

____ **17.** A crime punishable by imprisonment in a state or federal penitentiary for more than 1 year

____ **18.** A wrong committed by a person against another person or his/her property that generally results in a civil trial

____ **19.** A person who receives money or property from a will

***Match the type of law listed in Part A with an example of the law listed in Part B.***

**PART A**

**a.** Administrative law
**b.** Common law
**c.** Public law
**d.** Private law
**e.** Criminal law
**f.** Constitutional law
**g.** Statutory law

**PART B**

____ **20.** Laws regulating relationships between people and the government

____ **21.** Nurse practice acts

____ **22.** Rules and regulations of boards of nursing

____ **23.** Malpractice law

____ **24.** Laws regulating relationships among people

____ **25.** Laws involving murder, manslaughter, criminal negligence, theft, and illegal possession of drugs

**SHORT ANSWER**

**1.** Give an example of how nurses could avoid the following common allegations of malpractice.

**a.** Failure to ensure patient safety: ____________

____________

**b.** Improper treatment or performance of treatment: ____________

____________

**c.** Failure to monitor and report: ____________

____________

**d.** Medication errors and reactions: ____________

____________

**e.** Failure to follow facility procedure: ____________

____________

f. Equipment misuse: ______

g. Adverse incidents: ______

h. Improper use of infection control techniques: ______

2. Explain the difference between voluntary standards of nursing practice and legal standards and give an example of each.
   a. Voluntary standards: ______
      Example: ______
   b. Legal standards: ______
      Example: ______

3. List four cases in which informed consent is needed from a patient:
   a. ______
   b. ______
   c. ______
   d. ______

4. Give three examples of invasion of privacy in a nurse–patient relationship:
   a. ______
   b. ______
   c. ______

5. List three strengths a nurse must possess to testify competently as an expert witness:
   a. ______
   b. ______
   c. ______

6. What conditions are necessary for a contract to be valid?

______

7. Describe what conditions you, as a nurse, would require to accept a telephone order from a health care provider:

______

8. List two cases in which it would be appropriate to question a health care provider's order:
   a. ______
   b. ______

9. Mrs. Toole, age 85, is recovering from a hip replacement at home. When bathing Mrs. Toole, a visiting nurse practitioner forgets to replace her bed rails, and Mrs. Toole falls out of bed. Mrs. Toole is shaken up and sore from her fall, but there appears to be no further damage to her hip.
   a. What is the nurse's liability in this situation?

   ______

   b. What information should be included in the incident report?

   ______

   c. Do you feel the patient has a case for negligence? Explain why or why not, using the four elements of liability that must be present to prove that negligence has occurred (duty, breach of duty, causation, damages).

   ______

## APPLYING YOUR KNOWLEDGE

### CRITICAL THINKING QUESTIONS

1. Think about how you would respond in the following situation and discuss your responsibilities with your classmates. Are there ever differences between the legally prudent and morally right response?
   a. Another student tells you she inadvertently gave medications to the wrong patient. She is terrified of your nurse supervisor and has decided not to inform anyone.
   b. An older adult resident in a long-term care facility tells you that the evening nurses are mean and sometimes push and hit her, but she begs you not to tell anyone.
   c. You observe a surgeon contaminate a sterile field; when you inform him, he tells you not to be so squeamish.

2. Watch a TV show or movie that depicts a courtroom drama. Write down all the legal jargon you hear and see if you can define it. Note whether the jury delivers the same verdict that you would deliver. Describe your reaction to the proceedings and verdict, and state how your conscience would dictate your resolution of the conflict.
3. Stage a mock jury with your peers. Have each person take a turn suggesting a legal issue. Let the jury deliberate and return a verdict in each case.
4. Interview someone in the legal department of the institution where you will be practicing. Ask them about the legal issues that face novice nurse practitioners and what the hospital does to prevent problems from arising. Discuss with this administrator what you perceive to be your legal responsibilities to patients in terms of patient safety, informed consent, equipment use, incident reports, and medication errors.

### REFLECTIVE PRACTICE: CULTIVATING QSEN COMPETENCIES

***Use the following expanded scenario from Chapter 7 in your textbook to answer the questions below.***

*Scenario:* Meredith Bedford is the mother of a terminally ill young boy diagnosed with a brain tumor who is admitted to the pediatric oncology unit for a pain management program. One morning she comes out to the nurses' station and firmly says, "I'm very unhappy with the care my son is receiving. I'm going to talk with my attorney as soon as possible to press charges against the hospital." The nurse currently in charge of the boy's care is under investigation for malpractice in another case.

1. How might the nurses involved in this scenario respond to Ms. Bedford's disclosure that she will be pressing charges against the hospital?

______________________________

______________________________

______________________________

2. What intellectual, technical, interpersonal, and/or ethical/legal competencies are most likely to be used in this situation?

______________________________

______________________________

______________________________

3. What resources might be helpful for the nurses in this case?

______________________________

______________________________

______________________________

## PRACTICING FOR NCLEX

### MULTIPLE CHOICE QUESTIONS

***Circle the letter that corresponds to the best answer for each question.***

1. A nurse fails to alert a health care provider of a change in a patient's condition for the worse. This is an example of what aspect of malpractice?
   a. Duty
   b. Breach of duty
   c. Causation
   d. Damages
2. A nurse who obtains a license to practice nursing by misrepresenting him- or herself is guilty of what tort?
   a. Slander
   b. Fraud
   c. Libel
   d. Assault
3. Nurses practicing in a critical care unit must acquire specialized skills and knowledge to provide care to the critically ill patient. These nurses can validate this specialty competence through what process?
   a. Certification
   b. Accreditation
   c. Licensure
   d. Litigation

4. Nurses complete incident reports as dictated by the facility protocol. What is the primary reason nurses fill out an incident report?
   a. To document everyday occurrences
   b. To document the need for disciplinary action
   c. To improve quality of care
   d. To initiate litigation
5. In some cases, the act of providing nursing care in unexpected situations is covered by the Good Samaritan laws. Which nursing actions would most likely be covered by these laws?
   a. Any emergency care where consent is given
   b. Negligent acts performed in an emergency situation
   c. Medical advice given to a neighbor regarding her child's rash
   d. Emergency care for a choking victim in a restaurant
6. A student nurse is assisting an older adult patient to ambulate following hip replacement surgery, and the patient falls and reinjures the hip. Who is potentially responsible for the injury to this patient?
   a. The student nurse
   b. The nurse instructor
   c. The hospital
   d. All of the above
7. A nurse who comments to her coworkers at lunch that her patient with a sexually transmitted disease has been sexually active in the community may be guilty of what tort?
   a. Slander
   b. Libel
   c. Fraud
   d. Assault
8. A nurse is named as a defendant in a malpractice lawsuit. Which action would be recommended for this nurse?
   a. Discuss the case with the plaintiff to ensure understanding of each other's positions.
   b. If a mistake was made on a chart, change it to read appropriately.
   c. Be prepared to tell your side to the press, if necessary.
   d. Do not volunteer any information on the witness stand.

## ALTERNATE-FORMAT QUESTIONS

### Multiple Response Questions

***Circle the letters that correspond to the best answers for each question.***

1. A nurse is writing an email to a U.S. Congressman to support the promotion of health care issues. Which guidelines would ensure a properly written email? *(Select all that apply.)*
   a. The nurse should state the purpose of the email briefly and clearly in the first paragraph.
   b. The nurse should name the city and state where he or she lives and votes.
   c. The nurse should avoid using specific examples from the workplace to support the position.
   d. The nurse should ask the legislator to vote for/support what is being asked.
   e. The nurse should try to keep the email to two pages and include a cover page with contact information.
   f. The nurse should address the email to as many legislators as possible.
2. A lawyer is describing the litigation process to a nurse named in a malpractice lawsuit. Which statements by the lawyer accurately describe this process? *(Select all that apply.)*
   a. "The defendant is the person who is initiating the lawsuit."
   b. "The process of bringing and trying this lawsuit is called litigation."
   c. "As the defendant, you will be presumed guilty until proven innocent."
   d. "We will start litigation in the first-level court known as the appellate court."
   e. "The opinions of appellate judges are published and become common law."
   f. "Malpractice is the term generally used to describe negligence by professional personnel."
3. Nurses practice within the legal and mandatory standards of the nursing profession. What are examples of voluntary standards in nursing? *(Select all that apply.)*
   a. State nurse practice acts
   b. Rules and regulations of nursing
   c. American Nurses Association Standards of Practice

d. Professional standards for certification of individual nurses in general practice
e. Process of certification
f. Process of licensure

4. Nurses follow nursing practice rules when working within the profession. What are examples of state-mandated rules? *(Select all that apply.)*
   a. Nurse practice acts
   b. Medicare and Medicaid provisions for reimbursement of nursing services
   c. Nursing educational requirements
   d. Delegation trees
   e. Composition and disciplinary authority of board of nursing
   f. Medication administration

5. Nurses may commit both intentional and unintentional torts when practicing within the profession. What are examples of intentional torts in nursing practice? *(Select all that apply.)*
   a. A nurse forgets to put the side rails up on a crib and the toddler falls out.
   b. A nurse does not report a change in patient's condition in a timely manner.
   c. A nurse threatens to hit an older adult patient who has dementia and is wailing.
   d. A nurse seeks employment in a hospital after falsifying credentials on a resume.
   e. A nurse places a patient who is a fall risk in restraints without the proper order.
   f. A nurse makes disparaging remarks to the staff about a patient who has an STI.

6. A nurse is being sued for malpractice in a court of law. What elements must be established to prove that malpractice or negligence has occurred? *(Select all that apply.)*
   a. Duty
   b. Intent to harm
   c. Breach of duty
   d. Causation
   e. Punitive damages
   f. Fraud

7. Legal safeguards are in place in the nursing practice to protect the nurse from exposure to legal risks as well as protect the patient from harm. What are examples of legal safeguards for the nurse? *(Select all that apply.)*
   a. The nurse obtains informed consent from a patient to perform a procedure.
   b. The health care provider is responsible for administration of a wrongly prescribed medication.
   c. The nurse educates the patient about the Patient Bill of Rights.
   d. The nurse executes health care provider orders without questioning them.
   e. The nurse documents all patient care in a timely manner.
   f. The nurse claims management is responsible for inadequate staffing leading to negligence.

**Prioritization Question**

1. Place the following steps involved in malpractice litigation in the order in which they would normally occur:
   a. Decision or verdict is reached.
   b. The basis for the claim is appropriate and timely; all elements of liability are present.
   c. Trial takes place.
   d. Pretrial discovery activities and review of medical records and deposition of plaintiff, defendants, and witnesses are performed.
   e. All parties named as defendants, as well as insurance companies and attorneys, work toward a fair settlement.
   f. If the verdict is not accepted by both sides, it may be appealed to an appellate court.
   g. The case is presented to a malpractice arbitration panel. The panel's decision is either accepted or rejected, in which case a complaint is filed in trial court.
   h. The defendants contest allegations.

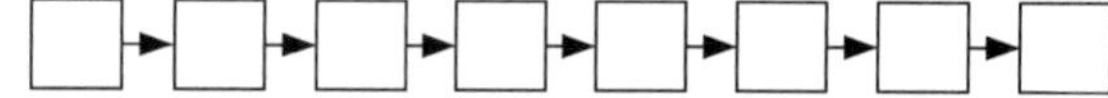

CHAPTER 8

# Communication

## ASSESSING YOUR UNDERSTANDING

### FILL IN THE BLANKS

1. A nurse initiates the communication process by addressing a patient need. This patient need becomes a(n) ____________ for conversation.
2. When a doctor communicates with a nurse by telephone to prescribe pain medication for a patient, the telephone is considered to be the ____________ of this communication.
3. A patient who verbally acknowledges understanding of discharge instructions is providing ____________ to the caregiver.
4. A patient who expresses anger at a diagnosis by slamming a food tray on the table is using ____________ communication.
5. When a nurse helps a patient achieve goals that allow his or her human needs to be satisfied, the nurse and patient are involved in a(n) ____________ relationship.
6. When a nurse and patient meet and learn to identify each other by name and clarify their roles, they are in the ____________ phase of the helping relationship.
7. A nurse is using a(n) ____________ comment/question when she says to her patient, "You have been following a diet high in fiber at home. Are you continuing to get enough fiber in the foods you've been eating since you've been here?"
8. Anger and aggressive behavior between nurses, or nurse-to-nurse hostility, has been labeled ____________.

### MATCHING EXERCISES

***Match the elements of the communication process in Part A with the appropriate definition in Part B.***

**PART A**

a. Source
b. Message
c. Channel
d. Receiver
e. Noise
f. Communication
g. Feedback

**PART B**

____ 1. The actual product of the encoder
____ 2. He or she must translate and make a decision about the product.
____ 3. Verbal and nonverbal evidence that the patient received and understood the product.
____ 4. He or she prepares and sends the product.
____ 5. The medium selected to convey the product.
____ 6. Factors that distort the quality of the product.

***Match the examples of patient goals in Part B with the appropriate phase in which they should occur listed in Part A. Answers may be used more than once.***

**PART A**

a. Orientation phase
b. Working phase
c. Termination

**PART B**

____ **7.** The patient will demonstrate ability to maneuver on crutches.

____ **8.** The patient will acknowledge the goals he or she has accomplished in physical therapy.

____ **9.** The patient will learn the name of the physical therapist and address him or her by name.

____ **10.** A patient with anorexia will establish an agreement with his or her health care professional to return gradually to a normal eating pattern.

____ **11.** The patient will express a desire to go home despite the excellent care he or she received at the facility.

____ **12.** The patient will attend a counseling session dealing with smoking.

____ **13.** The patient will verbalize the goals set forth in his or her transition to a home health care setting.

____ **14.** The patient will establish an agreement with the home health care worker about the frequency and length of contacts.

____ **15.** The patient will express his or her concerns about pending surgery to the nurse.

***Match the interviewing questions in Part B with the interviewing techniques useful in nurse–patient interactions listed in Part A. Answers may be used more than once.***

**PART A**

**a.** Validating question/comment
**b.** Clarifying question/comment
**c.** Reflective question/comment
**d.** Sequencing question/comment
**e.** Directing question/comment

**PART B**

____ **16.** "You say you've always been healthy and active; is this the first time you've been hospitalized?"

____ **17.** "You expressed concern about your children at home..."

____ **18.** "At home you've been treating your ulcer with an antacid. Did you take any today?"

____ **19.** "You've been on your present medication for 3 years. Did you experience any side effects?"

____ **20.** "Your chest pain began after exercising on a bicycle?"

____ **21.** "You've been upset about taking medication..."

**SHORT ANSWER**

**1.** Give an example of the following nonverbal forms of communication and explain how they can provide clues to the patient's health status.

**a.** Touch: ________________________________

________________________________

**b.** Eye contact: ________________________________

________________________________

**c.** Facial expressions: ________________________________

________________________________

**d.** Posture: ________________________________

________________________________

**e.** Gait: ________________________________

________________________________

**f.** Gestures: ________________________________

________________________________

**g.** General physical appearance: ________________________________

________________________________

**h.** Mode of dress and grooming: ________________________________

________________________________

**i.** Sounds: ________________________________

________________________________

**j.** Silence: ________________________________

________________________________

**2.** Briefly describe how you would alter your explanation of a surgical procedure to take into account the developmental considerations of the following patients:

**a.** An 8-year-old boy: ________________________________

________________________________

**b.** A 16-year-old girl: ________________________________

________________________________

**c.** A 65-year-old man with a hearing impairment: ________________________________

________________________________

**3.** What clues to a person's identity can sometimes be determined by knowing that person's occupation? ______________________

______________________

**4.** Briefly explain the role that communication plays in the following steps of the nursing process.

**a.** Assessing: ______________________

______________________

**b.** Diagnosing: ______________________

______________________

**c.** Planning: ______________________

______________________

**d.** Implementing: ______________________

______________________

**e.** Evaluating: ______________________

______________________

**f.** Documenting: ______________________

______________________

**5.** Explain why the following variables must be considered when establishing rapport between a nurse and a patient.

**a.** Having specific objectives: ______________________

______________________

**b.** Providing a comfortable environment: ______

______________________

**c.** Providing privacy: ______________________

______________________

**d.** Maintaining confidentiality: ______________________

______________________

**e.** Maintaining patient focus: ______________________

______________________

**f.** Using nursing observations: ______________________

______________________

**g.** Using optimal pacing: ______________________

______________________

**h.** Providing personal space: ______________________

______________________

**i.** Developing therapeutic communication skills: ______________________

______________________

**j.** Developing listening skills: ______________________

______________________

**k.** Using silence as a tool: ______________________

______________________

**6.** Rewrite the following questions/statements to promote more effective communication with the patient.

**a.** "Did you have a good night?" ______________________

______________________

**b.** "Are you ready to try walking on that foot?"

______________________

______________________

**c.** "I can't believe you stopped taking your insulin!"______________________

______________________

**d.** "You aren't afraid of taking that test, are you?"______________________

______________________

**e.** "No one should be afraid of that procedure; it's been done a million times!"______________________

______________________

**f.** "Don't worry; everything will be all right."

______________________

______________________

**7.** Underline the nonverbal communication in the following paragraph:

Mrs. Clarke, age 42, underwent a mastectomy. She has a husband and two children, ages 10 and 5. When the nurse enters Mrs. Clarke's room, she finds her patient's eyes are teary and there is a worried expression on her face. When asked how she is feeling, Mrs. Clarke replies "fine," although her face is rigid and her mouth is drawn in a firm line. She is moving her foot back and forth under the covers. On further investigation, the nurse finds that Mrs. Clarke is worried about her children and her own ability to be a healthy, functioning wife and mother again. After prompting, Mrs. Clarke says, "I don't know if my husband will still love me like this." She sighs and falls silent, reflecting upon her recovery. The nurse tries to make Mrs. Clarke comfortable and puts her hand over Mrs. Clarke's hand. She establishes eye contact with Mrs. Clarke and reassures her that things have a way of working out and suggests that she give her situation some time.

**8.** Mr. Uhl is a 72-year-old man with early signs of Alzheimer's disease. He is living with his daughter and son-in-law in a large city, where he is functioning well under supervision. His doctor suggests a daycare center to fill in the gaps when the daughter is away at her part-time job. Nurse Parish, employed by the day-care center, enters into a helping relationship with Mr. Uhl, even though she knows she will be starting a new job at the end of the month that will force them to terminate their relationship. Write two patient goals the nurse may prepare for Mr. Uhl in the following phases of their short helping relationship.

**a.** Orientation phase: ______

**(1)** ______

**(2)** ______

**b.** Working phase: ______

**(1)** ______

**(2)** ______

**c.** Termination phase: ______

**(1)** ______

**(2)** ______

**9.** Give an example of the following interpersonal skills necessary for the promotion of a healthy nurse–patient relationship. Rate your own skills in these areas on a scale of 1 to 10.

**a.** Warmth and friendliness: ______

**b.** Openness and respect: ______

**c.** Empathy: ______

**d.** Competence: ______

**e.** Consideration of patient variables: ______

______

**10.** List five common blocks to communication and describe nursing's role in overcoming these obstacles.

**a.** ______

______

**b.** ______

______

**c.** ______

______

**d.** ______

______

**e.** ______

______

**11.** Discuss how bullying may impact nursing care in health care facilities and the organizational response to these disruptive behaviors:

**a.** Bullying: ______

______

**b.** Organizational response: ______

______

## APPLYING YOUR KNOWLEDGE

### CRITICAL THINKING QUESTIONS

**1.** Write a general script for communicating with patients beginning with, "Hello, my name is..." to the end of the conversation. Make your script specific to the needs of the following patients:

**a.** A 4-year-old boy is admitted to the hospital with multiple fractures following a car accident.

**b.** A teenage girl is admitted to the burn unit with third-degree burns following a fire in her home.

**c.** A 29-year-old rape victim is brought to the emergency room for treatment and testing.

**d.** A 60-year-old man with a history of strokes is brought to the emergency room with left-sided paralysis.

How competent and comfortable are you in each situation? What skills do you need to develop?

**2.** Pick a partner and try to communicate the following messages using only nonverbal communication:

**a.** I'm thirsty.

**b.** I have a pain in my stomach.

**c.** It's too hot in here.

**d.** I'd like you to read me a story.

**e.** I'd like to go home now.

**f.** Where is the bathroom?

**g.** Can I have another pain reliever?

**h.** I'd like to go to sleep now.

**i.** It's too noisy in here.

**j.** I can't fall asleep.

Reflect on the importance of nonverbal communication.

3. Observe and interpret a patient's nonverbal communication and then ask the patient if your interpretation was correct; for example, "You seem to be in a lot of pain; is that correct?"
4. Ask a friend who has been a close confidante of yours to rate you on the following attributes that stimulate a healthy nurse–patient relationship: warmth and friendliness, openness, empathy, competence, and consideration of patient variables. See if this evaluation is consistent with your own feelings when practicing patient care. Work on the areas on which you had a lower score the next time you are with patients.

### REFLECTIVE PRACTICE: CULTIVATING QSEN COMPETENCIES

***Use the following expanded scenario from Chapter 8 in your textbook to answer the questions below.***

***Scenario:*** Mrs. Irwina Russellinski is a 75-year-old woman transferred from the emergency department, diagnosed with pneumonia. Her chart reveals that she is hard of hearing, "slightly confused" at times, and speaks "broken English." Mrs. Russellinski has a daughter living nearby who is listed as a contact person. Mrs. Russellinski tells the nurse not to call her daughter because "she is too busy with her own family and shouldn't have to bother with a sick mother." A nursing assessment is needed.

1. What communication skills might the nurse use to complete an assessment of Mrs. Russellinski?

   ______________________________

   ______________________________

   ______________________________

2. What would be a successful outcome for this patient?

   ______________________________

   ______________________________

   ______________________________

3. What intellectual, technical, interpersonal, and/or ethical/legal competencies are most likely to bring about the desired outcome?

   ______________________________

   ______________________________

   ______________________________

4. What resources might be helpful for Mrs. Russellinski?

   ______________________________

   ______________________________

   ______________________________

## PRACTICING FOR NCLEX

### MULTIPLE CHOICE QUESTIONS

***Circle the letter that corresponds to the best answer for each question.***

1. Nurses use social media to share ideas, develop professional connections, access educational offerings and forums, receive support, and investigate evidence-based practices. What is an example of the proper use of social media by a nurse?
   **a.** A nurse describes a patient on Twitter by giving the room number rather than the name of the patient.
   **b.** A nurse posts pictures of a patient who accomplished a goal of losing 100 lb and later deletes the photo.
   **c.** A nurse describes a patient on Twitter by giving the patient's diagnosis rather than the patient's name.
   **d.** A nurse uses a disclaimer to verify that any views expressed on Facebook are his or hers alone and not the employer's.
2. A home care nurse discusses with a patient when visits will occur and how long they will last. In what phase of the helping relationship is this type of agreement established?
   **a.** Orientation phase
   **b.** Working phase
   **c.** Termination phase
   **d.** All of the above

3. A nurse states the following to another nurse who is constantly forgetting to wash her hands between patients: "It looks like you keep forgetting to wash your hands between patients. It's really not safe for your patients. Let's think of some type of reminder we can use to help you remember." This communication is an example of what type of speech?
   a. Aggressive
   b. Assertive
   c. Nonassertive
   d. Therapeutic
4. A nurse is attempting to communicate with a patient who speaks a different language and does not understand what is being communicated. Which nursing action would best facilitate the communication process?
   a. Speaking slowly and distinctly but not loudly
   b. Repeating the message in the same manner many times until understood
   c. Using medical terms and abbreviations more frequently
   d. Avoiding using a dictionary to help maintain focus on the patient
5. In a helping relationship, the nurse would most likely perform what action?
   a. Encourage the patient to independently explore goals that allow his or her human needs to be satisfied.
   b. Set up a reciprocal relationship in which patient and nurse are both helper and person being helped.
   c. Establish communication that is continuous and reciprocal.
   d. Establish goals for the patient that are not set in a specific time frame.
6. Which technique would a nurse employ when using listening skills appropriately?
   a. The nurse would try to avoid body gestures when listening to the patient.
   b. The nurse would not allow conversation to lapse into periods of silence.
   c. The nurse would listen to the themes in the patient's comments.
   d. The nurse would stand close to the patient and maintain eye contact.
7. A nurse who is caring for newborn infants delivers care by using the sense that is most highly developed at birth. Which example of nursing care achieves this goal?
   a. The nurse speaks to the infant in a loud voice to get attention.
   b. The nurse plays "peek-a-boo" with the infant.
   c. The nurse wears colorful clothing to stimulate the infant.
   d. The nurse gently strokes the baby's cheek to facilitate breastfeeding.
8. A nurse who "unblocks" and "clears" congested areas of energy in a patient's body to promote comfort is applying the phenomenon known as:
   a. "Unruffling" touch
   b. Interpersonal touch
   c. Tactile manipulation
   d. Therapeutic touch
9. A 36-year-old patient who underwent a hysterectomy 4 days ago says to the nurse, "I wonder if I'll still feel like a woman." Which response would most likely encourage the patient to expand on this and express her concerns in more specific terms?
   a. "When did you begin to wonder about this?"
   b. "Do you want more children?"
   c. "Feel like a woman…"
   d. Remaining silent
10. When attending a staff meeting, a nurse is participating in what type of communication?
    a. Intrapersonal communication
    b. Interpersonal communication
    c. Small-group communication
    d. Organizational communication

## ALTERNATE-FORMAT QUESTIONS

### Multiple Response Questions

***Circle the letters that correspond to the best answers for each question.***

1. A nurse is communicating the care plan to a patient who is cognitively impaired. Which nursing actions facilitate this process? *(Select all that apply.)*
   - **a.** The nurse maintains eye contact with the patient.
   - **b.** The nurse is patient and gives the patient time to respond.
   - **c.** The nurse communicates in a busy environment to hold the patient's attention.
   - **d.** The nurse keeps communication simple and concrete.
   - **e.** The nurse gives lengthy explanations of the care that will be given.
   - **f.** If there is no response, the nurse does not repeat what is said and takes a break.
2. A nurse is communicating the care plan for a patient who is unconscious. Which nursing actions best facilitate this process? *(Select all that apply.)*
   - **a.** The nurse speaks to the patient in a louder-than-normal voice.
   - **b.** The nurse is careful about what is said in the patient's presence since hearing is the last sense to go.
   - **c.** The nurse assumes the patient can hear and discusses things that would ordinarily be discussed.
   - **d.** The nurse raises environmental noises to help stimulate the patient.
   - **e.** The nurse does not use touch to communicate with the patient.
   - **f.** The nurse speaks with the patient before touching him or her.
3. Nurses on a hospital burn unit meet as a group to discuss procedures. Which statements accurately describe the functions of group dynamics? *(Select all that apply.)*
   - **a.** Ideally, a group leader is selected who alone uses his or her talents and interpersonal strengths to assist the group to accomplish goals.
   - **b.** Effective groups possess members who elicit mutually respectful relationships.
   - **c.** The group's ability to function at a high level depends on only the group leader's sensitivity to the needs of the group and its individual members.
   - **d.** If a group member dominates or thwarts the group process, the leader or other group members must confront him or her to promote the needed collegial relationship.
   - **e.** In an effective group, power is used to "fix" immediate problems without considering the needs of the powerless.
   - **f.** In an effective group, members support, praise, and critique one another.
4. A nurse is using the SBAR technique for hand-off communication when transferring a patient. What are examples of the use of this process? *(Select all that apply.)*
   - **a.** S: The nurse handling the transfer describes the patient's situation to the new nurse.
   - **b.** S: The nurse discusses the patient's symptoms with the new nurse in charge.
   - **c.** B: The nurse gives the background of the patient by explaining the patient's history.
   - **d.** A: The nurse presents an assessment of the patient to the new nurse.
   - **e.** R: The nurse explains the rules of the new facility to the patient.
   - **f.** R: The nurse gives recommendations for future care to the new nurse in charge.
5. Nurses develop helping relationships with patients when caring for them. Which statements describe qualities of a helping relationship? *(Select all that apply.)*
   - **a.** The helping relationship occurs spontaneously.
   - **b.** The helping relationship is characterized by an equal sharing of information.
   - **c.** The helping relationship is built on the patient's needs, not on those of the helping person.
   - **d.** A friendship must develop from an effective helping relationship.
   - **e.** A helping relationship is dynamic.
   - **f.** A helping relationship is purposeful and time limited.

**6.** Which nursing actions would most likely help improve communications with patients and achieve a more effective helping relationship? *(Select all that apply.)*

**a.** The nurse controls the tone of his or her voice so that it conveys exactly what is meant.

**b.** The nurse remains focused on the topic at hand and does not allow the patient to diverge to another topic.

**c.** The nurse makes statements that are as simple as possible, gearing conversation to the patient's level.

**d.** The nurse feels free to use words that might have different interpretations when using the same language as the patient.

**e.** The nurse never admits a lack of knowledge to the patient to avoid undermining the patient's confidence in the helping relationship.

**f.** The nurse takes advantage of any available opportunities to communicate information to patients in routine caregiving situations.

**7.** Which nursing actions help improve listening skills when conversing with patients? *(Select all that apply.)*

**a.** The nurse sits with the patient in a comfortable environment with arms and legs crossed in a relaxed position.

**b.** The nurse always maintains eye contact with the patient in a face-to-face pose.

**c.** The nurse uses appropriate facial expressions and body gestures to indicate that he or she is paying attention to what the patient is saying.

**d.** The nurse thinks before responding to the patient, even if this creates a lull in the conversation.

**e.** The nurse listens for themes in the patient's comments.

**f.** If an action being performed does not allow for conversation, the nurse pretends to listen to the patient rather than interrupting the patient's conversation.

CHAPTER 9

# Teaching and Counseling

## ASSESSING YOUR UNDERSTANDING

### FILL IN THE BLANKS

1. The aim of patient education for a nurse who counsels an overweight teenager to eat a healthy diet and exercise is to ___________.
2. When a nurse and a patient form a relationship in which mutual respect and trust are established, they have developed a(n) ___________ relationship.
3. ___________ learning is the process by which a person acquires or increases knowledge in a measurable way as a result of teaching.
4. A patient who expresses a desire to control binge eating and to return to eating a healthy diet has experienced the ___________ domain of learning.
5. Generally, ___________ are considered the best source of assessment information.
6. ___________ is an internal impulse (such as emotion or physical pain) that encourages the patient to take action or change behavior.
7. Content that is supported by nursing research and reflects the most accurate and clinically supported information is called ___________.
8. When a nurse assists a patient to decide to quit smoking, the nurse is fulfilling the role of ___________.
9. A nurse ___________ establishes a partnership with a patient and uses discovery to identify the patient's personal goals and agenda in a way that will result in change rather than using teaching and education strategies directed by the nurse as the expert.

### MATCHING EXERCISES

***Match the examples in Part B with the appropriate teaching strategy listed in Part A. Answers may be used more than once.***

**PART A**

**a.** Role modeling
**b.** Lecture
**c.** Discussion
**d.** Demonstration
**e.** Discovery
**f.** Role-playing
**g.** Audiovisual materials
**h.** Printed material
**i.** Computer-assisted instruction programs

**PART B**

____ **1.** A nurse speaks to a group of patients about the dangers of smoking.

____ **2.** A nurse chooses a low-calorie meal for herself when having lunch with an obese patient.

____ **3.** A nurse performs a bathing procedure on a newborn in front of several new mothers.

____ **4.** A nurse obtains pamphlets for a 16-year-old that describe how STIs are transmitted.

____ **5.** One student pretends to be a patient while another student conducts a nursing interview.

____ **6.** A nurse uses a videotape to teach a patient about heart disease.

____ **7.** A nurse describes the symptoms of an anxiety attack to a patient with panic disorder and lets him choose measures to take during and after the attack.

____ **8.** A nurse shows a film on relaxation techniques to a cardiac patient.

____ **9.** A nurse shows a patient with diabetes how to give herself insulin by injecting an orange.

____ **10.** A nurse talks to a patient about the patient's feelings of powerlessness following a transient ischemic attack.

***Match the examples of teaching strategies in Part B with the aims of nursing listed in Part A. Answers may be used more than once.***

**PART A**

**a.** Promoting health

**b.** Preventing illness

**c.** Restoring health

**d.** Facilitating coping

**PART B**

____ **11.** A nurse demonstrates to a postoperative patient the proper way to bandage his incision.

____ **12.** A nurse explains to a new mother the importance and availability of immunizations for her baby.

____ **13.** A nurse counsels a woman in her first trimester on proper nutrition.

____ **14.** A nurse refers a recovering alcoholic to a local group meeting.

____ **15.** A nurse presents a lecture on babyproofing a home to a group of parents.

____ **16.** A nurse teaches a young athlete stretching exercises to be used before running track.

____ **17.** A nurse refers the daughter of a terminally ill patient to a counseling session on coping with death and dying.

____ **18.** A nurse introduces a patient recovering from a broken hip to the physical therapy staff.

____ **19.** A nurse refers a 42-year-old woman to a clinic providing free mammograms.

____ **20.** A nurse teaches relaxation techniques to a patient recovering from coronary bypass surgery.

***Match the learning domain listed in Part A with the example of the domain listed in Part B. Answers may be used more than once.***

**PART A**

**a.** Cognitive learning

**b.** Psychomotor learning

**c.** Affective learning

**PART B**

____ **21.** A patient learns how to care for his surgical wound.

____ **22.** A patient explains how eating a proper diet will lower his cholesterol level.

____ **23.** A patient learns how to perform range-of-motion exercises after surgery.

____ **24.** A patient expresses self-confidence after she completes a class to stop smoking.

____ **25.** A patient decides to get dressed in the morning following treatment for depression.

____ **26.** A patient reiterates the need for prenatal and infant care to her social worker.

## SHORT ANSWER

**1.** Briefly explain how teaching and counseling patients can facilitate the following nursing aims.

**a.** Promoting health: ________________________

________________________________

**b.** Preventing illness: ________________________

________________________________

**c.** Restoring health: ________________________

________________________________

**d.** Facilitating coping: ________________________

________________________________

2. How would you modify your teaching plan to motivate the following patients to learn a new skill?
   a. An adult who has a fear of failure: ________

   ________
   b. An adult who resists learning because of preconceived ideas about the process and your expectations of him or her: ________

   ________
   c. An older adult who is afraid to learn something new: ________

   ________
3. Mr. Lang is a 75-year-old man recovering from a stroke in a home care setting. He has partial paralysis of his left side and must be taught exercises for rehabilitation. List three teaching strategies you would use in treating this patient and give an example of each.
   a. ________

   ________
   b. ________

   ________
   c. ________

   ________
4. List two solutions to the problem that time constraints place on the nurse when planning patient learning.
   a. ________

   ________
   b. ________

   ________
5. Briefly describe the following types of teaching and give an example of each.
   a. Formal: ________

   ________
   b. Informal: ________

   ________
6. Give an example of a method that could be used to evaluate the following types of learning.
   a. Cognitive domain: ________
   b. Affective domain: ________
   c. Psychomotor domain: ________
7. How would you document successfully teaching a new mother how to bathe her infant?

   ________

   ________
8. Define the following types of counseling, and give an example of a case in which each type would be used by the nurse.
   a. Short-term counseling: ________

   ________
   b. Long-term counseling: ________

   ________
   c. Motivational counseling: ________

   ________
9. List four elements that should be considered in each assessment of patient learning needs.
   a. ________
   b. ________
   c. ________
   d. ________
10. Give an example of the following teaching strategies that you have experienced in your personal/student life. Which of these strategies do you feel were most effective for you?
    a. Role modeling: ________

    ________
    b. Lecture: ________

    ________
    c. Discussion: ________

    ________
    d. Panel discussion: ________

    ________
    e. Demonstration: ________

    ________
    f. Discovery: ________

    ________
    g. Role-playing: ________

    ________
    h. Audiovisual materials: ________

    ________

i. Programmed instruction: ______________

______________________________

j. Computer-assisted instruction: __________

______________________________

11. List four measures that promote patient and family compliance.

a. ______________________________

b. ______________________________

c. ______________________________

d. ______________________________

12. List five common mistakes that hinder patient teaching.

a. ______________________________

b. ______________________________

c. ______________________________

d. ______________________________

e. ______________________________

## APPLYING YOUR KNOWLEDGE

### CRITICAL THINKING QUESTIONS

1. As a child, you learned many things from your parents. Consider the types of teaching that you experienced and think about how you could use both formal and informal teaching to help children accomplish the following goals.

   a. Avoiding drugs and alcohol

   b. Learning how to cook a healthy meal

   c. Dealing with peer pressure

2. Observe nurses teaching and counseling patients and family members to promote health, prevent illness, restore health, or facilitate coping. What methods did the nurse use to identify each patient's learning needs? Was the nurse successful in teaching this patient? How would you have handled the teaching process differently? Assess each patient's knowledge, attitudes, and skills needed to independently manage his or her own health care.

3. Devise a plan to teach a woman how to lose weight by reducing the fat content in her diet and developing an exercise routine using the following methods:

   a. Lecture

   b. Discussion

   c. Demonstration

   d. Role-playing

   What was the advantage/disadvantage of each method?

### REFLECTIVE PRACTICE: CULTIVATING QSEN COMPETENCIES

***Use the following expanded scenario from Chapter 9 in your textbook to answer the questions below.***

***Scenario:*** Marco García Ramírez accompanies his wife, Claudia, to the antepartal clinic for a routine visit. They are expecting their first child in 5 months. He reports that they are happy and excited but also scared and very nervous. They are planning for a home birth and ask the nurse what she thinks of this method of childbirth. They are also asking lots of questions about childbirth and their new responsibilities as parents. Mr. Ramírez says, "We're both wondering if we'll be good parents." They also ponder whether they will have the resources to provide for a new child.

1. What should be the focus of patient teaching for this couple?

______________________________

______________________________

______________________________

2. What would be a successful outcome for Mr. and Mrs. Ramirez?

______________________________

______________________________

______________________________

3. What intellectual, technical, interpersonal, and/or ethical/legal competencies are most likely to bring about the desired outcome?

______________________________

______________________________

______________________________

4. What resources might be helpful for this couple?

_______________________________________________

_______________________________________________

_______________________________________________

## PRACTICING FOR NCLEX

### MULTIPLE CHOICE QUESTIONS

***Circle the letter that corresponds to the best answer for each question.***

1. Which developmental consideration is a nurse assessing when he or she determines that an 8-year-old boy is not equipped to understand the scientific explanation of his disease?
   a. Intellectual development
   b. Motor development
   c. Emotional maturity
   d. Psychosocial development
2. A nurse is documenting assessment data for a new patient. What is the best source of assessment information for the nurse?
   a. Nursing care plan
   b. Health care provider
   c. Patient
   d. Family and friends
3. Which diagnosis would best describe a situation in which a woman has a knowledge deficit concerning child safety for her toddler who is currently being treated for burns and was previously treated for a fracture from a fall?
   a. Deficient knowledge: Child safety, related to inexperience with the active developmental stage of a toddler
   b. Risk for injury, related to mother's lack of knowledge about child safety
   c. Readiness for enhanced parenting, related to child safety knowledge deficit
   d. Deficient knowledge: Child safety, related to mother's lack of experience and socioeconomic level
4. A nurse is writing learner objectives for a patient who was recently diagnosed with type 2 diabetes. Which statement describes the proper method for writing objectives?
   a. The nurse writes one or two broad objectives rather than several specific objectives.
   b. The nurse writes general statements for learner objectives that could be accomplished in any amount of time.
   c. The nurse plans learner objectives with another nurse before obtaining input from the patient and family.
   d. The nurse writes one long-term objective for each diagnosis, followed by several specific objectives.
5. When deciding what information the patient needs to meet the learner objectives successfully, the nurse is planning which part of the teaching plan?
   a. Content
   b. Teaching strategies
   c. Learning activities
   d. Learning domains
6. A nurse may attempt to help a patient solve a situational crisis during what type of counseling session?
   a. Long-term counseling
   b. Motivational counseling
   c. Short-term counseling
   d. Professional counseling
7. When a patient says, "I don't care if I get better; I have nothing to live for, anyway," which type of counseling would be appropriate?
   a. Long-term counseling
   b. Motivational counseling
   c. Short-term counseling
   d. Professional counseling
8. When teaching an adult patient how to control stress through relaxation techniques, the nurse should consider what assumption concerning adult learners?
   a. As an adult matures, his or her self-concept becomes more dependent; therefore, this patient must be made aware of the importance of reducing stress.

b. The adult learner is not as concerned with the immediate usefulness of the material being taught as he/she is with the quality of the material.
c. As patients, adults are the least likely to resist learning because of preconceived ideas about the teaching–learning process.
d. The nurse should be able to draw from the previous experience of the patient to emphasize the importance of stress reduction.

9. Which principle of teaching–learning is an accurate guideline for the nurse/teacher?
   a. Patient teaching should occur independently of the nursing process.
   b. Past life experience should not be a factor when helping patients assimilate new knowledge.
   c. The teaching–learning process can be facilitated by a helping relationship.
   d. Planning learner objectives should be done by the teacher alone.

10. When a nurse is planning for learning, who must decide who should be included in the learning sessions?
   a. The health care team
   b. The doctor and nurse
   c. The nurse and the patient
   d. The patient and the patient's family

## ALTERNATE-FORMAT QUESTIONS

### Multiple Response Questions

***Circle the letters that correspond to the best answers for each question.***

1. A nurse is providing teaching to patients in a short-term rehabilitation facility. Which examples are common teaching mistakes made by health care professionals? *(Select all that apply.)*
   a. The nurse fails to accept that patients have the right to change their minds.
   b. The nurse negotiates goals with the patient.
   c. The nurse uses medical jargon frequently when discussing the teaching plan.
   d. The nurse ignores the restrictions of the patient's environment.
   e. The nurse evaluates what the patient has learned.
   f. The nurse reviews educational media when planning learner objectives.

2. Which topics would the nurse be most likely to explore with a patient with the aim of restoring health? *(Select all that apply.)*
   a. Immunizations
   b. Patient and nurse's expectations of one another
   c. Community resources
   d. Hygiene
   e. Orientation to treatment center and staff
   f. The medical and nursing regimens and how the patient can participate in care

3. The nurse uses the acronym TEACH when planning care for patients on a busy hospital ward. Which intervention accurately represents an aspect of this acronym? *(Select all that apply.)*
   a. T—The nurse turns to the health care provider for support.
   b. E—The nurse educates the patient before treatment.
   c. A—The nurse acts on every teaching moment.
   d. C—The nurse clarifies often.
   e. H—The nurse helps the patient cope when education fails.
   f. H—The nurse honors the patient as a partner in the education process.

4. A nurse is using the teaching–learning process to teach new parents how to care for their infants. Which nursing actions reflect recommended steps of this process? *(Select all that apply.)*
   a. The nurse uses critical thinking skills to assess the learning needs and learning readiness of the parents.
   b. The nurse identifies general, attainable, measurable, and long-term goals for patient learning when developing learning objectives.
   c. The nurse includes group teaching and formal teaching in every teaching plan.
   d. The nurse does not allow time constraints, schedules, and the physical environment to influence the choice of teaching strategies.
   e. The nurse formulates a verbal or written contract with the patient.
   f. The nurse relates new learning material to the patient's past life experiences to help him or her to assimilate new knowledge.

5. Nurses plan patient learning based on the patient's developmental stage. Which nursing actions best reflect this consideration? *(Select all that apply.)*
   a. The nurse directs the health teaching for a 3-year-old to the parents.
   b. The nurse provides lengthy explanations of a procedure to a preschool child.
   c. The nurse includes a school-aged child in the teaching–learning process.
   d. The nurse uses the same learning strategies for an adolescent as for an adult.
   e. The nurse avoids relating teaching for an adult to a social role.
   f. The nurse provides material that is useful immediately to adult patients.

6. A nurse caring for patients in a skilled nursing facility assesses patient motivation to participate in care. Based on the health belief model, which patients would be most motivated? *(Select all that apply.)*
   a. A patient who does not view himself as susceptible to the disease
   b. A patient who views a disease as a serious threat
   c. A patient who believes there are actions that will reduce the probability of contracting the disease
   d. A patient who believes that the threat of taking actions against a disease is not as great as the disease itself
   e. A patient who believes that noncompliance is not an option
   f. A patient who believes that doing nothing is preferable to painful treatments

CHAPTER 10

# Leading, Managing, and Delegating

## ASSESSING YOUR UNDERSTANDING

### FILL IN THE BLANKS

1. A nurse unit manager displays power that is attained by virtue of the position. This type of power is known as ___________ power.
2. A charge nurse who makes all the decisions for the nursing team without considering their feelings or ideas is using the ___________ style of leadership.
3. In hospitals, the autocratic style of leadership is gradually being replaced by the ___________ style of leadership.
4. In the current "___________ age," change is conceived as dynamic, ever present, and continually unfolding.
5. A nurse influences other nurses in a hospital to become involved in community politics affecting the hospital. This ability to influence others to achieve a desired effect is known as ___________.
6. When an experienced nurse advises a less experienced nurse regarding patient care without receiving financial reward, their relationship is known as a(n) ___________.

### MATCHING EXERCISES

***Match the examples of leadership in Part B with the types of leadership they imply listed in Part A. Some answers may be used more than once.***

**PART A**

**a.** Autocratic leadership
**b.** Democratic leadership
**c.** Laissez-faire leadership
**d.** Transformational leadership
**e.** Transactional leadership
**f.** Quantum leadership
**g.** Servant leadership

**PART B**

____ **1.** A nurse unites with other nurses to create a shelter for battered women in their neighborhood.

____ **2.** A nurse opens a discussion among health care team members to determine the best care plan for a patient.

____ **3.** A nurse takes control during a "code blue" and directs all activities to resuscitate the patient.

____ **4.** A nurse leads other nurses in developing a schedule to cook meals for the homeless.

____ **5.** A nurse manager uses a reward and punishment system for employees to meet pre-established goals and work deadlines.

____ **6.** A nurse in charge of scheduling suggests that the nurses meet and work out the schedule on their own.

____ **7.** A nurse seeks input from coworkers to solve a problem of understaffing.

____ **8.** A head nurse makes schedules of ANA meetings available to any staff members who are interested.

____ **9.** A head nurse directs the triage unit after several earthquake victims arrive at the emergency room.

____ **10.** A head nurse issues a memo describing step-by-step documentation procedures that she wants initiated in the emergency room.

____ **11.** A head nurse openly seeks critiques of his work.

____ **12.** A head nurse desires to serve the population; to enrich the lives of people, build better organizations, and ultimately create a more just and caring world.

## SHORT ANSWER

**1.** Describe what the following leadership qualities mean to you and how they would help motivate patients in your practice to achieve their goals.

Leaders should:

**a.** Be dynamic: ____________________

____________________

**b.** Be enthusiastic: ____________________

____________________

**c.** Be self-directed: ____________________

____________________

**d.** Have a positive self-image: ____________________

____________________

**e.** Be a role model: ____________________

____________________

**f.** Have vision: ____________________

____________________

**2.** Mr. Eng is a 75-year-old man dying of lung cancer in a hospice. Give an example of how a nurse could use each of the following leadership skills to help relieve his suffering.

**a.** Communication skills: ____________________

____________________

**b.** Problem-solving skills: ____________________

____________________

**c.** Management skills: ____________________

____________________

**d.** Self-evaluation skills: ____________________

____________________

**3.** List the steps you would employ to change a nursing unit from paper records to a computerized method of record keeping. How would you handle people who resist the change?

____________________

____________________

____________________

____________________

**4.** Briefly describe the following reasons why people resist change and state how you would confront the problem in your own practice.

**a.** Threat to self: ____________________

____________________

____________________

**b.** Lack of understanding: ____________________

____________________

____________________

**c.** Limited tolerance to change: ____________________

____________________

____________________

**d.** Disagreements about the benefits of change: ____________________

____________________

____________________

**e.** Fear of increased responsibility: ____________________

____________________

____________________

5. Explain how you, as a nurse leader, can help change the negative portrayals of nursing in the media. ________________

6. Describe how you would use the following management functions to organize fellow students to form a group to help control binge drinking on campus.
   a. Planning: ________________
   b. Organizing: ________________
   c. Staffing: ________________
   d. Directing: ________________
   e. Controlling: ________________

7. Give an example from your present situation (home, school, work) where you feel that you may have the power to influence change. Explain what steps you would take to overcome resistance to this change.

   ________________

8. Explain how a nurse manager might accomplish the following leadership goals.
   a. Identifying strengths: ________________
   b. Evaluating work accomplishment: ________________
   c. Clarifying values: ________________
   d. Determining where he or she belongs and what he or she can contribute: ________________
   e. Assuming responsibility for relationships:

   ________________

9. Briefly describe four factors a nurse should consider before planning to make a change:
   a. ________________
   b. ________________
   c. ________________
   d. ________________

10. List six factors a nurse should consider before delegating a nursing intervention.
   a. ________________
   b. ________________
   c. ________________
   d. ________________
   e. ________________
   f. ________________

## APPLYING YOUR KNOWLEDGE

### CRITICAL THINKING QUESTIONS

1. Imagine you are the team leader on a busy intensive care unit. After giving the team members their patient assignments for the day, you notice that several RNs and float nurses are upset with their assignments. The unit is currently understaffed, and all team members are required to take on more responsibility than usual in order to keep the unit running efficiently. You overhear one RN say she'd rather quit than start taking on additional duties.
   a. As a leader, how would you handle this situation?
   b. What type of leadership style would you feel most comfortable using?
   c. How might your response to this situation differ depending on whether you were working in a Magnet hospital or a non-Magnet hospital?

2. Review the leadership styles of the people who have been authority figures in your life. What makes them effective or ineffective leaders? Which leadership styles have you tried? Which do you feel will be most helpful to you as you try to help patients/families and health care teams achieve health goals?

### REFLECTIVE PRACTICE: CULTIVATING QSEN COMPETENCIES

***Use the following scenario from Chapter 10 in your textbook to answer the questions below.***

*Scenario:* Rehema Kohls is a college sophomore who comes to the health care center requesting information about sexually transmitted infections (STIs). She says, "So many of my friends are concerned about STIs. They all say we should start a group on campus to discuss this problem, and they want me to set it up and be the leader. But I wouldn't know where to start or what to do!"

1. How might the nurse empower Ms. Kohls with the knowledge and ability to be a leader of her peers?

_______________

_______________

_______________

2. What would be a successful outcome for Ms. Kohls?

_______________

_______________

_______________

3. What intellectual, technical, interpersonal, and/or ethical/legal competencies are most likely to bring about the desired outcome?

_______________

_______________

_______________

4. What resources might be helpful for Ms. Kohls?

_______________

_______________

_______________

## PRACTICING FOR NCLEX

### MULTIPLE CHOICE QUESTIONS

***Circle the letter that corresponds to the best answer for each question.***

1. A nurse manager values group satisfaction and tries to motivate the staff to be the best nurses possible. In which style of leadership are group satisfaction and motivation primary benefits?
   a. Democratic
   b. Autocratic
   c. Laissez-faire
   d. Transformational
2. Which style of leadership is rarely used in a hospital setting because of the difficulty of task achievement by independent nurses?
   a. Democratic
   b. Autocratic
   c. Laissez-faire
   d. Transformational
3. A nurse arranges all the resources available to teach a teenage girl how to manage her asthma. Which role is this nurse performing?
   a. Planning role
   b. Organizing role
   c. Directing role
   d. Controlling role
4. A nurse manager of a hospital unit is working within a decentralized management structure. Which nursing action best exemplifies this type of system?
   a. Senior managers make all the decisions.
   b. Nurses are not intimately involved in decisions involving patient care.
   c. Decisions are made by those who are most knowledgeable about the issue.
   d. Nurse managers are not accountable for patient, staffing, supplies, or budgets.

5. A nurse manager is attempting to change the policy for scheduling staff on a critical care unit. The nurse is in the process of changing the schedules and announcing the changes. Based on Lewin's change theory, in what stage of change is this nurse participating?
   a. Moving
   b. Freezing
   c. Unfreezing
   d. Transforming

## ALTERNATE-FORMAT QUESTIONS

### Multiple Response Questions

***Circle the letters that correspond to the best answers for each question.***

1. Members of a hospital staff working together on a pediatric unit may have explicit or implied power. What are examples of people with implied power? *(Select all that apply.)*
   a. A nurse mentor
   b. A nurse manager
   c. A popular nurse
   d. A unit leader
   e. A prankster
   f. A veteran nurse with 20 years' experience
2. A nurse graduate applies for a job working in a hospital that achieved Magnet status. Which conditions would this nurse expect? *(Select all that apply.)*
   a. Focus on positive patient care outcomes
   b. Centralized decision making
   c. Autonomous, accountable professional nursing practice
   d. Higher staff turnover
   e. Higher levels of staff burnout and exodus from the bedside
   f. Supportive nurse managers
3. A nurse manager of a health care provider's office uses the laissez-faire style of leadership with the staff. Which nursing actions exemplify this management style? *(Select all that apply.)*
   a. The nurse manager is the authority on all issues.
   b. The nurse manager allows the staff to choose their own schedules.
   c. The nurse manager allows dominant staff members to direct the group activities.
   d. Manager and staff work independently, making task accomplishment difficult.
   e. The manager views staff as equal partners in the practice.
   f. The nurse manager inspires and motivates staff to provide excellent patient care.
4. A registered nurse is delegating activities to unlicensed assistive personnel (UAPs) on a hospital unit. Which activities could this nurse normally delegate? *(Select all that apply.)*
   a. The determination of a nursing diagnosis for a patient with breast cancer
   b. Giving a bed bath to a patient
   c. Planning patient education for a patient with a colostomy
   d. Taking routine vital signs
   e. Administering medications to patients
   f. Transferring a patient to another floor
5. A registered nurse checks the American Nurses Association (ANA) regulations prior to delegating tasks to UAPs on a burn unit. Which principles regarding the regulation, education, and use of the UAP are recommended by the ANA? *(Select all that apply.)*
   a. It is the health care institution that determines the scope of nursing practice.
   b. It is the LPN who supervises any assistant involved in providing direct patient care.
   c. It is the purpose of assistive personnel to work in a supportive role to the registered nurse.
   d. It is the role of the assistive personnel to carry out tasks to enable the professional nurse to concentrate on nursing care for the patient.
   e. It is the role of the LPN to assign nursing duties to the UAP.
   f. It is the registered nurse who is responsible and accountable for nursing practice.

CHAPTER 11

# The Health Care Delivery System

## ASSESSING YOUR UNDERSTANDING

### FILL IN THE BLANKS

1. A person enters a hospital for an operation and stays there for 3 days. This patient is a(n) ____________.
2. ____________ centers are often located in convenient areas, such as shopping malls, often offer walk-in services without appointments, and are often open at times other than traditional office hours.
3. ____________ care is a type of care provided for caregivers of homebound ill, disabled, or older adults.
4. ____________ is a program of palliative and supportive care services providing physical, psychological, social, and spiritual care for dying people and their families and loved ones.
5. Alcoholics Anonymous is an example of a(n) ____________ facility.
6. A(n)____________ is a member of the collaborative team trained in techniques that improve pulmonary function and oxygenation.

### MATCHING EXERCISES

***Match the type of health care listed in Part A with its definition in Part B.***

**PART A**

**a.** Respite care
**b.** Hospice services
**c.** Mental health centers
**d.** Voluntary facilities
**e.** Rehabilitation centers
**f.** Daycare centers
**g.** Parish nursing centers
**h.** Ambulatory care centers
**i.** Homeless shelters
**j.** Public health facilities
**k.** Long-term care facilities
**l.** Rural health centers
**m.** Hospitals
**n.** Schools
**o.** Home care
**p.** Industry
**q.** Primary care centers

**PART B**

____ **1.** Care for infants and children whose parents work, older adults who cannot be home alone, and patients with special needs who do not need to be in a health care institution

____ **2.** Not-for-profit community facilities financed by private donations, grants, or fundraisers

____ **3.** Community health nursing practice that emphasizes holistic health care, health promotion, and disease prevention, with the aim of reaching people before they are sick; often volunteer- and church-oriented

____ **4.** Special services available to terminally ill people and their families, providing inpatient and home care committed to maintaining quality of life and dignity in the dying person

____ **5.** Provides services for patients requiring physical or emotional rehabilitation and for treatment of chemical dependency

____ **6.** Local, state, or federal facilities that provide public health services to communities of various sizes

____ **7.** Urgent care center that provides walk-in emergency care services

____ **8.** Often located in geographically remote areas with few health care providers; many of these centers are run by nurse practitioners

____ **9.** Provide 24-hour services and hotlines for people who are suicidal, who are abusing drugs or alcohol, and who require psychological or psychiatric counseling

____ **10.** Living units that provide housing for people who do not have regular shelter

____ **11.** The traditional acute care provided for people who were too ill to care for themselves at home, who were severely injured, who required surgery or complicated treatments, or who were having babies

____ **12.** Health care services are provided by physicians and advanced practice nurses in offices and clinics offering the diagnosis and treatment of minor illnesses, minor surgical procedures, obstetric care, well-child care, counseling, and referrals

____ **13.** The type of care provided to homebound ill, disabled, or older adult patients to allow the primary caregiver to have some time away from the responsibilities of day-to-day care

____ **14.** Nurses in this setting are often the major source of health assessment, health education, and emergency care for the nation's children

____ **15.** Occupational health nurses practicing in these settings focus on preventing work-related illnesses and injuries by conducting health assessments, teaching health promotion, and caring for minor injuries and illnesses

***Match the team member in Part A with their role in the health care system listed in Part B.***

**PART A**

**a.** Health care provider
**b.** Physician assistant
**c.** Physical therapist
**d.** Respiratory therapist
**e.** Occupational therapist
**f.** Speech therapist
**g.** Dietitian
**h.** Pharmacist
**i.** Social worker
**j.** Unlicensed assistive personnel
**k.** Chaplain

**PART B**

____ **16.** Licensed to formulate and dispense medications

____ **17.** Trained to help hearing-impaired patients speak more clearly

____ **18.** Responsible for the diagnosis of illness and medical or surgical treatment of that illness

____ **19.** Help nurses provide direct care to patients; titles include nursing assistants, orderlies, attendants, or technicians

____ **20.** Responsible for managing and planning for dietary needs of patients

____ **21.** Licensed to assist physically challenged patients to adapt to limitations

____ **22.** Has completed a specific course of study and a licensing examination in preparation for providing support to the health care provider

____ **23.** Seeks to restore function or prevent further disability in a patient after an injury or illness

____ **24.** Counsels patients and family members and informs them of, and refers them to, various community resources

____ **25.** Has been trained in techniques that improve pulmonary function and oxygenation

### SHORT ANSWER

**1.** List four factors that have influenced the need for increased home health care.

**a.** ____________________

**b.** ____________________

**c.** ____________________

**d.** ____________________

**2.** Describe the role of the nurse in the following health care centers:

**a.** Primary care offices: ____________________

**b.** Ambulatory care centers and clinics: ____________________

**c.** Mental health centers: ____________________

**d.** Rehabilitation centers: ____________________

**e.** Long-term care centers: ____________________

**3.** How have recent changes in the health care system affected the role of the hospital as a provider of health care services?

____________________

**4.** List six services that can be performed during outpatient care.

**a.** ____________________

**b.** ____________________

**c.** ____________________

**d.** ____________________

**e.** ____________________

**f.** ____________________

**5.** Explain the term *DRG* and how it is implemented in hospitals:

____________________

**6.** Define the term *fragmentation of care* and its effect on the health care system:

____________________

## APPLYING YOUR KNOWLEDGE

### CRITICAL THINKING QUESTIONS

**1.** Think about a group of people in your community that is underserved and lacks access to nursing resources. How might the needs of this group be addressed?

**2.** Visit a health care clinic in your community. Find out what types of services are performed and the backgrounds of the patients seeking these services. Research how the clinic is funded and how the staff is reimbursed for its services. Would you feel comfortable being cared for in this clinic? Explain why or why not.

**3.** Look at the promotional materials for a local health care plan and interview people on the plan. Which features of the plan are most important for the insured? What does the plan lack? Is the insured party free to choose his/her own doctors or treatment plans?

**4.** Compare the roles and responsibilities of a physical therapist versus an occupational therapist, a physician versus a physician assistant, and a social worker versus a chaplain. Write down the responsibilities of each professional, where they overlap to provide continuity of care for the patient, and where they diverge to meet the specific needs of each patient. How will this information help you as a nurse to coordinate the efforts of the interdisciplinary team?

### REFLECTIVE PRACTICE: DEVELOPING QSEN COMPETENCIES

***Use the following expanded scenario from Chapter 11 in your textbook to answer the questions below.***

*Scenario:* Margaret Ritchie, age 63, is caring at home for her 67-year-old husband, who is diagnosed with amyotrophic lateral sclerosis (ALS, or Lou Gehrig's disease). She says, "All the help from the home care facility has been a blessing, but I need more help and some other equipment now, and our insurance company doesn't cover these things. Plus, now the doctor says that his condition has really worsened and he probably has 6 months or less to live." On further assessment, the nurse notes that Mrs. Ritchie appears overwhelmed with her home situation and may be suffering from "caregiver burnout."

1. What nursing interventions might the nurse employ to assist Mrs. Ritchie with her caregiver duties?

______________________________________

______________________________________

______________________________________

2. What would be a successful outcome for this patient?

______________________________________

______________________________________

______________________________________

3. What intellectual, technical, interpersonal, and/or ethical/legal competencies are most likely to bring about the desired outcome?

______________________________________

______________________________________

______________________________________

4. What resources might be helpful for Mrs. Ritchie?

______________________________________

______________________________________

______________________________________

## PRACTICING FOR NCLEX

### MULTIPLE CHOICE QUESTIONS

***Circle the letter that corresponds to the best answer for each question.***

1. A nurse is helping a patient choose a new health care plan. The patient states that he would prefer to be able to choose his own health care provider. Which plan would be the least appropriate for this patient based on his stated preferences?
   a. HMO
   b. PPO
   c. POS
   d. LTC
2. A nurse is caring for a patient who has a PPO health care plan. What is the greatest advantage of this type of plan?
   a. Ease of referrals
   b. Cost effectiveness
   c. Care coordination
   d. Improved health outcomes
3. A home health care nurse is providing visits for a 65-year-old widower who needs some assistance with ADLs but is living independently. What option might the nurse recommend that would enable the patient to maintain independence for as long as possible?
   a. Aging in place
   b. Medical home
   c. Long-term care facility
   d. Transitional subacute care facility
4. A nurse is discharging a patient who was admitted for observation following a motor vehicle accident. The patient is a single parent who is living in a new community. What service would be an appropriate referral for this patient?
   a. Respite care
   b. Hospice care
   c. Medical home
   d. Parish nursing

5. A nurse works with patients in a crisis intervention center. What ability would be most important for this nurse to develop?
   a. Technical skills
   b. Decision-making ability
   c. Communication and counseling skills
   d. Relating to coworkers on a professional level
6. A nurse recommends palliative care for a patient who is being discharged following a diagnosis of cancer. What is the chief focus of this type of care?
   a. Provision of a dignified death experience
   b. Physical rehabilitation
   c. Relief from physical, mental, and spiritual distress
   d. Occupational therapy
7. Nurses in various health care settings provide services to prevent the fragmentation of care that is occurring as a health care trend in today's society. What role of the nurse is most important in preventing this effect?
   a. Care provision
   b. Counselor
   c. Teacher
   d. Care coordinator
8. A nurse is a manager of an ambulatory care facility. What nursing function would be most commonly found in this type of facility?
   a. Serving as an administrator or manager
   b. Providing direct patient care
   c. Educating individual people or groups
   d. Assessing the home environment
9. Which patient would a nurse correctly refer to Medicare services?
   a. A patient with cancer
   b. A low-income family with infants needing immunizations
   c. A patient with a disability
   d. A 66-year-old patient with diabetes
10. A nurse is helping patients access the health insurance marketplace. What is the goal of this health insurance coverage concept?
   a. Comparison of available health care plans
   b. Insurance for older adults
   c. Insurance assistance for women and children
   d. Insurance coverage for people needing orphan drugs

## ALTERNATE-FORMAT QUESTIONS

### Multiple Response Questions

***Circle the letters that correspond to the best answers for each question.***

1. Nurses provide care for patients as they move throughout the health care system. What are methods used to ensure continuity of care and cost-effective care during this process? *(Select all that apply.)*
   a. Managed care
   b. Case management
   c. Rural health centers
   d. Parish nursing
   e. Primary health care
   f. Primary care centers
2. A nurse provides care for patients in a primary care center. What are typical roles of a nurse in this type of facility? *(Select all that apply.)*
   a. Managing members of the health care team
   b. Performing in-service education
   c. Making health assessments
   d. Performing technical procedures
   e. Researching nursing issues
   f. Providing health education
3. Home health care is one of the most rapidly growing areas of the health care system. What are chief tasks of the home health care nurse? *(Select all that apply.)*
   a. Developing a nursing care plan
   b. Providing for a dignified death at home
   c. Providing patient teaching and counseling
   d. Providing continuity of care
   e. Administering medications
   f. Collecting payment for nursing care
4. Nurses provide care for patients in a program called "Hospital at Home." What are the characteristics of this program? *(Select all that apply.)*
   a. Higher average patient length of stay
   b. Lower overall costs
   c. Better patient outcomes
   d. Lower chance of developing delirium
   e. Higher use of sedatives and restraints
   f. Higher satisfaction with care

CHAPTER 12

# Collaborative Practice and Care Coordination Across Settings

## ASSESSING YOUR UNDERSTANDING

### FILL IN THE BLANKS

1. A nurse is providing health care for people in a small neighborhood clinic. This type of care is termed ______ nursing.
2. A nurse is careful to protect the privacy of hospitalized patients. Federal mandates that protect patient privacy rights are provided under the ______ Act.
3. A patient who refuses treatment and leaves a hospital must sign a form releasing the health care provider and institution from legal responsibility for his/her health status. This patient is said to be leaving the hospital ______.
4. A nurse plans for continuity of care for a patient who is moving from an acute care setting to home health care. This planning process is known as ______.

### CORRECT THE FALSE STATEMENTS

***Circle the word "true" or "false" that follows the statement. If you circled "false," change the underlined word or words to make the statement true. Place your answer in the space provided.***

1. The <u>health care provider</u> is the person who most often is responsible for helping the patient make a smooth transition from one type of care setting to another.
   a. True
   b. False ______
2. <u>Discharge planning</u> is the coordination of services provided to patients before they enter a health care setting, during the time they are in the setting, and after they leave the setting.
   a. True
   b. False ______
3. People who enter a health care setting must take on the role of <u>patient</u>.
   a. True
   b. False ______

4. Ambulatory facilities are those in which the patient receives health care services but does not remain overnight.
   a. True
   b. False ______

5. The admitting diagnosis is generally included on the identification wristband that is placed on the patient's wrist during treatment at a health care facility.
   a. True
   b. False ______

6. Hospital admissions and lengths of hospital stay are increasing.
   a. True
   b. False ______

7. Discharge planning is not indicated when a patient is to be placed in a long-term care facility or other continuing care setting.
   a. True
   b. False ______

8. When goals are established with the patient, compliance with the treatment regimen is more likely.
   a. True
   b. False ______

9. When transferring a patient to a long-term facility for care, the original chart is sent with the patient.
   a. True
   b. False ______

10. Your patient says, "I'm going home today!" You verify this by checking the nursing care plan.
    a. True
    b. False ______

## SHORT ANSWER

1. Describe how a nurse could help reduce anxiety for a patient who expresses the following concerns on being admitted to a health care facility:
   a. "Who will take care of my children when I'm in here?"

   ______

   b. "Will the procedure be painful?"

   ______

   c. "Will I be able to afford this?"

   ______

   d. "Who will take care of me after my surgery?"

   ______

2. Briefly describe how a nurse should instruct a patient in the following areas of care before discharge:
   a. Medications: ______
   b. Procedures and treatments: ______
   c. Diet: ______
   d. Referrals: ______
   e. Health promotion: ______

3. Describe how the following methods help provide continuity of care for patients:
   a. Discharge planning: ______
   b. Collaboration with other members of the health care team: ______
   c. Involving patient and family in planning: ______

4. List five guidelines that should be followed when admitting and discharging a patient from a hospital, according to the standards established by The Joint Commission.
   a. ______
   b. ______
   c. ______
   d. ______
   e. ______

5. List four factors the nurse should assess before discharge planning for a 38-year-old woman hospitalized for a miscarriage in her second month of pregnancy, as well as for her husband; she has been trying to conceive a child for 2 years.
   a. ____________________
   b. ____________________
   c. ____________________
   d. ____________________

6. Describe the appropriate nursing actions that would be performed during the following patient transfers:
   a. Transfer within the hospital setting: ____________________
   b. Transfer to a long-term facility: ____________________
   c. Discharge from a health care setting: ____________________

7. What is the proper procedure for discharging a patient against medical advice (AMA)?
   ____________________

8. Describe how you would prepare a hospital room for a patient who is arriving on a stretcher and is receiving oxygen. ____________________

9. Give an example of the following skills needed to practice community-based nursing:
   a. Knowledgeable and skilled: ____________________
   b. Independent in making decisions: ____________________
   c. Accountable: ____________________

10. A nurse is using the ISBARQ approach to transfer an 82-year-old patient who was hospitalized for a week with pneumonia to a long-term care facility. Describe what actions would occur in the following steps of this process:
   a. I: ____________________
   b. S: ____________________
   c. B: ____________________
   d. A: ____________________
   e. R: ____________________
   f. Q: ____________________

## APPLYING YOUR KNOWLEDGE

### CRITICAL THINKING QUESTIONS

1. More and more hospital services are being performed on an outpatient basis. Although this practice is cost efficient, in many cases, patients are being sent home without the knowledge they need to care for themselves. Think about what can be done to bridge the gap between hospital and home health care. How would you use this knowledge to discharge a 59-year-old woman who lives alone and is recovering from back surgery?
2. Imagine that your older adult mother is being discharged from the hospital with a stroke that left her partially paralyzed, and she is no longer able to live alone. Community living options include a life-care community, a live-in companion, living with you, or living in a long-term care facility. Think about the information and support you would need to make this decision. How might this knowledge influence your nursing practice?

### REFLECTIVE PRACTICE: CULTIVATING QSEN COMPETENCIES

***Use the following expanded scenario from Chapter 12 in your textbook to answer the questions below.***

***Scenario:*** Jeff Hart is a 9-year-old with severe intellectual disability. He is being transferred from the state home for children to the hospital for respiratory complications associated with pneumonia. His grandmother is present and is anxious about her grandson's condition. She asks the nurse if she is responsible for admitting him.

1. How might the admitting nurse respond to the grandmother's anxiety regarding her grandson's admission and condition?

_______________________________________

_______________________________________

_______________________________________

2. What would be a successful outcome for this patient?

_______________________________________

_______________________________________

_______________________________________

3. What intellectual, technical, interpersonal, and/or ethical/legal competencies are most likely to bring about the desired outcome?

_______________________________________

_______________________________________

_______________________________________

4. What resources might be helpful for the nurse working with this family?

_______________________________________

_______________________________________

_______________________________________

## PRACTICING FOR NCLEX

### MULTIPLE CHOICE QUESTIONS

***Circle the letter that corresponds to the best answer for each question.***

1. A nurse is caring for a patient who is in acute respiratory distress from pneumonia but refuses to stay for treatment. It is the nurse's responsibility to:
   - **a.** restrain the patient until a social worker can explain the possible results of the patient's actions.
   - **b.** call for a psychological consultation to see if the patient is mentally stable.
   - **c.** notify the health care provider, discuss the outcomes of the patient's decision, and have the patient sign a release form.
   - **d.** call the patient's family and have them discharge her.

2. A nurse is preparing to discharge a patient from an acute care facility. Which action must be performed by the nurse upon discharge of this patient?
   - **a.** Coordinating future care for the patient
   - **b.** Writing a discharge order for the patient
   - **c.** Writing any orders for future home visits that may be necessary for the patient
   - **d.** Sending the patient's records to the health care provider

3. A nurse is transferring a patient from a hospital setting to an extended care facility. What action is most important to ensure continuity of care for this patient?
   - **a.** Notifying all departments of the room change
   - **b.** Carefully moving all the patient's personal items
   - **c.** Asking family members to take home the patient's jewelry, money, or other valuables
   - **d.** Providing accurate and complete communication to the new facility

4. A nurse sits down with a patient and explains the "Patient Care Partnership." This action best exemplifies what role of the community-based nurse?
   - **a.** Patient advocate
   - **b.** Coordinator of services
   - **c.** Patient educator
   - **d.** Care provider

5. A nurse is preparing for handoff communication for a patient who is being discharged from the hospital to home health care. Which example is not an action performed during this process?
   - **a.** The nurse determines who should be involved in the handoff communication.
   - **b.** The nurse prepares the new room for the patient.
   - **c.** The nurse asks the other health care professionals if they have any questions.
   - **d.** The nurse uses the SBAR technique during the handoff.

6. A nurse coordinator for a busy hospital provides for continuity of care for patients using the hospital services. What cognitive skill would this nurse need to ensure continuity of care?
   a. The ability to provide the technical nursing assistance to meet the needs of patients and their families
   b. The ability to establish trusting professional relationships with patients, family caregivers, and health care professionals in different practice settings
   c. The knowledge of how to communicate patient priorities and the related plan of care as a patient is transferred between different settings
   d. Commitment to securing the best setting for care to be provided for patients and the best coordination of resources to support the level of care needed

## ALTERNATE-FORMAT QUESTIONS

### Multiple Response Questions

***Circle the letters that correspond to the best answers for each question.***

1. A nurse is using the ISBARQ (introduction, situation, background, assessment, recommendation, and question and answer) framework for handoff communication. Which examples accurately represent this process? *(Select all that apply.)*
   a. The people involved in the process identify themselves, their roles, and their jobs.
   b. The nurse introduces the patient to the health care professionals who will be involved in the new facility.
   c. The nurse reports the patient's vital signs, mental and code status, medications, and lab results.
   d. The nurse makes arrangements for future home health care visits for the patient who is being discharged from the hospital.
   e. The nurse explains the patient's chief complaint, diagnosis, treatment plan, and patient wants and needs.
   f. The nurse reports the current provider's assessment of the patient and need for further services.
2. A nurse is preparing a room for patient admission. Which actions follow recommended guidelines for this process? *(Select all that apply.)*
   a. Keep the room always open and position the bed in the highest position.
   b. Fold back the top bed linens.
   c. Assemble the necessary equipment and supplies, including a hospital admission pack.
   d. Do not supply pajamas or hospital gowns until it is determined whether the patient will wear his or her own.
   e. Ask the health care provider to assemble special equipment needed by the patient (such as oxygen, cardiac monitors, or suction equipment).
   f. Adjust the physical environment of the room, including lighting and temperature.
3. A nurse is admitting a patient to a hospital. Which actions would the nurse perform initially upon this admission? *(Select all that apply.)*
   a. The nurse makes sure the patient's name and address and the name of his/her closest relative are printed on an identification wristband.
   b. The nurse informs the patient that he or she will be asked to sign consent forms that give consent to treatment and allow the hospital to contact insurance companies as needed.
   c. The nurse obtains patient information, which is printed on an admission sheet and becomes part of the patient's permanent record.
   d. The nurse asks the patient about advance directives that he or she may have already made; if none has been made, the nurse gives the appropriate form to the patient.
   e. The nurse clearly describes how the patient information will be used and disclosed to other parties.
   f. The nurse gives the patient a form explaining the Patient Care Partnership.

**4.** A nurse working in a hospital setting is responsible for transferring patients. Which recommended nursing actions would the nurse perform during this process? *(Select all that apply.)*

**a.** The nurse informs the patient's family of the change and asks them to remove the patient's personal belongings.

**b.** The nurse asks the family of a patient moved to a critical care unit to take home the patient's personal belongings.

**c.** The nurse does not formally discharge a patient who is being transferred from the hospital to a long-term care facility.

**d.** The nurse sends the original chart to the new facility when a patient is being transferred to a long-term care facility.

**e.** The nurse carefully packs the belongings of a patient being discharged and sends them to the new facility.

**f.** The hospital nurse prepares a detailed assessment and care plan to send to the long-term facility to which a patient is transferred.

**5.** A nurse is discharging a patient from the hospital. Which nursing actions should occur when a patient is discharged from a health care setting? *(Select all that apply.)*

**a.** The nurse performs discharge planning, which begins upon admission to the facility to ensure continuity of care.

**b.** A hospital administrator coordinates and performs an approved handoff for the patient to a new facility.

**c.** The nurse assesses the patient to ensure that the patient does not require any complicated treatment or care performed by family members.

**d.** The nurse ensures that the family members are taught the knowledge and skills needed to care for the patient.

**e.** The health care provider ensures that referrals are made to such facilities as home health care or social services to provide support and assistance during the recovery period.

**f.** Preferably, the nurse who conducts the initial nursing assessment will determine the special needs of the patient being discharged.

CHAPTER 13

# Blended Competencies, Clinical Reasoning, and Processes of Person-Centered Care

## ASSESSING YOUR UNDERSTANDING

### FILL IN THE BLANKS

1. A nurse who is committed to providing ____________ care develops caring professional relationships based on respect and mutual trust and uses a holistic approach to promote humanism, health, and quality of living.

2. When a nurse assists a patient to achieve desired goals such as promoting wellness, preventing disease and illness, restoring health, or facilitating coping with altered functioning, he or she is using the ____________ step of the nursing process.

3. The overall goal of the ____________ project is to meet the challenge of preparing future nurses who will have the knowledge, skills, and attitudes (KSAs) necessary to continuously improve the quality and safety of the health care systems within which they work.

4. A nurse who is considerate and compassionate and who keeps the person at the center of all deliberations in order to promote the humanity, dignity, and well-being of the person being cared for is practicing ____________ practice.

5. In Gibbs' Model of Reflection, making value judgments about what was good or bad about an experience occurs in the ____________ step.

### MATCHING EXERCISES

***Match the step of the nursing process listed in Part A with the related task listed in Part B. Answers will be used more than once.***

#### PART A

**a.** Assessing
**b.** Diagnosing
**c.** Planning
**d.** Implementing
**e.** Evaluating

#### PART B

____ **1.** A nurse performs an initial patient interview.

____ **2.** A home care nurse helps the physical therapist exercise the patient's limbs.

____ **3.** A nurse sits down with the health care team halfway through treatment of a patient to see how effective the treatment has been.

____ **4.** A nurse analyzes data to determine what health problems might exist.

____ **5.** A nurse sets a goal for an obese teenager to lose 2 lb a week.

____ **6.** A nurse consults with a patient's support people and other health care professionals to learn more about a patient's problem.

____ **7.** A nurse decides whether to continue, modify, or terminate the health care plan.

____ **8.** A nurse identifies the strengths a patient with cancer possesses.

____ **9.** A home care nurse determines how much nursing care is needed by an older adult stroke patient living with her daughter.

____ **10.** A nurse weighs a patient after 3 weeks to determine whether his or her new diet has been effective.

____ **11.** A nurse documents respiratory care performed on a patient.

____ **12.** A nurse reviews a patient's past medical records.

***Match the competencies listed in Part A with the appropriate example of competencies listed in Part B. Answers will be used more than once.***

**PART A**

**a.** Cognitive competencies
**b.** Technical competencies
**c.** Interpersonal competencies
**d.** Ethical/legal competencies

**PART B**

____ **13.** A nurse conducts a patient interview in such a way that the patient relaxes and "opens up" to her.

____ **14.** A nurse skillfully attaches a heart monitor to a patient.

____ **15.** A nurse carefully fills out an incident report documenting a fall.

____ **16.** A nurse understands the need for palpating the lungs of a patient with pneumonia.

____ **17.** A nurse checks the side rails on a bed of an older adult patient with a history of falls.

____ **18.** A nurse successfully performs a catheterization of a patient.

____ **19.** A nurse is familiar with the various types of medications for high blood pressure and their side effects.

____ **20.** A nurse calms the mother of an infant brought to the emergency room with a high fever.

____ **21.** A nurse competently starts an IV drip on a patient.

____ **22.** A nurse checks a patient's bracelet before administering medications.

## SHORT ANSWER

**1.** List three patient and three nursing benefits of using the nursing process correctly.

Patient:

**a.** ____________________
**b.** ____________________
**c.** ____________________

Nursing:

**a.** ____________________
**b.** ____________________
**c.** ____________________

**2.** Describe how the nurse and patient work together to accomplish the following tasks of the nursing process:

**a.** Determining the need for nursing care:

____________________

____________________

**b.** Planning and implementing the care:

____________________

____________________

**c.** Evaluating the results of the nursing care:

____________________

____________________

**3.** Define the nursing process:

___

___

What are the primary goals of the nursing process?

___

___

What skills are necessary to use the nursing process successfully?

___

___

Which of these skills do you personally possess, and which do you need to develop in your practice?

___

___

**4.** Describe what the following words mean to you and how they apply to your use of the nursing process:

**a.** Systematic: ___

___

**b.** Dynamic: ___

___

**c.** Interpersonal: ___

___

**d.** Outcome oriented: ___

___

**e.** Universally applicable in nursing situations: ___

___

**5.** Briefly explain how the following considerations are relevant to the successful use of critical thinking competencies:

**a.** Purpose of thinking: ___

___

**b.** Adequacy of knowledge: ___

___

**c.** Potential problems: ___

___

**d.** Helpful resources: ___

___

**e.** Critique of judgment/decision: ___

___

**6.** List four good habits nurses should develop to help them master the psychomotor skills essential to quality nursing process.

**a.** ___

**b.** ___

**c.** ___

**d.** ___

**7.** Think of three people you know personally, of different ages, professions, or cultures. What is it about each of these people that causes you to respect his or her human dignity? Are some people more deserving of respect than others? How do you show respect for them in your daily contact with them?

___

___

___

___

**8.** Follow three different nurses on their daily rounds of patients, noticing how they relate to their patients. Does their attitude say "drop dead," "you mean nothing to me," or "I care about you"? Note what each nurse said or did to display this attitude.

**a.** Nurse 1: ___

___

**b.** Nurse 2: ___

___

**c.** Nurse 3: ___

___

**9.** Nurses skilled in developing caring relationships often need to direct the conversations with their patients. Develop four opening statements/questions designed to elicit information from a patient that you could use in your own practice.

**a.** ___

**b.** ___

**c.** ___

**d.** ___

**10.** List four areas a nurse should consider when seeking to develop a sense of legal and ethical accountability to a patient.

**a.** ____________________

**b.** ____________________

**c.** ____________________

**d.** ____________________

**11.** Give an example of how the following personal attributes of the professional nurse assist the nurse in planning and delivering patient-centered care. Consider how each personal attribute affects each step of the nursing process.

**a.** Open-mindedness: ____________________

**b.** Profound sense of the value of the person: ____________________

**c.** Self-awareness and knowledge of own beliefs and values: ____________________

**d.** Sense of personal responsibility for actions: ____________________

**e.** Caring about well-being of patients and acting accordingly: ____________________

**f.** Leadership skills: ____________________

**g.** Bravery to question the "system": ____________________

## APPLYING YOUR KNOWLEDGE

### CRITICAL THINKING QUESTIONS

**1.** Assess your personal blend of the skills nurses need: cognitive, technical, interpersonal, and ethical/legal. Would you want you to be your nurse? What skills do you need to develop to meet the needs of those entrusted to your care?

**2.** Think about major health problems on campus. How might the school of nursing use the nursing process to address one or more of these problems? Do you as a nursing student have an obligation to address the health problems you encounter?

**3.** Think about a stressful situation you had to deal with, such as changing a course of study, accepting a job in another city, dealing with a sick relative, deciding on a life partner, and so on. What methods did you use to weigh all your options in making this decision? Where did you turn for information or assistance? How did you reach your final decision? Relate the method you used in your life to the models of problem solving listed in this chapter. Which process most accurately describes your personal process of problem solving? Compare this process to the nursing process.

**4.** Write down all the qualities you admire in your friends. What is it about them that makes you respect them? What attributes of their personality don't you like? How might this knowledge help you to understand your responses to patients with different personality traits? Are some patients more worthy of your respect than others? Do you feel your attitude toward a patient affects the outcome of treatment?

### REFLECTIVE PRACTICE: CULTIVATING QSEN COMPETENCIES

***Use the following expanded scenario from Chapter 13 in your textbook to answer the questions below.***

***Scenario:*** Charlotte Horvath is a single mother whose 5-year-old daughter is to be discharged soon. Ms. Horvath is scheduled to learn how to perform wound care for her daughter at home but has missed every planned teaching session thus far. When questioned by the nurse, Ms. Horvath says she doesn't have enough time to put a decent meal on the table, let alone learn how to take care of a wound at home. Ms. Horvath works in the evening shift and has a babysitter stay with her children from immediately after school until midnight.

**1.** How might the nurse use blended nursing skills to respond to this patient situation?

____________________

____________________

____________________

2. What would be a successful outcome for this patient and her family?

______________________________________

______________________________________

______________________________________

3. What intellectual, technical, interpersonal, and/or ethical/legal competencies are most likely to bring about the desired outcome?

______________________________________

______________________________________

______________________________________

4. What resources might be helpful for Ms. Horvath?

______________________________________

______________________________________

______________________________________

## PRACTICING FOR NCLEX

### MULTIPLE CHOICE QUESTIONS

***Circle the letter that corresponds to the best answer for each question.***

1. A nurse is using the QSEN competency of evidence-based practice when caring for patients. What is an example of this competency?
   - **a.** The nurse works with other health care team members to provide care for a patient diagnosed with Alzheimer's disease.
   - **b.** The nurse manager holds an in-service for staff to teach them the safe operation of a new piece of equipment.
   - **c.** The nurse researches best current practices for prevention of the spread of infection in health care provider offices.
   - **d.** The nurse uses computer-generated care plans for patient care.

2. A nurse takes the vital signs of a new hospital patient admitted for severe abdominal pain. What initial step of the nursing process is this nurse performing?
   - **a.** Assessment
   - **b.** Diagnosis
   - **c.** Implementation
   - **d.** Evaluation

3. When using the nursing process, the nurse notes that there is a great deal of overlapping of the steps, with each step flowing into the next. What is the term for this characteristic of the nursing process?
   - **a.** Interpersonal
   - **b.** Dynamic
   - **c.** Systematic
   - **d.** Universally applicable

4. A nurse administers medications to a patient as part of the implementation step of the nursing care plan. What step of the nursing process would the nurse perform next?
   - **a.** Assessing
   - **b.** Diagnosing
   - **c.** Evaluating
   - **d.** Planning

5. Nurses use the nursing process to plan care for patients. In which case is the nursing process applicable?
   - **a.** When nurses work with patients who are able to participate in their care
   - **b.** When families are clearly supportive and wish to participate in care
   - **c.** When patients are totally dependent on the nurse for care
   - **d.** In all the nursing situations listed above

6. What interpersonal skill is displayed by a nurse who is attentive and responsive to the health care needs of individual patients and ensures the continuity of care when leaving the patient?
   - **a.** Establishing caring relationships
   - **b.** Enjoying the rewards of mutual interchange
   - **c.** Developing accountability
   - **d.** Developing ethical/legal skills

7. The nurse uses the QSEN competency of Informatics when planning care for patients. What is an example of the use of this skill?
   - **a.** The nurse works collaboratively with a dietician to devise a patient meal plan.
   - **b.** The nurse orients a visually impaired patient to the hospital room.
   - **c.** The nurse checks with the patient for priorities when planning patient care.
   - **d.** The nurse researches new technologic advances in the treatment of cancer.

## ALTERNATE-FORMAT QUESTIONS

### Multiple Response Questions

***Circle the letters that correspond to the best answers for each question.***

1. Nurses are expected to have the KSAs necessary to continually improve the quality and safety of the health care system within which they work. Which KSAs are examples of nursing actions based on the QSEN competency of quality improvement? *(Select all that apply.)*
   - **a.** The nurse manager schedules a meeting of staff to review patient outcomes on the hospital ward.
   - **b.** The nurse schedules a meeting with the nurse manager to review and update the policies for patient admissions.
   - **c.** The nurse administrator sets up a committee to review the procedure manual and recommend any needed changes.
   - **d.** The nurse coordinator calls a meeting of all the health care professionals involved in the care of a patient.
   - **e.** The nurse uses the Internet to find new nursing techniques for the care of a patient with cystic fibrosis.
   - **f.** The nurse listens to a patient who is having trouble adjusting to a long-term care facility and treats the patient with compassion and respect.

2. Nurses use the nursing process to solve problems in their practices. Which statements describe the common use of problem solving in the nursing process? *(Select all that apply.)*
   - **a.** The trial-and-error problem-solving method is used extensively in the nursing process.
   - **b.** The trial-and-error problem-solving method is recommended as a guide for nursing practice.
   - **c.** The scientific problem-solving method is closely related to the more general problem-solving process (the nursing process) commonly used by health care professionals as they work with patients.
   - **d.** Nurse theorists and educators advocate basing clinical judgments on data alone in an attempt to establish nursing as a science, worthy of the respect of other professions.
   - **e.** Today, nurses acknowledge the positive role of intuitive thinking in clinical decision making.
   - **f.** Critical thinking in nursing can be intuitive or logical or a combination of both.

3. The ability to communicate clearly through documentation is a critical nursing skill. Which statements accurately describe the role of documenting in the nursing process? *(Select all that apply.)*
   - **a.** The patient record is the chief means of communication among members of the interdisciplinary team.
   - **b.** If a nurse is accused of negligent care, the nurse's word that he or she faithfully assessed the patient's needs, diagnosed problems, and implemented and evaluated an effective plan of care is his or her best defense.
   - **c.** Legally speaking, a nursing action not documented is a nursing action not performed.
   - **d.** It is helpful to practice documentation while learning any given nursing activity.
   - **e.** The content of the patient report and nursing documentation helps to establish nursing priorities in a practice setting.
   - **f.** Because data collection is ongoing and responsive to changes in the patient's condition, it should be documented in the final step of the nursing process.

4. Nurses who prize their role in securing patient well-being are sensitive to the ethical and legal implications of nursing practice. What are examples of these ethical/legal skills? *(Select all that apply.)*
   - **a.** Working collaboratively with the health care team as a respected and credible colleague to reach valued goals
   - **b.** Being trusted to act in ways that advance the interests of patients
   - **c.** Using technical equipment with sufficient competence and ease to achieve goals with minimal distress to patients
   - **d.** Selecting nursing interventions that are most likely to yield the desired outcomes
   - **e.** Being accountable for practice to oneself, the patient, the caregiving team, and society
   - **f.** Acting as an effective patient advocate

5. Cognitively skilled nurses are critical thinkers. What are characteristics of a critical thinker? *(Select all that apply.)*
   a. Thinking based on the opinions of others
   b. Being open to all points of view
   c. Acting like a "know-it-all"
   d. Resisting "easy answers" to patient problems
   e. Thinking "outside the box"
   f. Accepting the status quo

**Prioritization Questions**

1. Place the nursing activities in the order that they would most likely occur when a health care professional uses the nursing process:
   a. Modifying the plan of care (if indicated)
   b. Carrying out the plan of care
   c. Establishing the database
   d. Interpreting and analyzing patient data
   e. Establishing priorities
   f. Measuring how well the patient has achieved desired outcomes

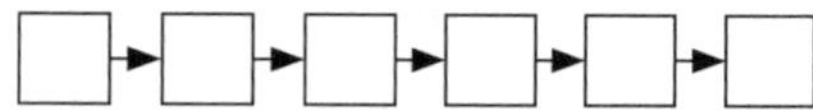

2. Place the steps of scientific problem solving in the order in which they occur in the process:
   a. Hypothesis formulation
   b. Plan of action
   c. Evaluation
   d. Interpretation of results
   e. Problem identification
   f. Data collection
   g. Hypothesis testing

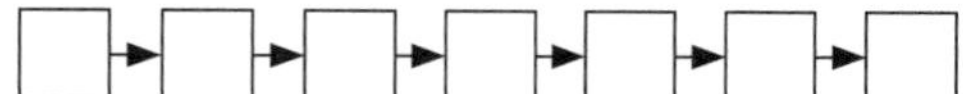

CHAPTER 14

# Assessing

## ASSESSING YOUR UNDERSTANDING

### FILL IN THE BLANKS

1. The primary source of patient data is the patient, but two other sources of patient data are ____________ and ____________.
2. The type of nursing assessment that is performed during the nurse's initial contact with the patient and involves collecting data about all aspects of the patient's health is called the ____________.
3. When a nurse confirms or verifies the data collected upon assessment to keep it free of error, bias, or misinterpretation, he or she is performing the act of ____________.
4. The ____________ is a health care tool practitioners can use to assess patient complexity using the social determinants of health, which affect the person's ability to manage his or her health.
5. A nurse who gathers data about a newly diagnosed case of hypertension in a 52-year-old patient is performing a(n) ____________ type of assessment.
6. When the nurse compares the current status of a patient to the initial assessment performed during the admitting process, he or she is performing a(n) ____________ type of assessment.
7. Most schools of nursing and health care institutions establish the specific information that must be collected from every patient in a structured assessment form. This information is known as a(n) ____________.

### MATCHING EXERCISES

***Match the term in Part A with the definition in Part B.***

**PART A**

- **a.** Database
- **b.** Focused assessment
- **c.** Interview
- **d.** Health assessment
- **e.** Nursing history
- **f.** Objective data
- **g.** Physical assessment
- **h.** Subjective data
- **i.** Validation
- **j.** Observation
- **k.** Time-lapsed assessments

**PART B**

____ **1.** Observable and measurable information that can be seen, heard, or felt by someone other than the person experiencing it

____ **2.** The conscious and deliberate use of the five physical senses to gather information

____ **3.** Clearly identifies patient strengths and weaknesses, health risks, and potential and existing health problems

____ **4.** A planned communication to obtain patient data

____ **5.** The examination of a patient for objective data that may better define the patient's condition and help the nurse in planning care

____ **6.** The act of confirming or verifying data

____ **7.** Compares a patient's current status to baseline data obtained earlier

____ **8.** Includes all the pertinent patient information collected by the nurse and other health care professionals, enabling a comprehensive and effective plan of care to be designed and implemented for the patient

____ **9.** The gathering of data about a specific problem that has already been identified

____ **10.** May be used by nurses to help patients identify potential and actual health risks and to explore the habits, behaviors, beliefs, attitudes, and values that influence their health

***Match the examples of data in Part B with the type of data in Part A. Answers will be used more than once.***

**PART A**

**a.** Objective data

**b.** Subjective data

**PART B**

____ **11.** Redness and swelling are noticed at the site of an incision.

____ **12.** A patient complains of pain in his left arm.

____ **13.** A patient has a violent spell of coughing.

____ **14.** A patient recovering from knee surgery favors his impaired leg when walking.

____ **15.** A patient is nauseated at the sight of food.

____ **16.** A patient worries about her children during her hospital stay.

**SHORT ANSWER**

**1.** List the five functions of the initial comprehensive nursing assessment.

**a.** ____________________

**b.** ____________________

**c.** ____________________

**d.** ____________________

**e.** ____________________

**2.** Identify eight sources of patient data and give an example of each.

**a.** ____________________

**b.** ____________________

**c.** ____________________

**d.** ____________________

**e.** ____________________

**f.** ____________________

**g.** ____________________

**h.** ____________________

**3.** Briefly describe why the following characteristics of data are important when collecting and recording patient data.

**a.** Purposeful: ____________________

**b.** Prioritized: ____________________

**c.** Complete: ____________________

**d.** Systematic: ____________________

**e.** Accurate: ____________________

**f.** Relevant: ____________________

**g.** Recorded in a standard manner: ____________________

**4.** Give an example of three observations nurses should make each time they encounter a patient.

**a.** ____________________

**b.** ____________________

**c.** ____________________

5. Give two examples of open-ended questions that could be used to elicit information from your patient, a 42-year-old mother of three young children who has recently been diagnosed with diabetes; she is admitted to the hospital overnight for observation.
   a. ____________________

   ____________________
   b. ____________________

   ____________________

6. Explain how the following factors affect assessment priorities when collecting patient data.
   a. Patient's health orientation: ____________________

   ____________________
   b. Patient's developmental stage: ____________________

   ____________________
   c. Patient's culture: ____________________

   ____________________
   d. Patient's need for nursing: ____________________

   ____________________

7. Give two examples of when data need to be validated.
   a. ____________________
   b. ____________________

8. Explain when the immediate communication of data is indicated.

   ____________________

   ____________________

# APPLYING YOUR KNOWLEDGE

## CRITICAL THINKING QUESTIONS

1. Role-play the following nursing interviews with your classmates:
   a. A 50-year-old woman with diabetes and diabetic foot ulcers is admitted to the emergency room for observation after she experienced a blackout.
   b. An 85-year-old man is admitted to the coronary care unit after experiencing a possible stroke.
   c. A teenage boy is admitted to the hospital with severe stomach pains and a possible ruptured appendix.

   Talk about which approaches and types of questions resulted in the best interviews.

2. Recall the last time you went to a doctor's office for a checkup or medical problem. How were you treated by the doctor's staff? Did they do anything to make you feel comfortable or uncomfortable? What did they do to include you in the process? How did it feel to be a patient at the mercy of others? What would you do to incorporate this learning into your own nursing practice?

## REFLECTIVE PRACTICE: CULTIVATING QSEN COMPETENCIES

***Use the following expanded scenario from Chapter 14 in your textbook to answer the questions below.***

***Scenario:*** Susan Morgan is a 34-year-old woman newly diagnosed with multiple sclerosis. She was recently married to a man she met while hiking the Appalachian Trail. While educating Ms. Morgan about her disease, the nurse notices that she appears distressed and angry. Ms. Morgan says, "How am I going to tell my husband? We were just married last year and planned to do lots of hiking and outdoor sports. It's not fair for him to be tied down to me if I can't be the wife and partner that he thought he married."

1. How might the nurse facilitate Ms. Morgan's ability to cope with disability?

   ____________________

   ____________________

   ____________________

2. What would be a successful outcome for this patient?

   ____________________

   ____________________

   ____________________

3. What intellectual, technical, interpersonal, and/or ethical/legal competencies are most likely to bring about the desired outcome?

   ____________________

   ____________________

   ____________________

4. What resources might be helpful for Ms. Morgan?

______________________________

______________________________

______________________________

## PRACTICING FOR NCLEX

### MULTIPLE CHOICE QUESTIONS

***Circle the letter that corresponds to the best answer for each question.***

1. Nurses collect objective and subjective data when performing patient assessments. What is an example of objective data?
   a. A patient receiving chemotherapy complains of nausea.
   b. A patient states that she is feeling very anxious about her tests.
   c. A patient with inner ear infections complains of dizziness.
   d. The skin of a patient who has liver failure has a yellowish tint.
2. A nurse is conducting an interview with a patient who complains of abdominal distress. What is an appropriate interview question for this patient?
   a. "You haven't eaten anything that could have been spoiled, have you?"
   b. "Do you think you might have appendicitis?"
   c. "Are you feeling poorly besides your stomachache?"
   d. "What is your problem as you see it?"
3. A nurse is interviewing a hospitalized patient. Which nurse–patient positioning facilitates an easy exchange of information?
   a. If the patient is in bed, the nurse stands at the foot of the bed.
   b. If both the nurse and patient are seated, their chairs are at right angles to each other, 1 foot apart.
   c. If the patient is in bed, the nurse sits in a chair placed at a 45-degree angle to the bed.
   d. If the patient is in bed, the nurse stands at the side of the bed.
4. A nurse is interviewing a new patient admitted to the hospital for surgery. Which action would the nurse perform in the introductory phase of the interview?
   a. The nurse assesses the patient's comfort and ability to participate in the interview.
   b. The nurse recapitulates the interview, highlighting important points.
   c. The nurse ensures the environment for the interview is comfortable and private.
   d. The nurse gathers all the information needed to form the subjective database.
5. A nurse is assessing a patient admitted to the hospital with complaints of left-sided weakness and difficulty speaking. Which assessment contains the data that best represent a nursing assessment?
   a. Neurologic examination reveals partial paralysis and aphasic speech.
   b. Brain scan shows evidence of a clot in the middle cerebral artery.
   c. Patient is unable to communicate basic needs and cannot perform hygiene measures with left hand.
   d. Left-sided weakness and speech deficit indicate probable stroke.
6. A nurse is assessing an energetic 80-year-old admitted to the hospital with complaints of difficulty urinating, bloody urine, and burning on urination. What is a priority assessment for this patient?
   a. Assessing only the urinary system
   b. Focusing on altered patterns of elimination common in older adults
   c. Obtaining a detailed assessment of the patient's sexual history
   d. Conducting a thorough systems review to validate data on the patient's record
7. During the nursing examination, the nurse notices that the patient, an older adult female, becomes very tired, but there are still questions that need to be addressed in order to have data for planning care. Which action would be most appropriate in this situation?
   a. Ask the patient to wake up and try to answer the interview questions.
   b. Ask the patient's husband to come in and answer the interview questions.
   c. Wait until the next day to obtain the answers to the interview questions.

d. Ask the patient if it is okay to interview her husband for the answers to the interview questions.

8. A 50-year-old female patient is admitted to a hospital unit with the diagnosis of scleroderma. The nurse is unfamiliar with this condition. What is the nurse's best source of information?
   a. Consult with the patient.
   b. Consult with the patient's doctor.
   c. Read the patient's chart.
   d. Consult nursing and medical literature.

## ALTERNATE-FORMAT QUESTIONS

### Multiple Response Questions

***Circle the letters that correspond to the best answers for each question.***

1. Nurses perform nursing assessments on patients as part of their routine care. Which statements accurately describe the unique focus of these nursing assessments? *(Select all that apply.)*
   a. Nursing assessments duplicate medical assessments.
   b. Nursing assessments target data pointing to pathologic conditions.
   c. Nursing assessments focus on the patient's responses to health problems.
   d. The findings from a nursing assessment may contribute to the identification of a medical diagnosis.
   e. The focus of nursing assessment is on actual, not potential, health problems.
   f. An initial assessment establishes a complete database for problem solving and care planning.
2. Following a patient interview, the nurse is organizing data obtained according to Gordon's functional health pattern model. Which statements reflect the focus of this model? *(Select all that apply.)*
   a. Data are clustered or organized according to a hierarchy of basic human needs.
   b. Data are collected regarding the health perception/health management of the patient.
   c. The perception of the major roles and responsibilities in the patient's life is explored.
   d. The major body systems are assessed and data are collected.
   e. Data related to human response patterns are collected and organized.
   f. Elimination, activity, sleep, and sexuality are components of the assessment and data collection.
3. Nurses collect objective and subjective data during the patient interview. Which patient data is subjective data? *(Select all that apply.)*
   a. A nurse observes a patient wringing her hands before signing consent for surgery.
   b. A nurse observes redness and swelling at an IV site.
   c. A patient describes his pain as an 8 on the pain assessment scale.
   d. A patient feels nauseated after eating his breakfast.
   e. A patient's blood pressure is elevated following physical activity.
   f. A patient complains of being cold and requests an extra blanket.

### Prioritization Question

1. Place the following actions performed by a nurse during a patient interview in the order in which they would most likely occur. Keep in mind the four distinct phases of the interview process: preparatory phase, introduction, working phase, and termination.
   a. The nurse gathers all the information needed to form the subjective database.
   b. The nurse prepares to meet the patient by reading current and past records and reports.
   c. The nurse recapitulates the interview, highlighting the key points.
   d. The nurse initiates the interview by stating his or her name, identifying the purpose of the interview, and clarifying the roles of the nurse and patient.
   e. The nurse ensures that the environment in which the interview is to be conducted is private and relaxed.
   f. The nurse assesses the patient's comfort and ability to participate in the interview.

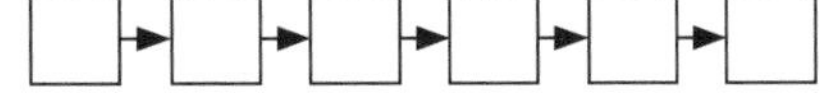

CHAPTER 15

# Diagnosing

## ASSESSING YOUR UNDERSTANDING

### FILL IN THE BLANKS

1. When a nurse writes a patient outcome that requires pain medication for goal achievement, the situation is a(n) ____________ problem.
2. Patient complaints of chills and nausea are considered significant data or ____________.
3. When determining the significance of a patient's urinalysis, the normative values to which the data can be compared are termed a(n) ____________.
4. When a nurse groups patient cues that point to the existence of a patient health problem, the cues form what is known as a(n) ____________.
5. When a nurse recognizes a cluster of significant patient data indicating that patient teaching and counseling for a colostomy is needed, a(n) ____________ should be written.
6. What part of the following nursing diagnosis would be considered the etiology: Spiritual distress related to inability to accept the death of newborn child? ____________
7. Two cues that must be present for a valid wellness diagnosis include ____________ and ____________.
8. A(n) ____________ is a clinical judgment concerning a specific cluster of nursing diagnoses that occur together and are best addressed together and through similar interventions.

### MATCHING EXERCISES

***Match the examples listed in Part B with the four steps involved in the interpretation and analysis of data listed in Part A. Answers will be used more than once.***

**PART A**

**a.** Recognizing significant data
**b.** Recognizing patterns or clusters
**c.** Identifying strengths and problems
**d.** Reaching conclusions

**PART B**

____ **1.** A nurse notes that a patient's refusal to stop smoking will adversely affect his recovery from cardiac surgery.

____ **2.** A nurse compares a 15-month-old child's motor abilities with the norms for that age group.

____ **3.** A nurse recognizes an unhealthy situation developing when her patient, recovering from a mastectomy, cries at night, refuses to eat, and sleeps all day.

____ **4.** A nurse decides no further nursing response is indicated for a woman who recovered from gallbladder surgery according to schedule.

____ **5.** A maternity nurse notices a newborn's skin tone is markedly different from that of the other babies and checks for jaundice.

____ **6.** A nurse determines that a man with a history of diabetes is highly motivated to develop a healthy pattern of nutrition in response to his problem.

____ 7. A nurse notices that a patient with AIDS has an adverse reaction to a drug and consults the prescribing health care provider.

## CORRECT THE FALSE STATEMENTS

***Circle the word "true" or "false" that follows the statement. If you circled "false," change the underlined word or words to make the statement true. Place your answers in the space provided.***

1. Actual or potential health problems that can be prevented or resolved by independent nursing intervention are termed collaborative problems.
   a. True
   b. False ____________________

2. Medical diagnoses represent situations that are the primary responsibility of nurses.
   a. True
   b. False ____________________

3. A cue is a generally accepted rule, measure, pattern, or model that can be used to compare data in the same class or category.
   a. True
   b. False ____________________

4. A data cluster is a grouping of patient data or cues that points to the existence of a patient health problem.
   a. True
   b. False ____________________

5. Nursing diagnoses should be derived from a single cue.
   a. True
   b. False ____________________

6. The NANDA-I list is a beginning list of suggested terms for health problems that may be identified and treated by nurses.
   a. True
   b. False ____________________

7. The problem statement of a nursing diagnosis identifies the physiologic, psychological, sociologic, spiritual, and environmental factors believed to be related to the problem as either a cause or a contributing factor.
   a. True
   b. False ____________________

8. The etiology of nursing diagnoses directs nursing intervention.
   a. True
   b. False ____________________

9. A possible nursing diagnosis is written when the nurse suspects that a health problem exists but needs to gather more data to confirm the diagnosis.
   a. True
   b. False ____________________

10. A wellness diagnosis is a clinical judgment about an individual, family, or community in transition from a specific level of wellness to a higher level of wellness.
   a. True
   b. False ____________________

11. In the diagnosing step, the nurse collects patient data.
   a. True
   b. False ____________________

12. A possible nursing diagnosis is a clinical judgment that an individual, family, or community is more likely to develop the problem than others in the same or similar situation.
   a. True
   b. False ____________________

## SHORT ANSWER

1. Place a check next to the nursing diagnoses that are written correctly, and identify the errors in the incorrect diagnoses on the lines that follow.
   a. __________ Risk for injury related to absence of restraints and side rails __________
   ____________________
   b. __________ Impaired skin integrity related to mobility deficit __________
   ____________________
   c. __________ Grieving related to loss of breast __________
   ____________________
   d. __________ Bathing self-care deficit related to immobility __________
   ____________________

e. ____________ Disturbed sleep pattern related to insomnia ____________

f. ____________ Imbalanced nutrition: less than body requirements related to loss of appetite ____________

g. ____________ Powerlessness related to poor family support system ____________

h. ____________ Anxiety: mild, related to changing lifestyle/diet ____________

i. ____________ Ineffective airway clearance related to 20-year smoking habit ____________

j. ____________ Constipation related to cancer of bowel ____________

k. ____________ Nausea and Vomiting related to medication side effects ____________

l. ____________ Deficient knowledge related to noncompliance with diet ____________

m. ____________ Impaired parenting related to knowledge deficit: child growth and development, discipline ____________

n. ____________ Acute pain related to discomfort in abdomen ____________

o. ____________ Impaired physical mobility: amputation of left leg related to gangrene ____________

p. ____________ Overweight related to obesity ____________

q. ____________ Ineffective health management related to unresolved hostility ____________

r. ____________ Needs assistance walking to bathroom: related to immobility ____________

2. What questions would you ask a patient to validate the following nursing diagnoses?
   a. Impaired urinary elimination: ____________
   b. Impaired social interaction: ____________
   c. Ineffective coping: ____________
   d. Disturbed sleep pattern: ____________

3. Describe the appropriate nursing response to each of the following basic conclusions after interpreting and analyzing patient data.
   a. No problem: ____________
   b. Possible problem: ____________
   c. Actual or potential nursing diagnosis: ____________
   d. Clinical problem other than nursing diagnosis: ____________

4. Give three examples of how standards may be used to identify significant cues.
   a. ____________
   b. ____________
   c. ____________

5. List nine questions a nurse should consider when using critical thinking in diagnostic reasoning.
   a. ____________
   b. ____________
   c. ____________
   d. ____________
   e. ____________
   f. ____________
   g. ____________
   h. ____________
   i. ____________

6. In her book on the nursing process, Alfaro-LeFevre (2014) describes the shift from Diagnose and Treat (DT) to Predict, Prevent, Manage, and Promote (PPMP). The latter approach focuses on early evidence-based intervention to prevent and manage problems and their potential complications. Describe the three activities nurses need to perform to follow this approach in daily nursing care.
   a. ____________________
   b. ____________________
   c. ____________________

7. Read the three mini-cases that follow. In each one, underline the cues that form a data cluster indicating a nursing diagnosis and write the appropriate nursing diagnosis as a three-part statement.
   a. Mr. Klinetob, age 86, has been seriously depressed since the death, 6 months ago, of his wife of 52 years. Although he suffers from degenerative joint disease and has talked for years about having "just a touch of arthritis," this never kept him from being up and about. Recently, however, he spends all day sitting in a chair and seems to have no desire to engage in self-care activities. He tells the visiting nurse that he doesn't get washed up anymore because he's "too stiff" in the morning to bathe and "I just don't seem to have the energy." The visiting nurse notices that his hair is matted and uncombed, his face has traces of previous meals, and he has a strong body odor. His children have complained that their normally fastidious father seems not to care about personal hygiene any longer.

      Nursing Diagnosis: ____________________

      ____________________

      ____________________

   b. Ms. Adams sustained a right-sided cerebral infarct that resulted in left hemiparesis (paralysis on the left side of the body) and left "neglect." She ignores the left side of her body and actually denies its existence. When asked about her left leg, she stated that it belonged to the woman in the next bed—this while she was in a private room. This patient was previously quite active: she walked for 45 to 60 minutes four or five times a week and was an avid swimmer. At present, she cannot move either her left arm or leg.

      Nursing Diagnosis: ____________________

      ____________________

      ____________________

   c. After trying to conceive a child for 11 years, Ted and Rosemary Hines sought the assistance of a fertility specialist who was highly recommended by a friend. It was determined that Ted's sperm was inadequate, and Rosemary was inseminated with sperm from an anonymous donor. The couple was told that the donor was healthy and that he was selected because he resembled Ted. Rosemary became pregnant after the second in vitro fertilization attempt and delivered a healthy baby girl named Sarah.

      Sarah is now 7 years old, and Ted and Rosemary have learned from blood tests that their fertility specialist is the biologic father of their child. It seems that he lied to some couples about using sperm from anonymous donors and deceived others into thinking their wives had become pregnant when he had simply injected them with hormones. Ted and Rosemary have joined other couples in pressing charges against this health care provider.

      Rosemary tells the nurse in her pediatrician's office that she is concerned about how all this is affecting her family. "Ted and I both love Sarah and would do nothing to hurt her, but I'm so angry about this whole situation I'm afraid I may be taking it out on her," she says. Questioning reveals that Rosemary has found herself yelling at Sarah for minor disobedience and spanking her, something she rarely did before. Both Ted and Rosemary had commented before about Sarah's striking physical resemblance to the fertility specialist but attributed this to coincidence. Rosemary says, "Whenever I see her now, I can't help but see Dr. Clowser, and everything inside me clenches up and I want to scream." Both Ted and Rosemary express great remorse that Sarah, who is innocent, is bearing the brunt of something that is in no way her fault.

      Nursing Diagnosis: ____________________

      ____________________

      ____________________

## APPLYING YOUR KNOWLEDGE

### CRITICAL THINKING QUESTIONS

1. With a partner or several classmates, write appropriate nursing diagnoses for the following patient. Be sure to include actual, potential, and possible diagnoses. Compare your diagnoses with your partner's and note similarities and differences. Decide which diagnoses best suit the patient's situation.

   A 35-year-old woman presents with chills, fever, and severe vaginal bleeding. She tells you she is 2 months pregnant and has had two previous miscarriages. She is overwrought and says she feels God is punishing her for an abortion she had when she was in college. She and her husband have been trying to have children for years and were counting on this pregnancy to come to term.

2. Interview members of your family or several close friends. Identify wellness diagnoses for each person. What factors contributed to these diagnoses?

### REFLECTIVE PRACTICE: CULTIVATING QSEN COMPETENCIES

***Use the following expanded scenario from Chapter 15 in your textbook to answer the questions below.***

***Scenario:*** Martin Prescott, age 46, comes to the clinic for a routine physical examination. During the assessment, he says, "I've had problems with constipation, and I've seen some blood when I wipe myself after a bowel movement. It's just hemorrhoids, right? Nothing to worry about?" Upon further questioning, the nurse discovers that Mr. Prescott's father and an uncle both died in their early 50s from colon cancer.

1. What nursing diagnosis would be appropriate for Mr. Prescott? How might the nurse advocate for Mr. Prescott to ensure that he gets tested for colon cancer?

   ______________________________

   ______________________________

   ______________________________

2. What would be a successful outcome for this patient?

   ______________________________

   ______________________________

   ______________________________

3. What intellectual, technical, interpersonal, and/or ethical/legal competencies are most likely to bring about the desired outcome?

   ______________________________

   ______________________________

   ______________________________

4. What resources might be helpful for Mr. Prescott?

   ______________________________

   ______________________________

   ______________________________

## PRACTICING FOR NCLEX

### MULTIPLE CHOICE QUESTIONS

***Circle the letter that corresponds to the best answer for each question.***

1. The formulation of nursing diagnoses is unique to the nursing profession. Which statement accurately represents a characteristic of diagnosing?
   a. Nursing diagnoses remain the same for as long as the disease is present.
   b. Nurses formulate nursing diagnoses to identify diseases.
   c. Nurses write nursing diagnoses to describe patient problems that nurses can treat.
   d. Nursing diagnoses focus on identifying healthy responses to health and illness.

2. A nurse documents the following in the patient chart: Risk for decreased cardiac output related to myocardial ischemia. This is an example of what aspect of patient care?
   a. Nursing diagnosis
   b. Nursing assessment
   c. Medical diagnosis
   d. Collaborative problem

3. A nurse is caring for a toddler who has been treated on two different occasions for lacerations and contusions due to the parents' negligence in providing a safe environment. What is an appropriate nursing diagnosis for this patient?
   a. Risk for injury related to abusive parents
   b. Risk for injury related to impaired home management
   c. Child abuse related to unsafe home environment
   d. Risk for injury related to unsafe home environment
4. A nurse suspects that a patient has a Self-Care Deficit but needs more data to confirm this diagnosis. What nursing diagnosis would the nurse write for this patient?
   a. Actual
   b. Potential
   c. Possible
   d. Apparent
5. Which example of patient care is not the responsibility of the nurse?
   a. Monitoring for changes in health status
   b. Promoting safety and preventing harm; detecting and controlling risks
   c. Tailoring treatment and medication regimens for each person
   d. Confirming a medical diagnosis

## ALTERNATE-FORMAT QUESTIONS

### Multiple Response Questions

***Circle the letters that correspond to the best answers for each question.***

1. A student nurse is learning how to write a nursing diagnosis for a patient. Which actions are accurate guidelines when formulating nursing diagnoses? *(Select all that apply.)*
   a. Include the medical diagnosis in the nursing diagnosis.
   b. Make sure the patient problem precedes the etiology.
   c. Write the diagnosis in legally advisable terms.
   d. Phrase the nursing diagnosis as a patient need rather than alteration.
   e. Be sure the problem statement indicates what is unhealthy about the patient.
   f. Make sure defining characteristics follow the etiology.
2. Nurses write various types of nursing diagnoses depending on the patient's condition. Which statements accurately describe types of NANDA nursing diagnoses? *(Select all that apply.)*
   a. A wellness diagnosis has four components: label, definition, defining characteristics, and related factor.
   b. A possible diagnosis is a clinical judgment about an individual, group, or community in transition from a specific level of wellness to a higher level of wellness.
   c. A risk nursing diagnosis is a clinical judgment that an individual, family, or community is more likely to develop the problem than others in the same or similar situation.
   d. An actual diagnosis represents a problem that has been validated by the presence of major defining characteristics.
   e. A potential nursing diagnosis is a statement describing a suspected problem for which additional data are needed.
   f. A syndrome nursing diagnosis comprises a cluster of actual or risk nursing diagnoses that are predicted to be present because of certain events or situations.
3. A nurse is writing nursing diagnoses for patients on a busy hospital ward. Which nursing diagnoses are written correctly? *(Select all that apply.)*
   a. Deficient fluid volume related to abnormal fluid loss
   b. Risk for impaired skin integrity
   c. Grieving related to disturbed body image
   d. Risk for chronic low self-esteem
   e. Imbalanced nutrition related to inability to eat a balanced diet
   f. Deficient knowledge related to noncompliance with physical therapy routine

4. Nurses use approved NANDA-I nursing diagnoses when writing diagnoses for patients. Which diagnoses represent domain 1: health promotion as established by NANDA?
   a. Ineffective health management
   b. Risk for disuse syndrome
   c. Impaired Environmental Interpretation Syndrome
   d. Sedentary lifestyle
   e. Decreased diversional activity engagement
   f. Readiness for enhanced coping

5. The electronic health record enables the nurse to facilitate which nursing actions related to diagnosing? *(Select all that apply.)*
   a. Viewing the patient's ongoing risks
   b. Deciding on and documenting new nursing diagnoses
   c. Facilitating communication of the patient's actual problems
   d. Making decisions about mutual patient goals and interventions
   e. Determining and documenting when the nursing diagnoses are resolved
   f. Preparing a patient for discharge from a health care facility

CHAPTER 16

# Outcome Identification and Planning

## ASSESSING YOUR UNDERSTANDING

### FILL IN THE BLANKS

1. A(n) ____________ is an expected conclusion to a patient health problem or, in the event of a wellness diagnosis, an expected conclusion to a patient's health expectation.
2. While driving to a restaurant for lunch, a nurse contemplates how to help a young cancer patient accept the loss of a limb. This nurse is using the process of ____________ planning.
3. In acute care settings, the three basic stages of planning that are critical to comprehensive nursing care are ____________, ____________, and ____________.
4. From what part of the nursing diagnosis "Pain related to delayed healing of surgical incision" would outcomes be derived?

   ____________
5. The ____________, developed by the Iowa Outcomes Project, presents the first comprehensive standardized language used to describe the patient outcomes that are responsive to nursing intervention.
6. A nurse writes the following statement on a patient's chart: "Goal partially met; patient ate approximately one half of food offered for lunch." This nurse has written a(n) ____________ statement.
7. A(n) ____________ is any treatment based on clinical judgment and knowledge that a nurse performs to enhance patient outcomes.
8. When a nurse supplies education to an obese teenager regarding the fat content in food and helps him choose a nutritious diet, he or she is performing a(n) ____________ intervention.
9. When a nurse administers health care provider–prescribed pain medication to a patient after surgery, he or she is performing a(n) ____________ intervention.
10. A(n) ____________ is a set of steps (typically embedded in a branching flowchart) that approximates the decision process of an expert clinician and is used to make a decision.
11. The ____________ is the written guide that directs the efforts of the nursing team as the nurses work with patients to meet health goals.

### MATCHING EXERCISES

***Match the definition in Part B with the type of care plan listed in Part A. Answers may be used more than once.***

#### PART A

**a.** Initial care plan
**b.** Ongoing, problem-solving care plan
**c.** Discharge care plan
**d.** Standardized care plan

**e.** Computerized care plan
**f.** Case management care plan
**g.** Clinical pathways
**h.** Concept map care plan

**PART B**

____ **1.** A care plan developed by the nurse who performs the admission nursing history and physical assessment

____ **2.** Benefits of this type of care plan include ready access to an expanded knowledge base, improved record keeping and documentation, and decreased paperwork.

____ **3.** The chief purpose of this type of planning is to keep the plan up to date.

____ **4.** Prepared plans of care that identify the nursing diagnoses, outcomes, and related nursing interventions common to a specific population or health problem.

____ **5.** This type of plan for leaving the institution is best prepared by the nurse who has worked most closely with the patient, in conjunction with a social worker familiar with the patient's community.

____ **6.** The emphasis of this care plan is to clearly state expected patient outcomes and the specific times by which it is reasonable to achieve these outcomes.

____ **7.** The emphasis of this type of care plan is to individualize the plan to meet unique patient needs.

____ **8.** This diagram of patient problems and interventions is used to organize data, analyze data, and take a holistic view of the patient situation.

***Match the patient goals in Part B with the type of goal listed in Part A. Answers may be used more than once.***

**PART A**

**a.** Cognitive goals
**b.** Psychomotor goals
**c.** Affective goals

**PART B**

____ **9.** By 3/30/20, the patient will successfully navigate the length of the hallway with walker.

____ **10.** By 3/30/20, the patient will list five low-fat snacks to replace high-fat foods.

____ **11.** By 3/30/20, the patient will bathe infant on her own.

____ **12.** By 3/30/20, the patient will value her health sufficiently to stop smoking.

____ **13.** By 3/30/20, the patient will list three reasons to continue taking blood pressure medication.

____ **14.** By 3/30/20, the patient will show concern for his well-being and participate in AA meetings.

***Match the descriptions in Part B with the type of planning being performed in Part A. Answers may be used more than once.***

**PART A**

**a.** Initial planning
**b.** Ongoing planning
**c.** Discharge planning

**PART B**

____ **15.** Used to keep the nursing care plan up to date

____ **16.** Addresses each problem listed in the prioritized nursing diagnoses and identifies appropriate patient goals and related nursing care

____ **17.** States nursing diagnoses more clearly and develops new diagnoses

____ **18.** Should be carried out by the nurse who has worked most closely with the patient and family

____ **19.** Involves teaching and counseling skills to help the patient and family carry out self-care behaviors at home

____ **20.** Standardized care plans provide an excellent basis for this type of planning if the nurse individualizes them.

## SHORT ANSWER

**1.** Give an example of an appropriate nursing order for the following patients:

**a.** A child with asthma who must be taught to use an inhaler: ______

**b.** An older adult woman recovering from hip surgery who must learn to ambulate with a walker: ______

**c.** An obese teenager who needs weight counseling: ______

**d.** A new mother who must ambulate after having a cesarean delivery: ______

**2.** Briefly define the following elements of planning. Explain why they are necessary to the planning step of the nursing process.

**a.** Setting priorities: ______

**b.** Writing goals/outcomes that determine the evaluative strategy: ______

**c.** Selecting appropriate evidence-based nursing interventions: ______

**d.** Communicating the nursing care plan: ______

**3.** List two examples of informal planning.

______

**4.** Explain how a formal plan of care benefits the nurse and patient.

______

**5.** Individualize the following standard plans to meet the patient's specific goals.

**a.** Manage pain for a terminally ill patient: ______

**b.** Explore support people for a patient with AIDS: ______

**c.** Provide sensory stimulation for an older adult man in a long-term care facility: ______

**d.** Teach self-help to a stroke patient in the home care setting: ______

**6.** Describe the following types of nursing care and give an example of each type.

**a.** Nursing care related to basic human needs: ______

Example: ______

**b.** Nursing care related to nursing diagnoses: ______

Example: ______

**c.** Nursing care related to the medical and interdisciplinary plan of care: ______

Example: ______

**7.** List four considerations a nurse should employ when planning nursing care for each day.

**a.** ______

**b.** ______

**c.** ______

**d.** ______

**8.** Place a check mark next to the patient goals that are written correctly, and, on the line below, rewrite those that are written incorrectly:

**a.** Teach Mrs. Myers one lesson per day on the nutritional value of foods.

______________________________

**b.** Mrs. Gray will know the dangers of smoking after viewing a film on smoking.

______________________________

**c.** By the end of the shift, the patient ambulates in the hallway using crutches.

______________________________

**d.** By 2/7/20, the patient correctly demonstrates subcutaneous injections using normal saline.

______________________________

**e.** By next visit, the patient will understand the benefits of psychotherapy.

______________________________

**f.** By 6/12/20, the patient correctly demonstrates application of wet-to-dry dressing on leg ulcer.

______________________________

______________________________

**9.** Identify a patient goal that shows a direct resolution of the health problem expressed in the nursing diagnoses below.

**a.** Nursing Diagnosis: Deficient fluid volume related to decreased fluid intake during fever

Patient goal: ______________________________

______________________________

**b.** Nursing Diagnosis: Sexual dysfunction: Loss of desire related to change in body image and feelings of unattractiveness following mastectomy

Patient goal: ______________________________

______________________________

**c.** Nursing Diagnosis: Stress urinary incontinence related to age-related degenerative changes and weak pelvic muscles and structural supports

Patient goal: ______________________________

______________________________

**d.** Nursing Diagnosis: Activity intolerance related to decreased amount of oxygenated blood available to tissues

Patient goal: ______________________________

______________________________

**e.** Nursing Diagnosis: Acute pain related to fear of taking prescribed analgesics

Patient goal: ______________________________

______________________________

**10.** List six measures nurses should consider to correctly plan health care for a patient.

**a.** ______________________________
**b.** ______________________________
**c.** ______________________________
**d.** ______________________________
**e.** ______________________________
**f.** ______________________________

**11.** Give four examples of questions a nurse should ask when thinking critically about setting priorities for a patient plan of care.

**a.** ______________________________
**b.** ______________________________
**c.** ______________________________
**d.** ______________________________

## APPLYING YOUR KNOWLEDGE

### CRITICAL THINKING QUESTIONS

**1.** Think about what type of goals would be appropriate in each of the three stages of planning (initial planning, ongoing planning, discharge planning) using the following patient data.

**a.** A mother brings her 5-year-old son to the emergency room. She says he has been running a low fever and complaining of abdominal pain and headache. You notice his skin is pale and there are several bruises on his arms and legs. On examination, you notice his spleen is enlarged and the abdominal area is tender. A medical diagnosis confirms the child has acute leukemia.

**b.** A 45-year-old man presents with low fever, weight loss, chronic fatigue, and heavy sweating at night. He has a productive cough with yellowish mucus and chest pain. A TB skin test comes back positive.

c. A 12-year-old girl presents with fatigue, weight loss, excessive thirst, and frequent urination. Laboratory tests confirm a diagnosis of diabetes mellitus.

Why is the identification of goals in each stage necessary for optimal care and outcomes?

2. Some nurses may tell you that care plans are a waste of time. Think about what knowledge and experience you need to respond to this comment. If possible, interview nurses or search through the literature to discover how plans can make a difference.

### REFLECTIVE PRACTICE: CULTIVATING QSEN COMPETENCIES

***Use the following expanded scenario from Chapter 16 in your textbook to answer the questions below.***

*Scenario:* Glenda Kronk, age 35, comes to the health center for a routine checkup. Upon assessment, the nurse notes that she is 25 lb overweight and has high-normal blood pressure. During the visit, she verbalizes a strong motivation and desire to become physically fit, lose weight, increase her muscle tone, and improve her cardiorespiratory capacity. She says, "I know it'll involve some major lifestyle changes, including diet and exercise. What's with all these diets and diet supplements now?"

1. How might the nurse respond to Ms. Kronk's questions regarding fitness?

___________________________________

___________________________________

___________________________________

2. What would be a successful outcome for this patient?

___________________________________

___________________________________

___________________________________

3. What intellectual, technical, interpersonal, and/or ethical/legal competencies are most likely to bring about the desired outcome?

___________________________________

___________________________________

___________________________________

4. What resources might be helpful for Ms. Kronk?

___________________________________

___________________________________

___________________________________

## PRACTICING FOR NCLEX

### MULTIPLE CHOICE QUESTIONS

***Circle the letter that corresponds to the best answer for each question.***

1. A nurse is planning care for a patient who has just been diagnosed with type 2 diabetes. Which nursing action is performed during the planning step of the nursing process?
   a. The nurse interprets and analyzes the patient data.
   b. The nurse establishes a database for the patient.
   c. The nurse identifies patient strengths and weaknesses.
   d. The nurse selects nursing measures, including patient teaching.

2. A nurse is writing goals for a patient who is scheduled to ambulate following hip replacement surgery. What is a correctly written goal for this patient?
   a. Over the next 24-hour period, the patient will walk the length of the hallway assisted by the nurse.
   b. The nurse will help the patient ambulate the length of the hallway once a day.
   c. Offer to help the patient walk the length of the hallway each day.
   d. Patient will become mobile within a 24-hour period.

3. The nurse is caring for a 48-year-old male patient with a new colostomy. Which patient goal for Mr. Conner is written correctly?
   a. Explain to Mr. Conner the proper care of the stoma by 3/29/20.
   b. Mr. Conner will know how to care for his stoma by 3/29/20.
   c. Mr. Conner will demonstrate proper care of stoma by 3/29/20.
   d. Mr. Conner will be able to care for stoma and cope with psychological loss by 3/29/20.

4. When planning nursing interventions, the nurse must review the etiology of the problem statement. The etiology:
   a. Identifies the unhealthy response preventing desired change
   b. Identifies factors causing undesirable response and preventing desired change
   c. Suggests patient goals to promote desired change
   d. Identifies patient strengths
5. A nurse is caring for an overweight, highly stressed 50-year-old male executive who is being discharged from the hospital after undergoing coronary bypass surgery. What is an affective goal for this patient?
   a. By 6/30/20, the patient will list three benefits of daily exercise.
   b. By 6/30/20, the patient will correctly demonstrate breathing techniques to reduce stress.
   c. By 6/30/20, the patient will value his health sufficiently to reduce the cholesterol in his diet.
   d. By 6/30/20, the patient will be able to plan healthy weekly menus.
6. A nurse is planning nursing interventions for patients on a busy hospital ward. Which guideline would the nurse follow when designing the plan of care?
   a. Make sure the nursing interventions are a separate entity from the original goal/outcomes.
   b. Date the nursing interventions when written and when the plan of care is reviewed.
   c. Make sure the nursing interventions are approved of and signed by the attending health care provider.
   d. Make sure the nursing intervention does not describe the nursing action to be performed.
7. The nurse is aware that basic patient needs must be met before a patient can focus on higher ones. According to Maslow's hierarchy of human needs, which example would be the highest priority for a patient after physiologic needs have been met?
   a. A patient enrolls in art class after recovering from major surgery.
   b. A nurse arranges for a teenage patient to have visits from school friends.
   c. Grab bars are installed in a patient's bathroom to facilitate safe showering.
   d. A nurse identifies strengths in a patient who is scheduled for a mastectomy.

## ALTERNATE-FORMAT QUESTIONS

### Multiple Response Questions

***Circle the letters that correspond to the best answers for each question.***

1. A nurse is planning care for patients in a health care provider's office. Which actions will the nurse perform during this step of the nursing process? *(Select all that apply.)*
   a. Establishing priorities
   b. Collecting and interpreting patient data
   c. Identifying expected patient outcomes
   d. Selecting evidence-based nursing interventions
   e. Recording patient outcomes
   f. Communicating the nursing care plan
2. A nurse is performing initial care planning for a hospitalized patient. Which actions occur during the initial planning of patient care? *(Select all that apply.)*
   a. The nurse who performs the admission nursing history and physical assessment makes the initial plan.
   b. After the initial plan is developed, the nurse prioritizes nursing diagnoses.
   c. The nurse identifies patient goals and the related nursing care in the initial plan.
   d. The nurse uses tailored plans as opposed to standardized care plans as a basis for the initial plan.
   e. The nurse collects new data and analyzes it to make the plan more specific and effective.
   f. The nurse making the initial plan focuses on using teaching and counseling skills to help the patient carry out necessary self-care behaviors at home.
3. A nurse is writing outcomes for patients in a rehabilitation facility. Which guidelines should the nurse consider? *(Select all that apply.)*
   a. The nurse should derive each set of outcomes from a combination of nursing diagnoses.

**b.** At least one of the outcomes the nurse writes should show a direct resolution of the problem statement in the nursing diagnosis.

**c.** The nurse should not be concerned if patient and family do not value the outcomes as long as they support the plan of care.

**d.** The nurse should write outcomes that are brief and specific and support the overall plan of care.

**e.** The outcomes the nurse writes need not be supportive of the total treatment plan as long as they specify a goal.

**f.** The nurse may write outcomes that do not specify a time line as long as they are linked with other outcomes.

**4.** Nurses write outcomes that are categorized as cognitive, psychomotor, or affective. Which examples are cognitive outcomes? *(Select all that apply.)*

**a.** Within 1 week of teaching, the patient will list three benefits of quitting smoking.

**b.** By 6/8/20, the patient will correctly demonstrate injecting himself with insulin.

**c.** Before discharge, the patient will verbalize valuing health sufficiently to follow a healthy diet.

**d.** By 6/8/20, the patient will describe a meal plan that is high in fiber.

**e.** By 6/8/20, the patient will correctly demonstrate ambulating with a walker.

**f.** After viewing the film, the patient will verbalize four benefits of daily exercise.

**5.** The nurse is writing a measurable outcome for a patient with a new prosthesis to begin walking again. Which components must be included in the outcome? *(Select all that apply.)*

**a.** The action the patient will perform

**b.** Modifiers describing the end result

**c.** Description in subjective terms of the expected patient behavior

**d.** Particular circumstances in which the outcome is to be achieved

**e.** The patient or some part of the patient

**f.** Target time when the patient is expected to be able to achieve the outcome

**6.** The nurse is writing goals for patients being discharged from an acute care setting. Which goals are written correctly? *(Select all that apply.)*

**a.** Demonstrate the correct use of crutches to the patient prior to discharge.

**b.** The patient will know how to dress her wound after receiving a demonstration.

**c.** After attending an infant care class, the patient will correctly demonstrate the procedure for bathing her newborn.

**d.** By 4/5/20, the patient will demonstrate how to care for a colostomy.

**e.** The patient will list the dangers of smoking and quit.

**f.** After counseling, the patient will describe two coping measures to deal with stress.

**7.** A nurse is using the SMART acronym to plan outcomes for patients in a long-term care facility. Which criteria describe the use of this acronym? *(Select all that apply.)*

**a.** S = goals should be supportive

**b.** S = goals should be specific

**c.** M = goals should be measurable

**d.** A = goals should be accurate

**e.** R = goals should be realistic

**f.** T = goals should be temporary

CHAPTER 17

# Implementing

## ASSESSING YOUR UNDERSTANDING

### FILL IN THE BLANKS

1. When a nurse administers medications that were prescribed by the patient's doctor, he or she is carrying out a(n) ___________ intervention.
2. ___________ are written plans that detail the nursing activities to be executed in specific situations, such as might occur in the emergency department of a hospital.
3. ___________ are interventions targeted to promote and preserve the health of populations.
4. A(n) ___________ intervention is a treatment performed away from the patient but on behalf of a patient or group of patients.
5. McCloskey and Bulechek published a report of research to construct a taxonomy of nursing interventions known as ___________.
6. Interventions that are performed jointly by nurses and other members of the health care team are known as ___________.

### MATCHING EXERCISES

***Match the examples in Part B with the types of nursing interventions listed in Part A. Answers may be used more than once.***

#### PART A

a. Nurse-initiated independent intervention
b. Health care provider–initiated dependent intervention
c. Collaborative interdependent intervention

#### PART B

____ 1. A nurse notices that her patient is extremely anxious before surgery and recommends psychiatric evaluation by the psychiatric nurse specialist.

____ 2. A nurse administers the prescribed dosage of pain medication for a patient recovering from knee surgery.

____ 3. A nurse teaches the daughter of a patient who has leg ulcers how to apply the dressings.

____ 4. A nurse meets with a patient's health care provider to describe a patient's lack of response to prescribed therapy.

____ 5. A nurse prepares a patient for surgery by performing a bowel cleansing.

____ 6. A nurse meets in conference with a patient's health care provider, social worker, and psychiatrist to discuss the patient's failure to progress.

### CORRECT THE FALSE STATEMENTS

***Circle the word "true" or "false" that follows the statement. If you circled "false," change the underlined word or words to make the statement true. Place your answer in the space provided.***

1. The <u>health care provider</u> is legally responsible for the assessments nurses make and for their nursing responses.
   a. True
   b. False ___________________________

2. Nurse-initiated interventions involve carrying out nurse-prescribed orders written on the nursing care plan.
   a. True
   b. False ______________________

3. Standing orders are written plans that detail the nursing activities to be executed in specific situations.
   a. True
   b. False ______________________

4. The health care provider plays the role of coordinator within the health care team.
   a. True
   b. False ______________________

5. The nursing team carries out the nursing orders detailed in the nursing care plan.
   a. True
   b. False ______________________

6. When working with patients to achieve the goals/outcomes specified in the care plan, it is important to remember that everything about the care plan is fixed.
   a. True
   b. False ______________________

7. When choosing nursing interventions, it is important to consider the patient's background.
   a. True
   b. False ______________________

8. Sincere motivation to benefit the patient and conscientious attempts to implement nursing orders are sufficient to protect a nurse from legal action due to negligence.
   a. True
   b. False ______________________

9. When a patient fails to follow the care plan despite the nurse's best efforts, it is time to change the patient's attitude toward his care.
   a. True
   b. False ______________________

10. If a care plan is well written, carrying out its orders is the nurse's most important task and should receive top priority.
    a. True
    b. False ______________________

11. All nursing actions for implementing the care plan must be consistent with standards for practice.
    a. True
    b. False ______________________

## SHORT ANSWER

1. List three duties nurses perform when acting as coordinators for the health care team.
   a. ______________________
   b. ______________________
   c. ______________________

2. Give an example of a nurse variable, a patient variable, and a health care variable that might influence the implementation of the care plan.
   a. Nurse variable: ______________________
   b. Patient variable: ______________________
   c. Health care variable: ______________________

3. Explain why the following nursing actions are important to the continuity of nursing care.
   a. Promoting self-care: teaching, counseling, and advocacy ______________________
   ______________________
   ______________________
   b. Assisting patients to meet health goals
   ______________________
   ______________________

4. Mr. Franks, a new resident in a long-term care facility, is recovering from a minor surgery. He shows no interest in his condition and refuses to participate in self-care. You suspect an underlying problem of loneliness and boredom stemming from his admittance to the home, which was not mentioned in his original care plan. How would you reevaluate the nursing care plan and incorporate self-care for Mr. Franks, taking into consideration his mental state?
   ______________________
   ______________________
   ______________________

5. Your patient is a pregnant woman, living in a subsidized housing development. You believe she is not receiving proper nutrition. She has two other children and complains that there is not enough money to put three square meals a day on the table. When evaluating her care plan, you notice there is no mention of providing counseling in this area. How would you reevaluate the nursing care plan for this patient to include options for proper nutrition?

6. Give an example of the following types of interventions defined by the Nursing Intervention Classification (NIC).
   a. Direct care intervention:
   b. Indirect care intervention:
   c. Community (or public health) intervention:

## APPLYING YOUR KNOWLEDGE

### CRITICAL THINKING QUESTIONS

1. Work with your classmates to list all the factors (nurse, health care team, patient/family, health care setting, resources, and so on) that might interfere with the nurse's ability to implement a care plan for the following patients. Then identify facilitating factors. Think about how you can use this knowledge.
   a. A 5-year-old girl with cystic fibrosis is being discharged into the care of her family, which consists of a single working mother and two older brothers.
   b. A 17-year-old single mother who is living with her parents is being sent home with her newborn son. She is having difficulty nursing the baby, and the baby is being treated for jaundice.
2. Spend some time observing nurses as they care for patients. List all the nursing actions you observe. Determine whether these actions involved the use of the nurse's cognitive skills, interpersonal skills, technical skills, ethical/legal skills, or a blend of these skills. Rate your own skills in these areas and note in which areas you feel confident and in which areas you need improvement. Write a plan of action to help you improve these skills.

### REFLECTIVE PRACTICE: CULTIVATING QSEN COMPETENCIES

***Use the following expanded scenario from Chapter 17 in your textbook to answer the questions below.***

***Scenario:*** Antoinette Browne, a toddler, is brought to the well-child community clinic by her grandmother, who lives with the child and her mother. Physical examination reveals a negligible gain in height and weight, lethargy, and a delay in achieving developmental milestones. The grandmother says, "The baby keeps me awake all night with her crying. I can't take it anymore." Further questioning reveals that the mother is a single woman who works nights and sleeps most of the day, leaving the bulk of the childcare to the grandmother.

1. What might be the nurse's response when advocating for Antoinette and her family?

2. What would be a successful outcome for this patient?

3. What intellectual, technical, interpersonal, and/or ethical/legal competencies are most likely to bring about the desired outcome?

4. What resources might be helpful for this family?

## PRACTICING FOR NCLEX

### MULTIPLE CHOICE QUESTIONS

***Circle the letter that corresponds to the best answer for each question.***

**1.** The Joint Commission encourages patients to become active, involved, and informed participants on the health care team. What nursing action follows The Joint Commission recommendations for improving patient safety by encouraging patients to speak up?

- **a.** The nurse explains each procedure twice to prevent patient questions from wasting time.
- **b.** The nurse encourages the patient to participate in all treatment decisions as the center of the health care team.
- **c.** The nurse encourages patients to advocate for themselves instead of choosing a trusted family member or friend.
- **d.** The nurse assures the patient who questions a medication that it is the right medication prescribed for him and administers the medicine.

**2.** Nurses perform many independent nursing actions when caring for patients. Which action is considered an independent (nurse-initiated) action?

- **a.** Executing health care provider orders for a catheter
- **b.** Meeting with other health care professionals to discuss a patient
- **c.** Helping to allay a patient's fears about surgery
- **d.** Administering medication to a patient

**3.** A nurse follows set guidelines for administering pain medication to patients in a critical care unit. This nurse's authority to initiate actions that normally require the order or supervision of a health care provider is termed:

- **a.** Protocols
- **b.** Nursing interventions
- **c.** Collaborative orders
- **d.** Standing orders

**4.** As the nurse bathes a patient, she notes his skin color and integrity, his ability to respond to simple directions, and his muscle tone. Which statement best explains why such continuing data collection is so important?

- **a.** It is difficult to collect complete data in the initial assessment.
- **b.** It is the most efficient use of the nurse's time.
- **c.** It enables the nurse to revise the care plan appropriately.
- **d.** It meets current standards of care.

**5.** A patient, who presented with high blood pressure, is put on a low-salt diet and instructed to quit smoking. The nurse finds him in the cafeteria eating a cheeseburger and French fries. He also tells you there is no way he can quit smoking. What is the nurse's first objective when implementing care for this patient?

- **a.** Explain the effects of a high-salt diet and smoking on blood pressure.
- **b.** Identify why the patient is not following the therapy.
- **c.** Collaborate with other health care professionals about the patient's treatment.
- **d.** Change the nursing care plan.

### ALTERNATE-FORMAT QUESTIONS

#### Multiple Response Questions

***Circle the letters that correspond to the best answers for each question.***

**1.** Nurses implement care for patients in various health care settings. Which activities would typically be carried out during the implementation step of the nursing process? *(Select all that apply.)*

- **a.** Collecting additional patient data
- **b.** Modifying the patient care plan
- **c.** Performing an initial assessment of the patient
- **d.** Developing patient outcomes and goals
- **e.** Measuring how well the patient has achieved patient goals
- **f.** Collecting a database to enable an effective care plan

2. Nurses use the Nursing Outcomes Classifications (NOCs) when choosing nursing goals for patients. What are the goals of the research that is behind the NOCs? *(Select all that apply.)*
   a. To identify, label, and validate nursing-sensitive patient outcomes and indicators
   b. To teach decision making
   c. To ensure appropriate reimbursement for nursing services
   d. To communicate nursing to non-nurses
   e. To evaluate the validity and usefulness of the classification in clinical field testing
   f. To define and test measurement procedures for the outcomes and indicators

3. Nurses utilize the McCloskey, Dochterman, and Bulechek *Nursing Interventions Classification* (NIC) report of research when choosing nursing interventions for patients. What are the advantages of having standard NICs? *(Select all that apply.)*
   a. Limiting the amount of reimbursement allowed for nursing services
   b. Teaching decision making
   c. Allocating nursing resources
   d. Allowing the use of multiple systems of nomenclature
   e. Developing information systems
   f. Communicating nursing to non-nurses

4. What are examples of nursing actions listed in the ANA's *Nursing: Scope and Standards of Practice* for Standard 5: Implementation? *(Select all that apply.)*
   a. The nurse demonstrates quality by documenting the application of the nursing process in a responsible, accountable, and ethical manner.
   b. The nurse incorporates new knowledge to initiate changes in nursing practice if the desired outcomes are not achieved.
   c. The nurse develops expected outcomes that provide direction for the continuity of care.
   d. The nurse documents implementation and any modifications, including changes or omissions, of the identified plan.
   e. The nurse uses evidence-based interventions and strategies to achieve the mutually identified goals and outcomes specific to the problem or needs.
   f. The nurse integrates critical thinking and technology solutions to implement the nursing process to collect, measure, record, retrieve, trend, and analyze data and information to enhance nursing practice and health care consumer outcomes.

CHAPTER 18

# Evaluating

## ASSESSING YOUR UNDERSTANDING

### FILL IN THE BLANKS

1. During the evaluation step of the nursing process, based on the patient's responses to the care plan, the nurse decides to ____________, ____________, or ____________ the care plan.

2. Nurses are involved in many types of evaluations, but the ____________ is always the nurse's primary concern.

3. The most important act of evaluation performed by nurses is evaluating ____________ with the patient.

4. The nurse evaluates a patient's outcome by measuring the skills and knowledge that the patient has achieved. These measurable qualities, attributes, or characteristics are called ____________.

5. ____________ are the levels of performance accepted by and expected of the nursing staff or other health care team members established by authority, custom, or consent.

6. ____________ are recommendations for how care should be managed in specific diseases, problems, or situations.

7. The nurse manager of a hospital unit sets up a program to help improve teamwork on the unit. These types of specially designed programs that promote excellence in nursing are called ____________ programs.

8. An inspector is evaluating the physical facility and equipment of a health care provider's office. This type of evaluation that focuses on the environment in which care is provided is a(n) ____________ evaluation.

9. A person who evaluates nursing care by using post-discharge questionnaires, patient interviews (by telephone or face to face), or chart review (nursing audit) to collect data is conducting a(n) ____________ evaluation.

### MATCHING EXERCISES

***Match the term in Part A with the correct definition listed in Part B.***

**PART A**

a. Concurrent evaluation

b. Retrospective evaluation

c. Outcome evaluation

d. Process evaluation

e. Structure evaluation

f. Introspective evaluation

**PART B**

____ 1. An evaluation that focuses on the environment in which care is provided

____ 2. An evaluation that focuses on measurable changes in the health status of the patient

____ 3. An evaluation of nursing care and patient goals while the patient is receiving the care

____ **4.** An evaluation that focuses on the nature and sequence of activities carried out by the nurse implementing the nursing process

____ **5.** An evaluation to collect data after discharge usually by using post-discharge interviews and questionnaires and chart review

***Match the measurement tool in Part A with its appropriate example in Part B. Answers may be used more than once.***

**PART A**

**a.** Criteria

**b.** Standard

**PART B**

____ **6.** Patient will be able to walk the length of the hall by 5/15/20.

____ **7.** The admission database will be completed on all patients within 24 hours of admission to the unit.

____ **8.** All patients in active labor will have continuous external fetal heart monitoring.

____ **9.** Upon completion of an ECG course, the nurse will be able to recognize common arrhythmias when they appear on a heart monitor.

____ **10.** The student will be able to name and describe steps of the nursing procedure by the end of the semester.

## SHORT ANSWER

**1.** Explain how you would evaluate whether a patient has achieved the following outcomes.

**a.** Cognitive outcomes: ____________________

____________________

**b.** Psychomotor outcomes: ____________________

____________________

**c.** Affective outcomes: ____________________

____________________

**2.** Explain how the following elements of evaluation help to determine whether goals/outcomes have been met.

**a.** Identifying evaluative criteria: ____________________

____________________

**b.** Determining whether these criteria and standards are met: ____________________

____________________

**c.** Terminating, continuing, or modifying the plan: ____________________

____________________

**3.** Give an example of a variable that may influence goal/outcome achievement in the following areas.

**a.** Patient: ____________________

**b.** Nurse: ____________________

**c.** Health care system: ____________________

**4.** Mr. Bogash, a 28-year-old man with leukemia, recently had a bone marrow transplantation. His medical condition has improved, but he is unable to meet his goal of being up and alert during the daytime hours. What would be the appropriate step to take after evaluating Mr. Bogash? How would you document Mr. Bogash's failure to progress? How would you revise his care plan?

____________________

____________________

____________________

**5.** Explain the following three essential components of quality care and how nursing care is evaluated in each area.

**a.** Structure: ____________________

____________________

**b.** Process: ____________________

____________________

**c.** Outcome: ____________________

____________________

**6.** Explain why the following revisions may be made to a care plan.

**a.** Delete or modify the nursing diagnosis: ____

____________________

**b.** Make the goal statement more realistic: ____

____________________

**c.** Adjust the time criteria in the goal statement: ____________________

____________________

**d.** Change nursing interventions: ____________________

____________________

7. Would you rather work in an environment that ensures the quality of the profession using quality by inspection or quality as opportunity? Explain your answer. ____________

______________________________________________

8. Give four examples of the type of evaluations nurses are involved in as members of the health care team.

   a. ______________________________________________
   b. ______________________________________________
   c. ______________________________________________
   d. ______________________________________________

## APPLYING YOUR KNOWLEDGE

### CRITICAL THINKING QUESTIONS

1. Interview friends and family members who have experienced a stay in the hospital. Ask them if they were aware of specific nursing plans geared to their recovery. See if they were given goals and taught behaviors to accomplish them. Was goal attainment evaluated before they were discharged? Were further goals incorporated into their discharge plan? What do they feel could have been done to help them attain their health goals? How can you use this knowledge to help you develop the blended skills necessary to help patients achieve goals?
2. Reflect on the role that evaluation plays in promoting your scholastic achievement. Has it been positive or negative? Think of specific ways nurses can use evaluation to motivate patients to achieve healthy goals.
3. Give an example of each of the following "Seven Crucial Conversations in Health Care" and brainstorm with a friend or the class to provide a recommendation for solving the problems.
   a. Broken rules
   b. Mistakes
   c. Lack of support
   d. Incompetence
   e. Poor teamwork
   f. Disrespect
   g. Micromanagement

### REFLECTIVE PRACTICE: CULTIVATING QSEN COMPETENCIES

***Use the following expanded scenario from Chapter 18 in your textbook to answer the questions below.***

***Scenario:*** Mrs. Mioshi Otsuki, an older adult woman with a history of heart failure being treated with diuretics, is receiving home care. Mrs. Otsuki lives alone and has a daughter nearby who checks on her once a day. Questioned about her prescribed drug therapy regimen, the patient says, "I take this one labeled 'furosemide' every day in the morning, along with this other one labeled 'Lasix.'"

1. What should be the focus of an evaluation of Mrs. Otsuki's nursing care plan conducted by the home health care nurse?

   ______________________________________________

   ______________________________________________

   ______________________________________________

2. What would be a successful outcome for this patient?

   ______________________________________________

   ______________________________________________

   ______________________________________________

3. What intellectual, technical, interpersonal, and/or ethical/legal competencies are most likely to bring about the desired outcome?

   ______________________________________________

   ______________________________________________

   ______________________________________________

4. What resources might be helpful for Mrs. Otsuki?

   ______________________________________________

   ______________________________________________

   ______________________________________________

## PRACTICING FOR NCLEX

### MULTIPLE CHOICE QUESTIONS

***Circle the letter that corresponds to the best answer for each question.***

1. A nurse evaluates patients prior to discharge from a hospital setting. Which action is the most important act of evaluation performed by the nurse?
   - **a.** The nurse evaluates the patient's goal/outcome achievement.
   - **b.** The nurse evaluates the care plan.
   - **c.** The nurse evaluates the competence of nurse practitioners.
   - **d.** The nurse evaluates the types of health care services available to the patient.
2. A nurse caring for an older adult patient who has dementia observes another nurse putting restraints on the patient without a health care provider's order. The patient is agitated and not cooperating. What would be the best initial action of the first nurse in this situation?
   - **a.** Report the nurse applying the restraints to the supervisor.
   - **b.** File an incident report and have the second nurse sign it.
   - **c.** Confront the nurse and explain how this could be dangerous for the patient.
   - **d.** Contact the health care provider for an order for the restraints.
3. Nurses formulate different types of goals for patients when planning patient care. What is considered a psychomotor patient goal?
   - **a.** By 8/18/20, patient will value his health sufficiently to quit smoking.
   - **b.** By 8/18/20, patient will demonstrate improved motion in left arm.
   - **c.** By 8/18/20, patient will list three foods that are low in salt.
   - **d.** By 8/18/20, patient will learn three exercises designed to strengthen leg muscles.
4. A nurse is evaluating nursing care and patient outcomes by using a retrospective evaluation. Which action would the nurse perform in this approach?
   - **a.** The nurse directly observes the nursing care being provided.
   - **b.** The nurse reviews the patient chart while the patient is being cared for.
   - **c.** The nurse interviews the patient while he or she is receiving the care.
   - **d.** The nurse devises a post-discharge questionnaire to evaluate patient satisfaction.
5. Which action should the nurse take when patient data indicate that the stated goals have not been achieved?
   - **a.** Collect more data for the database.
   - **b.** Review each preceding step of the nursing process.
   - **c.** Implement a standardized care plan.
   - **d.** Change the nursing orders.
6. For a patient with self-care deficit, the long-term goal is that the patient will be able to dress himself by the end of the 6-week therapy. For best results, when should the nurse evaluate the patient's progress toward this goal?
   - **a.** When the patient is discharged
   - **b.** At the end of the 6-week therapy
   - **c.** Only when the patient shows some progress
   - **d.** As soon as possible
7. The quality assurance model of the ANA identifies three essential components of quality care. Which one of these components does the nurse use when determining whether a patient has met the goals stated on the care plan?
   - **a.** Structure
   - **b.** Process
   - **c.** Retrospect
   - **d.** Outcome
8. Which action is appropriate when evaluating a patient's responses to a care plan?
   - **a.** Reinforce the care plan when each expected outcome is achieved.
   - **b.** Terminate the plan if there are difficulties achieving the goals/outcomes.
   - **c.** Terminate the care plan upon patient discharge.
   - **d.** Continue the care plan if more time is needed to achieve the goals/outcomes.

## ALTERNATE-FORMAT QUESTIONS

### Multiple Response Questions

***Circle the letters that correspond to the best answers for each question.***

1. Nurses formulate physiologic goals for patients when providing patient care. What are examples of physiologic goals? *(Select all that apply.)*
   a. By 4/6/20, the baby will demonstrate adequate sleep–wakefulness patterns
   b. Before discharge, the parents of the baby will verbalize decreased anxiety about taking care of a newborn.
   c. By 4/6/20, the parents will list appropriate resources in case questions arise after discharge.
   d. By 4/6/20, the baby will show an adequate comfort level indicating satisfactory parenting.
   e. Before discharge, the baby will have reached a target weight gain of 8 lb (birth weight: 7 lb, 6 oz).
   f. Before discharge, the parents will demonstrate confidence in bathing and feeding their baby.

2. A nurse is documenting evaluation of the care provided for an infant born with Down's syndrome. Which nursing actions exemplify the appropriate documentation process? *(Select all that apply.)*
   a. After the data have been collected to determine patient outcome achievement, the nurse writes an evaluative statement to summarize the findings.
   b. The nurse writes a two-part evaluative statement that includes a decision about how well the outcome was met, along with patient data that support the decision.
   c. The nurse has three decision options for how goals have been met.
   d. The nurse determines whether a patient goal has been met or not met. In each case, the goal is discontinued.
   e. The nurse does not increase the complexity of a goal after it has been achieved to prevent patient anxiety and distrust.
   f. If a nurse writes a properly written goal, it is not affected by patient, nurse, or health care variables.

3. A nurse is following the rules recommended by the Institute of Medicine's Committee on Quality of Health Care in America to help redesign and improve patient care. Which nursing actions are based on these rules? *(Select all that apply.)*
   a. The nurse bases patient care on established nursing needs and values.
   b. The nurse becomes the source of control for patient care.
   c. The nurse bases care on evidence-based decision making.
   d. The nurse customizes care based on availability of resources.
   e. The nurse promotes shared knowledge and the free flow of information.
   f. The nurse acknowledges that continuous decrease in waste improves patient care.

4. A nurse manager attempts to achieve performance improvement in the emergency department of a busy inner-city hospital. Which nursing actions follow Haase and Miller's recommended steps in performance improvement? *(Select all that apply.)*
   a. The nurse discovers that there is a problem with the triage system that is in place in the emergency department.
   b. The nurse calls a meeting of the emergency department interdisciplinary team to affect change in the triage process.
   c. The nurse organizes a task force to implement change in the triage process of a busy emergency department.
   d. The nurse meets with the emergency department staff to assess changes made to the triage process.
   e. When the goal of making changes to the triage process in the emergency department is not met, the nurse discontinues efforts to force change.
   f. When met with resistance to change from the emergency department staff, the nurses involves management to force the changes.

CHAPTER 19

# Documenting and Reporting

## ASSESSING YOUR UNDERSTANDING

### FILL IN THE BLANKS

1. The Joint Commission specifies that nursing care data related to patient assessments, nursing diagnoses or patient needs, nursing interventions, and patient outcomes are permanently integrated into the ___________.

2. A nurse documents healthcare-associated pneumonia in a postsurgical patient by using ___________ charting, which documents the unexpected event, the cause of the event, actions taken in response to the event, and discharge planning if appropriate.

3. A nurse documents care in a long-term care facility by using ___________, a core set of screening, clinical, and functional status elements that forms the foundation of the comprehensive assessment of all residents in long-term care facilities certified to participate in Medicare or Medicaid.

4. The ___________ is a group of data elements that represent core items of a comprehensive assessment for an adult home care patient and form the basis for measuring patient outcomes for purposes of outcome-based quality improvement.

5. Nurses document care in long-term care settings as specified by the ___________, which helps the staff gather definitive information on a resident's strengths and needs and address these in an individualized care plan.

6. A nurse who communicates oral, written, or audiotaped patient data to the nurse replacing him or her on the next shift is giving a(n) ___________ report.

7. A nurse uses a(n) ___________ form to document the injury that occurred to a patient by improper use of medical equipment.

8. A(n) ___________ is a meeting of nurses to discuss some aspect of a patient's care.

### MATCHING EXERCISES

***Match the formats of nursing documentation listed in Part A with their appropriate example listed in Part B.***

#### PART A

a. Initial nursing assessment
b. Nursing care plan
c. Critical/collaborative pathways
d. Progress notes
e. Graphic record
f. Fluid intake and output
g. Medication record
h. 24-hour nursing care record
i. Discharge and transfer summary
j. Home care documentation
k. Long-term care documentation

**PART B**

____ 1. The nurse documents the case management plan for a patient population with a designated diagnosis that includes expected outcomes, interventions to be performed, and the sequence and timing of these interventions.

____ 2. The nurse documents a diabetic patient's intake and output of fluids.

____ 3. The nurse summarizes a patient's reason for treatment, significant findings, procedure performed and treatment rendered, and any specific instructions for the patient/family.

____ 4. The nurse uses this form to record a patient's pulse, respiratory rate, blood pressure, body temperature, weight, and bowel movements.

____ 5. The nurse records the database obtained from the nursing history and physical assessment.

____ 6. The nurse documents the administration of ciprofloxacin IV, 400 mg every 12 hours.

____ 7. The nurse documents a patient's diagnosis of AIDS, expected outcomes, and specific nursing interventions.

____ 8. A nurse documents that a patient is homebound and still needs nursing care.

____ 9. A nurse uses RAI to document care.

**SHORT ANSWER**

1. List four areas of nursing care data that, according to The Joint Commission, must be permanently integrated into the patient record.
   a. ____
   b. ____
   c. ____
   d. ____

2. Briefly describe the following methods of reporting patient data.
   a. Change-of-shift/hand-off reports: ____
   b. Telephone/telemedicine reports: ____
   c. Telephone orders: ____
   d. Transfer and discharge reports: ____
   e. Reports to family members and significant others: ____
   f. Incident reports: ____
   g. Conferring about care: ____
   h. Consultations and referrals: ____
   i. Nursing and interdisciplinary team care conference: ____
   j. Nursing care rounds: ____

3. Briefly explain the following purposes of the patient record.
   a. Communication: ____
   b. Care planning: ____
   c. Quality process and performance improvement: ____
   d. Research: ____
   e. Decision analysis: ____
   f. Education: ____
   g. Credentialing, regulation, and legislation: ____
   h. Legal documentation: ____
   i. Reimbursement: ____
   j. Historical document: ____

4. List five guidelines nurses should follow when reporting a significant change in a patient's condition to other health care professionals by telephone.
   a. ______
   b. ______
   c. ______
   d. ______
   e. ______

5. List four benefits of using the Resident Assessment Instrument (RAI).
   a. ______
   b. ______
   c. ______
   d. ______

6. Complete the chart below listing the purpose (description), advantages, and disadvantages of the various methods of documentation.

| Documentation Method | Description/Advantages/Disadvantages |
|---|---|
| *SOURCE-ORIENTED RECORD* | Description:<br>Advantages:<br>Disadvantages: |
| *PROBLEM-ORIENTED MEDICAL RECORDS* | Description:<br>Advantages:<br>Disadvantages: |
| *PIE—PROBLEM, INTERVENTION, EVALUATION* | Description:<br>Advantages:<br>Disadvantages: |
| *FOCUS CHARTING* | Description:<br>Advantages:<br>Disadvantages: |
| *CHARTING BY EXCEPTION* | Description:<br>Advantages:<br>Disadvantages: |
| *CASE MANAGEMENT MODEL* | Description:<br>Advantages:<br>Disadvantages: |
| *OCCURRENCE OR VARIANCE CHARTING* | Description:<br>Advantages:<br>Disadvantages: |
| *ELECTRONIC HEALTH RECORDS* | Description:<br>Advantages:<br>Disadvantages: |

## APPLYING YOUR KNOWLEDGE

### CRITICAL THINKING QUESTIONS

1. Consider the following patient: A 79-year-old woman with Alzheimer's disease is admitted to a long-term care unit. She has a history of falls and has fractured her left hip in the past. She no longer recognizes her daughter, who was taking care of her. The daughter states she can no longer handle her mother's condition. The daughter insists that the nurses restrain her mother physically to prevent falls.

   Think about the information the team will need to provide safe, quality care for this patient. What types of data should the admitting nurse record, and what system of documentation is most likely to bring the information to the attention of everyone who needs it?

2. How would you go about scheduling a consultation for a male amputee who needs physical therapy? Write a brief summary of the patient's condition and how you would present his case to the referred facility.

3. Make an appointment to interview the risk manager of a health care system. Find out how important the documentation of patient care is to the patient, nurse, and health facility when legal questions arise. How can this knowledge help to safeguard your practice?

### REFLECTIVE PRACTICE: CULTIVATING QSEN COMPETENCIES

***Use the following expanded scenario from Chapter 19 in your textbook to answer the questions below.***

***Scenario:*** Phillippe Baron, age 52, is being discharged from the outpatient surgery department after undergoing a colonoscopy for removal of three polyps. Upon admittance, Mr. Baron stated that he was allergic to a pain medication but couldn't remember the name of it. The RN phoned the health care provider's office to check his medical record. His attending gave an order via phone for a PRN analgesic that worked in the past. He will be going home with his wife, who is a nurse, and they require discharge teaching.

1. What should be the focus of discharge teaching for Mr. Baron and his wife?

   ______________________________

   ______________________________

   ______________________________

2. What would be a successful outcome for this patient?

   ______________________________

   ______________________________

   ______________________________

3. What intellectual, technical, interpersonal, and/or ethical/legal competencies are most likely to bring about the desired outcome?

   ______________________________

   ______________________________

   ______________________________

4. What resources might be helpful for Ms. Baron?

   ______________________________

   ______________________________

   ______________________________

## PRACTICING FOR NCLEX

### MULTIPLE CHOICE QUESTIONS

***Circle the letter that corresponds to the best answer for each question.***

1. A patient accuses a nurse of negligence when he trips when ambulating for the first time since hip replacement surgery. Which action is the best defense against allegations of negligence?
   a. Notifying the nursing team of the patient condition
   b. Documenting patient data on the flow sheet
   c. Keeping an accurate medication record
   d. Accurately documenting patient care on the patient record

2. Which nursing action is an example of properly handling the patient record?
   a. A nurse shares the patient record with a close family member.
   b. A nurse does not share the patient record with other health care team members.
   c. A nurse does not allow a patient to update his health record.
   d. A nurse allows a patient to see and copy her own health record.
3. A nurse documents the following patient data in the patient record according to the SOAP format: Patient complains of unrelieved pain; patient is seen clutching his side and grimacing; patient pain medication does not appear to be effective; call in to primary care provider to increase dosage of pain medication or change prescription. This is an example of what charting method?
   a. Source-oriented method
   b. PIE charting method
   c. Problem-oriented method
   d. Focus charting method
4. A nurse documents hypertension in a woman who is 5 months pregnant and then writes a narrative describing the situation. This type of abnormal status can be seen immediately with narrative easily retrieved in what documentation format?
   a. Charting by exception
   b. PIE
   c. Narrative notes
   d. SOAP notes
5. A nurse helps a patient who has cystic fibrosis prepare a standalone personal health record. Which statement by the nurse best explains this type of information?
   a. "You can fill in information from your own records and store it on your computer or the Internet."
   b. "You can link your record to a specific health care organization's electronic health record system."
   c. "Your health care provider is obligated to read your personal health record and share it with your insurance provider."
   d. "Your entire health care team may access and securely share your vital medical information electronically."
6. The nurse is finding it difficult to plan and implement care for a patient and decides to have a nursing care conference. What action would the nurse take to facilitate this process?
   a. The nurse consults with someone in order to exchange ideas or seek information, advice, or instructions.
   b. The nurse meets with nurses or other health care professionals to discuss some aspect of patient care.
   c. The nurse, along with other nurses, visits patients with similar problems individually at each patient's bedside in order to plan nursing care.
   d. The nurse sends or directs someone to take action in a specific nursing care problem.
7. A nurse is documenting the effectiveness of a patient's pain management on the patient record. Which documentation is written correctly?
   a. Mr. Gray is receiving sufficient relief from pain medication.
   b. Mr. Gray appears comfortable and is resting adequately.
   c. Mr. Gray reports that on a scale of 1 to 10, the pain he is experiencing is a 3.
   d. Mr. Gray appears to have a low tolerance for pain and complains frequently about the intensity of his pain.
8. A nurse is arranging for home care for patients and reviews the Medicare reimbursement requirements. Which patient meets one of these requirements?
   a. A patient who is homebound and needs skilled nursing care
   b. A patient whose rehabilitation potential is not good
   c. A patient whose status is stabilized
   d. A patient who is not making progress in expected outcomes of care
9. A nurse takes a patient's pulse, respiratory rate, blood pressure, and body temperature. On which form would the nurse most likely document the results?
   a. Progress notes
   b. Flow sheets
   c. Graphic sheets
   d. Medical records

10. A nurse has a two-way video communication with the specialist involved in the care of a patient in a long-term care facility. This is an example of what nursing informatics technology?
    a. Patient engagement technology
    b. Data aggregation technology
    c. Telemedicine and mobile technology
    d. Population health management technology

## ALTERNATE-FORMAT QUESTIONS

### Multiple Response Questions

***Circle the letters that correspond to the best answers for each question.***

1. A nurse is documenting care for an older adult patient who is recovering from a mild stroke. Which documentation entries follow the recommended guidelines for communicating and documenting patient information? *(Select all that apply.)*
    a. The patient rates pain as 2 compared to a 7 yesterday.
    b. The patient seems comfortable today.
    c. The patient drank an average amount of fluids.
    d. Vital signs returned to normal.
    e. The patient appears anxious about having another stroke.
    f. Radial pulse is 72, strong and regular.
2. A nurse manager of a health care provider's office is responsible for obtaining signed authorizations for releasing patient information to third parties. In which situations would the nurse not need an authorization from the patient? *(Select all that apply.)*
    a. Reporting the incidence of an infectious disease to the Centers for Disease Control and Prevention
    b. Releasing a medical record to the court when a nurse is being sued for negligence
    c. Sharing information regarding home care with a patient's spouse
    d. Submitting charges for nursing services
    e. Facilitating organ donation of a deceased patient
    f. Providing statistics related to the use of a dangerous piece of equipment
3. A nurse is documenting care for patients in a hospital setting. Which documenting errors may potentially increase the nurse's risk for legal problems? *(Select all that apply.)*
    a. The content reflects patient needs.
    b. The content includes descriptions of situations that are out of the ordinary.
    c. The content is not in accordance with professional standards.
    d. There are lines between the entries.
    e. The documentation is not countersigned.
    f. Dates and times of entries are omitted.
4. HIPAA allows incidental disclosures of patient health information as long as it cannot reasonably be prevented, is limited in nature, and occurs as a byproduct of an otherwise permitted use or disclosure of PHI. What are examples of this type of PHI disclosure? *(Select all that apply.)*
    a. The nurse uses sign-in sheets that contain information about the reason for the patient visit.
    b. A visitor hears a confidential conversation between two nurses in surroundings that are appropriate and with voices that are kept low.
    c. The nurse uses white boards on an unlimited basis.
    d. The nurse uses x-ray light boards that can be seen by passersby; however, patient x-rays are not left unattended on them.
    e. The nurse calls out names in the waiting room, but does not disclose the reason for the patient visit.
    f. The nurse leaves a detailed appointment reminder message on a patient's voice mail.
5. The nurse is using the ISBARR format to report a surgical patient's deteriorating condition to a health care provider. Which actions would the nurse perform when using this guide? *(Select all that apply.)*
    a. The nurse asks the health care provider to describe the admitting diagnosis of the patient.
    b. After introductions, the nurse states the patient name, room number, and problem.
    c. The nurse asks the health care provider to estimate the discharge date for the patient.
    d. The nurse asks the health care provider to comment on the present situation before giving recommendations.
    e. The nurse states that the patient's condition "could be life threatening."
    f. The nurse reads back the health care provider's new orders at the conclusion of the call.

CHAPTER 20

# Nursing Informatics

## ASSESSING YOUR UNDERSTANDING

### FILL IN THE BLANKS

1. A(n)__________ is a computer-based system designed for collecting, storing, manipulating, and making available clinical information important to the health care delivery process.
2. A digital version of a patient's chart or medical history is called a(n) __________.
3. A nurse who integrates nursing science with multiple information management and analytical sciences into her nursing practice is employing the techniques of nursing __________.
4. An informatics nurse who helped to implement the use of an electronic health record (EHR) in her practice may become a(n) __________, or a system expert who can navigate the EHR with ease.
5. The extent to which a product can be used by specified users to achieve specified goals with effectiveness, efficiency, and satisfaction in a specified context of use is termed __________.
6. A patient may use a home computer to access a patient __________ to review lab results.
7. The ability of analysts to see analytics presented visually to identify new patterns or see difficult concepts is termed __________.
8. __________ comprises the accumulation of health care–related data from various sources, combined with new technologies that allow for the transformation of data to information, to knowledge, and ultimately to wisdom.

### MATCHING EXERCISES

***Match the standard of practice area for nursing informatics listed in Part A with the appropriate example listed in Part B.***

**PART A**

a. Assessment
b. Diagnosis, problem, and issue identification
c. Outcome identification
d. Planning
e. Implementation
f. Evaluation
g. Ethics
h. Education
i. Evidence-based practice and research
j. Quality of practice
k. Communication
l. Leadership
m. Collaboration
n. Professional practice evaluation
o. Resource utilization
p. Environmental health

**PART B**

____ 1. A nurse reviews the institution's protocols for hazardous spills in the workplace.

____ 2. A nurse analyzes data to improve nursing and informatics outcomes in the facility.

____ 3. A nurse uses effective communications skills to collect pertinent data to define an issue.

____ 4. A nurse integrates evidence-based practice and research into a patient care plan.

____ 5. A nurse coordinates health care provision based on availability of operational resources.

____ 6. A nurse uses a decision tree to define a new issue affecting a patient's care plan.

____ 7. A nurse teaches colleagues nursing informatics practices and helps to put them in use.

____ 8. A nurse uses informatics to help define the goals of a patient health care plan.

____ 9. A nurse employs informatics principles to promote consumer confidentiality.

____ 10. A nurse uses a variety of formats to share knowledge of informatics technology with colleagues.

____ 11. A nurse asks colleagues for feedback on her performance as head nurse.

____ 12. A nurse puts in place a plan to improve documentation based on the principles of informatics.

____ 13. A nurse schedules a teleconference with a patient's primary care provider and nutritionist.

____ 14. A nurse systematically reviews the outcomes of new policies instituted in the workplace.

____ 15. A nurse attends an in-service on new informatics techniques to advance his practice.

____ 16. A nurse uses available informatics resources to research evidence-based practices.

## SHORT ANSWER

1. List four meaningful uses of certified EHR technology as defined by HealthIT.gov.
   a. ____
   b. ____
   c. ____
   d. ____

2. List five positive results of the meaningful use of certified EHR technology.
   a. ____
   b. ____
   c. ____
   d. ____
   e. ____

3. Describe the Informatics Scope and Standards Definitions (DIKW) listed below:
   a. Data: ____
   b. Information: ____
   c. Knowledge: ____
   d. Wisdom: ____

4. Nurses who use a clinical information system should be involved in all phases of a system development lifecycle (SDLC) to ensure the best chance that the system will meet its intended need. Consider the scenario of an OB/GYN office converting to EHRs, and give an example of a nursing responsibility related to the following areas of focus of an SDLC:
   a. Analyze and plan: ____
   b. Design: ____
   c. Test: ____
   d. Train: ____
   e. Implement: ____
   f. Maintain: ____
   g. Evaluate: ____

5. Briefly define the following informatics concepts and state how they affect the implementation and maintenance of clinical information systems:
   a. Usability: ________________________
   b. Optimization: ________________________
   c. Standard terminologies: ________________________
   d. Interoperability: ________________________
   e. Security and privacy: ________________________

6. List five benefits of using a patient portal in a medical practice.
   a. ________________________
   b. ________________________
   c. ________________________
   d. ________________________
   e. ________________________

7. Give two examples of the following types of mobile technologies:
   a. Telehealth: ________________________
   b. Telecare: ________________________
   c. Telemedicine: ________________________

## APPLYING YOUR KNOWLEDGE

### CRITICAL THINKING QUESTIONS

1. Nurses handle sensitive patient information on a daily basis when using clinical information systems. Interview an informatics nurse specialist to discuss how to keep this information safe. Then research the Internet for Health Insurance Portability and Accountability Act (HIPAA) policies related to the use of EHRs. Based on your results, devise a plan detailing strategies to ensure the privacy and confidentiality of patient data. Consider what you would do if you encountered a coworker who placed a sticky note on a computer with his or her password written on it.

2. Nurses use analytics and big data to support population health. What can you as a nurse do to improve patient care by identifying patients at risk of needing additional assistance to manage their disease? Think about what types of patient conditions best respond to this type of analysis and what type of data can be retrieved from information systems to positively affect the patient care plan.

### REFLECTIVE PRACTICE: CULTIVATING QSEN COMPETENCIES

***Use the following expanded scenario from Chapter 20 in your textbook to answer the questions below.***

***Scenario:*** Frank is a 72-year-old patient who has chronic obstructive pulmonary disease. His wife, who has been his primary caretaker since his diagnosis 5 years ago, died last year and he now lives alone in their original two-level family home. He has been sleeping on the couch in the living room because he can no longer go upstairs. He has a daughter who lives across country who tries to get home once a month to be sure he has food and medications. When the nurse asks Frank if he takes his medication regularly, he states: "I try to take my medication, but I don't always remember, my wife used to always bring me my pills." Not surprisingly, Frank has had four hospital readmissions in the past year.

1. What should be the focus of an evaluation of Frank's nursing care plan. How can informatics be of help in this case?

   ________________________

2. What would be a successful outcome for this patient?

   ________________________

3. What intellectual, technical, interpersonal, and/or ethical/legal competencies are most likely to bring about the desired outcome?

   ________________________

4. What resources might be helpful for Frank?

________________________________________

________________________________________

________________________________________

## PRACTICING FOR NCLEX

### MULTIPLE CHOICE QUESTIONS

***Circle the letter that corresponds to the best answer for each question.***

1. The nurse reviews the list of drugs that have been prescribed for a patient based on pharmacogenomics. What is the basis for this emerging practice?
   a. The knowledge that each drug works essentially the same for everyone.
   b. The inclusion of personal preference in the drug choice.
   c. The choice of drugs based on economics or patient's ability to pay.
   d. The effect of genetic makeup on the drug prescribed.
2. The nurse using EHRs for patients decides upon a password to keep patient information safe. Which password guideline is recommended?
   a. Never use a password manager for EHR access.
   b. Use at least 6 characters for your password.
   c. Consider using multifactor authentication.
   d. Use the same password for all electronic needs to prevent password resetting.
3. The nurse is using the SDLC to implement the placement of new computers in the workplace. In what stage of this process would the nurse most likely consult with coworkers for their input in creating the new work stations?
   a. Analyze and plan
   b. Design
   c. Test
   d. Implement
4. The nurse meets with coworkers to discuss and make improvements to a new EHR reporting system being used in their office. What is the technical term for this core concept?
   a. Usability
   b. Optimization
   c. Interoperability
   d. Standard terminologies
5. The nurse is able to share patient data stored on an EHR with a specialist in another country. What is the term for this advantage of informatics use?
   a. Interoperability
   b. Data visualization
   c. Big data
   d. System usability
6. A nurse is reviewing data from EHRs that is transformed into pie charts. What is the term for this presentation of analytics?
   a. Data visualization
   b. Big data
   c. Graphic picture
   d. Predictive analytics

### ALTERNATE-FORMAT QUESTIONS

#### Multiple Response Questions

***Circle the letters that correspond to the best answers for each question.***

1. A nurse is using a drop-down menu to enter patient activity level on an EHR. Which entries are MOST likely to be presented? *(Select all that apply.)*
   a. Walks without assistance
   b. Nonambulatory
   c. Walks with a cane
   d. Able to walk short distances
   e. Requires an assistive device
   f. Sometimes uses a walker to walk
2. A nurse is using technology testing phases to evaluate the use of a new patient reporting system. Which actions would the nurse perform during integration testing? *(Select all that apply.)*
   a. Use test scripts to validate one particular function of the system.
   b. Ensure that there is proper functioning and communication among all systems.
   c. Perform an initial basic test to ensure all components are in place.
   d. Test whether the new system can handle high volumes of information.
   e. Use test script to validate that multiple components of the system are working.
   f. Test drive the system to ensure all components are working as designed.

## Prioritization Questions

1. Place the following steps in informatics evaluation in the order in which they would occur:
   a. Conduct a literature search.
   b. Determine the question.
   c. Determine the study type.
   d. Collect, analyze, and display data.
   e. Determine what will be evaluated.
   f. Determine the needed data.
   g. Document your outcome evaluation.
   h. Determine the data collection method and sample size.

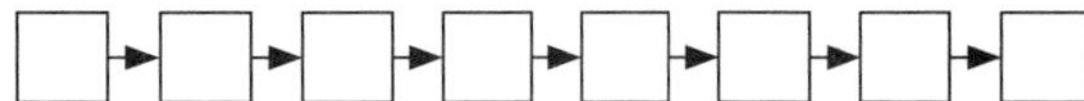

2. Place the following testing technology testing phases in the order in which they should be performed:
   a. Function testing
   b. Performance testing
   c. User acceptance testing
   d. Unit testing
   e. Integration testing

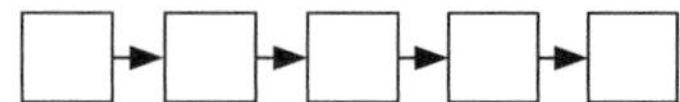

CHAPTER 21

# Developmental Concepts

## ASSESSING YOUR UNDERSTANDING

### FILL IN THE BLANKS

1. The nurse assessing infants and children in a pediatrician's office notes that growth progresses from gross motor movements, such as learning to crawl, to fine motor movements, such as drawing with a crayon. This trend in growth development is known as ___________ development.
2. A nurse is counseling a 16-year-old female who is seeking contraception at a local health clinic. According to developmental theorist Sigmund Freud, this patient is in the ___________ stage.
3. A 6-year-old child says bedtime prayers together with his parents at night. According to the developmental theorist Fowler, this child is in the ___________ stage of spiritual development.
4. According to Erik Erikson, during the ___________ years, a person desires to make a contribution to the world and, if this is not accomplished, stagnation may occur.
5. Freud identified the underlying stimulus for human behavior as sexuality, which he called ___________.
6. According to Jean Piaget, a child who enters preschool and integrates the experience into existing schemata is using the ___________ process of restructuring knowledge.
7. A 13-year-old female is using deductive reasoning to test beliefs regarding her sexuality. This female is in the ___________ stage of Piaget's theory of cognitive development.
8. Levinson and associates based their theory of human development on the organizing concept of "individual life structure." This theory centered on the belief that the pattern of life at any point in time is formed by the interaction of three components: the ___________, the social and cultural aspects of one's life, and the particular set of ___________ in which a person participates.

### MATCHING EXERCISES

***Match Erikson's stages of development listed in Part A with the appropriate example listed in Part B. Some answers will be used more than once.***

#### PART A

**a.** Trust versus mistrust
**b.** Autonomy versus shame and doubt
**c.** Initiative versus guilt
**d.** Industry versus inferiority
**e.** Identity versus role confusion
**f.** Intimacy versus isolation
**g.** Generativity versus stagnation
**h.** Ego integrity versus despair

**PART B**

____ **1.** A 10-year-old boy proudly displays his principal's award certificate.

____ **2.** An infant believes that his parents will feed him.

____ **3.** A 22-year-old woman picks a circle of friends with whom she spends her free time.

____ **4.** A 13-year-old girl fights with her mother about appropriate dress.

____ **5.** A long-term care facility resident reflects positively on her past life experiences.

____ **6.** A 15-year-old boy worries about how his classmates treat him.

____ **7.** A 45-year-old man meets a goal of guiding his two children into rewarding careers.

____ **8.** A kindergarten student learns the alphabet.

____ **9.** A 2-year-old boy expresses interest in dressing himself.

____ **10.** A 35-year-old woman volunteers Saturday mornings to work with the homeless.

***Match the stages of faith development listed in Part A with the appropriate definition listed in Part B. Note which of the following stages you have personally experienced in your lifetime. Give an example from your past that illustrates your passage through each stage on the lines provided at the end of the definitions.***

**PART A**

**a.** Stage 1: Intuitive–projective faith

**b.** Stage 2: Mythical–literal faith

**c.** Stage 3: Synthetic–conventional faith

**d.** Stage 4: Individuative–reflective faith

**e.** Stage 5: Conjunctive faith

**f.** Stage 6: Universalizing faith

**PART B**

____ **11.** This stage integrates other viewpoints about faith into one's understanding of truth. One is able to see the paradoxical nature of the reality of one's own beliefs. Personal example: ____________________

____________________

____ **12.** This is the characteristic stage for many adolescents. An ideology has emerged, but it has not been closely examined until now; attempts to stabilize own identity. Personal example:

____________________

____________________

____ **13.** This stage involves making tangible the values of absolute love and justice for humankind; total trust in principle of being and existence of future. Personal example: ____________________

____________________

____ **14.** In this stage, children imitate religious gestures and behaviors of others; they follow parental attitudes toward religious or moral beliefs without a thorough understanding of them. Personal example: ____________________

____________________

____ **15.** This stage is critical for older adolescents and young adults because the responsibility for their commitments, beliefs, and attitudes becomes their own. Personal example: ____________________

____________________

____ **16.** This stage predominates in the school-aged child with increased social interaction. Stories represent religious and moral beliefs, and the existence of a deity is accepted. Personal example:

____________________

____________________

## CORRECT THE FALSE STATEMENTS

***Circle the word "true" or "false" that follows the statement. If you circled "false," change the underlined word or words to make the statement true. Place your answer in the space provided.***

**1.** The human processes of growth and development result from two interrelated factors: heredity and environment.

**a.** True

**b.** False ____________________

**2.** Growth and development follow irregular and unpredictable trends.

**a.** True

**b.** False ____________________

3. Different aspects of growth and development occur at the same stages and rates.
   a. True
   b. False ______________________
4. In the third level of Carol Gilligan's theory of moral development, nonviolence governs all moral judgments and actions.
   a. True
   b. False ______________________
5. According to Freud, the ego is the part of the psyche concerned with self-gratification by the easiest and quickest available means.
   a. True
   b. False ______________________
6. In Freud's phallic stage, the child has increased interest in biological sex differences, curiosity about the genitals, and masturbation increases.
   a. True
   b. False ______________________
7. According to Havighurst, developing a conscience, morality, and a scale of values should occur in middle childhood.
   a. True
   b. False ______________________
8. In Kohlberg's preconventional level, stage 2, instrumental relativist orientation, the motivation for choices of action is fear of physical consequences or authority's disapproval.
   a. True
   b. False ______________________
9. According to Gould, between the ages of 22 and 28, self-acceptance increases as the person's need to prove his or her competence disappears.
   a. True
   b. False ______________________

## SHORT ANSWER

1. Complete the following chart, using the first theorist (Sigmund Freud) as an example.

| Theorist and Theory | Basic Concepts of Theory | Stages of Development |
|---|---|---|
| **Sigmund Freud**<br>Psychoanalytic theory | Stressed the impact of instinctual human drives on determining behavior: unconscious mind, the id, the ego, the superego, stages of development based on sexual motivation | Oral stage<br>Anal stage<br>Phallic stage<br>Latent stage<br>Genital stage |
| **Erik Erikson** | | |
| **Robert J. Havighurst** | | |
| **Roger Gould** | | |
| **Daniel Levinson** | | |
| **Jean Piaget** | | |
| **Lawrence Kohlberg** | | |
| **Carol Gilligan** | | |
| **James Fowler** | | |

**2.** Describe Lawrence Kohlberg's three levels of moral development, and give an example of behavior that would typify each level.

**a.** Preconventional level: ____________________

____________________

Example: ____________________

____________________

**b.** Conventional level: ____________________

____________________

Example: ____________________

____________________

**c.** Postconventional level: ____________________

____________________

Example: ____________________

____________________

**3.** A 6-year-old girl with leukemia is admitted to the hospital for her first session of chemotherapy. What insight into this patient's needs could be gained from the following theorists?

**a.** Freud: ____________________

____________________

**b.** Erikson: ____________________

____________________

**c.** Havighurst: ____________________

____________________

**d.** Piaget: ____________________

____________________

**e.** Kohlberg: ____________________

____________________

**f.** Gilligan: ____________________

____________________

**g.** Fowler: ____________________

____________________

**4.** Identify the stage of the theorists noted below that the nurse could use in responding to the following statements made by a 15-year-old boy who has been admitted to the hospital following an ATV accident. He has multiple fractures and several deep cuts in his face that require stitches.

**a.** Freud: ____________ "My dad told me not to ride that thing. I should have listened to him, and this never would have happened."

**b.** Erikson: ____________ "I'm going to be so ugly with these scars on my face. No girl will ever look at me again."

**c.** Piaget: ____________ "What's the best way to be sure I don't lose strength in my muscles? If I do those exercises you taught me, I'll be able to go back to school and play basketball next year."

**d.** Fowler: ____________ "I don't believe in God. If there were a God, He never would have let this happen to me."

**5.** What role does the family play in health promotion and illness prevention? How has your family affected your attitudes toward health and illness? ____________________

____________________

____________________

____________________

## APPLYING YOUR KNOWLEDGE

### CRITICAL THINKING QUESTIONS

**1.** Reflect on the nursing plan you would develop for a 3-year-old, a 10-year-old, and a 16-year-old undergoing heart surgery. How would your plan differ to take into consideration the age differences of the patients? How would you explain the procedure to each child? Give a rationale for each nursing intervention planned. Support your rationale by using a different developmental theory for each age group's nursing plan.

3-year-old:

10-year-old:

16-year-old:

2. Make a chart listing Freud's stages of psychosexual development, Piaget's psychosocial development of different ages, and Havighurst's developmental tasks. Observe children in different settings and find an example of each stage of development. Talk with classmates about how these findings would influence your nursing practice.

### REFLECTIVE PRACTICE: CULTIVATING QSEN COMPETENCIES

***Use the following expanded scenario from Chapter 21 in your textbook to answer the questions below.***

***Scenario:*** Joseph Logan, age 70, fell and fractured his hip while repairing the exterior of his home. He has a wife and two grown children. His son, age 42, is mentally challenged and lives at home with the couple. His wife tells you she is apprehensive about having to care for two people now. When the nurse comes into Mr. Logan's room to perform morning care, he says, "Go away and leave me alone. I'm a grown man; I can take care of myself. And get rid of this tray. I'm not hungry!" Further investigation reveals that Mr. Logan has been the traditional head of his household and is now troubled by needing others, including his wife, to care for him.

1. What developmental considerations may affect care planning for Mr. Logan?

_______________________________________

_______________________________________

_______________________________________

2. What would be a successful outcome for this patient?

_______________________________________

_______________________________________

_______________________________________

3. What intellectual, technical, interpersonal, and/or ethical/legal competencies are most likely to bring about the desired outcome?

_______________________________________

_______________________________________

_______________________________________

4. What resources might be helpful for Mr. Logan and his family?

_______________________________________

_______________________________________

_______________________________________

## PRACTICING FOR NCLEX

### MULTIPLE CHOICE QUESTIONS

***Circle the letter that corresponds to the best answer for each question.***

1. A nurse is caring for a 6-year-old boy who is hospitalized for observation following a motor vehicle accident. Based on Havighurst's developmental tasks, what would be the best choice for a diversional activity for this patient?
   a. Reading a story book
   b. Playing video games
   c. Watching television
   d. Speaking to school friends on the telephone

2. A nurse is assessing the psychosocial development of children in a day care center. Which child would the nurse expect to be experiencing the most intense period of speech development?
   a. A 2-year-old
   b. A 4-year-old
   c. A 6-year-old
   d. An 8-year-old

3. A nurse is teaching parents of preschoolers about growth and development of their children. Which teaching point would the nurse include?
   a. The pace of growth and development is specific for each person.
   b. Growth and development occur at similar stages and rates for each age group.
   c. Aspects of growth and development cannot be modified.
   d. Growth and development do not follow regular predictable trends.

4. A nurse is caring for a hospitalized 3-year-old female who is having surgery for a cleft palate repair. While in the hospital, the parents of the child tell the nurse that their child who was previously potty-trained has begun to wet her pants. What is the best response of the nurse?
   a. "We should have a child psychologist assess your child."
   b. "Just put a diaper on her while she is in the hospital."
   c. "This is normal; children often regress during difficult periods or crises."
   d. "You should offer her a reward for not wetting the bed."
5. A nurse is assessing older adults in a long-term care facility. According to Havighurst, what is a developmental task of this generation?
   a. Developing a conscious and morality
   b. Adjusting to decreasing physical status and health
   c. Becoming financially independent
   d. Depending on family for psychosocial needs
6. A child who learns that he must sit quietly during story hour in kindergarten, thereby integrating this new experience into his existing schemata, is applying the process of:
   a. Accommodation
   b. Dissemination
   c. Assimilation
   d. Orientation
7. A nurse is caring for a child who states: "I don't like the taste of this medicine, but my parents told me it will help me get better, so I'll take it." This example best exemplifies which stage of Piaget's cognitive development theory?
   a. Sensorimotor stage
   b. Preoperational stage
   c. Concrete operational stage
   d. Formal operational stage
8. The nurse observes a hospitalized 15-year-old male refuse his meal tray and state: "I usually eat pizza at home. I can't eat the food in here." This type of rebellious behavior is characteristic of which of Erik Erikson's stages of psychosocial development?
   a. Autonomy versus shame and doubt
   b. Initiative versus guilt
   c. Industry versus inferiority
   d. Identity versus role confusion
9. The nurse is counseling a woman who states: "I'm never going to find a husband, every time I start dating I end up getting hurt. I'm not even going to try anymore." This woman is in what stage of Carol Gilligan's theory of moral development?
   a. Level 1—selfishness
   b. Level 2—goodness
   c. Level 3—nonviolence
   d. Level 3—ethic of care

## ALTERNATE-FORMAT QUESTIONS

### Multiple Response Questions

***Circle the letters that correspond to the best answers for each question.***

1. A nurse assesses the effect of the environment and nutrition on patients visiting a walk-in clinic in a low-income community. Which statements accurately describe these effects? *(Select all that apply.)*
   a. Infants who are malnourished in utero develop the same amount of brain cells as infants who had adequate prenatal nutrition.
   b. Substance abuse by a pregnant woman increases the risk for congenital anomalies in her developing fetus.
   c. Failure to thrive cannot be linked to emotional deprivation.
   d. Abuse of alcohol and drugs is more prevalent in teenagers who have poor family relationships.
   e. An increased incidence of teenage pregnancy can be linked to substance abuse by adolescents.
   f. Child abuse can lead to deficits in physical development, but psychosocial development is not affected.

2. A nurse is using Freud's theory of psychoanalytic development to assess the development of children in the phallic stage of this theory. Which developmental milestones would the nurse expect in this age group? *(Select all that apply.)*
   a. The child becomes toilet trained.
   b. The child has increased interest in biological sex differences.
   c. The child is possessive of the opposite-sex parent.
   d. The child is curious about genitals and masturbation increases.
   e. The child prepares for adult roles and relationships.
   f. The child experiences sexual pressures and conflicts.

3. A school nurse is using Havighurst's developmental theory to teach parents of adolescents what to expect at this developmental stage. Which behaviors are typical of adolescents? *(Select all that apply.)*
   a. The adolescent learns physical skills necessary for games.
   b. The adolescent accepts his or her body and uses it effectively.
   c. The adolescent learns to get along with age-mates.
   d. The adolescent achieves emotional independences from parents.
   e. The adolescent acquires an ethical system as a guide to behavior.
   f. The adolescent achieves social and civic responsibility.

4. A nurse is assessing children using Kohlberg's theory of moral development. What are examples of milestones achieved in the preconventional level of this theory? *(Select all that apply.)*
   a. The child learns to follow parent's rules.
   b. The child identifies with family members and conforms to their expectations.
   c. The child is motivated by punishment for not conforming to rules.
   d. The child strives for approval in an attempt to be viewed as "good."
   e. The child develops moral judgment that is rational and internalized into self.
   f. The child develops a perception of goodness or badness.

## Prioritization Questions

1. Place the examples of stages of Sigmund Freud's theory of psychoanalytic development in the order in which they occur:
   a. The child has increased interest in biological sex differences and his or her own biological sex.
   b. The child increases sex-role identification with the parent of the same sex.
   c. The child uses his or her mouth as a major source of gratification and exploration.
   d. The child begins overt sexual relationships with others.
   e. The child develops neuromuscular control necessary for toilet training.

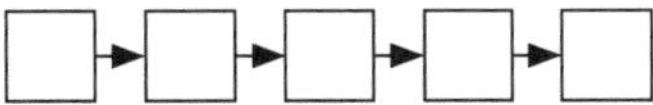

2. Place the stages of Havighurst's theory of development (developmental tasks) in the order in which they occur:
   a. Achieving biological sex–specific social role; achieving independence; acquiring a set of values and ethical system to guide behavior
   b. Learning sex differences; forming concepts; getting ready to read
   c. Learning to walk; learning to talk; learning to control body waste elimination
   d. Achieving social and civic responsibility; accepting and adjusting to physical changes
   e. Learning physical skills; learning to get along with others; developing conscience and morality
   f. Adjusting to decreasing physical status and health; adjusting to retirement

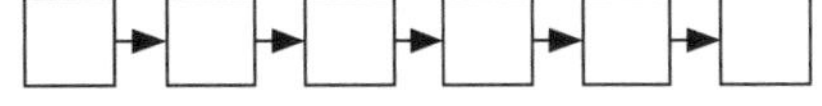

CHAPTER 22

# Conception Through Young Adult

## ASSESSING YOUR UNDERSTANDING

### FILL IN THE BLANKS

1. The nurse explains to a class of pregnant women that the __________ layer of the zygote will eventually become the respiratory system, the digestive system, the liver, and the pancreas.
2. The nurse is assessing a pregnant woman whose fetus is 6 weeks. This fetus is in the __________ stage of the development in which there is initiation of rapid growth and differentiation of the cell layers.
3. One minute and five minutes after birth, the nurse assesses the neonate using the most popular rating scale called the __________ rating scale.
4. A nurse encourages a new mother to cuddle and talk to her newborn. This intervention stimulates __________, which occurs when a mother forms an emotional link to her newborn.
5. A nurse documents inadequate growth in height and weight resulting from the infant's inability to obtain or use calories needed for growth. The term for this condition is __________.
6. The unexpected death of an infant under the age of 1 year in which postmortem examination fails to reveal a cause of death is known as __________.
7. A nurse uses the __________ tool to determine quickly and inexpensively atypical developmental patterns in infants and children.

### MATCHING EXERCISES

***Match the stage of development listed in Part A with the risk factor associated with that age listed in Part B.***

**PART A**

**a.** Neonate
**b.** Infant
**c.** Toddler
**d.** Preschooler
**e.** School-aged
**f.** Adolescent and young adult

**PART B**

____ **1.** Hormonal changes cause physical symptoms.

____ **2.** Communicable diseases and respiratory tract infections begin to develop in this stage.

____ **3.** Congenital disorders, such as hypospadias, inguinal hernias, and cardiac anomalies, require surgery at this stage.

____ **4.** The suicide rate is highest for this group.

____ **5.** A mother who smokes cigarettes, drinks alcohol, or uses drugs may cause developmental deficits in this stage.

____ **6.** Accidents, poisonings, burns, drowning, aspiration, and falls remain the major causes of death in this stage.

____ **7.** Gastroenteritis, food allergies, and skin disorders are common in this stage of development.

____ **8.** Scabies, impetigo, and head lice are more prevalent in this stage.

## SHORT ANSWER

**1.** Write down the age group in which the following physiologic characteristics and behaviors are commonly developed. Use *N* for neonate, *I* for infant, *T* for toddler, *P* for preschooler, *S* for school-aged, and *A* for adolescent/young adult.

____ Motor abilities include skipping, throwing and catching, copying figures, and printing letters and numbers.

____ Puberty begins.

____ Brain grows to about half the adult size.

____ Reflexes include sucking, swallowing, blinking, sneezing, and yawning.

____ Temperature control responds quickly to environmental temperatures.

____ Walks forward and backward, runs, kicks, climbs, and rides tricycle.

____ Drinks from a cup and uses a spoon.

____ Sebaceous and axillary sweat glands become active.

____ Height increases 2 to 3 in and weight increases 3 to 6 lb a year.

____ The feet, hands, and long bones grow rapidly, and muscle mass increases.

____ Alert to environment, sees color and form, hears and turns to sound.

____ Birthweight usually triples.

____ Full set of 20 deciduous teeth; baby teeth fall out and are replaced.

____ Body is less chubby and becomes leaner and more coordinated.

____ Primary and secondary development occurs with maturation of genitals.

____ Typically four times the birthweight and 23 to 37 inches in height.

____ Body temperature stabilizes.

____ Average weight is 45 lb.

____ Brain reaches 90% to 95% of adult size; nervous system is almost mature.

____ Head is close to adult size.

____ Motor abilities develop, allowing feeding self, crawling, and walking.

____ Can smell and taste and is sensitive to touch and pain.

____ Begins to eliminate stool and urine.

____ Deciduous teeth begin to erupt.

____ All permanent teeth are present except for second and third molars.

____ Attains bladder control during the day and sometimes during the night.

____ Holds a pencil and eventually writes in script and sentences.

____ Full adult size is reached.

____ Drinks breast milk, glucose water, and plain water.

____ Eyes begin to focus and fixate.

____ Turns pages in a book and by age 3 draws stick people.

____ Heart doubles in weight, heart rate slows, blood pressure rises.

____ Rapid brain growth; increase in length of long bones of the arms and legs.

____ Uses fingers to pick up small objects.

____ Sexual organs grow but are dormant until late in this period.

**2.** Write down the age group in which the following psychosocial characteristics and behaviors are commonly developed. Use *N* for neonate, *I* for infant, *T* for toddler, *P* for preschooler, *S* for school-aged, and *A* for adolescent/young adult.

____ Is in oral stage (Freud); strives for immediate gratification of needs; strong sucking need.

____ Developmental task of learning appropriate sex's social role.

____ In Freud's genital stage, libido reemerges in mature form.

____ Is in anal stage (Freud); focus on pleasure of sphincter control.

____ Self-concept is being stabilized, with peer group as greatest influence.

____ Develops trust (Erikson) if caregiver is dependable to meet needs.

____ Achieves personal independence; develops conscience, morality, and scale of values.

____ Tries out different roles, personal choices, and beliefs (identity versus role confusion).

____ Meets developmental tasks (Havighurst) by learning to eat, walk, and talk.

____ Develops skill in reading, writing, and calculating, as well as concepts for everyday living.

____ More mature relationships with both males and females of same age.

____ Enters Erikson's stage of autonomy versus shame and doubt.

____ Is in Erikson's stage of initiative versus guilt.

____ Inner turmoil/examination of propriety of actions by rigid conscience.

____ Getting ready to read and learning to distinguish right from wrong.

____ One's personal appearance accepted; set of values internalized.

____ Freud's latency stage; strong identification with own sex.

____ Developmental tasks of learning to control elimination; begins to learn sex differences, concepts, language, and right from wrong.

____ Focuses on learning useful skills with an emphasis on doing, succeeding, and accomplishing.

____ Developmental tasks of describing social and physical reality through concept formation and language development.

____ Is in phallic stage (Freud) with biologic focus on genitals.

____ Superego and conscience begin to develop.

____ Developmental tasks of learning sex differences and modesty.

____ Developmental task of learning physical game skills.

____ Is in Erikson's industry versus inferiority stage.

3. Briefly describe the growth and development of the fetus in the following three stages of fetal growth.
   a. Pre-embryonic stage: ____________________

   ____________________
   b. Embryonic stage: ____________________

   ____________________
   c. Fetal stage: ____________________

   ____________________

4. List four critical areas of development that are assessed by the Denver Developmental Screening test.
   a. ____________________
   b. ____________________
   c. ____________________
   d. ____________________

5. After observing infants in a neonatal unit, describe the physical symptoms of the following temperaments:
   a. "Easy": ____________________
   b. "Slow to warm": ____________________
   c. "Difficult": ____________________

6. Define the following infant health problems and the role of the nurse in treating/preventing them.
   a. Colic: ____________________

   ____________________
   b. Failure to thrive: ____________________

   ____________________
   c. Sudden infant death syndrome and sudden unexpected infant death syndrome: ____________________

   ____________________
   d. Child abuse and neglect: ____________________

   ____________________

7. Describe age-appropriate methods for preparing the following age groups for eye surgery; explain why you have chosen this method.
   a. Toddler: ____________________

   ____________________

   ____________________
   b. Preschooler: ____________________

   ____________________

   ____________________
   c. School-aged child: ____________________

   ____________________

   ____________________
   d. Adolescent and young adult: ____________________

   ____________________

   ____________________

**8.** The nurse plays an important role in health care for each stage of development. Explain how you would tailor your care plan for the various age groups listed below.

**a.** Infant: ______

**b.** Toddler: ______

**c.** Preschooler: ______

**d.** School-aged child: ______

**e.** Adolescent and young adult: ______

**9.** Briefly describe the following stages of puberty.

**a.** Prepubescence: ______

**b.** Pubescence: ______

**c.** Postpubescence: ______

## APPLYING YOUR KNOWLEDGE

### CRITICAL THINKING QUESTIONS

**1.** A child is admitted to the intensive care unit with third-degree burns. How would your nursing care plan differ for a child in each of the stages listed below? Be sure to include the type of dialog you would use to explain painful procedures to each age group.

**a.** Toddler: ______

**b.** Preschooler: ______

**c.** School-aged child: ______

**d.** Adolescent: ______

**2.** No two parents are the same in their methods of raising children. Although there aren't always clear-cut right or wrong ways to raise children, some parents just seem to do a better job of it than others. Interview some of your friends to find out how successful they feel their parents were in raising them. Ask them about their parents' methods of discipline, motivation, and encouragement. Compare their answers with your own thoughts about how you were raised by your parents. What is nursing's role in promoting good parenting?

### REFLECTIVE PRACTICE: CULTIVATING QSEN COMPETENCIES

***Use the following expanded scenario from Chapter 22 in your textbook to answer the questions below.***

***Scenario:*** Darlene Schneider, a pregnant 14-year-old in her third trimester, comes to the prenatal clinic for the first time. Her history reveals sexual activity with multiple partners, smoking two packs of cigarettes per day, beer "4 or 5 nights a week," and eating mostly "fast foods," or no food when she's nauseated. She has had no prenatal care and hasn't been taking any prenatal vitamins. She is homeless but occasionally stays with an older girlfriend since her parents "threw me out of the house." Darlene asks the nurse: "How will I be able to care for this child when he's born? I can't even take care of myself."

**1.** What should be the focus of the nursing care plan developed for Ms. Schneider?

______

**2.** What would be a successful outcome for this patient?

______

3. What intellectual, technical, interpersonal, and/or ethical/legal competencies are most likely to bring about the desired outcome?

_______________________________________________

_______________________________________________

_______________________________________________

4. What resources might be helpful for Ms. Schneider?

_______________________________________________

_______________________________________________

_______________________________________________

## PRACTICING FOR NCLEX

### MULTIPLE CHOICE QUESTIONS

***Circle the letter that corresponds to the best answer for each question.***

1. A nurse records a score of 3 for a newborn taken 1 minute after birth. What would be a priority intervention for this newborn?
   a. This is a normal Apgar score requiring no further interventions.
   b. Provide respiratory support.
   c. Provide immediate life-saving support.
   d. Report the Apgar score to the primary care provider.

2. After assessing a female adolescent, a nurse collects the following data: development of breast tissue, growth spurt in height and weight, appearance of axillary hair, and initiation of menarche. Which stage of sexual development does this data confirm?
   a. Prepubescence
   b. Pubescence
   c. Postpubescence
   d. Precocious puberty

3. The nurse observes a hospitalized preschooler who clings excessively to his mother and uses infantile speech patterns. This child is exhibiting what type of behavior?
   a. Regression
   b. Separation anxiety
   c. Negativism
   d. Self-expression

4. A nurse is assessing and diagnosing children in a pediatrician's office. Which diagnosis would be most appropriate for a school-aged child?
   a. Disturbed personal identity
   b. Risk for infection
   c. Risk-prone health behavior
   d. Risk for poisoning

5. A nurse is teaching a parenting class for parents with infants. What is an example of an appropriate teaching point for this developmental age?
   a. Place the infant on the side or stomach when sleeping.
   b. Line the crib with bumpers to keep the infant from hitting the posts.
   c. If choking occurs, give back blows and chest thrusts or CPR.
   d. Wean the infant from the breast or bottle when 9 months old.

6. A nurse is caring for children in a children's hospital. Which child would the nurse expect to develop separation anxiety?
   a. An infant who was abandoned by his parents
   b. A newly hospitalized toddler
   c. A preschooler who is on an isolation ward
   d. A school-aged child who has low self-esteem

7. A nurse is implementing a sex education program in a public school. With which grade level should the nurse begin the program?
   a. Kindergarten
   b. Elementary
   c. Middle school/junior high
   d. High school

8. A nurse is choosing activities for a toddler who is hospitalized for tests. Which toy would be most appropriate for this patient?
   a. Tricycle
   b. Basketball
   c. Building blocks
   d. Stuffed animal

9. The school nurse is teaching parents of adolescents about the development of self-concept in their children. What would the nurse state is most influential in stabilizing self-concept in this age group?
   a. Parents
   b. Siblings
   c. Peers
   d. Teachers

10. A nurse is counseling pregnant women about the detrimental effects of smoking and drinking on a fetus. During what stage of development is the fetus most susceptible to these teratogens?
   a. Pre-embryonic stage
   b. Embryonic stage
   c. Fetal stage
   d. Neonatal stage

11. When assessing the health of a neonate, the nurse should be aware that:
   a. The neonate has not yet developed reflexes that allow sucking, swallowing, or blinking.
   b. The neonate has labile temperature control that responds slowly to environmental temperatures.
   c. The neonate is alert to the environment but cannot distinguish color and form.
   d. The neonate hears and turns toward sound and can smell and taste.

## ALTERNATE-FORMAT QUESTIONS

### Multiple Response Questions

***Circle the letters that correspond to the best answers for each question.***

1. A nurse is assessing neonates in a hospital nursery. Which neonates are exhibiting normal characteristics? *(Select all that apply.)*
   a. A neonate displays the Moro and stepping reflex.
   b. A neonate's body temperature responds slowly to environmental temperature.
   c. A neonate's senses are not developed enough to feel pain from a heel-stick.
   d. A neonate eliminates urine and stool.
   e. A neonate exhibits both an active crying state and a quiet alert state.
   f. The neonate inherits a transient immunity from infections from the mother.

2. A nurse is assessing infants during regular visits to a pediatrician's office. What are normal physical characteristics of an infant? *(Select all that apply.)*
   a. Brain grows to about one-third the adult size.
   b. Body temperature stabilizes.
   c. Eyes begin to focus and fixate.
   d. Heart triples in weight.
   e. Heart rate slows and blood pressure rises.
   f. Birth weight usually doubles by 1 year.

3. A nurse is assessing toddlers in a community health care clinic. Which toddlers would the nurse refer for follow-up care? *(Select all that apply.)*
   a. A 2-year-old whose birth weight quadrupled.
   b. A 2-year-old who cannot kick a ball.
   c. A 3-year-old who is drawing stick figures.
   d. A 1½-year-old whose arms and legs are not increasing in length.
   e. A 1-year-old who does not pick up small objects with fingers.
   f. A 1-year-old who does not have bladder control during the day.

4. A nurse is teaching parents of preschoolers about normal development for this age group. Which teaching points would the nurse include? *(Select all that apply.)*
   a. By 6 years of age, the preschooler's head is close to adult size.
   b. The preschooler's body is less chubby and more coordinated.
   c. The preschooler still has baby teeth.
   d. The average weight of a preschooler is 60 lb.
   e. The preschooler is able to skip, jump, and throw a ball.
   f. The preschooler is more egocentric than the toddler.

5. A school nurse is assessing school-aged children for developmental milestones. Which students would be a concern for the nurse? *(Select all that apply.)*
   a. An 8-year-old student who is not writing with a pencil
   b. A 10-year-old student who has not begun puberty
   c. A 12-year-old student who still has baby teeth

**d.** A 9-year-old student who has not developed a set of values

**e.** An 8-year-old student whose height hasn't changed since preschool

**f.** An 11-year-old student who is not developing skills for physical games

**6.** A nurse is counseling adolescents in a group home setting. Which statements accurately describe the cognitive and psychosocial development of this age group? *(Select all that apply.)*

**a.** The concept of time and its passage enables the adolescent to set long-term goals.

**b.** According to Piaget, adolescence is the stage when the cognitive development of formal operations is developed.

**c.** In the adolescent, egocentrism diminishes and is replaced by an awareness of the needs of others.

**d.** Based on Erikson's theory, the adolescent tries out different roles and personal choices and beliefs in the stage called generativity versus stagnation.

**e.** The parents act as the greatest influence on the adolescent.

**f.** According to Havighurst, more mature relationships with boys and girls are achieved by the adolescent.

### Chart/Exhibit Question

***Use the chart below to determine the 5-minute Apgar score of the following neonates:***

**1.** A neonate has a pink skin tone on the body with blue extremities, displays minimum resistance to having extremities extended, has a hearty cry, and has a heart rate of 105 beats/min. Score ____________

**2.** A neonate has a pale skin tone, heart rate of 96 beats/min, respiratory rate of 20 breaths/min, a weak cry, and no response to being slapped on the sole. Score ____________

**3.** A neonate has a pink skin color, cries vigorously, clenches fists and flexes knees, and has a heart rate of 130 beats/min. Score ____________

**Apgar Scoring Chart**

| Category[a] | 0 | 1 | 2 |
|---|---|---|---|
| Heart rate | Absent | Slow (less than 100 beats/min) | More than 100 beats/min |
| Respiratory effort | Absent | Slow, irregular | Good, crying |
| Muscle tone | Flaccid | Some flexion of extremities | Active motion |
| Reflex irritability | No response | Weak cry or grimace | Vigorous cry |
| Color | Blue, pale | Body pink, extremities blue | Completely pink |

[a]Each category is rated as 0, 1, or 2. The rating for each category is then totaled to a maximum score of 10. Normal neonates score between 7 and 10. Neonates who score between 4 and 6 require special assistance; those who score below 4 are in need of immediate life-saving support.

CHAPTER 23

# The Aging Adult

## ASSESSING YOUR UNDERSTANDING

### FILL IN THE BLANKS

1. According to the ____________ theory, a chemical reaction produces damage to the DNA and cell death and, as one ages, ____________ accumulate, leading to essential molecules in the cell binding together and interfering with normal cell function.
2. The nurse is assessing a 50-year-old female patient during a regular checkup. This patient's age category is termed ____________ adult.
3. The nurse is examining a 57-year-old female who states: "I'm so busy lately between watching my grandson and taking care of my mother who is disabled." The term ____________ describes the middle adult who is involved in relationships with his or her own children and aging family members.
4. The older adult period is often further divided into the young-old, ages ____________; the middle-old, ages ____________; and the old-old, ages ____________.
5. A nurse who believes that all older adults take more time to answer interview questions due to slowed mental processes is guilty of a form of stereotyping known as ____________.
6. The ____________ theory of aging assumes that healthy aging is related to the older adult's ability to continue similar patterns of behavior from young and middle adulthood.
7. When an older adult tells the nurse about his successes on the golf course, he is engaging in what is termed ____________ or ____________.
8. ____________ is the most common degenerative neurologic illness and the most common cause of cognitive impairment.
9. ____________ is the scientific and behavioral study of all aspects of aging and its consequences.

### SHORT ANSWER

1. Briefly describe the following characteristics of middle and older adulthood.
   a. Middle adulthood
      Physiologic development: ____________
      ____________
      Psychosocial development: ____________
      ____________
      Cognitive, moral, and spiritual development:
      ____________
      ____________
   b. Older adulthood
      Physiologic development: ____________
      ____________
      Psychosocial development: ____________
      ____________
      Cognitive, moral, and spiritual development:
      ____________
      ____________

2. List five health-promotion activities recommended for all older adults.
   a. ______
   b. ______
   c. ______
   d. ______
   e. ______

3. Briefly describe the following theories on aging.
   a. Genetic theory: ______
   b. Immunity theory: ______
   c. Cross-linkage theory: ______
   d. Free radical theory: ______
   e. Disengagement theory: ______
   f. Activity theory: ______
   g. Identity-continuity theory: ______

4. You are a visiting nurse for a patient with Alzheimer's disease (AD). Describe what physical and psychological changes you would expect to occur in this patient over time.

______

5. Give an example of how older adulthood may affect the following body systems.
   a. Integumentary: ______
   b. Musculoskeletal: ______
   c. Neurologic: ______
   d. Cardiopulmonary: ______
   e. Gastrointestinal: ______
   f. Genitourinary: ______

## APPLYING YOUR KNOWLEDGE

### CRITICAL THINKING QUESTIONS

1. Because of advances in medical technology and the increased awareness of the need to eat right and exercise, there has been a dramatic increase in the number of active older adults. Although adults in this age group as a whole are healthier than the generations that preceded them, they still have specific health risks and needs that must be identified by the nursing process. Consider the older adults you know personally and identify nursing strategies that would enhance their cognitive development and overall functioning (physiologic, social, emotional, spiritual).

2. Identify healthy middle-aged adults and older adults among your family and friends. Interview them to learn about their physical, emotional, and spiritual selves. Compare their long- and short-range goals, life stressors, physical ability, and emotional stability. How have age factors affected their life experiences? What can you learn from this healthy group that will enable you to help others?

3. Take a look at the way older adults are portrayed on TV dramas. Are these dramas a realistic representation of this age group? Identify several health risks for older adults and preventive methods to promote health and safety.

### REFLECTIVE PRACTICE: CULTIVATING QSEN COMPETENCIES

***Use the following expanded scenario from Chapter 23 in your textbook to answer the questions below.***

*Scenario:* Larry Jenkins is a 67-year-old man with diabetes who lives with his wife, Mary. Mrs. Jenkins brings her husband to the clinic for a checkup and says she is worried about her husband's physical and emotional health. She reports that their three children live in different states and don't visit often. Mr. and Mrs. Jenkins moved to Florida 5 months ago when Mr. Jenkins retired, and Mrs. Jenkins says they have had trouble finding friends "as good as the ones we had at home." During the nursing interview, Mr. Jenkins says, "Everything's gone downhill since I retired." He reports that he is "bored out of my mind" and is drinking more alcohol, "simply because there's nothing else to do!"

1. How might the nurse use blended nursing skills to provide holistic, developmentally sensitive care for Mr. and Mrs. Jenkins?

_______________________________________

_______________________________________

_______________________________________

2. What would be a successful outcome for this patient?

_______________________________________

_______________________________________

_______________________________________

3. What intellectual, technical, interpersonal, and/or ethical/legal competencies are most likely to bring about the desired outcome?

_______________________________________

_______________________________________

_______________________________________

4. What resources might be helpful for Mr. and Mrs. Jenkins?

_______________________________________

_______________________________________

_______________________________________

## PRACTICING FOR NCLEX

### MULTIPLE CHOICE QUESTIONS

***Circle the letter that corresponds to the best answer for each question.***

1. A nurse is assessing middle adults living in a retirement community. What behavior would the nurse typically see in the middle adult?
   a. Believes in establishment of self but fears being pulled back into the family
   b. Usually substitutes new roles for old roles and perhaps continues formal roles in a new context
   c. Looks inward, accepts life span as having definite boundaries, and has special interest in spouse, friends, and community
   d. Looks forward but also looks back and begins to reflect on his or her life

2. A nurse encourages residents of a long-term care facility to continue a similar pattern of behavior and activity that existed in their middle adulthood years to ensure healthy aging. This intervention is based on which aging theory?
   a. Identity-continuity theory
   b. Disengagement theory
   c. Activity theory
   d. Life review theory

3. Based on an understanding of the cognitive changes that normally occur with aging, what might the nurse expect a newly hospitalized older adult to do?
   a. Talk rapidly but be confused
   b. Withdraw from strangers
   c. Interrupt with frequent questions
   d. Take longer to respond and react

4. Which nursing action would help maintain safety in the older adult?
   a. Treat each patient as a unique person.
   b. Orient the patient to new surroundings.
   c. Encourage independence.
   d. Provide planned rest and activity times.

5. Erikson identified ego integrity versus despair and disgust as the last stage of human development, which begins at about 60 years of age. Which intervention would best foster older adults' ego integrity?
   a. Distracting the patient
   b. Praising the patient
   c. Encouraging life review
   d. Promoting independent living

6. Based on Havighurst's theory of human development, which nursing intervention would best facilitate the accomplishment of a developmental task of older adulthood?
   a. Helping a patient move independently using a walker
   b. Helping a patient accept a move to live with a daughter
   c. Helping a patient cope with living alone after the death of a spouse
   d. Helping a patient become established in the community

7. Gould viewed the middle years as a time when adults increase their feelings of self-satisfaction, value their spouse as a companion, and

become more concerned with health. Which nursing action best facilitates this process?

a. Counseling a patient who complains of being depressed
b. Providing entertainment for a patient on bedrest
c. Arranging for social services to assist with meals for a homebound patient
d. Encouraging a patient to have regular checkups

8. A nurse is caring for a 52-year-old male patient who is being treated for depression following the death of his spouse. Which action best facilitates the accomplishment of a developmental task of this middle adult?
   a. Encouraging him to start dating again to find a life partner
   b. Helping him to see the value of guiding his children to become responsible adults
   c. Helping him to establish a social network within the community
   d. Encouraging the formation of a personal philosophical and ethical structure

9. A nurse caring for older adults in a long-term care facility is teaching a novice nurse characteristic behaviors of older adults. Which statement is not considered ageism?
   a. Old age begins at age 65.
   b. Personality is not changed by chronologic aging.
   c. Most older adults are ill and institutionalized.
   d. Intelligence declines with age.

## ALTERNATE-FORMAT QUESTIONS

### Multiple Response Questions

***Circle the letters that correspond to the best answers for each question.***

1. A nurse is assessing a 55-year-old female patient. What is a normal physical change in the middle adult? *(Select all that apply.)*
   a. Skin moisture increases.
   b. Hormone production increases.
   c. Hearing acuity diminishes.
   d. Cognitive ability diminishes.
   e. Cardiac output begins to decrease.
   f. There is a loss of calcium from bones.

2. A nurse working in a community clinic assists middle adult patients to follow guidelines for health-related screenings and immunizations. What preventive measures would the nurse recommend for this population? *(Select all that apply.)*
   a. A physical exam every year from age 40 on
   b. Clinical skin examination every 3 years
   c. Breast self-examination every month for women
   d. Pelvic examination and Pap exam at least every 5 years for women
   e. Prostate-specific antigen (PSA) test every 5 years for men
   f. Zoster vaccine, live for adults 50 years and older

3. A nurse is screening for AD in patients in a long-term care facility. Which facts regarding AD are accurate? *(Select all that apply.)*
   a. AD accounts for about one-third of the cases of dementia in the United States.
   b. AD primarily affects young to middle adults.
   c. Scientists estimate that more than 5 million people have AD.
   d. Nearly half of 85-year-old adults have AD.
   e. AD affects brain cells and is characterized by the formation of amyloid plaques and tangles of tau proteins.
   f. AD is a progressively serious but not a life-threatening disease.

4. When caring for older adults, nurses must be aware of common conditions found in this population. Which statements accurately describe these conditions? *(Select all that apply.)*
   a. Sundowning syndrome is a condition in which an older adult habitually becomes confused, restless, and agitated after dark.
   b. Delirium is a permanent state of confusion occurring in older adulthood.
   c. Depression is a prolonged or extreme state of sadness occurring in a small percentage of older adults.
   d. Researchers have shown no link between delirium and hospitalization of the older adult.
   e. Polypharmacy is a term that is used to describe the habit of older adults to use many pharmacies to obtain their prescription drugs.
   f. A significant percentage of older adults limit their activities because of fear of falling that might result in serious health consequences.

CHAPTER 24

# Asepsis and Infection Control

## ASSESSING YOUR UNDERSTANDING

### FILL IN THE BLANKS

1. The __________ initiative has identified safety as one of the leading issues in health care and focuses on effective infection control practices.
2. Nurses caring for patients in health care institutions see __________ as the most significant and most commonly observed infection-causing agents in these facilities.
3. Most bacteria require oxygen to live and grow and are, therefore, referred to as __________; those that can live without oxygen are __________ bacteria.
4. The nurse caring for children in a pediatrician's office assesses patients for athlete's foot, ringworm, and yeast infections caused by __________.
5. Microorganisms that commonly inhabit various body sites and are part of the body's natural defense system are referred to as __________.
6. The natural habitats of organisms, such as humans, animals, soil, and food, are examples of __________.
7. A nurse who fails to properly sterilize equipment exposes patients to infection by introducing microorganisms at the __________, or the point at which organisms enter a new host.
8. During the immune response, the body responds to an antigen by producing a(n) __________.
9. A(n) __________ is an infection, not present on admission, that certain patients in health agencies develop during the course of treatment for other conditions.
10. A nurse who causes an infection in a patient during a diagnostic procedure has exposed the patient to what is referred to as a(n) __________ infection.

### MATCHING EXERCISES

***Match the terms in Part A with their definitions listed in Part B.***

#### PART A

a. Infection
b. Pathogen
c. Bacteria
d. Gram-positive bacteria
e. Gram-negative bacteria
f. Aerobic bacteria
g. Anaerobic bacteria
h. Host
i. Fungi
j. Normal flora
k. Opportunists
l. Virus
m. Antigen
n. Antibody

**PART B**

____ **1.** Normal flora that becomes potentially harmful by taking advantage of a susceptible host

____ **2.** Bacteria that require oxygen to live

____ **3.** A disease state that results from the presence of pathogens in or on the body

____ **4.** A general term for a disease-producing microorganism

____ **5.** Microorganisms that commonly inhabit various body sites and are part of the body's natural defense system

____ **6.** Plant-like organisms that can cause infection

____ **7.** An invading foreign protein such as bacteria, or in some cases the body's own proteins

____ **8.** Most significant and commonly observed infection-causing agents in health care institutions

____ **9.** Bacteria that have chemically more complex cell walls and can be decolorized by alcohol

____ **10.** Bacteria that can live without oxygen

____ **11.** Bacteria that have thick cell walls that resist colorization and are stained violet

____ **12.** The body responds to an antigen by producing this

***Match the type of infection in Part A with its definition listed in Part B.***

**PART A**

**a.** Health care–associated infection (HAI)
**b.** Exogenous
**c.** Endogenous
**d.** Iatrogenic

**PART B**

____ **13.** An infection that occurs as a result of treatment or a diagnostic procedure

____ **14.** A hospital-acquired infection

____ **15.** An infection in which the causative organism is normally harbored within the patient

____ **16.** An infection caused by an organism acquired from other people

**CORRECT THE FALSE STATEMENTS**

***Circle the word "true" or "false" that follows the statement. If you circled "false," change the underlined word or words to make the statement true. Place your answer in the space provided.***

**1.** <u>Gram-negative bacteria</u> have chemically complex walls and can be decolorized by alcohol.
**a.** True
**b.** False ____________________

**2.** Methicillin-resistant *Staphylococcus aureus* and vancomycin-resistant enterococci are most often transmitted by <u>the hands of health care providers</u>.
**a.** True
**b.** False ____________________

**3.** <u>Wearing gloves</u> is the most effective way to help prevent the spread of organisms.
**a.** True
**b.** False ____________________

**4.** <u>Resident bacteria</u>, normally picked up by the hands in the course of usual activities of daily living, are relatively few on clean and exposed areas of the skin.
**a.** True
**b.** False ____________________

**5.** <u>Nonantimicrobial agents</u> are considered adequate for routine mechanical cleansing of the hands and removal of most transient microorganisms.
**a.** True
**b.** False ____________________

**6.** <u>Sterilization</u> is the process by which all microorganisms, including spores, are destroyed.
**a.** True
**b.** False ____________________

**7.** In a home environment, contaminated items may be disinfected by placing them in boiling water for <u>10 minutes</u>.
**a.** True
**b.** False ____________________

**8.** When observing <u>medical asepsis</u>, areas are considered contaminated if they are touched by any object that is not also sterile.
**a.** True
**b.** False ____________________

9. Using body substance isolation precautions eliminates the need for category-specific or disease-specific systems, except for certain airborne diseases that require special precautions.
   a. True
   b. False ______

## SHORT ANSWER

1. List four factors that influence an organism's potential to produce disease.
   a. ______
   b. ______
   c. ______
   d. ______
2. Give an example of a disease that is transmitted by organisms from the following reservoirs.
   a. Other humans: ______
   b. Animals: ______
   c. Soil: ______
3. List three portals of exit in the human body.
   a. ______
   b. ______
   c. ______
4. Give an example of the following means of transmission.
   a. Direct contact: ______
   b. Indirect contact: ______
   c. Vectors: ______
   d. Fomite: ______
   e. Airborne: ______
5. Briefly describe the following body defenses against infection.
   a. Inflammatory response: ______
   b. Immune response: ______
6. List four factors that influence the susceptibility of a host.
   a. ______
   b. ______
   c. ______
   d. ______
7. Briefly describe the nurse's role in controlling or treating infection in the following stages of the nursing practice.
   a. Assessing: ______
   b. Diagnosing: ______
   c. Planning: ______
   d. Implementing: ______
   e. Evaluating: ______
8. Give two examples of how you would practice medical asepsis in the following areas.
   a. Patient's home: ______
   b. Public facilities: ______
   c. Community: ______
   d. Health care facility: ______
9. List three measures that health care agencies have found to be successful in reducing the incidence of hospital-acquired infections.
   a. ______
   b. ______
   c. ______
10. Explain why the following factors should be considered when selecting sterilization and disinfection methods.
    a. Nature of organisms present: ______
    b. Number of organisms present: ______

c. Type of equipment: ____________________

____________________

d. Intended use of equipment: ____________

____________________

e. Available means for sterilization and disinfection: ____________________

____________________

f. Time: ____________________

____________________

11. Describe the role of the infection control nurse in the following situations.

a. Hospital: ____________________

____________________

b. Home care setting: ____________________

____________________

12. Zelen is a 35-year-old fireman who sustained third-degree burns on his upper body.

a. Write a nursing diagnosis that relates to his increased risk for skin infection.

____________________

____________________

b. Describe how the nurse can help to control or prevent infection for this patient.

____________________

____________________

13. In the emergency department, a patient you are treating for lacerations tells you that he was recently diagnosed with TB. Would you use different precautions for this patient than for another emergency department patient? Why?

____________________

____________________

____________________

## APPLYING YOUR KNOWLEDGE

### CRITICAL THINKING QUESTIONS

1. Try to imagine what it must feel like to be in strict isolation. Then interview a patient whose medical condition necessitated the use of isolation precautions. Find out how it felt to be isolated and, in some cases, feared by health care workers. See if anything was done to help alleviate the disorientation and meet the patient's basic needs of love and belonging. What did you learn that would help you to direct your future nursing care for patients in isolation?

2. A nurse is obligated to provide nursing care to all patients regardless of race, creed, religion, and so forth. Should this code also include "regardless of the medical condition of the patient"? Should nurses be able to choose whether or not to take care of a patient who has a contagious disease? Do you believe the precautions being taken with these patients offer adequate protection for the health care provider? Should there be consequences for medical personnel who refuse to take care of these patients? Share your responses with your classmates and see if you agree.

### REFLECTIVE PRACTICE: CULTIVATING QSEN COMPETENCIES

***Use the following expanded scenario from Chapter 24 in your textbook to answer the questions below.***

***Scenario:*** Giselle Turheis, age 38, is undergoing chemotherapy treatment for leukemia in the hospital. The staff has placed Ms. Turheis on neutropenic precautions and restricted visitors to her room. The flowers she received from her family were sent home to avoid having standing water in her room. Health care workers regularly appear at her bedside in masks and gowns. When the nurse explains the reason for these precautions to Ms. Turheis and her family, Ms. Turheis says, "I know my risk for infection is really high because of my poor immune status, but I feel so out of touch with reality now. And when I get home, how will I respond to my Sunday school students who are used to greeting me with a big hug? I want to be safe, but I know that I need these hugs too!"

1. How might the nurse respond to Ms. Turheis in a manner that respects her human dignity, while at the same time maintaining a safe environment for her?

____________________

____________________

____________________

2. What would be a successful outcome for Ms. Turheis?

______________________________________

______________________________________

______________________________________

3. What intellectual, technical, interpersonal, and/or ethical/legal competencies are most likely to bring about the desired outcome?

______________________________________

______________________________________

______________________________________

4. What resources might be helpful for Ms. Turheis?

______________________________________

______________________________________

______________________________________

## PRACTICING FOR NCLEX

### MULTIPLE CHOICE QUESTIONS

***Circle the letter that corresponds to the best answer for each question.***

1. The nurses on a busy surgical ward use hand hygiene when caring for postsurgical patients. Which action represents the appropriate use of hand hygiene?
   a. The nurse uses gloves in place of hand hygiene.
   b. The nurse keeps fingernails less than ¼ in long.
   c. The nurse uses hand hygiene instead of gloves when in contact with blood.
   d. The nurse refrains from using hand moisturizer following hand hygiene.
2. A nurse is caring for a patient who is diagnosed with tuberculosis. Which nursing intervention promotes infection control based on the QSEN competency of safety?
   a. The nurse places the patient in a private room with the door open.
   b. The nurse uses droplet precautions when providing care for the patient.
   c. The nurse keeps visitors 3 ft away from the infected person.
   d. The nurse places the patient in a private room with monitored negative air pressure.
3. The nurse performs hand hygiene using soap and water before and after providing patient care. Which nursing action is performed correctly according to the procedure?
   a. The nurse uses soap and cold water to wash hands.
   b. The nurse uses about 2 teaspoons of liquid soap to wash hands.
   c. The nurse washes at least 1 in above the area of contamination if present.
   d. The nurse rinses thoroughly with water flowing away from the fingertips.
4. Which patient would the nurse consider the most infectious?
   a. A patient who is in the incubation period
   b. A patient who is in the prodromal stage
   c. A patient who is in the full stage of illness
   d. A patient who is in the convalescent period
5. A nurse prefers to use an alcohol-based handrub when providing care for patients. In which case is this practice contraindicated?
   a. The nurse is changing the dressing on a surgical wound.
   b. The nurse performs routine care and is moving to another patient.
   c. The nurse finishes cleaning a patient's table.
   d. The nurse finishes patient care and hands are not visibly soiled.
6. The nurse is setting up a sterile field to perform a catheterization when the patient touches the end of the sterile field. What would be the nurse's next appropriate action?
   a. Change the sterile field, but reuse the sterile equipment.
   b. Proceed with the procedure since it was only touched by the patient.
   c. Discard the sterile field and the supplies and start over.
   d. Call for help and ask for new supplies.
7. A patient is to have an indwelling urinary catheter inserted. Which precaution is followed during this procedure?
   a. Surgical asepsis technique
   b. Medical asepsis technique
   c. Droplet precautions
   d. Strict reverse isolation

## ALTERNATE-FORMAT QUESTIONS

### Multiple Response Questions

***Circle the letter that corresponds to the best answer for each question.***

1. A nurse is following medical asepsis when caring for patients in a critical care unit. Which nursing actions follow these principles? *(Select all that apply.)*
   a. The nurse carries soiled items away from the body.
   b. The nurse places soiled bed linen on the floor.
   c. The nurse moves soiled equipment away from the body when cleaning it.
   d. The nurse opens a window and dusts the room in the direction of the window.
   e. The nurse cleans least soiled areas first and then moves to more soiled ones.
   f. The nurse pours discarded liquids into a basin then pours them into the drain.

2. A nurse practitioner is setting up a sterile field to perform a biopsy on a patient. Which actions follow recommended guidelines for this procedure? *(Select all that apply.)*
   a. The nurse considers the outer 1-in edge of the sterile field to be contaminated.
   b. The nurse places the cap of an opened solution on the table with edges down.
   c. The nurse discards a sterile field when a portion of it becomes contaminated.
   d. The nurse calls for help when realizing a supply is missing.
   e. The nurse drops a sterile item on a sterile field from the height of 12 in.
   f. The nurse holds a facility-wrapped item with top flap opening toward the body.

3. An operating room nurse is putting on sterile gloves to assist with patient surgery. Which actions are performed correctly in this procedure? *(Select all that apply.)*
   a. The nurse places the sterile gloves on a clean dry surface at or below waist level.
   b. The nurse opens the outside wrapper by carefully peeling the top layer back.
   c. The nurse places the inner package on the work surface with the side labeled "cuff end" furthest from body.
   d. The nurse carefully opens the inner package by folding open the top flap, then the bottom and sides.
   e. The nurse lifts and holds the glove up and off the inner package with fingers down and carefully inserts hand palm up into glove.
   f. The nurse touches only the inner surface of the package and the gloves.

4. The nurse is removing soiled gloves after assisting with a sterile procedure. Which actions follow recommended guidelines for this procedure? *(Select all that apply.)*
   a. Using the dominant hand to grasp the opposite glove near cuff end on the outside exposed area
   b. Removing the glove by pulling it off, inverting it as it is pulled, and keeping the contaminated area on the inside
   c. Sliding the fingers of the ungloved hand between the remaining glove and the wrist
   d. Removing the second glove by pulling the cuff up, inverting it as it is pulled, and keeping the contaminated area on the outside
   e. Securing the second glove inside the first glove while keeping the contaminated area on the outside
   f. Discarding the gloves in appropriate container, removing additional protective personal equipment (PPE), if used, and performing hand hygiene

5. Nurses wear personal protective equipment to protect themselves and patients from infectious materials. Which examples accurately represent the proper use of personal protective equipment in a health care facility? *(Select all that apply.)*
   a. Nurses need only apply clean gloves when performing or assisting with invasive patient procedures.
   b. During some care activities for an individual patient, nurses may need to change gloves more than once.
   c. Nurses may use a waterproof gown more than one time.
   d. Nurses should remove PPE at the doorway or in an anteroom except for the respirator.
   e. To remove a gown, nurses should unfasten ties, if at the neck and back, and allow the gown to fall away from shoulders.

f. Nurses may lower a mask around the neck when not being worn and bring it back over the mouth and nose for reuse.

6. For which patients would the nurse be required to use droplet precautions? *(Select all that apply.)*
   a. A patient with rubella
   b. A patient with tuberculosis
   c. A patient with SARS
   d. A patient with mumps
   e. A patient with MRSA
   f. A patient with diphtheria

**Prioritization Questions**

1. Place the steps for removing protective equipment in the order in which they should occur when the nurse has completed patient care:
   a. Remove gown.
   b. Remove mask/respirator.
   c. Remove gloves.
   d. Remove goggles/face shield.

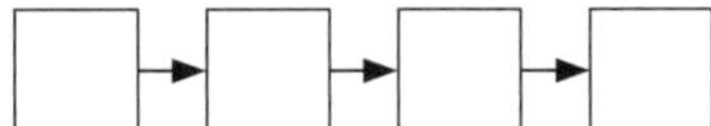

2. Place the steps of the infection cycle in the order in which an infection would occur:
   a. Portal of exit
   b. Infectious agent
   c. Means of transmission
   d. Reservoir
   e. Portal of entry
   f. Susceptible host

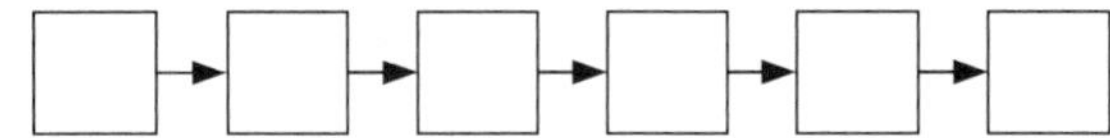

CHAPTER 25

# Vital Signs

## ASSESSING YOUR UNDERSTANDING

### FILL IN THE BLANKS

1. Stroke volume and ___________ determine cardiac output.
2. The nurse is choosing a bladder width and length to measure the blood pressure of an older child with an arm circumference of 20 cm. The bladder width and length (in centimeters) that would typically be used for this child is: width: ___________ and length: ___________.
3. A nurse is documenting the pulse amplitude for a patient with a weak pulse. The number that would describe this patient's pulse is ___________.
4. A nurse measures a patient's oral temperature at 101°F; therefore, the axillary temperature would most likely be ___________.
5. A nurse converts a patient's temperature of 39°C to ___________°F.
6. A nurse converts a patient's temperature of 99.5°F to ___________°C.

## DEVELOPING YOUR KNOWLEDGE BASE

### IDENTIFICATION

1. Identify the pulse assessment sites on the figure below by placing your answers on the lines provided.

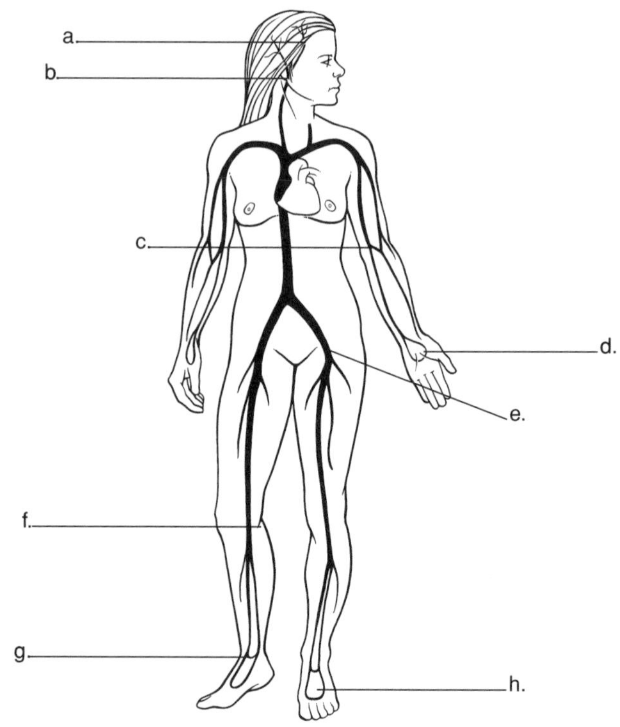

## MATCHING EXERCISES

***Match the following definitions related to pulse in Part B with the appropriate term listed in Part A.***

**PART A**

**a.** Pulse
**b.** Pulse rate
**c.** Tachycardia
**d.** Palpitation
**e.** Bradycardia
**f.** Pulse rhythm
**g.** Pulse amplitude
**h.** Arrhythmia
**i.** Stroke volume
**j.** Cardiac output
**k.** Ventricular contraction
**l.** Pulse deficit

**PART B**

____ **1.** Number of pulsations felt in a minute

____ **2.** Quantity of blood forced out of the left ventricle with each contraction

____ **3.** Person is aware of own heartbeat without having to feel for it

____ **4.** Quality of the pulse in terms of fullness; reflects strength of left ventricular contraction

____ **5.** Light tap caused by expansion of the aorta sending a wave through the walls of the arterial system

____ **6.** Irregular pattern of heartbeats

____ **7.** Heart rate below 60 beats/min in an adult

____ **8.** The amount of blood pumped per minute

____ **9.** A rapid heart rate

____ **10.** The pattern of pulsations and pauses between them

____ **11.** The difference between the apical and radial pulse rates

***Match the term in Part A with the correct definition in Part B.***

**PART A**

**a.** Inspiration
**b.** Expiration
**c.** Apnea
**d.** Dyspnea
**e.** Orthopnea
**f.** Diffusion
**g.** Eupnea
**h.** Tachypnea
**i.** Ventilation
**j.** Bradypnea

**PART B**

____ **12.** A fast respiratory rate

____ **13.** Difficult or labored breathing

____ **14.** The act of breathing in

____ **15.** The exchange of oxygen and carbon dioxide between the alveoli of the lungs and the circulating blood

____ **16.** Movement of air in and out of the lungs

____ **17.** Normal respirations with equal rate and depth

____ **18.** Being able to breathe more easily in an upright position

____ **19.** Periods during which there is no breathing

____ **20.** Slow breathing

***Match the definitions of body temperatures and variations in Part B with the appropriate term listed in Part A.***

**PART A**

**a.** Pyrexia
**b.** Febrile
**c.** Afebrile
**d.** Hyperpyrexia
**e.** Hypothermia
**f.** Hyperthermia
**g.** Ineffective thermoregulation

**PART B**

____ **21.** Body temperature below limit of normal

____ **22.** State in which temperature fluctuates between above-normal and below-normal ranges

____ **23.** Fever caused by extreme heat exposure

____ **24.** Fever caused by pyrogens

____ **25.** Person with normal body temperature

____ **26.** High fever, usually above 106°F

## SHORT ANSWER

1. Briefly describe how the following factors affect body temperature.
   a. Circadian rhythms: ______________________________
   ______________________________
   ______________________________
   b. Age: ______________________________
   ______________________________
   ______________________________
   c. Biological sex: ______________________________
   ______________________________
   ______________________________
   d. Stress: ______________________________
   ______________________________
   ______________________________
   e. Environmental temperature: ______________________________
   ______________________________
   ______________________________

2. Complete the table below describing the types of thermometers used to assess body temperature.

| Type of Thermometer | Brief Description | Contraindication | Normal Reading |
|---|---|---|---|
| ***A. ELECTRONIC AND DIGITAL*** | | | |
| ***B. TYMPANIC MEMBRANE*** | | | |
| ***C. DISPOSABLE SINGLE USE*** | | | |
| ***D. TEMPORAL ARTERY*** | | | |
| ***E. AUTOMATED MONITORING DEVICE*** | | | |

**3.** List three methods that can be used to assess the pulse by palpating or auscultating.

**a.** ______________________

**b.** ______________________

**c.** ______________________

**4.** Briefly describe how the following variables may affect a patient's blood pressure.

**a.** Pumping action of the heart: ______________________

**b.** Blood volume: ______________________

**c.** Viscosity of blood: ______________________

**d.** Elasticity of vessel walls: ______________________

**5.** Briefly define the following NANDA nursing diagnoses for altered respirations.

**a.** Impaired gas exchange: ______________________

**b.** Ineffective airway clearance: ______________________

**c.** Ineffective breathing pattern: ______________________

**d.** Impaired spontaneous ventilation: ______________________

**6.** Briefly define the following NANDA nursing diagnoses for alterations in pulse and blood pressure.

**a.** Ineffective peripheral tissue perfusion: ______________________

**b.** Risk for deficient fluid volume: ______________________

**c.** Excess fluid volume: ______________________

**d.** Deficient fluid volume: ______________________

**e.** Decreased cardiac output: ______________________

**7.** Describe the use of the following equipment to assess the pulse and blood pressure.

**a.** Stethoscope: ______________________

**b.** Sphygmomanometer: ______________________

## APPLYING YOUR KNOWLEDGE

### CRITICAL THINKING QUESTIONS

**1.** Using a partner, locate the nine sites for pulse assessment. Practice the technique for obtaining radial and apical pulses. Then practice the technique for measuring respirations and assessing blood pressure. Why is it important to be proficient in assessing and reporting vital sign measurements? If you were unsure of one of your vital sign assessments, what would you do?

**2.** An obese woman in the clinic needs a large blood pressure cuff, and one is not available. The resident tells you, "Just use the cuff you have." What do you do, and why?

**3.** Using a mannequin in your nursing laboratory, practice taking oral, rectal, and axillary temperatures. Research any new devices for taking temperature, and familiarize yourself with their use. Why do nurses need to be competent in using different methods and devices?

### REFLECTIVE PRACTICE: CULTIVATING QSEN COMPETENCIES

***Use the following expanded scenario from Chapter 25 in your textbook to answer the questions below.***

***Scenario:*** Noah Shoolin is a 2-year-old who is brought to the emergency department by his mother. His mother says he has been running a high fever and has refused to take food or fluids for the past 24 hours. When you attempt to obtain a tympanic temperature, the child begins to scream uncontrollably, crying and pushing the device away from his ear.

1. What might be causing Noah's reaction to the nurse's attempt to assess a tympanic temperature?

_______________________________________

_______________________________________

_______________________________________

2. What would be a successful outcome for Noah?

_______________________________________

_______________________________________

_______________________________________

3. What intellectual, technical, interpersonal, and/or ethical/legal competencies are most likely to bring about the desired outcome?

_______________________________________

_______________________________________

_______________________________________

4. What resources might be helpful for the nurse caring for Noah?

_______________________________________

_______________________________________

_______________________________________

## PRACTICING FOR NCLEX

### MULTIPLE CHOICE QUESTIONS

***Circle the letter that corresponds to the best answer for each question.***

1. A nurse documents the following assessment for an infant: temperature 98.2, pulse 90 beats/min, respirations 50 breaths/min, and blood pressure 73/55. What is the next appropriate action of the nurse based on these assessments?
   a. Report an abnormal temperature.
   b. Report abnormal pulse and respirations.
   c. Report low blood pressure reading.
   d. No action is needed; these are normal assessments.

2. A nurse is taking the vital signs of a 9-year-old child who is anxious about the procedures. Which nursing action would be appropriate when assessing this child?
   a. Make sure the child does not touch the assessment equipment.
   b. Perform as many tasks as possible with the child lying on the examining table.
   c. Perform the blood pressure measurement last.
   d. Perform the assessments quickly while maintaining a serious demeanor.

3. A nurse is calculating the cardiac output of an adult with a stroke volume of 75 mL and a pulse of 78 beats/min. What number would the nurse document for this assessment?
   a. 5,000 mL
   b. 5,550 mL
   c. 5,850 mL
   d. 6,000 mL

4. The nurse is assessing an adult who has a pulse rate of 180 beats/min. Which condition would the nurse document?
   a. Bradycardia
   b. Arrhythmia
   c. Pulse amplitude
   d. Tachycardia

5. The nurse is taking a rectal temperature on a patient who reports feeling light-headed during the procedure. What would be the nurse's priority action in this situation?
   a. Leave the thermometer in and notify the health care provider.
   b. Remove the thermometer and assess the blood pressure and heart rate.
   c. Remove the thermometer and assess the temperature via another method.
   d. Call for assistance and anticipate the need for CPR.

6. The nurse is assessing the apical pulse of a patient using auscultation. What action would the nurse perform after placing the diaphragm over the apex of the heart?
   a. Listen for heart sounds.
   b. Count the heartbeat for 2 minutes.
   c. Count each "lub-dub" as 2 beats.
   d. Palpate the space between the fifth and sixth ribs.

7. A nurse is assessing the respirations of a 60-year-old female patient and finds that the patient is breathing so shallowly that the respirations cannot be counted. What would be the appropriate initial nursing intervention in this situation?
   a. Notify the primary care provider.
   b. Perform a pain assessment.
   c. Administer oxygen.
   d. Auscultate the lung sounds and count respirations.
8. Which patient would the nurse consider at risk for low blood pressure?
   a. A patient with high blood viscosity
   b. A patient with low blood volume
   c. A patient with decreased elasticity of walls of arterioles
   d. A patient with a strong pumping action of blood into the arteries
9. After taking vital signs, the nurse writes down findings as T = 98.6, P = 66, R = 18, BP = 124/82. Which of these numbers represents the systolic blood pressure?
   a. 98.6
   b. 124
   c. 82
   d. 66

## ALTERNATE-FORMAT QUESTIONS

### Multiple Response Questions

***Circle the letters that correspond to the best answers for each question.***

1. The nurse is assessing a patient's blood pressure and obtains a falsely low pressure reading. Which nursing actions might have contributed to this false reading? *(Select all that apply.)*
   a. The nurse performed the assessment in a noisy environment.
   b. The nurse misplaced the bell beyond the direct area of the artery.
   c. The nurse used a manometer not calibrated at the zero mark.
   d. The nurse viewed the meniscus from below eye level.
   e. The nurse failed to pump the cuff 20 to 30 mm Hg above disappearing pulse.
   f. The nurse applied a cuff that is too narrow.
2. A nurse is taking a blood pressure measurement to assess for orthostatic hypotension in a patient. Which signs and symptoms might occur related to this condition? *(Select all that apply.)*
   a. Dizziness
   b. Palpitations
   c. Erythema
   d. Fever
   e. Lightheadedness
   f. Pallor
3. A nurse is assessing patients in the Emergency Department for body temperature. Which nursing actions reflect proper technique when assessing body temperature by various methods? *(Select all that apply.)*
   a. When assessing tympanic membrane temperature, wipe the tympanic probe cover with alcohol before inserting it snugly into the ear.
   b. When assessing an oral temperature with an electronic thermometer, place the probe beneath the patient's tongue in the posterior sublingual pocket.
   c. When assessing rectal temperature with an electronic thermometer, lubricate about 1 in of the probe with a water-soluble lubricant.
   d. When assessing axillary temperature using a glass thermometer, place the bulb in the center of the axilla and bring the patient's arm down close to the body. Leave the thermometer in place for 3 minutes.
   e. When assessing temperature with an electronic thermometer, hold the thermometer in place in the assessment site until you hear a beep.
   f. Note the assessment site used because axillary temperatures are generally about 1° more than oral temperatures and rectal temperatures are generally about 1° less than oral temperatures.

4. The nurse is providing discharge teaching for a patient diagnosed with hypertension. Which teaching points about monitoring blood pressure should the nurse include in the plan? *(Select all that apply.)*
   a. Use the blood pressure devices in public places to measure BP whenever possible.
   b. Use manual cuffs over digital BP monitoring equipment.
   c. Recommend taking the blood pressure every day at the same time.
   d. Recommend a cuff size appropriate for the patient's limb size.
   e. Recommend the use of lower extremities when monitoring BP.
   f. If using a wrist monitor, tell the patient to keep wrist at heart level when using it.
5. The nurse is assessing a patient's brachial artery blood pressure. Which nursing actions are performed correctly? *(Select all that apply.)*
   a. The nurse centers the bladder of the cuff over the brachial artery about midway on the arm.
   b. The nurse places the cuff over the patient's clothing and fastens it snugly.
   c. The nurse notes the point on the gauge at which the first faint but clear sound appears and increases in intensity as the diastolic pressure.
   d. The nurse has the patient lying or sitting down with the forearm supported at the level of the heart and the palm of the hand upward.
   e. The nurse wraps the cuff around the arm smoothly and snugly and fastens it.
   f. The nurse repeats any suspicious reading before 1 minute has passed since the last reading.
6. The nurse is assessing the blood pressure of a hospitalized patient using a Doppler ultrasound device. Which actions are performed correctly? *(Select all that apply.)*
   a. The nurse places the patient in a comfortable lying or sitting position.
   b. The nurse centers the bladder of the cuff over the artery lining.
   c. The nurse wraps the cuff around the limb smoothly and snugly and fastens it.
   d. The nurse checks that the needle on the aneroid gauge is within the zero mark.
   e. The nurse checks to see that the manometer is in the horizontal position.
   f. The nurse opens the valve to the sphygmomanometer once the pulse is found.

CHAPTER 26

# Health Assessment

## ASSESSING YOUR UNDERSTANDING

### IDENTIFICATION QUESTIONS

1. Locate the organs listed below that are found in the anterior section of the abdominal cavity. Place your answers on the lines provided on the illustration below.

   Sigmoid colon
   Small intestine
   Stomach
   Appendix
   Bladder
   Spleen
   Transverse colon
   Ascending colon
   Cecum
   Liver
   Descending colon

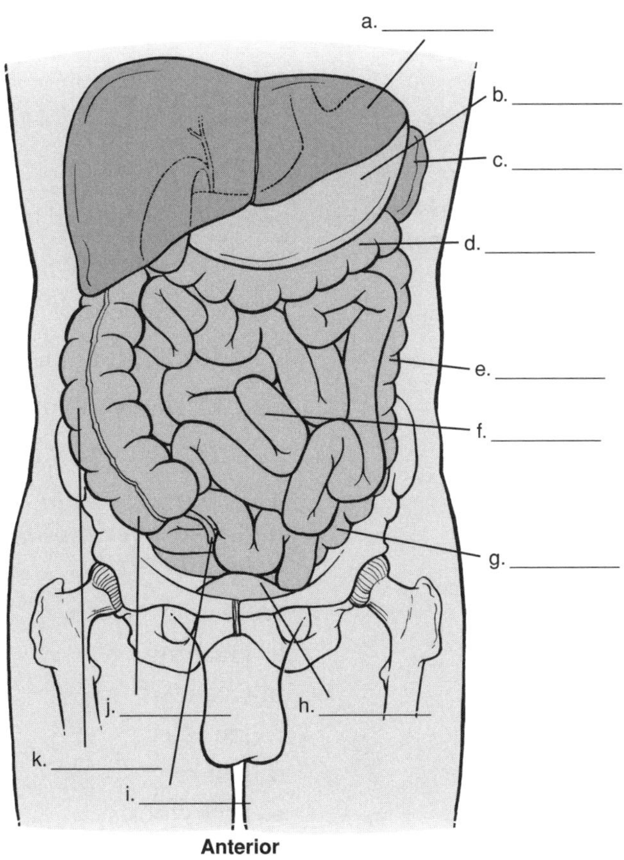

2. Locate the following list of internal structures of the ear and place your answers on the lines provided on the illustration below.

Incus
Facial nerve
Cochlea
Semicircular canals
Malleus
Tympanic membrane
Stapes and footplate
Cochlear and vestibular branch
Oval window
Eustachian tube
Round window

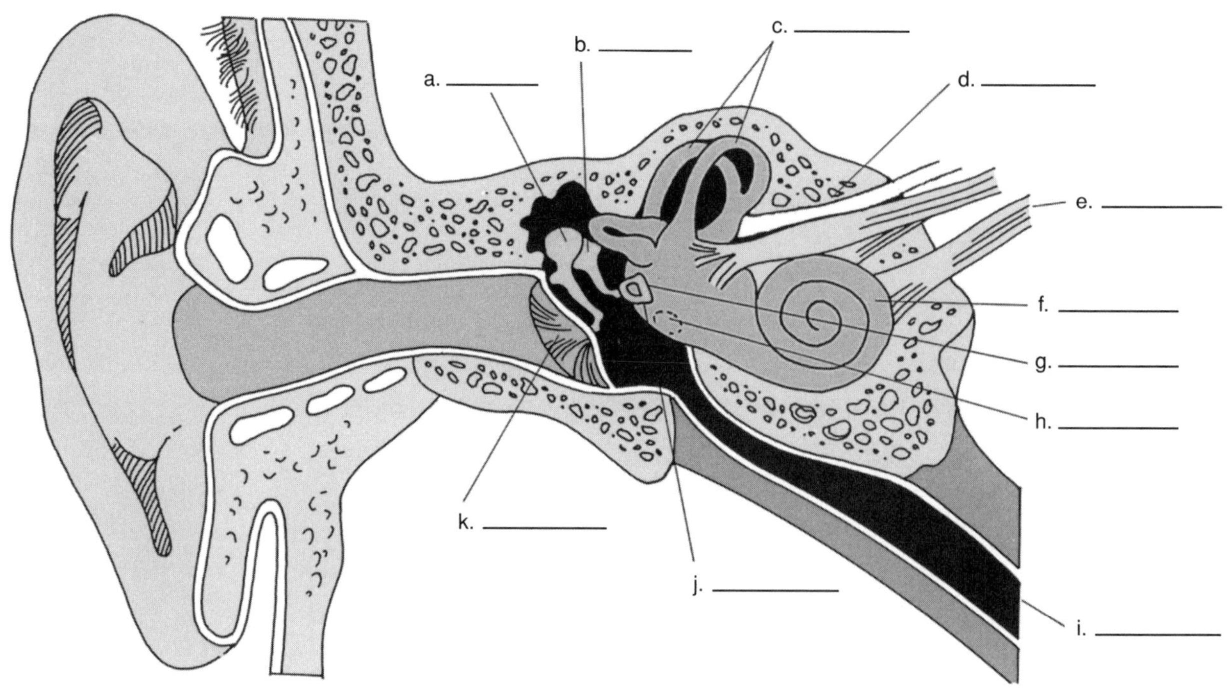


## MATCHING EXERCISES

***Match the organs listed in Part B with their proper location listed in Part A. Answers may be used more than once.***

**PART A**

**a.** Right upper quadrant
**b.** Left upper quadrant
**c.** Right lower quadrant
**d.** Left lower quadrant
**e.** Midline

**PART B**

____ **1.** Liver
____ **2.** Stomach
____ **3.** Gallbladder
____ **4.** Sigmoid colon
____ **5.** Cecum
____ **6.** Spleen
____ **7.** Urinary bladder
____ **8.** Left ureter and lower kidney pole
____ **9.** Appendix
____ **10.** Right kidney and adrenal gland
____ **11.** Body of pancreas
____ **12.** Left ovary and fallopian tube

***Match the terms in Part A with the correct definitions for findings during skin assessment listed in Part B.***

**PART A**

**a.** Flushing
**b.** Cyanosis
**c.** Jaundice
**d.** Pallor
**e.** Ecchymosis

**f.** Petechiae
**g.** Lesion
**h.** Turgor
**i.** Bruits

**PART B**

____ **13.** Yellow color

____ **14.** Redness

____ **15.** Dusky, blue color

____ **16.** Purplish discoloration

____ **17.** Diseased or injured tissue

____ **18.** Paleness

____ **19.** Elasticity of the skin

____ **20.** Very small hemorrhagic spots

***Match each nerve listed in Part A with its function listed in Part B.***

**PART A**

**a.** Olfactory (I) nerve
**b.** Optic (II) nerve
**c.** Oculomotor (III), trochlear (IV), and abducens (VI) nerves
**d.** Trigeminal (V) nerve
**e.** Facial (VII) nerve
**f.** Acoustic (VIII) nerve
**g.** Glossopharyngeal (IX) nerve
**h.** Accessory (XI) nerve
**i.** Hypoglossal (XII) nerve

**PART B**

____ **21.** A sensory nerve that is tested by assessing hearing ability

____ **22.** A sensory nerve whose function is vision; vision is tested for acuity and visual fields

____ **23.** A sensorimotor nerve that is assessed by observing the facial muscles for deviation of the jaw to one side and by palpating facial muscles for tone while the patient clenches the jaw

____ **24.** A motor nerve that affects the movement and strength of the tongue

____ **25.** A sensory nerve whose function is the sense of smell

____ **26.** Motor nerves that control the movement of the eyes through the cardinal fields of gaze; pupil size, shape, response to light, and accommodation; and opening of the upper eyelids

____ **27.** A sensorimotor nerve that innervates the muscles of the face and functions to provide the taste sensation of the anterior two thirds of the tongue

____ **28.** A motor nerve that is assessed by asking the patient to open the mouth and say "aaah" as the upward movement of the soft palate is observed

____ **29.** A motor nerve that controls the movement of the head and shoulders

***Match the positions listed in Part A with their description and function listed in Part B.***

**PART A**

**a.** Sitting position
**b.** Supine position
**c.** Dorsal recumbent position
**d.** Sims' position
**e.** Prone position
**f.** Lithotomy position
**g.** Knee–chest position
**h.** Standing position

**PART B**

____ **30.** The patient kneels, with the body at a 90-degree angle to the hips, back straight, arms above the head. The position is used to assess the rectal area.

____ **31.** The patient lies on the left or right side with the lower arm behind the body and the upper arm flexed at the shoulder and elbow. The knees are both flexed, with the uppermost leg more acutely flexed. The position is used to assess the rectum or vagina.

____ **32.** The patient is in the dorsal recumbent position with the buttocks at the edge of the examining table and the heels in stirrups. This position is used to assess the female rectum and genitalia.

____ **33.** The patient may sit upright in a chair or on the side of the examining table or bed or remain in bed with the head elevated. This position allows visualization of the upper body and facilitates lung expansion. It is used to take vital signs and assess the head, neck, posterior and anterior thorax and lungs, breasts, heart, and upper extremities.

____ **34.** The patient lies on the back with legs separated, knees bent, and soles of the feet flat on the bed. This position is used to assess the head and neck, anterior thorax and lungs, breasts, heart, extremities, and peripheral pulses.

____ **35.** The patient lies flat on the back with legs extended and knees slightly flexed. This position is used to assess the head and neck, anterior thorax and lungs, breasts, heart, abdomen, extremities, and peripheral pulses.

____ **36.** The patient lies on the abdomen, flat on the bed, with the head turned to one side. This position is used to assess the hip joint and posterior thorax.

## SHORT ANSWER

**1.** Identify five purposes of performing a health assessment.

**a.** ____________________

**b.** ____________________

**c.** ____________________

**d.** ____________________

**e.** ____________________

**2.** Briefly describe how the following instruments are used in a health assessment.

**a.** Ophthalmoscope: ____________________

**b.** Otoscope: ____________________

**c.** Snellen chart: ____________________

**d.** Nasal speculum: ____________________

**e.** Vaginal speculum: ____________________

**f.** Tuning fork: ____________________

**g.** Percussion hammer: ____________________

**h.** Thermometer and sphygmomanometer: ____________________

**i.** Scale: ____________________

**j.** Flashlight or penlight: ____________________

**k.** Stethoscope: ____________________

**l.** Tape measure and ruler: ____________________

**3.** List four factors that should be considered when deciding on a position for the physical assessment of a patient.

**a.** ____________________

**b.** ____________________

**c.** ____________________

**d.** ____________________

**4.** Describe how you would prepare a patient and the environment for a physical assessment.

**a.** Patient: ____________________

**b.** Environment: ____________________

5. Complete the table below listing the four assessment techniques; give a brief description of each technique and the types of assessments made.

| Technique | Definition | Assessment/Observation |
|---|---|---|
| a. Inspection: | | |
| b. Palpation: | | |
| c. Percussion: | | |
| d. Auscultation: | | |

6. List and describe the four characteristics of sound assessed by auscultation.

   a. ____________________

   b. ____________________

   c. ____________________

   d. ____________________

7. Briefly describe how you would assess a patient for the following conditions.

   a. Edema: ____________________

   ____________________

   b. Dehydration: ____________________

   ____________________

8. Describe the procedure for assessing the pupils of a patient for the following.

   a. Pupillary reaction: ____________________

   ____________________

   ____________________

   b. Accommodation: ____________________

   ____________________

   ____________________

   c. Convergence: ____________________

   ____________________

   ____________________

9. You are asked to perform a neurologic assessment on a patient. List the equipment you would assemble before performing the assessment. In what position would you place your patient?

   ____________________

   ____________________

10. Give an example of a question you may ask to assess a patient's mental status in the following areas.

    a. Orientation: ____________________

    ____________________

    b. Immediate memory: ____________________

    ____________________

    c. Past memory: ____________________

    ____________________

    d. Abstract reasoning: ____________________

    ____________________

    e. Language: ____________________

    ____________________

**11.** Complete the following paragraph by filling in the blanks with the correct word.

During auscultation of the heart, the first heart sound heard is the (a) ___________ of "lub-dub." This sound occurs when the (b) ___________ and (c) ___________ valves close and corresponds with the onset of (d) ___________ contraction. This sound is called (e) ___________ and is heard best in the (f) ___________ area. The second heart sound, (g) ___________, occurs at the end of (h) ___________ and represents the closure of the (i) ___________ and (j) ___________ valves. It is the (k) ___________ of "lub-dub." These two sounds occur within (l) ___________ second(s) or less.

**12.** Give an example of an interview question you would ask a patient to elicit the following eight components of the health history.

**a.** Biographical data: ___________

**b.** Reason for seeking health care:

___________

**c.** Present health history: ___________

**d.** Past health history: ___________

**e.** Family history: ___________

**f.** Functional health: ___________

**g.** Psychosocial and lifestyle factors:

___________

**h.** Review of systems: ___________

## APPLYING YOUR KNOWLEDGE

### CRITICAL THINKING QUESTIONS

**1.** Being prepared is a key factor in conducting a competent health assessment. The nurse must display well-developed cognitive, interpersonal, technical, and ethical skills. Describe what you would do to prepare the patient, the room, and the environment for an examination. How and why would you modify these preparations for the following patients?

**a.** A patient who is comatose

**b.** A patient who is uncooperative

**c.** A patient who does not understand your language

**d.** A small child

**2.** Make a list of all the instruments you would use to perform a health assessment. Arrange the instruments according to the order in which they will be used. Write a definition of each instrument and how it is to be used during the assessment. Rate yourself on your technical ability to use each instrument and technique. Practice using the instruments on a partner until you feel confident. Reflect on:

**a.** How confident you need to be before you can assess a patient independently

**b.** When it is safe to "practice" on a patient

### REFLECTIVE PRACTICE: DEVELOPING QSEN COMPETENCIES

***Use the following expanded scenario from Chapter 26 in your textbook to answer the questions below.***

***Scenario:*** Billy Collins, a 9-year-old with a history of allergies, including an allergy to insect stings, is spending a week at a summer camp. He suddenly reports to the camp counselor that he was just stung by a bee. The counselor rushes Billy to the nearest emergency health center after helping him self-inject epinephrine. He presents with itching and hives, difficulty breathing, nausea, and palpitations. When his parents arrive, they ask you what more they can do, if anything, to prevent this situation from occurring in the future.

**1.** What type of health assessments would the nurse caring for Billy conduct?

___________

___________

___________

**2.** What would be a successful outcome for Billy and his family?

___________

___________

___________

**3.** What intellectual, technical, interpersonal, and/or ethical/legal competencies are most likely to bring about the desired outcome?

___________

___________

___________

4. What resources might be helpful for this family?

______________________________________

______________________________________

______________________________________

## PRACTICING FOR NCLEX

### MULTIPLE CHOICE QUESTIONS

***Circle the letter that corresponds to the best answer for each question.***

1. A nurse is performing eye assessments at a community clinic. Which assessment would the nurse document as normal?
   a. The patient's eyes do not converge when the nurse moves a finger toward his nose.
   b. The patient's pupils are black, equal in size, and round and smooth.
   c. An older adult's pupils are pale and cloudy.
   d. The patient's pupils dilate when looking at a near object and constrict when looking at a distant object.
2. Which assessment measure would the nurse use to assess the location, shape, size, and density of a tumor?
   a. Observation
   b. Palpation
   c. Percussion
   d. Auscultation
3. What assessment technique would the nurse use to assess a patient's chest for color, shape, or contour?
   a. Inspection
   b. Palpation
   c. Percussion
   d. Auscultation
4. A nurse uses observation to examine a patient's skin. Which patient would the nurse document as having cyanosis?
   a. A patient who presents with redness in the facial area
   b. A patient whose skin has a yellowish tint
   c. A patient whose skin is a dusky, bluish color
   d. A patient whose skin is pale
5. A nurse is assisting with assessment of the internal eye structures of patients in an ophthalmologist's office. What would the nurse document as a normal finding?
   a. A uniform yellow reflex
   b. A clear, reddish optic nerve disc
   c. Dark-red arteries and light-red veins
   d. A reddish retina
6. A nurse is assessing the lungs of a patient and auscultates soft, low-pitched sounds over the base of the lungs during inspiration. What would be the nurse's next action?
   a. Suspect an inflamed pleura rubbing against the chest wall
   b. Document normal breath sounds
   c. Recommend testing for pneumonia
   d. Assess for asthma
7. The nurse is palpating the skin of a patient and documents that when picked up in a fold, the skin fold slowly returns to normal. What would be the next action of the nurse based on this finding?
   a. Document a normal skin finding on the patient chart.
   b. Assess the patient for cardiovascular disorders.
   c. Report the finding as a positive sign for cystic fibrosis.
   d. Assess the patient for dehydration.
8. The nurse is assessing the ear canal and tympanic membrane of a patient using an otoscope. Which finding would the nurse document as normal?
   a. The tympanic membrane is translucent, shiny, and gray.
   b. The ear canal is rough and pinkish.
   c. The tympanic membrane is reddish.
   d. The ear canal is smooth and white.
9. A nurse is assessing the bowel sounds of a patient who has Crohn's disease. What assessment technique would the nurse use?
   a. Auscultation
   b. Palpation
   c. Percussion
   d. Inspection

10. The nurse is using a bed scale to weigh a patient, and the patient becomes agitated as the sling rises in the air. What would be the priority nursing intervention in this situation?
    a. Reassure the patient that the procedure will only take a few minutes.
    b. Stop lifting the patient and reassess him or her.
    c. Administer a sedative to the patient and try again when the sedative takes effect.
    d. Enlist the help of another nurse to hold the patient steady during the procedure.
11. A nurse asks a patient to raise her eyebrows, smile and show her teeth, and puff out her cheeks. This nurse is most likely assessing which cranial nerve?
    a. Facial (VII)
    b. Vagus (X)
    c. Hypoglossal (XII)
    d. Accessory (XI)
12. A nurse is testing the function of the spinal cord of a patient who presents in the emergency department following a motorcycle accident. What would be the focus of this assessment?
    a. Motor ability
    b. Balance and gait
    c. Reflexes
    d. Sensory abilities
13. The nurse is assessing a child for an underactive thyroid gland. Which assessment technique would the nurse use?
    a. Palpation
    b. Inspection
    c. Percussion
    d. Auscultation
14. A weak, thready pulse found after the nurse palpates peripheral pulses may indicate what condition?
    a. Hypertension and circulatory overload
    b. Decreased cardiac output
    c. Impaired circulation
    d. Inflammation of a vein

## ALTERNATE-FORMAT QUESTIONS

### Multiple Response Questions

***Circle the letters that correspond to the best answers for each question.***

1. A nurse assesses patient breath sounds for patients presenting at a local clinic with difficulty breathing. Which sounds would the nurse document as normal? *(Select all that apply.)*
    a. Musical or squeaking sounds or high-pitched continuous sounds auscultated during inspiration and expiration
    b. Sonorous or coarse sounds with a snoring quality auscultated during inspiration and expiration
    c. Soft, low-pitched, whispering sounds heard over most of the lung fields
    d. Medium-pitched, medium-intensity, blowing sounds; auscultated over the first and second interspaces anteriorly and the scapula posteriorly
    e. Blowing, hollow sounds; auscultated over the larynx and trachea
    f. Bubbling, crackling, or popping sounds auscultated during inspiration and expiration
2. The nurse is testing the peripheral vision of a patient. Which actions are recommended guidelines for this test? *(Select all that apply.)*
    a. Have the patient stand or sit about 3 ft away.
    b. Have the patient cover one eye with a hand or index card.
    c. Ask the patient to look directly at a predetermined spot on the wall behind you.
    d. Cover your own eye opposite the patient's closed eye.
    e. Hold one arm outstretched to one side equidistant from you and the patient, and move your fingers into the visual fields from various peripheral points.
    f. Ask the patient to tell you when the fingers are first seen (you should see the fingers a second before the patient).

3. The nurse testing a patient's eyes asks the patient to focus on a finger from 2 ft away and moves the patient's eyes through the six cardinal positions of gaze. Which cranial nerve is this nurse testing using this procedure? *(Select all that apply.)*
   a. III: Oculomotor
   b. II: Optic
   c. V: Trigeminal
   d. IV: Trochlear
   e. VII: Facial
   f. VI: Abducens

4. A nurse is assessing the thorax and lungs of patients visiting a health care provider's office. Which findings would the nurse document as normal, age-related thorax and lung variations? *(Select all that apply.)*
   a. Softer auscultated breath sounds found in newborns and children
   b. Children under 10 having a slower respiratory rate than an adult
   c. Newborns and children using abdominal muscles during respirations
   d. Older adults having an increased anteroposterior chest diameter
   e. Older adults having an increase in the dorsal spinal curve (kyphosis)
   f. Older adults having increased thoracic expansion

**Hot Spot Question**

1. Place an X on the figure below to mark the spot where the nurse would auscultate to best hear the $S_1$ heart sound.

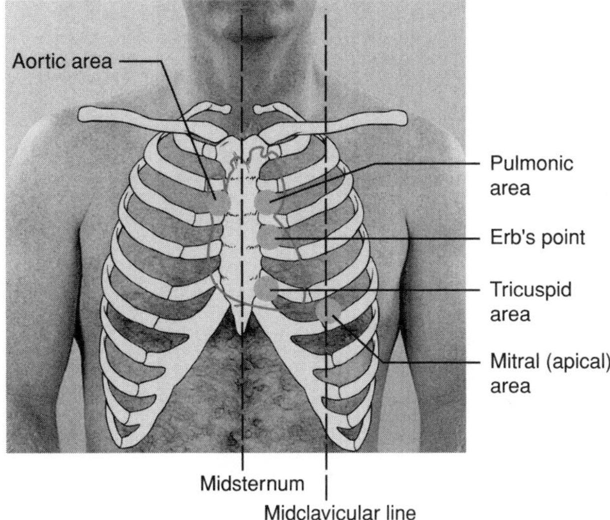

CHAPTER 27

# Safety, Security, and Emergency Preparedness

## ASSESSING YOUR UNDERSTANDING

### MATCHING EXERCISES

***Match the type of poisonous agent in Part A with its description listed in Part B.***

**PART A**

**a.** Biotoxins

**b.** Blister agents/vesicants

**c.** Blood agent

**d.** Caustics (acids)

**e.** Choking/lung/pulmonary agents

**f.** Incapacitating agents

**g.** Nerve agent

**h.** Organic solvents

**i.** Toxic alcohols

**PART B**

____ **1.** Chemicals that burn or corrode people's skin, eyes, and mucous membranes on contact

____ **2.** Agents that may cause damage the heart, kidneys, and nervous system

____ **3.** Chemicals that may cause severe irritation or swelling of the respiratory tract

____ **4.** Poisons from plants or animals that can cause harm to body systems

____ **5.** Agents that cause harm by being absorbed into the blood

____ **6.** Chemicals that severely burn the eyes, respiratory tract, and skin on contact

____ **7.** Agents that damage the tissues of living things by dissolving fats and oils

____ **8.** Highly poisonous chemicals that work by preventing the nervous system from working properly

____ **9.** Drugs that make people unable to think clearly or that cause an altered state of consciousness or even unconsciousness

***Match the safety precaution listed in Part B with the appropriate age group listed in Part A. Some answers may be used more than once.***

**PART A**

**a.** Fetus

**b.** Infant

**c.** Toddler and preschooler

**d.** School-aged child

**e.** Adolescent

**f.** Adult

**g.** Older adult

**PART B**

____ **10.** This age group needs assistance to evaluate activities that are potentially dangerous and to discuss specific interventions that provide for safety at home, at school, and in the neighborhood.

____ **11.** Falls, fires, and motor vehicle crashes are significant hazards for this age group, and safety measures should be directed toward preventing these injuries.

____ **12.** Education for this group must focus on safe driving skills, the dangers of drug and alcohol use, and creation of a healthy lifestyle as a way to respond to the stress of daily living.

____ **13.** A pregnant student requires reinforcement about the risks associated with alcohol consumption, smoking, drug use, and exposure to dangers in the environment.

____ **14.** This group needs education about ways to handle the stresses of daily life (e.g., raising a family, handling a demanding career) without relying on drugs and alcohol.

____ **15.** Vigilant supervision by parents and guardians is required to anticipate hazards and provide protection for this group, with precautionary devices.

____ **16.** Safety care for this group entails never leaving them unattended, using crib rails, and monitoring objects that may be placed in the mouth and swallowed.

## CORRECT THE FALSE STATEMENTS

***Circle the word "true" or "false" that follows the statement. If you circled "false," change the underlined word or words to make the statement true. Write your answer in the space provided.***

**1.** An example of a modifiable intrinsic fall risk factor is postural hypotension.

**a.** True

**b.** False ____________________

**2.** In the older adult population, one out of five falls causes a serious injury such as broken bones or a head injury, with falls being the most common cause of traumatic brain injuries.

**a.** True

**b.** False ____________________

**3.** Dosing errors comprise 5% of medication poisoning cases and involve giving the medication twice by mistake, giving the medication doses too close together, giving the incorrect dose, confusing the units of measurement, and using the dispensing cup incorrectly.

**a.** True

**b.** False ____________________

**4.** Most exposures to toxic fumes occur in the workplace.

**a.** True

**b.** False ____________________

**5.** Asphyxiation may occur in any age group, but the incidence is greatest among older adults.

**a.** True

**b.** False ____________________

**6.** Keeping a gun in the home increases the risk for domestic homicide.

**a.** True

**b.** False ____________________

**7.** The American Academy of Pediatrics (AAP) now recommends that infants and toddlers up to 2 years of age (or up to the maximum height and weight for the seat) remain in a rear-facing safety seat.

**a.** True

**b.** False ____________________

**8.** For the school-aged child, the focus of parental responsibility is on childproofing the environment.

**a.** True

**b.** False ____________________

**9.** As the primary reason for applying restraints, nurses consistently cite the risk for injury to patients and health care workers from irrational behavior.

**a.** True

**b.** False ____________________

**10.** Using a restraint on an older adult who tends to wander is justified to ensure his or her safety.

**a.** True

**b.** False ____________________

**11.** Approximately one in five people who die from drowning are children aged 5 or younger.

**a.** True

**b.** False ____________________

12. The number of deaths from accidental poisoning has decreased over the years.
    a. True
    b. False ____________________

13. Physical restraints decrease the possibility of serious injury due to a fall.
    a. True
    b. False ____________________

## SHORT ANSWER

1. Identify two safety risks for each of the following age groups.
   a. Neonates and infants: ____________________
   b. Toddler and preschooler: ____________________
   c. School-aged child: ____________________
   d. Adolescent: ____________________
   e. Adult: ____________________
   f. Older adult: ____________________

2. List two examples of how the following factors can affect safety.
   a. Developmental considerations: ____________________
   b. Lifestyle: ____________________
   c. Limitation in mobility: ____________________
   d. Limitation in sensory perception: ____________________
   e. Limitation in knowledge: ____________________
   f. Limitation in ability to communicate: ____________________
   g. Limitation in health status: ____________________
   h. Limitation in psychosocial state: ____________________

3. Briefly explain why the following information is necessary when assessing the patient for safety.
   a. Nursing history: ____________________
   b. Physical assessment: ____________________
   c. Accident-prone behavior: ____________________
   d. The environment: ____________________

4. Mrs. Vogel, age 72, fell when getting out of bed to use the bathroom in her nursing home. List four characteristics that should be assessed to determine whether this patient is at a greater risk for falls.
   a. ____________________
   b. ____________________
   c. ____________________
   d. ____________________

5. You are visiting a homebound patient who is staying with her daughter, who also has a toddler at home. You notice that the house is not childproofed and watch in horror as the toddler pulls a bottle of disinfectant out from under the sink while the mother is busy caring for her own mother. How would you prepare and present a plan for this mother to childproof her home?

   ____________________

6. List three questions you could ask a patient to assess for hazards that may cause a child to asphyxiate or choke.
   a. ____________________
   b. ____________________
   c. ____________________

**7.** Write a sample nursing diagnosis for each of the following situations.

**a.** A mother refuses to use a car seat for her child: ______________________

______________________

**b.** An older adult has poor vision and cannot read the label on her medication bottle:

______________________

______________________

**c.** A mother leaves her child unattended in the bathtub while she answers the phone:

______________________

**d.** A patient tells you she is "clumsy" and has fallen several times in the past few years:

______________________

**e.** The windows and doors do not operate properly in the home of an older couple, but they cannot afford repairs: ______________________

______________________

**8.** List three opportunities a nurse can use to teach students about safety.

**a.** ______________________

**b.** ______________________

**c.** ______________________

**9.** List five risks associated with the use of restraints.

**a.** ______________________

**b.** ______________________

**c.** ______________________

**d.** ______________________

**e.** ______________________

**10.** Mrs. Bender is a patient who has been placed in restraints to protect her from falling after other methods have failed. She refused to listen to information about the dangers of falling and repeatedly attempted to go to the bathroom on her own. How would you document the use of restraints on this patient?

______________________

______________________

______________________

______________________

______________________

**11.** List the information that should be included on a safety event report, when it should be filled out, and who is responsible for recording the event.

______________________

______________________

______________________

______________________

**12.** Describe how you would assess a patient for risk for falling by using the Get Up and Go test (Hendrich, 2007). State the time parameters for full mobility, almost complete independence, and impaired mobility.

______________________

______________________

______________________

______________________

______________________

## APPLYING YOUR KNOWLEDGE

### CRITICAL THINKING QUESTIONS

**1.** Visit the homes of friends or relatives who have children of different ages living with them. Ask for permission to inspect their home for safety features that are appropriate to the ages of the children. Check for poison control, fire prevention, fall protection, burn and shock protection, and so on. Share your results with the family, and explain to them what they need to do (if anything) to improve safety in their home. Reflect on the importance that different families attach to safety and its implication for your nursing practice.

**2.** Many people tend to take safety measures for granted. Draw on your experiences in conversations with nurses to identify safety risks for both nurses and patients in different practice settings. What can you do to minimize these risks?

### REFLECTIVE PRACTICE: CULTIVATING QSEN COMPETENCIES

***Use the following expanded scenario from Chapter 27 in your textbook to answer the questions below.***

***Scenario:*** Bessie Washington, age 77, was recently discharged to her home after suffering a cerebrovascular accident (brain attack). She lives alone in a small one-bedroom apartment and uses a walker to ambulate. A visiting nurse performing a safety assessment notes that she has hardwood floors with throw rugs covering the traffic areas, and old newspapers and magazines are stacked in piles close to heating vents. There are no fire alarms visible in the room. Mrs. Washington tells you, "I have so much stuff crammed into this apartment, I almost fell this morning going from my bedroom to the kitchen."

1. What safety interventions might the nurse implement for this patient?

______________________________

______________________________

______________________________

2. What would be a successful outcome for Mrs. Washington?

______________________________

______________________________

______________________________

3. What intellectual, technical, interpersonal, and/or ethical/legal competencies are most likely to bring about the desired outcome?

______________________________

______________________________

______________________________

4. What resources might be helpful for Mrs. Washington?

______________________________

______________________________

______________________________

## PRACTICING FOR NCLEX

### MULTIPLE CHOICE QUESTIONS

***Circle the letter that corresponds to the best answer for each question.***

1. A school nurse is preparing a teaching session on safety for parents of school-aged children. What would be an appropriate topic for this age group?
   - **a.** Selecting toys for the developmental level
   - **b.** Providing drug, alcohol, and sexuality education
   - **c.** Teaching stress reduction techniques
   - **d.** Providing close supervision to prevent injuries
2. A nurse follows the universal patient compact principles for partnership when providing care for patients. Which nursing action does not reflect this philosophy?
   - **a.** The nurse includes the patient as a member of the health care team.
   - **b.** The nurse asks for family input from the assigned advocate of the patient.
   - **c.** The nurse makes health care decisions for a patient who is uncooperative.
   - **d.** The nurse allows the patient to review his own medical information.
3. A nurse is filing a safety event report for an older adult patient who tripped and fell when getting out of bed. Which action exemplifies an accurate step of this process?
   - **a.** The nurse adds the information in the safety event report to the patient medical record.
   - **b.** The nurse calls the primary health care provider to fill out and sign the safety event report.
   - **c.** The nurse provides an opinion of the physical and mental condition of the patient that may have precipitated the incident.
   - **d.** The nurse details the patient's response and the examination and treatment of the patient after the incident.

4. The nurse is performing a safety belt fit test for a young patient at a well-child checkup. What criteria confirm that the child may sit in the back seat of a vehicle with a lap and shoulder belt in place?
   a. The knees do not bend at the edge of the seat when back is against vehicle's seat back.
   b. The seat belt stays low on the hips and is not resting on the soft part of the stomach.
   c. The shoulder belt does not lay on the collarbone or shoulder when fastened.
   d. The child's feet touch the floor of the car when belted in with the lap and shoulder belt.
5. A nurse is assessing a patient who was exposed to botulism from contaminated food supplies. Which symptom would the nurse expect to find in this patient?
   a. Skeletal muscle paralysis that progresses symmetrically and in a descending manner
   b. Flu-like symptoms
   c. Skin lesion with local edema that progresses, enlarges, ulcerates, and becomes necrotic
   d. Petechial hemorrhages
6. The nurse is caring for an 80-year-old patient who was admitted to the hospital in a confused and dehydrated state. After the patient got out of bed and fell, restraints were applied. She began to fight and was rapidly becoming exhausted. She has black-and-blue marks on her wrists from the restraints. What would be the most appropriate nursing intervention for this patient?
   a. Sedate her with sleeping pills and leave the restraints on.
   b. Take the restraints off, stay with her, and talk gently to her.
   c. Leave the restraints on and talk with her, explaining that she must calm down.
   d. Talk with the patient's family about taking her home because she is out of control.
7. A nurse working in a long-term care facility institutes interventions to prevent falls in the older adult population. Which intervention would be an appropriate alternative to the use of restraints for ensuring patient safety and preventing falls?
   a. Involve family members in the patient's care.
   b. Allow the patient to use the bathroom independently.
   c. Keep the patient sedated with tranquilizers.
   d. Maintain a high bed position so the patient will not attempt to get out unassisted.

## ALTERNATE-FORMAT QUESTIONS

### Multiple Response Questions

***Circle the letters that correspond to the best answers for each question.***

1. A nurse is teaching the RACE acronym to a student nurse as a guide for a fire safety plan in the facility. Which statements accurately reflect steps in this procedure? *(Select all that apply.)*
   a. R—Race to the front of the building to call for help.
   b. R—Rescue anyone in immediate danger.
   c. A—Activate the fire code system and notify the appropriate person.
   d. C—Check if the fire is contained or spreading to the hallways.
   e. C—Confine the fire by closing doors and windows.
   f. E—Extinguish the fire with an appropriate fire extinguisher.
2. A nurse is performing safety assessments in a health care facility. Which statements reflect considerations a nurse should keep in mind when assessing a patient for safety? *(Select all that apply.)*
   a. A person with a history of falls is likely to fall again.
   b. Some people are more prone to have accidents than others.
   c. Fires are responsible for most hospital incidents.
   d. Between 15% and 25% of falls result in fractures or soft tissue injury.
   e. A medication regimen that includes diuretics or analgesics places a person at risk for falls.
   f. A nurse whose behavior is reasonable and prudent and similar to what would be expected of another nurse in a similar circumstance is still likely to be found liable if a patient falls, especially if an injury results.

3. The nurse is teaching parents of toddlers how to prevent accidents and promote safety for their children. What are age-appropriate safety interventions for this age group? *(Select all that apply.)*
   a. Supervise the child closely to prevent injury.
   b. Childproof the house to ensure that poisonous products and small objects are out of reach.
   c. Instruct the child to wear proper safety equipment when riding bicycles or scooters.
   d. Do not leave the child alone in the bathtub or near water.
   e. Provide drug, alcohol, and sexuality education.
   f. Practice emergency evacuation measures with the child.
4. A nurse is applying restraints to a confused patient who has threatened the safety of a roommate. Which actions would the nurse perform when properly applying restraints to a patient? *(Select all that apply.)*
   a. Check facility policy for the application of restraints and secure a health care provider's order.
   b. Choose the most restrictive type of device that allows the least amount of mobility.
   c. Pad bony prominences.
   d. For a restraint applied to an extremity, ensure that the restraint is tight enough that a finger cannot be inserted between the restraint and the patient's wrist or ankle.
   e. Fasten the restraint to the side rail.
   f. Remove the restraint at least every 2 hours or according to facility policy and patient need.

**Prioritization Question**

1. Place the following steps for applying restraints to a patient in the order in which they should occur:
   a. Explain the reason for use of restraints to the patient and family.
   b. Determine the need for restraints and assess patient's physical condition, behavior, and mental status.
   c. Fasten restraint to the bed frame, not the bed rail.
   d. Apply restraints according to manufacturer's directions.
   e. Perform hand hygiene; document reason for restraining patient.
   f. Perform hand hygiene.
   g. Remove restraint at least every 2 hours; reassure patient at regular intervals and assess for signs of sensory deprivation.
   h. Confirm facility policy for application of restraints and secure health care provider's order.

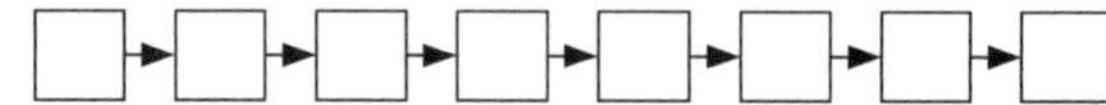

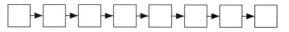

CHAPTER 28

# Complementary and Integrative Health

## ASSESSING YOUR UNDERSTANDING

### FILL IN THE BLANKS

1. The nurse planning care for a patient who believes in traditional Chinese medicine (TCM) incorporates the ____________ theory of two opposing, yet complementary, forces that shape the world and all life and are central to TCM.
2. A nurse's philosophy of patient care focuses on the connections and interactions between the parts of the whole in order to heal the whole person. This nurse is incorporating the ____________ theory into practice.
3. ____________ consists of placing very thin, short, sterile needles at particular points believed to be centers of nerve and vascular tissue.
4. The nurse teaches a patient to use all five senses to depict a plan of healing. This nurse is guiding the patient to use ____________.
5. The nurse recommends the use of chemical compounds that contain ingredients believed to promote health called ____________ for a patient diagnosed with anorexia.
6. A nurse who massages a patient's back using scented oils is using the complementary health approach (CHA) modality known as ____________.

### MATCHING EXERCISES

***Match the CHA in Part A with its description listed in Part B.***

**PART A**

a. Ayurveda
b. Yoga
c. Traditional Chinese medicine
d. Acupuncture
e. Qi gong
f. Homeopathy
g. Naturopathy

**PART B**

____ 1. Uses thin, short, sterile needles, placed at centers of nerve and vascular tissue

____ 2. Based on the belief of supporting the body while the symptoms are allowed to run their course

____ 3. Consists of a set of exercises that promote health through various physical postures

____ 4. A system of postures, exercises (gentle and dynamic), breathing techniques, and visualization

____ 5. Key concepts include universal interconnectedness among people, their health, and the universe; and the body's constitution and life forces

____ 6. Qi (energy) is the central theme

### SHORT ANSWER

1. Define the following concepts and their basic philosophy of medicine.
   a. Allopathy: ______
   b. Holism: ______
   c. Integrative care: ______
2. Briefly describe the following CHAs and related nursing considerations.
   a. Ayurveda: ______
      Nursing considerations: ______
   b. Yoga: ______
      Nursing considerations: ______
   c. Traditional Chinese medicine: ______
      Nursing considerations: ______
   d. Qi gong: ______
      Nursing considerations: ______
3. Describe three mind–body therapies you might use for a patient experiencing unrelieved pain due to chemotherapy.
   a. ______
   b. ______
   c. ______
4. Describe the four scientific principles used in Therapeutic Touch.
   a. ______
   b. ______
   c. ______
   d. ______
5. Describe how the nursing care plan would differ for a patient diagnosed with leukemia when using the following different spiritual approaches.
   a. Shamanism: ______
   b. Relaxation response: ______
6. Explain why the following therapies might be used to heal patients.
   a. Nutritional therapy: ______
   b. Aromatherapy: ______
   c. Music: ______
   d. Humor: ______
7. List and give an example of the four types or domains of CHA described by the National Center for Complementary and Alternative Medicine.
   a. ______
   b. ______
   c. ______
   d. ______

## APPLYING YOUR KNOWLEDGE

### CRITICAL THINKING QUESTIONS

1. Discuss how you might change your nursing plan to include CHA when treating the following patients.
   a. A 42-year-old man with end-stage AIDS who is receiving hospice care at home
   b. A 7-year-old girl diagnosed with juvenile diabetes who must learn to self-administer insulin
   c. A 75-year-old man with Alzheimer's disease who is living in a long-term care facility

2. Discuss the blended skills you would need to care for a patient when incorporating the following spiritual approaches into the plan of care.
   a. Shamanism
   b. TCM

### REFLECTIVE PRACTICE: CULTIVATING QSEN COMPETENCIES

***Use the following expanded scenario from Chapter 28 in your textbook to answer the questions below.***

***Scenario:*** Sylvia Puentes is a middle-aged woman scheduled to undergo abdominal surgery next week. She comes to the outpatient clinic for preoperative evaluation and laboratory testing. During the nursing interview, she says, "I'm really anxious about the surgery, but I don't want to take any medicines. Is there anything I can do to help me relax?" She also says she would like to learn about new therapies for treating her pain postoperatively.

1. What type of CHA might the nurse suggest to promote relaxation for Ms. Puentes?

______________________________________________

______________________________________________

______________________________________________

2. What would be a successful outcome for Ms. Puentes?

______________________________________________

______________________________________________

______________________________________________

3. What intellectual, technical, interpersonal, and/or ethical/legal competencies are most likely to bring about the desired outcome?

______________________________________________

______________________________________________

______________________________________________

4. What resources might be helpful for Ms. Puentes?

______________________________________________

______________________________________________

______________________________________________

## PRACTICING FOR NCLEX

### MULTIPLE CHOICE QUESTIONS

***Circle the letter that corresponds to the best answer for each question.***

1. A nurse works in an office that follows the allopathic philosophy of medicine. For which patient would this type of medicine be most effective?
   a. A patient whose spinal cord was severed in a motor vehicle accident
   b. A patient diagnosed with juvenile diabetes
   c. A patient who has chronic obstructive pulmonary disease
   d. A patient who has rheumatoid arthritis

2. The nurse is caring for a patient whose treatment has been based on the Ayurveda medical system. Which nursing intervention incorporates this patient's beliefs into the nursing plan?
   a. Basing practice on the Yin–Yang theory
   b. Preparing the patient for exercises that help the patient regulate *qi*
   c. Helping the patient to balance his body, mind, and spirit
   d. Including the patient's shaman in the plan of care

3. The nurse is caring for a 48-year-old Native American man hospitalized following a myocardial infarction who asks to see his medicine man. What would be the nurse's best response to this patient?
   a. Inform the patient that he may visit with his medicine man when he is discharged.
   b. Arrange for a visit with the medicine man in the hospital.
   c. State that while in the hospital, it is necessary to follow traditional medicine.
   d. Ask the patient to concentrate on getting better and following his care plan.

4. For which patient might the nurse need to alter the plan of care based on the principles of the patient's chosen medical system?
   a. A patient who visits a chiropractor
   b. A patient who believes in a strong mind–body connection
   c. A patient who is being treated by a naturopathic provider
   d. A patient who is being treated by an allopathic provider

5. A nurse is teaching a patient meditation techniques to provide mental calmness and physical relaxation. Which nursing intervention facilitates this process?
   a. Helping the patient to assume a specific, comfortable posture
   b. Providing a stimulating environment in which to conduct the meditation
   c. Teaching the patient to have multiple focal points
   d. Promoting a closed attitude to avoid judgments and distractions

6. A nurse is caring for a hospitalized patient who states: "I feel so sick all the time, my aura must be disturbed by all of these bad force fields." What is an appropriate NANDA diagnosis for this patient?
   a. Social isolation
   b. Ineffective coping
   c. Hopelessness
   d. Imbalanced energy field

## ALTERNATE-FORMAT QUESTIONS

### Multiple Response Questions

***Circle the letters that correspond to the best answers for each question.***

1. A nurse who has incorporated complementary health approaches (CHAs) into nursing practice is caring for a patient in a short-term care facility. Which examples of nursing interventions are based on CHA? *(Select all that apply.)*
   a. The nurse investigates herbs that may stimulate the patient's immune system.
   b. The nurse encourages the patient to join a yoga class.
   c. The nurse administers pain medication prescribed by the primary care provider.
   d. The nurse schedules diagnostic tests for the patient.
   e. The nurse teaches the patient how to meditate.
   f. The nurse uses guided imagery to relieve patient anxiety.

2. A nurse uses healing touch to care for patients on a hospital ward. For which patients would this practice be most appropriate? *(Select all that apply.)*
   a. A patient with a surgical wound
   b. A patient who has unrelenting pain
   c. A patient whose energy field is unbalanced
   d. A patient who is overweight
   e. A patient who leaves the hospital against medical advice
   f. A patient who is being prepared for a surgical procedure

3. In today's environment, nurses must be prepared to use CHA in their nursing practices. Which statements accurately represent the role of CHA in nursing today? *(Select all that apply.)*
   a. The nursing profession is expanding its knowledge base to include information that explains selected CHA.
   b. Certification is available for nurses wishing to practice holistic nursing.
   c. Graduate-level specialization in holistic nursing is available at some universities.
   d. The development of CHA is market and patient driven.
   e. It is expected that CHA will eventually replace traditional nursing in many health care facilities.
   f. Practitioners of CHA are strictly regulated by the government.

4. The nurse is teaching a patient how to use herbs and supplements as part of an integrated treatment plan. Which teaching points would the nurse include? *(Select all that apply.)*
   a. Use the Internet to buy herbs and supplements.
   b. Whenever possible, buy products with more than one ingredient.
   c. Buy herbs and supplements that are standardized.
   d. Give the product adequate time to work.
   e. Be knowledgeable about the product and its therapeutic actions.
   f. Take a higher than recommended dose of herbs to initiate the therapeutic effect.

**5.** A nurse is explaining the method of allopathic medicine to a patient. Which statements describe this approach to medicine? *(Select all that apply.)*

**a.** "Curing is accomplished by internal agents."

**b.** "Illness occurs in either the mind or the body, which are separate entities."

**c.** "Illness is a manifestation of imbalance or disharmony and is a process."

**d.** "Curing occurs quickly and seeks to destroy the invading organism or repair the affected part."

**e.** "Healing is done by the patient."

**f.** "Health is the absence of disease."

**6.** A nurse is teaching an overweight patient the holistic approach to choosing foods. Which teaching points would the nurse include? *(Select all that apply.)*

**a.** Eat foods that are in season.

**b.** Avoid organically grown foods.

**c.** Reduce intake of refined and natural sugars.

**d.** Consider adopting a vegetarian diet.

**e.** Increase intake of dairy products.

**f.** Replace refined sugars with artificial sweeteners.

CHAPTER 29

# Medications

## ASSESSING YOUR UNDERSTANDING

### FILL IN THE BLANKS

***A health care provider has ordered medications in certain amounts. You have them on hand but in different quantities. Make the necessary conversions and write what you will give to each patient on the line provided.***

1. Order: gentamicin 60 mg. On hand: gentamicin 80 mg/2 mL. Give patient: ______________

______________________________

2. Order: Mestinon 30 mg. On hand: Mestinon 60 mg/tab. Give patient: ______________

______________________________

3. Order: amitriptyline 75 mg. On hand: amitriptyline 25 mg/tab. Give patient: ______________

______________________________

4. Order: phenylbutazone 250 mg. On hand: phenylbutazone 500 mg/tab. Give patient:

______________________________

______________________________

5. Order: Pro-Banthine 15 mg. On hand: Pro-Banthine 5 mg/tab. Give patient: ______________

______________________________

6. Order: penicillin V 250 mg. On hand: penicillin V 500 mg/tab. Give patient: ______________

______________________________

7. Order: Lanoxin 0.125 mg. On hand: Lanoxin 0.250 mg/tab. Give patient: ______________

______________________________

8. Order: metaproterenol sulfate 20 mg. On hand: metaproterenol sulfate 10 mg/tab. Give patient: ______________

______________________________

9. Order: ACTH 40 mg. On hand: ACTH 10 mg/mL. Give patient: ______________

______________________________

### MATCHING EXERCISES

***Match the types of drug preparations in Part A with their descriptions listed in Part B.***

**PART A**

a. Capsule
b. Elixir
c. Liniment
d. Lotion
e. Ointment
f. Tablet
g. Pill
h. Powder
i. Solution
j. Suppository
k. Suspension
l. Syrup
m. Enteric coated

**PART B**

____ **1.** Small, solid dose of medication; compressed or molded; may be any size or shape, or enteric coated

____ **2.** Powder or gel form of an active drug enclosed in a gelatinous container

____ **3.** Medication mixed with alcohol, oil, or soap, which is rubbed on the skin

____ **4.** Finely divided, undissolved particles in a liquid medium; should be shaken before use

____ **5.** Medication in a clear liquid containing water, alcohol, sweeteners, and flavoring

____ **6.** An easily melted medication preparation in a firm base, such as gelatin, that is inserted into the body

____ **7.** Drug particles in a solution for topical use

____ **8.** Mixture of a powdered drug with a cohesive material; may be round or oval

____ **9.** A drug dissolved in another substance

____ **10.** Single drug or mixture of finely ground drugs

____ **11.** Medication combined with water and sugar solution

____ **12.** Tablet or pill that prevents stomach irritation

***Match the types of injections listed in Part A with their injection site listed in Part B.***

**PART A**

**a.** Subcutaneous injection
**b.** Intramuscular injection
**c.** Intradermal injection
**d.** Intravenous injection
**e.** Intra-arterial injection
**f.** Intracardial injection
**g.** Intraperitoneal injection
**h.** Intraspinal injection
**i.** Intraosseous injection

**PART B**

____ **13.** Corium

____ **14.** Bone

____ **15.** Muscle tissue

____ **16.** Artery

____ **17.** Heart tissue

____ **18.** Vein

____ **19.** Peritoneal cavity

____ **20.** Subcutaneous tissue

**SHORT ANSWER**

**1.** List two categories for drug classification.

**a.** ________________________________

**b.** ________________________________

**2.** Explain the following processes by which drugs alter cell physiology.

**a.** Drug–receptor interactions: ________________

________________________________

**b.** Drug–enzyme interactions: ________________

________________________________

**3.** Give an example of how the following factors affect drug action.

**a.** Developmental stage of patient: ________

________________________________

**b.** Weight: ________________________

________________________________

**c.** Sex: ____________________________

________________________________

**d.** Genetic and cultural factors: __________

________________________________

**e.** Psychological factors: ______________

________________________________

**f.** Pathology: ______________________

________________________________

**g.** Environment: ____________________

________________________________

**h.** Time of administration: ______________

________________________________

4. Give three examples of situations in which you would question a medical order.
   a. ___
   b. ___
   c. ___
5. Briefly describe the following four types of medication supply systems.
   a. Stock supply system (computerized automated dispensing cabinets [ADCs]): ___
   b. Unit dose dispensing system: ___
   c. Medication cart: ___
   d. Bar code-enabled medication administration (BCMA): ___
6. List the three checks and eleven rights of administering medication.
   a. Three checks: ___
   b. Eleven rights: ___
7. Your patient tells you she refuses to take the medication prescribed for her because it tastes "disgusting." List three techniques you could use to mask the taste.
   a. ___
   b. ___
   c. ___
8. Explain how the following factors would affect the type of equipment a nurse would choose for an injection.
   a. Route of administration: ___
   b. Viscosity of the solution: ___
   c. Quantity to be administered: ___
   d. Body size: ___
   e. Type of medication: ___
9. List four steps that should be followed when a medication error occurs.
   a. ___
   b. ___
   c. ___
   d. ___
10. Describe the use of the following types of prepackaged medications.
   a. Ampules: ___
   b. Vials: ___
   c. Prefilled cartridges: ___

11. Transcribe the following medication orders on the patient medication record below and sign for the medications you would administer in a 24-hour period. Be prepared to discuss administration guidelines.

    Tenormin, 50 mg, PO OD

    HydroDIURIL, 50 mg, PO OD

    NPH insulin U100, 45 units SQ daily in AM

    Regular insulin U100, 10 units SQ stat

    Cipro, 500 mg, PO q12h

    Timoptic 0.25% GTT OD BID

    Dalmane, 30 mg, PO hs, PRN

    Nitro-paste ½ in, q8h to chest wall

    Tylenol with codeine #2, PO q4h, PRN

    Colace, 100 mg, PO OD

**Medical Administration Record**

| ORD DATE | PRN MEDS. | |
|---|---|---|
| | | Date |
| | | Time |
| | | Init / Site |
| | | Date |
| | | Time |
| | | Init / Site |

**SINGLE ORDERS—PREOPERATIVES**

| ORD DATE | MEDICATION—DOSAGE—ROUTE OF ADMIN | DATE/TIME | SITE/INITIALS |
|---|---|---|---|
| | | | |
| | | | |

**INJECTION SITES MUST BE CHARTED**

**ROUTINE MEDICATIONS**

| ORD DATE | MEDICATION—DOSAGE—ROUTE OF ADMIN | HR | DATE/TIME | | | | | | |
|---|---|---|---|---|---|---|---|---|---|
| | | | | | | | | | |
| | | | | | | | | | |
| | | | | | | | | | |
| | | | | | | | | | |
| | | | | | | | | | |
| | | | | | | | | | |
| | | | | | | | | | |
| | | | | | | | | | |
| | | | | | | | | | |
| | | | | | | | | | |
| | | | | | | | | | |
| | | | | | | | | | |
| | | | | | | | | | |
| | | | | | | | | | |
| | | | | | | | | | |
| | | | | | | | | | |
| | | | | | | | | | |
| | | | | | | | | | |
| | | | | | | | | | |
| | | | | | | | | | |
| | | | | | | | | | |

**12.** You are preparing Jim Toole for discharge. He will be taking the following medications at home: alprazolam, ranitidine, and ciprofloxacin. Use the chart below to identify the information you will need to teach him about these medications. Use a pharmacology for medication information.

| Method | Alprazolam | Ranitidine | Ciprofloxacin |
|---|---|---|---|
| Dosage range | | | |
| Possible route of administration | | | |
| Frequency/schedule | | | |
| Desired effects | | | |
| Possible adverse effects | | | |
| Signs and symptoms of toxic drug effects | | | |
| Special instructions | | | |
| Nursing/collaborative management of adverse effects | | | |

## APPLYING YOUR KNOWLEDGE

### CRITICAL THINKING QUESTIONS

1. Think about your responsibilities when administering medication and then describe how you would respond in the following situations:
   a. A health care provider who is in a hurry prescribes a medication for your patient. After he leaves, you read the order and don't understand why your patient would need the medication prescribed. Because you are legally responsible for medications administered, what would you do?
   b. You bring a medication to a patient, who tells you, "That's not my pill." What would you do?
2. Medication errors are not uncommon and may be lethal. Interview several nurses about their experiences with errors and what contributes to them. Think about how nurses individually and collectively can act to reduce errors. Develop a plan with your classmates to help minimize these errors.

### REFLECTIVE PRACTICE: CULTIVATING QSEN COMPETENCIES

***Use the following expanded scenario from Chapter 29 in your textbook to answer the questions below.***

*Scenario:* François Baptiste is an older adult with a wound infection requiring intravenous antibiotic therapy. He is scheduled to receive his next dose at 1000. The medication delivered by the pharmacy is labeled with the correct drug and dose, but with another patient's name. The nurse checks the patient identification band, and notes that it does not match the medication label.

1. How might the nurse use blended nursing skills to respond to this medication error?

   ______________________________________________

   ______________________________________________

   ______________________________________________

2. What would be a successful outcome for this patient?

   ______________________________________________

   ______________________________________________

   ______________________________________________

3. What intellectual, technical, interpersonal, and/or ethical/legal competencies are most likely to bring about the desired outcome?

   ______________________________________________

   ______________________________________________

   ______________________________________________

## PRACTICING FOR NCLEX

### MULTIPLE CHOICE QUESTIONS

***Circle the letter that corresponds to the best answer for each question.***

1. A nurse is administering an intradermal injection to a patient for a skin allergy test. When the nurse is finished, there is no sign of a wheal or blister at the site of injection. What is the nurse's best action in this situation?
   a. Choose another site and reinject the medication.
   b. Prepare another syringe and administer it to the patient at the same site.
   c. Document the administration as correctly administered.
   d. Document the administration and inform the primary care provider.
2. The nurse is administering a subcutaneous injection of insulin to a patient. Which action would the nurse take after choosing the appropriate administration site?
   a. Identify the appropriate landmarks for the site chosen.
   b. Cleanse the area around the injection site with alcohol.
   c. Use a firm, back and forth motion to cleanse the site.
   d. Remove the needle cap with the dominant hand pulling it straight off.
3. When administering a subcutaneous injection to a patient, the needle pulls out of the skin when the skin fold is released. What would be the appropriate next action of the nurse in this situation?
   a. Pull out and discard the needle.
   b. Discard the equipment and start the procedure from the beginning.

c. Engage safety shield on needle guard and discard needle appropriately.
d. Document the incident and inform the primary care provider.

4. A nurse is administering an injection of insulin to a 5-year-old who has juvenile diabetes. Which statement by the nurse would take into consideration this child's developmental level?
   a. "Don't worry, this won't hurt a bit."
   b. "If you are brave and don't cry, I will give you a sticker."
   c. "Try not to move, or this will hurt more."
   d. "You will just feel a little pinch."
5. A health care provider prescribes a PRN order for a postsurgical patient. When would the nurse administer the medication?
   a. Every hour
   b. As needed
   c. One time only
   d. Immediately
6. A home care nurse is teaching a patient with diabetes how to self-administer insulin. Which teaching point would the nurse include in the teaching plan?
   a. Use the same area of the body at the same time every day.
   b. Use the same site on the body for each injection.
   c. Reuse syringes and needles up to three times.
   d. Store needles and syringes in a glass container.
7. While injecting a needle into a patient for an intramuscular injection, the nurse hits the patient's bone. What would be the appropriate initial response of the nurse to this situation?
   a. Remove the needle and have another nurse stay with the patient while informing the primary care provider.
   b. Withdraw the needle, apply a new needle to syringe, and administer the injection in an alternate site.
   c. Document the incident according to facility policy and then remove the needle and syringe and discard it.
   d. Remove the needle and discard the needle and syringe; call the primary care provider.
8. A nurse preparing medication for a patient is called away to an emergency. What should the nurse do?
   a. Have another nurse guard the preparations.
   b. Put the medications back in the containers.
   c. Have another nurse finish preparing and administering the medications.
   d. Lock the medications in a room and finish them upon return.
9. A nurse is administering an antihypertensive drug to a hospitalized patient. What action should the nurse take to identify the patient prior to administration?
   a. Call the patient by name.
   b. Check the patient's ID bracelet.
   c. Check the patient's record.
   d. Check the patient's name with family or significant others.
10. A nurse is ordered to administer epinephrine to a child who was stung by a bee and is allergic to insect bites. Which means of drug administration would the nurse use to achieve rapid absorption and quicker results in this emergency situation?
    a. Injection
    b. Oral
    c. Patch
    d. Inhalation
11. A nurse is administering a hepatitis B shot to an adult patient. Which site would the nurse choose for this injection?
    a. Vastus lateralis site
    b. Deltoid muscle site
    c. Ventrogluteal site
    d. Dorsogluteal site
12. A nurse is administering medication to an older adult patient who experienced symptoms of stroke. When administering the medication prescribed, the nurse should be aware that this patient has an increased possibility of drug toxicity due to which age-related factor?
    a. Decreased adipose tissue and increased total body fluid in proportion to total body mass
    b. Increased number of protein-binding sites
    c. Increased kidney function, resulting in excessive filtration and excretion
    d. Decline in liver function and production of enzymes needed for drug metabolism

13. How would the nurse convert 0.8 grams to milligrams?
    a. Move the decimal point 2 places to the right.
    b. Move the decimal point 3 places to the right.
    c. Move the decimal point 2 places to the left.
    d. Move the decimal point 3 places to the left.

14. A nurse administers a dose of gentamicin, and the patient has an immediate reaction of hypotension, bronchospasms, and rapid, thready pulse. What is the next appropriate action of the nurse?
    a. Administer antibiotic, antihistamines, and isoproterenol.
    b. Administer bronchodilators, antihistamines, and vasodilators.
    c. Administer epinephrine, antihistamines, and bronchodilators.
    d. Administer antihistamines, vasodilators, and bronchoconstrictors.

15. A patient has an order for chloramphenicol, 500 mg every 6 hours. The drug comes in 250-mg capsules. What would the nurse administer?
    a. 1 tab
    b. 2 tabs
    c. 3 tabs
    d. 4 tabs

16. An oral medication has been ordered for a patient who has a nasogastric tube in place. Which nursing activity would increase the safety of medication administration?
    a. Check the tube placement before administration.
    b. Have the patient swallow the pills around the tube.
    c. Flush the tube with 30 to 40 mL saline before medication administration.
    d. Bring the liquids to room temperature before administration.

17. What action should the nurse take when giving an intramuscular injection using the Z-track method?
    a. Use a needle at least 1 in long.
    b. Apply pressure to the injection site.
    c. Inject the medication quickly, and steadily withdraw the needle.
    d. Do not massage the site because it may cause irritation.

## ALTERNATE-FORMAT QUESTIONS

### Multiple Response Questions

***Circle the letters that correspond to the best answers for each question.***

1. A nurse is administering intramuscular injections to patients on a hospital ward. What needle sizes has the nurse used correctly? *(Select all that apply.)*
    a. 5/8-in needle for the vastus lateralis site
    b. 5/8-in needle for an adult in the ventrogluteal site
    c. 1¼-in needle for a child in the deltoid site
    d. 1½-in needle for an adult in the deltoid site
    e. 5/8-in needle for a child in the deltoid site
    f. 5/8-in needle for an adult in the ventrogluteal site

2. The nurse is teaching a patient how to use an insulin pen. Which steps reflect recommended procedure? *(Select all that apply.)*
    a. After administering injection, keep button depressed; count to 3 before removal.
    b. Hold the pen upright and tap to force any air bubbles to the top.
    c. Check that dose selector is at 2 before dialing units of insulin for the dose.
    d. After administering the injection, push the button on the pen half-way in.
    e. Dial the dose selector to 2 units to perform an "air shot" to get rid of bubbles.
    f. Administer injection by holding pen in palm of hand perpendicular to the forearm.

3. The nurse is administering medication to a patient through a drug-infusion lock using the saline flush. During the process, the patient complains of pain at the site. Which interventions are appropriate in this situation? *(Select all that apply.)*
    a. Stop the medication and assess the site for signs of infiltration and phlebitis.
    b. Flush the medication lock with normal saline again to recheck patency.
    c. If site is within normal limits, resume medication administration at a slower rate.
    d. Immediately stop the medication, remove medication lock, and restart at new site.
    e. Notify the primary care provider that the site has been infiltrated.
    f. Finish administering medication and then change the medication lock.

4. A nurse who is administering a piggyback intermittent intravenous infusion of medication to a patient observes that there is a cloudy, white substance forming in the IV tubing. What actions should the nurse take in this situation? *(Select all that apply.)*
   a. Assess the IV site for signs of infiltration or phlebitis.
   b. Stop the IV from flowing and stop administering the medication.
   c. Prime the secondary tubing by "backfilling" it.
   d. Clamp the IV at the site nearest to the patient.
   e. Replace tubing on primary and secondary infusions.
   f. Check literature regarding incompatibilities of medications after administering.

5. Which actions would the nurse take when instilling eye drops correctly? *(Select all that apply.)*
   a. Perform hand hygiene and put on gloves.
   b. Clean the eyelids and eyelashes using a cotton ball soaked in water moving from the outer to the inner canthus.
   c. Tilt the patient's head back slightly if sitting or place the head on a pillow if lying down.
   d. Have the patient look up and focus on something on the ceiling.
   e. Place the thumb near the margin of the lower eyelid and exert pressure upward over the bony prominence of the cheek.
   f. Squeeze the container and allow the prescribed number of drops to fall into the cornea.

6. Which actions would a nurse perform when instilling ear drops correctly? *(Select all that apply.)*
   a. Make sure the solution to be instilled is at room temperature.
   b. Clean the external ear with cotton balls moistened with water or normal saline solution.
   c. Place the patient on the affected side in bed.
   d. Draw up the amount of solution needed in the dropper and return any excess medication to the stock bottle.
   e. Straighten the auditory canal by pulling the cartilaginous portion of the pinna up and back in an adult and down and back in an infant or child under 3 years.
   f. Invert and hold the dropper in the ear with its tip above the auditory canal.

7. Which actions would the nurse perform when administering a subcutaneous injection correctly? *(Select all that apply.)*
   a. Cleanse the area around the injection site with an antimicrobial swab using soft up and down motions.
   b. Remove the needle cap with the dominant hand, pulling it straight off.
   c. Pinch the area surrounding the injection site or spread the skin taut at the site.
   d. Inject the needle quickly at an angle of 45 to 90 degrees.
   e. If blood appears when aspirating, withdraw the needle and reinject it at another site.
   f. Withdraw the needle quickly at the same angle at which it was inserted.

8. What are components of a medication order? *(Select all that apply.)*
   a. Patient's name and a secondary identifier (date of birth, medical record number)
   b. The date and the time when the order is written
   c. Preferably the brand name of the drug to be administered
   d. The dosage of the drug, stated in either the apothecary or metric system
   e. The route by which the drug is to be administered, only if there is more than one route possible
   f. The signature of the nurse carrying out the order

CHAPTER 30

# Perioperative Nursing

## ASSESSING YOUR UNDERSTANDING

### FILL IN THE BLANKS

1. Nurses carry out a wide variety of nursing interventions prior to, during, and after surgery. This type of nursing is known as _______________ nursing.
2. A patient who presents at the emergency department with internal bleeding following a motor vehicle accident is scheduled for surgery. This type of surgery is classified as surgery based on _______________.
3. A patient who schedules knee replacement surgery is having a planned surgery classified as _______________ surgery.
4. Surgery is classified as minor or major based on _______________.
5. A patient is scheduled for jaw surgery. An appropriate choice for regional anesthesia for this patient is _______________.
6. A surgeon makes an incision in a patient undergoing gall bladder surgery. At this point in the surgical experience, the patient is in the _______________ phase of general anesthesia.
7. A patient who is scheduled for a colonoscopy would most likely receive what type of sedation? _______________
8. _______________ is a patient's voluntary agreement to undergo a particular procedure or treatment after receiving the appropriate information from the health care provider.
9. _______________ allow patients to specify instructions for health care treatment should they be unable to communicate these wishes postoperatively.
10. During The Joint Commission protocol known as the _______________, the surgical team members agree on the identity of the patient, the correct surgical site, and the procedure that will be performed.

### MATCHING EXERCISES

***Match the type of nurse listed in Part A with the role he or she performs listed in Part B. Answers may be used more than once.***

#### PART A

**a.** Scrub nurse

**b.** Circulating nurse

**c.** RNFA

**d.** APRN

**e.** PA

#### PART B

____ **1.** Member of the sterile team who maintains surgical asepsis while draping and handling instruments and supplies

____ **2.** Actively assists the surgeon by providing exposure, hemostasis, and wound closure

____ **3.** Coordinates care activities and collaborates with health care providers and nurses in all phases of perioperative and postanesthesia care

____ 4. Assesses the patient on admission to the operating room and collaborates in safely positioning the patient on the operating bed

____ 5. Integrates case management, critical paths, and research into care of the surgical patient

____ 6. Assists with monitoring the patient during surgery, provides additional supplies, and maintains environmental safety

**SHORT ANSWER**

1. Briefly describe the time period for the following stages of the perioperative period.
   a. Preoperative phase: ____
   b. Intraoperative phase: ____
   c. Postoperative phase: ____
2. Give a brief description of the following types of surgery.
   a. Based on urgency: ____
   b. Based on degree of risk: ____
   c. Based on purpose: ____
3. Describe the following three phases of anesthesia.
   a. Induction: ____
   b. Maintenance: ____
   c. Emergence: ____
4. Your patient is undergoing surgery to remove a lump from her breast. List six areas of information that should be given to the patient when securing informed consent.
   a. ____
   b. ____
   c. ____
   d. ____
   e. ____
   f. ____
5. Indicate how each of the following diseases places the patient at greater risk for postoperative complications.
   a. Cardiovascular disease: ____
   b. Pulmonary disorders: ____
   c. Kidney and liver function disorders: ____
   d. Endocrine disorders: ____
6. Explain how you would help your patient overcome the following fears experienced in the preoperative phase.
   a. Fear of the unknown: ____
   b. Fear of pain and death: ____
   c. Fear of changes in body image and self-concept: ____

7. Describe the nurse's role in providing screening tests for the preoperative patient.

8. Describe how you would prepare a preoperative patient for the following conditions.
   a. Surgical events and sensations:
   b. Pain management:

9. Describe how you would prepare a patient on the day of surgery in the following areas.
   a. Hygiene and skin preparation:
   b. Elimination:
   c. Nutrition and fluids:
   d. Rest and sleep:

10. Give three examples of expected outcomes for a patient during the intraoperative phase.
    a.
    b.
    c.

11. List the five phases that signify the return of CNS function.
    a.
    b.
    c.
    d.
    e.

12. Prepare a teaching plan for a postoperative patient who is moving into a home health care setting. Include the family in your planning.

13. Give an example of how the following factors may present a greater surgical risk for some patients.
    a. Developmental considerations:
    b. Medical history:
    c. Medications:
    d. Previous surgery:
    e. Perceptions and knowledge of surgery:
    f. Lifestyle:
    g. Nutrition:
    h. Use of alcohol, illicit drugs, nicotine:
    i. Activities of daily living:
    j. Occupation:
    k. Coping patterns:
    l. Support systems:
    m. Sociocultural needs:

14. Explain what a nurse in the PACU would assess when checking a patient in the postoperative phase using the following guidelines.
    a. Vital signs: ______________________
    b. Color and temperature of skin: ______________________
    c. Level of consciousness: ______________________
    d. Intravenous fluids: ______________________
    e. Surgical site: ______________________
    f. Other tubes: ______________________
    g. Pain management: ______________________
    h. Position and safety: ______________________
    i. Comfort: ______________________

15. Give an example of two nursing interventions you would institute for a postoperative patient to help alleviate the following problems that interfere with comfort.
    a. Nausea and vomiting: ______________________
    b. Thirst: ______________________
    c. Hiccups: ______________________
    d. Surgical pain: ______________________

## APPLYING YOUR KNOWLEDGE

### CRITICAL THINKING QUESTIONS

1. Prepare a preoperative assessment for the patients described below. Develop a nursing care plan for each patient based on the data collected. Be sure to include preoperative care, intraoperative care, and postoperative care in your planning.
    a. A 52-year-old man who smokes a pack of cigarettes a day is scheduled to undergo heart bypass surgery. The patient is overweight and says he rarely finds time to exercise.
    b. A 35-year-old woman is scheduled to undergo surgery to remove a colon tumor. She underwent radiation therapy 6 weeks before the surgery date. She has a family history of colon cancer.

   Reflect on how individual differences in patients influence their need for nursing and nursing's perioperative priorities.

2. Make a list of common postoperative complications. Describe how you would monitor the patient for these complications and what nursing measures you would take to prevent them. Be sure to include cardiovascular complications, shock, hemorrhage, thrombophlebitis, respiratory complications, pneumonia, atelectasis, and wound complications. Think of personal and system variables that might influence your effectiveness.

### REFLECTIVE PRACTICE: CULTIVATING QSEN COMPETENCIES

***Use the following expanded scenario from Chapter 30 in your textbook to answer the questions below.***

***Scenario:*** Molly Greenbaum is a 38-year-old woman diagnosed with recurring vaginal cysts. Her health care provider recommends a vaginal hysterectomy to be performed on an outpatient basis. She arrives at the hospital at 6:30 AM and is scheduled for surgery later in the day. The patient, with tears in her eyes and wringing her hands, says, "I really didn't sleep very much last night. I kept thinking about the surgery." She tells you she has been unable to sleep or eat properly since receiving the news, 2 weeks ago, that she needed a hysterectomy. She asks the nurse, "What if I don't feel like a woman anymore? What will this do to my sex life? Is this operation really necessary?"

1. How might the nurse use blended nursing skills to implement the perioperative plan of care in a manner that respects Ms. Greenbaum's human dignity and addresses her fears and concerns about the surgical experience?

______________________

______________________

______________________

2. What would be a successful outcome for this patient?

______________________________

______________________________

______________________________

3. What intellectual, technical, interpersonal, and/or ethical/legal competencies are most likely to bring about the desired outcome?

______________________________

______________________________

______________________________

4. What resources might be helpful for Ms. Greenbaum?

______________________________

______________________________

______________________________

## PRACTICING FOR NCLEX

### MULTIPLE CHOICE QUESTIONS

***Circle the letter that corresponds to the best choice for each question.***

1. A nurse administers regional anesthesia to a patient being prepared for facial surgery. What type of regional anesthesia would be the appropriate choice for this patient?
   - a. Nerve block
   - b. Subdural block
   - c. Surface anesthesia
   - d. Local infiltration with lidocaine
2. Which fact should the nurse keep in mind when obtaining consent forms from patients scheduled to undergo surgery?
   - a. A consent form is legal, even if the patient is confused or sedated.
   - b. The form that is signed is not a legal document and would not hold up in court.
   - c. In emergency situations, the doctor may obtain consent over the telephone.
   - d. The responsibility for securing informed consent from the patient lies with the nurse.
3. A 9-month-old baby is scheduled for heart surgery. When preparing this patient for surgery, the nurse should consider which surgical risk associated with infants?
   - a. Prolonged wound healing
   - b. Potential for hypothermia or hyperthermia
   - c. Congestive heart failure
   - d. Gastrointestinal upset
4. A patient is scheduled for elective hernia surgery. While taking a medical history, the nurse learns that the patient is taking antibiotics for an infection. Which surgical risk should the nurse monitor based on this antibiotic use?
   - a. Hemorrhage
   - b. Electrolyte imbalances
   - c. Cardiovascular collapse
   - d. Respiratory paralysis
5. When preparing a patient who has diabetes mellitus for surgery, the nurse should be aware of what surgical risk associated with this disease?
   - a. Fluid and electrolyte imbalance
   - b. Slow wound healing
   - c. Respiratory depression from anesthesia
   - d. Altered metabolism and excretion of drugs
6. The nurse is assessing an obese patient scheduled for heart surgery. Which surgical risk related to obesity should the nurse monitor?
   - a. Delayed wound healing and wound infection
   - b. Alterations in fluid and electrolyte balance
   - c. Respiratory distress
   - d. Hemorrhage
7. The nurse is providing teaching for a postoperative patient regarding pain management. Which teaching point should the nurse include?
   - a. "Be sure to ask for your PRN medication when the pain becomes severe."
   - b. "If your pain is not relieved, ask your nurse to order a different medication."
   - c. "You will receive pain medication by injection as long as you are NPO."
   - d. "All postoperative pain control methods will be given by injection."

8. Which nursing action should the PACU nurse take to prevent postoperative complications in patients?
   a. Instruct the patient to avoid coughing to prevent injury to the incision.
   b. Encourage the patient to breathe shallowly to prevent collapse of the alveoli.
   c. Assist the patient to do leg exercises to increase venous return.
   d. Avoid turning the patient in bed until the incision is no longer painful.
9. The nurse is assessing patients for postoperative complications. What is the most commonly assessed postanesthesia recovery emergency?
   a. Respiratory obstruction
   b. Cardiac distress
   c. Wound infection
   d. Dehydration
10. A nurse is monitoring a patient post cardiac surgery. What action would help to prevent cardiovascular complications for this patient?
    a. Position the patient in bed with pillows placed under his knees to hasten venous return.
    b. Keep the patient from ambulating until the day after surgery.
    c. Implement leg exercises and turn the patient in bed every 2 hours.
    d. Keep the patient cool and uncovered to prevent elevated temperature.
11. A nurse caring for patients in a PACU assesses a patient who is displaying signs and symptoms of shock. What is the priority nursing intervention for this patient?
    a. Remove extra coverings on the patient to keep temperature down.
    b. Place the patient in a flat position with legs elevated 45 degrees.
    c. Do not administer any further medication.
    d. Place the patient in the prone position.
12. What intervention would a nurse perform when physically preparing a patient undergoing surgery?
    a. Shave the area of the incision with a razor.
    b. Empty the patient's bowel of feces.
    c. Do not allow the patient to eat or drink anything for 8 to 12 hours before surgery.
    d. Ensure that the patient is well nourished and hydrated.
13. A nurse administers anticholinergics to a patient as a postoperative medication. What condition does this medication help to prevent?
    a. Cardiovascular complications
    b. Laryngospasm
    c. Nausea
    d. Shock
14. In which position would the surgical nurse place a patient undergoing minimally invasive surgery of the lower abdomen or pelvis?
    a. Trendelenburg position
    b. Sims' position
    c. Lithotomy position
    d. Prone position
15. A nurse is assessing a patient who is experiencing pulmonary embolus. What would be the priority nursing intervention for this patient?
    a. Attempt to overhydrate the patient with fluids.
    b. Instruct the patient to perform Valsalva's maneuver.
    c. Place the patient in semi-Fowler's position.
    d. Assist the patient to ambulate every 2 to 3 hours.
16. A postsurgical patient is experiencing decreased lung sounds, dyspnea, cyanosis, crackles, restlessness, and apprehension. Which condition would the nurse suspect?
    a. Atelectasis
    b. Pneumonia
    c. Pulmonary embolus
    d. Thrombophlebitis

## ALTERNATE-FORMAT QUESTIONS

### Multiple Response Questions

***Circle the letters that correspond to the best answers for each question.***

1. A nurse is assessing patients in a PACU. Which nursing actions would the nurse perform in this phase of the perioperative period? *(Select all that apply.)*
   a. Prepare the patient for home care.
   b. Inform the patient that surgical intervention is necessary.
   c. Transfer the patient to the recovery room.
   d. Admit the patient to the recovery area.
   e. Assess for complications as the patient emerges from anesthesia.
   f. Arrange for a rehabilitative program for the patient.
2. Which patients would the nurse schedule for surgery based on purpose? *(Select all that apply.)*
   a. A patient who has uncontrolled bleeding
   b. A patient undergoing a breast biopsy
   c. A patient needing a cleft palate repair
   d. A patient needing a bowel resection
   e. A patient in respiratory distress who needs a tracheostomy
   f. A patient post mastectomy who decides to have breast reconstruction
3. Which methods would the nurse use when administering regional anesthesia to surgical patients? *(Select all that apply.)*
   a. Inhalation
   b. Spinal block
   c. Intravenous
   d. Oral route
   e. Nerve block
   f. Epidural block
4. What information must be provided to a patient to obtain informed consent? *(Select all that apply.)*
   a. A description of the procedure or treatment, along with potential alternative therapies
   b. The name and qualifications of the nurse providing perioperative care
   c. The underlying disease process and its natural course
   d. Explanation of the risks involved and how often they occur
   e. Explanation that a signed consent form is binding and cannot be withdrawn
   f. Customary insurance coverage for the procedure
5. Which factors would the nurse consider when assessing surgical patients following surgery? *(Select all that apply.)*
   a. Infants are at a greater risk from surgery than are middle-aged adults.
   b. Infants experience a slower metabolism of drugs that require renal biotransformation.
   c. Muscle relaxants and narcotics have a shorter duration of action in infants.
   d. Older adults have decreased renal blood flow and a reduced bladder capacity, necessitating careful monitoring of fluid and electrolyte status and input and output.
   e. Older adults have an increased gastric pH and require monitoring of nutritional status during the perioperative period.
   f. Older adults have an increased hepatic blood flow, liver mass, and enzyme function that prolongs the duration of medication effects.
6. Which factors should the nurse consider when assessing patients for postsurgical risks? *(Select all that apply.)*
   a. Cardiovascular diseases increase the risk for dehydration after surgery.
   b. Patients with respiratory disease may experience alterations in acid–base balance after surgery.
   c. Kidney and liver diseases influence the patient's response to anesthesia.
   d. Endocrine diseases increase the risk for hyperglycemia after surgery.
   e. Endocrine diseases increase the risk for slow surgical wound healing.
   f. Pulmonary disorders increase the risk for hemorrhage and hypovolemic shock after surgery.
7. Which effects of medications should the nurse consider when assessing patients for surgical risks? *(Select all that apply.)*
   a. Diuretics may precipitate hemorrhage.
   b. Anticoagulants may cause electrolyte imbalances.

c. Diuretics may cause respiratory depression from anesthesia.
d. Tranquilizers may increase the hypotensive effect of anesthetic agents.
e. Adrenal steroids may cause respiratory paralysis.
f. Abrupt withdrawal from adrenal steroids may cause cardiovascular collapse in long-term users.

8. Which examples accurately describe significant abnormal findings related to presurgical screening tests that the nurse should report to the surgeon? *(Select all that apply.)*
   a. An elevated white blood cell count, indicating an infection
   b. Decreased hematocrit and hemoglobin level, indicating bleeding or anemia
   c. Increased hyperkalemia or hypokalemia, indicating possible renal failure
   d. Elevated blood urea nitrogen or creatinine levels, indicating an increased risk for cardiac problems
   e. Abnormal urine constituents, indicating infection or fluid imbalances
   f. Increased hemoglobin level, indicating infection

9. Which nursing interventions would be appropriate for a patient recovering from a surgical procedure? *(Select all that apply.)*
   a. Teach the patient to suppress urges to cough in order to protect the incision.
   b. Encourage the patient to take frequent shallow breaths to improve lung expansion and volume.
   c. Place the patient in a semi-Fowler's position to perform deep-breathing exercises every 1 to 2 hours for the first 24 to 48 hours after surgery and as necessary thereafter.
   d. Encourage the patient to lie still in bed with the incision facing upward to prevent putting pressure on the stitches.
   e. Teach the patient the appropriate leg exercises to increase venous blood return from the legs.
   f. Encourage the patient to use incentive spirometry 10 times each waking hour for the first 5 days after surgery.

**Prioritization Questions**

1. Place the following guidelines for teaching a patient deep breathing in the order in which they would be performed:
   a. Ask the patient to inhale through the nose gently and completely.
   b. Place the patient in semi-Fowler's position with the neck and shoulders supported.
   c. Ask the patient to exhale gently and completely.
   d. Repeat this exercise three times every 1 to 2 hours.
   e. Ask the patient to place the hands over the rib cage so he or she can feel the chest rise as the lungs expand.
   f. Ask the patient to exhale as completely as possible through the mouth with lips pursed (as if whistling).
   g. Ask the patient to hold his or her breath for 3 to 5 seconds and mentally count "one, one thousand, two, one thousand, etc."

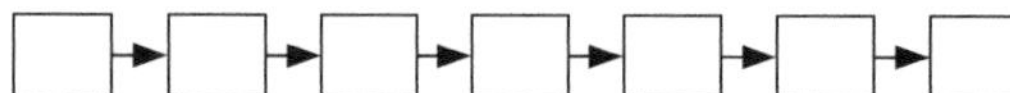

2. Place the following guidelines for teaching a patient effective coughing in the order in which they would be performed:
   a. Ask the patient to "hack out" for three short breaths.
   b. Repeat the exercise every 2 hours while awake.
   c. Place the patient in a semi-Fowler's position, leaning forward, and provide a pillow or bath blanket to splint the incision.
   d. Ask the patient to cough deeply once or twice and take another deep breath.
   e. Ask the patient to take a quick breath with mouth open.
   f. Ask the patient to inhale and exhale deeply and slowly through the nose three times.
   g. Ask the patient to take a deep breath and hold it for 3 seconds.

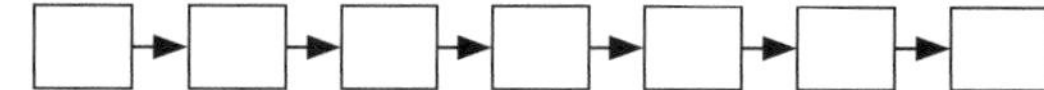

CHAPTER 31

# Hygiene

## ASSESSING YOUR UNDERSTANDING

### FILL IN THE BLANKS

1. A nurse assesses the mouth of a patient and documents ___________, which is an inflammation of the tissue that surrounds the teeth.
2. The nurse notes that a patient has patchy losses of hair on his head related to an infection. This hair loss is known as baldness or ___________.
3. Infestation with lice is called ___________.
4. The nursing care provided to a patient shortly before he or she retires to bed (assistance with toileting, washing face and hands, and oral care) is known as ___________ care.
5. The nurse uses a self-contained bathing system consisting of a plastic bag containing 8 to 10 premoistened washcloths to wash a patient. This type of bath is called a(n) ___________.

### MATCHING EXERCISES

***Match the oral diseases/conditions in Part A with their definitions listed in Part B.***

**PART A**

**a.** Stomatitis
**b.** Gingivitis
**c.** Periodontitis
**d.** Halitosis
**e.** Plaque
**f.** Tartar
**g.** Glossitis
**h.** Cheilosis
**i.** Dry oral mucosa
**j.** Oral malignancies
**k.** Caries
**l.** *Candida albicans*

**PART B**

____ **1.** A strong mouth odor
____ **2.** A marked inflammation of the gums involving the alveolar tissues
____ **3.** Ulceration of the lips, most often caused by vitamin B complex deficiencies
____ **4.** Lumps or ulcers
____ **5.** Inflammation of the oral mucosa with numerous causes (bacteria, virus, mechanical trauma, irritants, nutritional deficiencies, and systemic infection)
____ **6.** May be related to dehydration or may be caused by mouth breathing, an alteration in salivary functioning, or certain medications
____ **7.** Hard deposits at the gum lines that attack the fibers that fasten teeth to the gums and eventually attack bone tissue
____ **8.** An inflammation of the tissue that surrounds the teeth
____ **9.** An invisible, destructive bacterial film that builds up on everyone's teeth and eventually leads to the destruction of tooth enamel
____ **10.** An inflammation of the tongue
____ **11.** The formation of cavities

## CORRECT THE FALSE STATEMENTS

***Circle the word "true" or "false" that follows the statement. If you circled "false," change the underlined word or words to make the statement true. Place your answer in the space provided.***

1. The sebaceous glands secrete cerumen, which consists of a heavy oil and brown pigment, into the external ear canals.
   a. True
   b. False ____________________
2. Fluid loss through fever, vomiting, or diarrhea reduces the fluid volume of the body and is called dehydration.
   a. True
   b. False ____________________
3. Jaundice, a condition caused by excessive bile pigments in the skin, results in a grayish skin color.
   a. True
   b. False ____________________
4. A nurse ensures the patient's comfort after lunch and offers assistance to nonambulatory patients with toileting, handwashing, and oral care during afternoon care (PM care).
   a. True
   b. False ____________________
5. Before leaving the patient's bedside, the nurse should ensure that the bed is in its highest position.
   a. True
   b. False ____________________
6. The odor of perspiration occurs when bacteria act on the skin's normal secretions.
   a. True
   b. False ____________________
7. Dry skin is especially bothersome during adolescence.
   a. True
   b. False ____________________
8. Pressure ulcers are areas of cellular necrosis caused by increased blood circulation to the involved area.
   a. True
   b. False ____________________
9. Rigid gas permeable (RGP) lenses are more inflexible than soft lenses.
   a. True
   b. False ____________________
10. When providing perineal care for a female patient, the nurse should spread the labia and move the washcloth from the pubic area toward the anal area to prevent carrying organisms from the anal area back over the genital area.
    a. True
    b. False ____________________
11. Pediculus humanus capitis infests the body.
    a. True
    b. False ____________________
12. A health care provider who treats foot disorders is known as a pediatrician.
    a. True
    b. False ____________________
13. Depending on the patient's self-care abilities, the nurse offers assistance with toileting, oral care, bathing, back massage, special skin care measures, cosmetics, dressing, and positioning for comfort during the afternoon care schedule.
    a. True
    b. False ____________________

## SHORT ANSWER

1. Briefly describe how the following factors may influence personal hygiene behaviors.
   a. Culture: ____________________
   b. Socioeconomic class: ____________________
   c. Spiritual practices: ____________________
   d. Developmental level: ____________________
   e. Health state: ____________________
   f. Personal preference: ____________________

**2.** List four specific activities necessary to meet daily needs that may be addressed as self-care deficits.

**a.** ______________________

**b.** ______________________

**c.** ______________________

**d.** ______________________

**3.** A mother brings her 6-month-old baby to a well-baby clinic for immunizations. Upon examining the infant, you notice dirt accumulated in the skin folds and a scaly scalp. Write a sample diagnosis for the infant's hygiene deficit. Develop a nursing care plan for the infant and mother that includes teaching hygiene.

______________________

______________________

______________________

**4.** Describe the activities the nurse would perform in the following scheduled care time periods.

**a.** Early morning care: ______________________

______________________

______________________

**b.** Morning care: ______________________

______________________

______________________

**c.** Afternoon care: ______________________

______________________

______________________

**d.** Hour of sleep care: ______________________

______________________

______________________

**e.** As-needed care: ______________________

______________________

______________________

**5.** List five benefits of bathing.

**a.** ______________________

**b.** ______________________

**c.** ______________________

**d.** ______________________

**e.** ______________________

**6.** Describe how you would prepare a bed bath for a patient who is able to wash himself.

______________________

______________________

______________________

**7.** List four advantages of a towel bath.

**a.** ______________________

**b.** ______________________

**c.** ______________________

**d.** ______________________

**8.** List three benefits of a back rub.

**a.** ______________________

**b.** ______________________

**c.** ______________________

**9.** Describe how the following conditions should be controlled in order to provide a comfortable environment for the patient.

**a.** Ventilation: ______________________

______________________

______________________

**b.** Odors: ______________________

______________________

______________________

**c.** Room temperature: ______________________

______________________

______________________

**d.** Lighting and noise: ______________________

______________________

______________________

**10.** You are visiting a patient at home who is recovering from heart surgery. When you prepare a bed bath for the patient, you notice her skin is dry and flaky. List four interventions you could use for this patient to prevent injury and irritation.

**a.** ______________________

**b.** ______________________

**c.** ______________________

**d.** ______________________

**11.** Describe the conditions you would look for when assessing the following areas.

**a.** Lips: ______

**b.** Buccal mucosa: ______

**c.** Gums: ______

**d.** Tongue: ______

**e.** Hard and soft palates: ______

**f.** Eye: ______

**g.** Ear: ______

**h.** Nose: ______

**12.** Describe how you would clean the following areas for a patient.

**a.** Eye: ______

**b.** Ear: ______

**c.** Nose: ______

**13.** Briefly describe the care necessary for the following corrective devices.

**a.** Contact lenses: ______

**b.** Artificial eye: ______

**c.** Hearing aids: ______

**d.** Dentures: ______

**14.** List four variables known to cause nail and foot problems.

**a.** ______

**b.** ______

**c.** ______

**d.** ______

## APPLYING YOUR KNOWLEDGE

### CRITICAL THINKING QUESTIONS

**1.** Think about nurses' responsibility to assist patients with daily hygiene. Then reflect on how you would respond in the following situations. See if your classmates would respond as you do.

**a.** A same-age, opposite-sex patient requires total assistance with hygiene.

**b.** A patient confined to bed but able to assist with hygiene refuses to do so.

**c.** An older adult incontinent patient refuses your offer to assist her with perineal care.

**2.** Interview patients of different backgrounds or cultures to find out how they perform their daily hygiene routine. Note how their routine is similar to or different from your personal routine. What would you do to assist these people if they were placed in your care?

### REFLECTIVE PRACTICE: CULTIVATING QSEN COMPETENCIES

***Use the following expanded scenario from Chapter 31 in your textbook to answer the questions below.***

*Scenario:* Sonya Delamordo is an older Hispanic woman who has had a stroke, resulting in right-sided paralysis. She is being discharged from the hospital and will now live with her daughter, who will be her primary caretaker. Her daughter, who is eager to help her mother, asks numerous questions about how to keep her mother clean. She tells the nurse she is worried about being able to take care of her mother's fine hair, as well as her dentures and hearing aids.

**1.** What patient teaching should be implemented to help meet the hygienic needs of Ms. Delamordo?

**2.** What would be a successful outcome for this patient?

3. What intellectual, technical, interpersonal, and/or ethical/legal competencies are most likely to bring about the desired outcome?
4. What resources might be helpful for Ms. Delamordo and her daughter?

### PATIENT CARE STUDY

***Read the following patient care study and use your nursing process skills to answer the questions below.***

*Scenario:* Dominic Gianmarco, a 78-year-old retired man with a history of Parkinson's disease, lives alone in a small home. He was recently hospitalized for problems with cardiac rhythm, and a pacemaker was installed. The home health care nurse visits 1 week after he was discharged to monitor his recovery and compliance with his medication regimen. The nurse observes that Mr. Gianmarco is disheveled, and there are multiple stains on his clothing. Several food items are in various stages of preparation on the kitchen counter, and some appear to have spoiled. Mr. Gianmarco has several days' growth of beard, and a body odor is apparent. He is pleasant and oriented to place and person but cannot identify the time or day of the week: "I lose track of what day it is. Time is not important when you are my age. The most important thing to me right now is to be able to take care of myself and stay in this house near my friends." There is a walker visible in a corner of the living room, but Mr. Gianmarco ambulates slowly around the house with a minimum of difficulty and does not use the walker. He comments that he keeps busy "reading, watching old movies, and going to senior citizen activities with friends who stop by for me." His daughter, who lives several hours away, visits him every weekend and prepares his medications for the week in a plastic container that is easy for him to open. The nurse observes that all the medications appeared to have been taken to date: "I don't mess around with my medicines. One helps my ticker and the others keep me from shaking so much."

1. Identify pertinent patient data by placing a single underline beneath the objective data in the case study and a double underline beneath the subjective data.
2. Complete the Nursing Process Worksheet on page 194 to develop a three-part diagnostic statement and related plan of care for this patient.
3. Write down the patient and personal nursing strengths you hope to draw on as you assist this patient to better health.

   Patient strengths: ________________________

   ________________________________________

   ________________________________________

   Personal strengths: ________________________

   ________________________________________

   ________________________________________
4. Pretend that you are performing a nursing assessment of this patient after the plan of care is implemented. Document your findings.

   ________________________________________

   ________________________________________

   ________________________________________

## PRACTICING FOR NCLEX

### MULTIPLE CHOICE QUESTIONS

***Circle the letter that corresponds to the best answer for each question.***

1. The nurse is teaching an adolescent how to treat acne. What would the nurse include as a teaching point?
   a. Gently squeeze the infected areas to release the infection.
   b. Wash your face less frequently to avoid removing beneficial oils.
   c. Keep hair off the face and wash hair daily.
   d. Use cosmetics and emollients to cover the condition.
2. When caring for a patient with dentures, what should the nurse teach the patient?
   a. Keeping dentures out for long periods of time permits the gum line to change, affecting denture fit.
   b. Dentures should be wrapped in tissue or a disposable wipe when out of the mouth and stored in a disposable cup.
   c. Dentures should never be stored in water because the plastic material may warp.
   d. A brush and nonabrasive powder should be used to clean the dentures, and hot water should be used to rinse them.

3. The nurse is providing perineal care for patients in a hospital setting. What is an appropriate nursing action when providing this type of care?
   a. Always proceed from the most contaminated area to the least contaminated area.
   b. Do not retract the foreskin in an uncircumcised male.
   c. Dry the cleaned areas and apply an emollient as indicated.
   d. Powder the area to prevent the growth of bacteria.
4. Which nursing action is appropriate when providing foot care for a patient?
   a. Soak the feet in a solution of mild soap and tepid water.
   b. Rinse the feet, dry thoroughly, and apply moisturizer on the tops and bottoms.
   c. For diabetic patients, trim the nails with nail clippers.
   d. Cut off any corns or calluses.
5. When bathing a patient, the nurse notices that the patient has a rash on her arms. What would be an appropriate nursing intervention?
   a. Avoid washing the area because cleansing agents will only make the rash worse.
   b. Use a tepid bath to relieve inflammation and itching.
   c. Do not use over-the-counter products on unknown rashes.
   d. Use a moisturizing lotion on a wet rash to prevent itching.
6. A nurse caring for the skin of patients of different age groups should consider which accurately described condition?
   a. An infant's skin and mucous membranes are protected from infection by a natural immunity.
   b. Secretions from skin glands are at their maximum from age 3 on.
   c. The skin becomes thicker and more leathery with aging and is prone to wrinkles and dryness.
   d. An adolescent's skin ordinarily has enlarged sebaceous glands and increased glandular secretions.

## ALTERNATE-FORMAT QUESTIONS

### Multiple Response Questions

***Circle the letters that correspond to the best answers for each question.***

1. A nurse is making an unoccupied bed for a hospitalized patient. Which actions are appropriate steps for the nurse to perform? *(Select all that apply.)*
   a. First, adjust the bed to the high position and drop the side rails.
   b. Fold reusable linens on the bed in fourths and hang them over a clean chair.
   c. Snugly roll the soiled linens into the bottom sheet and place on the floor next to the bed.
   d. Place the bottom sheet with its center fold in the center of the bed and place the drawsheet with its center fold in the center of the bed.
   e. Tuck the bottom sheets securely under the head of the mattress, forming a corner according to facility policy.
   f. Place the pillow at the head of the bed with the closed end facing toward the window.
2. A nurse is preparing the environment in a hospital room for a newly admitted patient. Which actions are recommended? *(Select all that apply.)*
   a. Do not store patient's personal items in the bedside stand because nurses need to open and close the stand to obtain bath basin, lotion, and other items.
   b. Position patient beds at the appropriate height with the wheels unlocked.
   c. Follow principles of surgical asepsis at the bedside.
   d. Do not place soiled dressings or anything with a strong odor in the waste receptacle in the patient's room.
   e. In general, keep the room temperature between 20° and 23°C (68° and 74°F).
   f. Avoid carrying out conversations immediately outside the patient's room.

**3.** Which statements accurately describe findings the nurse would document when performing a physical assessment of the oral cavity? *(Select all that apply.)*

**a.** Caries may exist in the teeth, resulting from the failure to remove plaque.

**b.** Gingivitis may be present involving the alveolar tissues.

**c.** Hard deposits of tartar may be found on the teeth if plaque is allowed to build up.

**d.** Stomatitis may be noted as an inflammation of the tongue.

**e.** Cheilosis may present as reddened fissures at the angles of the mouth.

**f.** Oral malignancies may be present in the form of a dry oral mucosa.

**4.** Which nursing actions are recommended guidelines when performing oral care? *(Select all that apply.)*

**a.** Use a hard toothbrush to remove plaque from the teeth.

**b.** Ideally, brush teeth immediately after eating or drinking.

**c.** Never clean the tongue with a toothbrush.

**d.** If desired, use an automatic toothbrush to remove debris and plaque from teeth.

**e.** Never use water-spray units to assist with oral hygiene.

**f.** If desired, use salt and sodium bicarbonate as cleaning agents for short-term use.

**5.** What are appropriate nursing measures when caring for a patient's eyes and ears? *(Select all that apply.)*

**a.** Clean the eye from the inner canthus to the outer canthus using a wet, warm washcloth; cotton ball; or compress.

**b.** Use artificial tear solution or normal saline twice a day when the blink reflex is decreased or absent.

**c.** Use a protective shield if necessary to keep the lids closed when the blink reflex is absent.

**d.** Use boric acid to remove excess secretions from the eyes.

**e.** Clean the patient's external ear with a washcloth-covered finger.

**f.** Use cotton-tipped swabs to clean the inner ear and to remove cerumen.

## NURSING PROCESS WORKSHEET

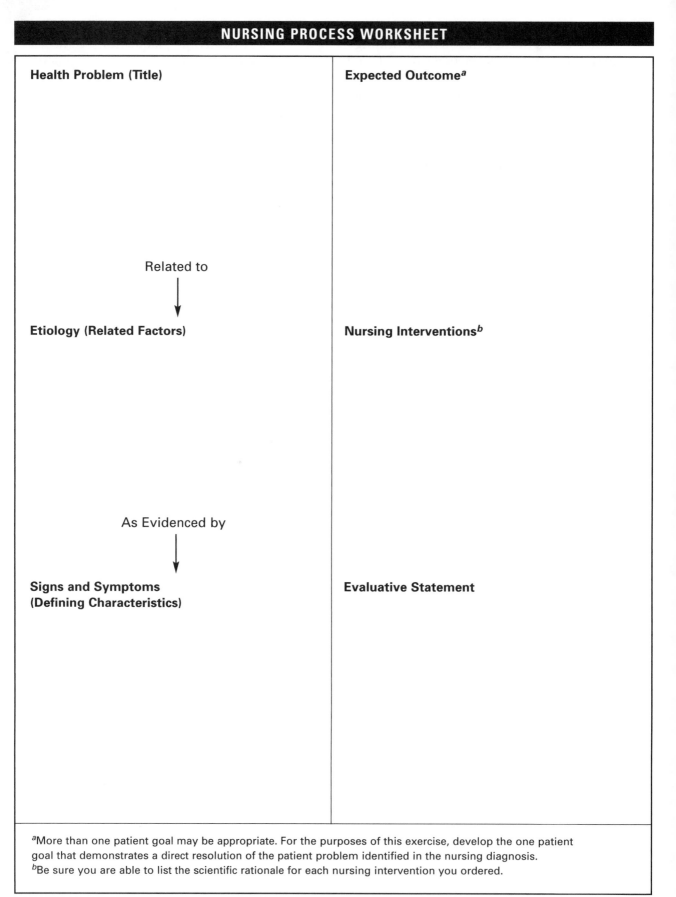

**Health Problem (Title)**

Related to

↓

**Etiology (Related Factors)**

As Evidenced by

↓

**Signs and Symptoms (Defining Characteristics)**

**Expected Outcome[a]**

**Nursing Interventions[b]**

**Evaluative Statement**

[a]More than one patient goal may be appropriate. For the purposes of this exercise, develop the one patient goal that demonstrates a direct resolution of the patient problem identified in the nursing diagnosis.
[b]Be sure you are able to list the scientific rationale for each nursing intervention you ordered.

CHAPTER 32

# Skin Integrity and Wound Care

## ASSESSING YOUR UNDERSTANDING

### FILL IN THE BLANKS

1. The nurse is changing the dressing on a patient's incision. This type of wound is commonly known as a(n) ____________ wound.
2. The nurse notes swelling and pain occurring from an incision. These symptoms are most likely caused by an accumulation of ____________.
3. A patient's wound is in the inflammatory cellular phase, meaning that ____________ or ____________ cells arrive first to ingest bacteria and cellular debris.
4. New tissue found in a wound that is highly vascular, bleeds easily, and is formed in the proliferative phase is known as ____________ tissue.
5. The nurse is measuring the depth of a patient's wound and discovers an abnormal passage from an internal organ to the skin. This wound condition is known as a(n) ____________.
6. When cleaning a wound, the nurse might choose sterile 9% ____________ as the cleansing solution.
7. The nurse anchors a bandage by wrapping it around the patient's body part with complete overlapping of the previous bandage turn. This procedure is the ____________ method of bandage wrapping.
8. A nurse assessing a patient's wound documents a localized area of tissue necrosis. This type of wound is known as a(n) ____________.

### MATCHING EXERCISES

***Match the term in Part A with the correct definition in Part B.***

**PART A**

a. Dehiscence
b. Ischemia
c. Eschar
d. Wound
e. Exudate
f. Granulation tissue
g. Epithelialization
h. Scar
i. Hemorrhage
j. Evisceration
k. Serous wound drainage
l. Sanguineous wound drainage
m. Purulent wound drainage
n. Red wounds
o. Yellow wounds
p. Black wounds
q. Dressing

**PART B**

____ **1.** The partial or total disruption of wound layers

____ **2.** New tissue, pink-red in color, composed of fibroblasts and small blood vessels that fill an open wound when it starts to heal

____ **3.** Natural act of healing of dermal and epidermal tissue in which a protective membrane forms over a wound

____ **4.** The protrusion of viscera through the incisional area

____ **5.** Composed of fluid and cells that escape from the blood vessels and are deposited in or on tissue surfaces

____ **6.** Wounds in the proliferative stage of healing that are the color of granulation tissue

____ **7.** Wound drainage that is composed of the clear, serous portion of the blood and drainage from serous membranes

____ **8.** Wounds that are covered with thick eschar, which is usually black but may be brown, gray, or tan

____ **9.** May occur from a slipped suture, a dislodged clot from stress at the suture line, infection, or the erosion of a blood vessel by a foreign body (such as a drain)

____ **10.** Wound drainage that is made up of white blood cells, liquefied dead tissue debris, and both dead and live bacteria

____ **11.** Wounds that are characterized by oozing from the tissue covering the wound, often accompanied by purulent drainage

____ **12.** Necrotic tissue

____ **13.** A disruption in the normal integrity of the skin

____ **14.** Avascular collagen tissue that does not sweat, grow hair, or tan in sunlight

____ **15.** Wound drainage that consists of large numbers of red blood cells and looks like blood

***Match the wound care dressings and wraps in Part A with their definition/indication listed in Part B. Some answers may be used more than once.***

**PART A**

**a.** Telfa

**b.** Gauze dressings

**c.** Sof-Wick

**d.** ABDs, Surgipads

**e.** Transparent films

**f.** Bandages

**g.** Binders

**h.** Roller bandages

**PART B**

____ **16.** Strips of cloth, gauze, or elasticized material used to wrap a body part

____ **17.** A special gauze that covers the incision line and allows drainage to pass through and be absorbed by the center absorbent layer

____ **18.** Wraps designed for a specific body part

____ **19.** Used to prevent outer dressings from adhering to the wound and causing further injury when removed

____ **20.** Commonly used to cover wounds; they come in various sizes and are commercially packaged as single units or in packs.

____ **21.** Placed over the smaller gauze to absorb drainage and protect the wound from contamination or injury

____ **22.** Precut halfway to fit around drains or tubes

____ **23.** Applied directly over a small wound or tube, these dressings are occlusive, decreasing the possibility of contamination while allowing visualization of the wound

____ **24.** They may be made of cloth (flannel or muslin) or an elasticized material that fastens together with Velcro

____ **25.** The type of dressing often used over intravenous sites, subclavian catheter insertion sites, and noninfected healing wounds

**SHORT ANSWER**

**1.** List six major functions of the skin.

**a.** ____________________

**b.** ____________________

**c.** ____________________

**d.** ____________________

**e.** ____________________

**f.** ____________________

**2.** Describe how the following mechanisms contribute to pressure injury development.

**a.** External pressure: ______

**b.** Friction and shearing forces: ______

**3.** Give an example of how the following factors affect the likelihood that a patient will develop a pressure injury.

**a.** Nutrition: ______

**b.** Hydration: ______

**c.** Moisture on the skin: ______

**d.** Mental status: ______

**e.** Age: ______

**f.** Immobility: ______

**4.** When visiting a patient recovering from a stroke in her home, you notice a pressure injury developing on her coccyx. Develop a nursing care plan for this patient that involves the family in the treatment of the injury.

______

**5.** Briefly describe the phases of wound healing.

**a.** Hemostasis: ______

**b.** Inflammatory phase: ______

**c.** Proliferative phase: ______

**d.** Maturation phase: ______

**6.** List three goals for patients who are at risk for impaired skin integrity.

**a.** ______

**b.** ______

**c.** ______

**7.** Give two examples of interview questions that could be asked to assess a patient's skin integrity in the following areas.

**a.** Overall appearance of the skin: ______

**b.** Recent changes in skin condition: ______

**c.** Activity/mobility: ______

**d.** Nutrition: ______

**e.** Pain: ______

**f.** Elimination: ______

**8.** Describe how you would assess the following aspects of wound healing.

**a.** Appearance: ______

**b.** Wound drainage: ______

**c.** Pain: ______

**d.** Sutures and staples: ______

9. List the purposes for wound dressings. ______

______

______

10. Describe the RYB color classification and care of open wounds.
    a. R = red = protect: ______

    ______

    ______

    b. Y = yellow = cleanse: ______

    ______

    ______

    c. B = black = debride: ______

    ______

    ______

11. Briefly describe the use of the following methods of applying heat and any advantages or disadvantages.
    a. Hot water bags or bottles: ______

    ______

    b. Electric heating pad: ______

    ______

    c. Aquathermia pad: ______

    ______

    d. Chemical heat packs: ______

    ______

    e. Warm moist compresses: ______

    ______

    f. Sitz baths: ______

    ______

    g. Warm soaks: ______

    ______

## APPLYING YOUR KNOWLEDGE

### CRITICAL THINKING QUESTIONS

1. Develop a nursing plan to assist the following patients who are at high risk for pressure injuries.
    a. A comatose 35-year-old man
    b. A frail older adult who is confined to bed
    c. A 20-year-old woman who is in a lower body cast
    d. A premature baby on life support

    What knowledge and skills do you need to prevent pressure injuries in these patients?

2. Follow the wound care for three patients with different types of wounds (e.g., gunshot wound, a wound from surgery, a pressure injury). Help the nurse assess the wound each day and apply the dressings. Interview the patients to see how the wound has affected their mobility, sensory perception, activity, nutrition, and exposure to friction and shear. Keep a log of the daily changes in the wound.

### REFLECTIVE PRACTICE: CULTIVATING QSEN COMPETENCIES

***Use the following expanded scenario from Chapter 32 in your textbook to answer the questions below.***

***Scenario:*** Sam Bentz is a 56-year-old man admitted to the hospital for aggressive treatment of a bone infection that has not responded to usual methods. His wife has been taking care of him at home for the past 3 weeks. She states that the medicines the doctor prescribed made her husband feel sick to his stomach and occasionally made him throw up. She says her husband spent most of his day in bed and had no energy to get up to wash or eat. Mr. Bentz is 5 ft 4 in tall and weighs more than 300 lb. During the nursing assessment, he says, “Last time I was here, my skin got really irritated and I developed several skin wounds.”

1. What nursing intervention would be appropriate to prevent skin irritation and the development of pressure injuries for Mr. Bentz?

______

______

______

2. What would be a successful outcome for this patient?

______

______

______

3. What intellectual, technical, interpersonal, and/or ethical/legal competencies are most likely to bring about the desired outcome?

______________________________________

______________________________________

______________________________________

4. What resources might be helpful for Mr. Bentz and his wife?

______________________________________

______________________________________

______________________________________

### PATIENT CARE STUDY

***Read the following patient care study and use your nursing process skills to answer the questions below.***

*Scenario:* Mrs. Chijioke, an 88-year-old woman who has lived alone for years, was brought to the hospital after neighbors found her lying at the bottom of her cellar steps. She had broken her hip and underwent hip repair surgery 3 days ago. The nurse assigned to care for Mrs. Chijioke noticed during the patient's bath that the skin of her coccyx, heels, and elbows was reddened. The skin returned to a normal color when pressure was relieved in these areas. There was no edema, nor was there induration or blistering. Although Mrs. Chijioke can be lifted out of bed into a chair, she spends most of the day in bed, lying on her back with an abductor pillow between her legs. At 5 ft tall and 89 lb, Mrs. Chijioke looks lost in the big hospital bed. Her eyes are bright, and she usually attempts a warm smile, but she has little physical strength and lies seemingly motionless for hours. Her skin is wrinkled and paper thin, and her arms are bruised from unsuccessful attempts at intravenous therapy. She was dehydrated on admission because she had spent almost 48 hours crumpled at the bottom of her steps before being found by her neighbors, and she was clearly in need of nutritional, fluid, and electrolyte support. A long-time diabetic, Mrs. Chijioke is now spiking a fever (39.0°C, or 102.2°F), which concerns her nurse.

1. Identify pertinent patient data by placing a single underline beneath the objective data in the patient care study and a double underline beneath the subjective data.

2. Complete the Nursing Process Worksheet on page 204 to develop a three-part diagnostic statement and related plan of care for this patient.

3. Write down the patient and personal nursing strengths you hope to draw upon as you assist this patient to better health.

   Patient strengths: ______________________

   ______________________________________

   ______________________________________

   Personal strengths: ______________________

   ______________________________________

   ______________________________________

4. Pretend that you are performing a nursing assessment of this patient after the plan of care is implemented. Document your findings.

______________________________________

______________________________________

______________________________________

## PRACTICING FOR NCLEX

### MULTIPLE CHOICE QUESTIONS

***Circle the letter that corresponds to the best answer for each question.***

1. A female patient who is being treated for self-inflicted wounds tells the nurse that she is anorexic. What criteria would alert the health care worker to her nutritional risk?
   a. Albumin level of 3.5 mg/dL
   b. Total lymphocyte count of 989/$mm^3$
   c. Body weight decrease of 5%
   d. Arm muscle circumference 90% of standard

2. The nurse is caring for a patient who has a pressure injury on his back. What nursing intervention would the nurse perform?
   a. The nurse places a foam wedge under his body to keep body weight off the patient's back.
   b. The nurse uses a ring cushion to protect reddened areas from additional pressure.
   c. The nurse increases the amount of time the head of the bed is elevated.
   d. The nurse uses positioning devices and techniques to maintain posture and distribute weight evenly for the patient in a chair.

3. The nurse caring for a postoperative patient is cleaning the patient's wound. Which nursing action reflects the proper procedure for wound care?
   a. The nurse works outward from the wound in lines parallel to it.
   b. The nurse uses friction when cleaning the wound to loosen dead cells.
   c. The nurse swabs the wound with povidone–iodine to fight infection in the wound.
   d. The nurse swabs the wound from the bottom to the top.
4. The nurse is changing the dressing of a patient with a gunshot wound. What nursing action would the nurse provide?
   a. The nurse uses wet-to-dry dressings continuously.
   b. The nurse keeps the intact, healthy skin surrounding the injury moist because it is susceptible to breakdown.
   c. The nurse selects a dressing that absorbs exudate, if it is present, but still maintains a moist environment.
   d. The nurse packs the wound cavity tightly with dressing material.
5. When giving a back rub to an older adult at home, the nurse notices a stage II pressure injury. What nursing interventions would the nurse perform next?
   a. Place a sterile dressing over the pressure injury.
   b. Use a wet-to-dry dressing on the pressure injury.
   c. Use a nonadherent dressing and changes it every 3 hours.
   d. Use normal saline to clean the pressure injury.
6. The nurse is caring for a Penrose drain for a patient post abdominal surgery. What nursing action reflects a step in the care of a Penrose drain that needs to be shortened each day?
   a. The nurse carefully cleans around the sutures with a swab and normal sterile saline solution prior to shortening the drain.
   b. The nurse empties and suctions the device, following the manufacturer's directions prior to shortening the drain.
   c. The nurse pulls the drain out a short distance using sterile forceps and a twisting motion and cuts off the end of the drain with sterile scissors.
   d. The nurse compresses the container while the port is open, then closes the port after the device is compressed to empty the system before shortening the drain.
7. A patient's pressure injury is superficial and presents clinically as an abrasion, blister, or shallow crater. How would the nurse document this pressure injury?
   a. Stage 1
   b. Stage 2
   c. Stage 3
   d. Stage 4
8. The nurse is applying a heating pad to a patient experiencing neck pain. Which nursing action is performed correctly?
   a. The nurse uses a safety pin to attach the pad to the bedding.
   b. The nurse covers the heating pad with a heavy blanket.
   c. The nurse places the heating pad under the patient's neck.
   d. The nurse keeps the pad in place for 20 to 30 minutes, assessing it regularly.
9. The nurse is performing pressure injury assessment for patients in a hospital setting. Which patient would the nurse consider to be at greatest risk for developing a pressure injury?
   a. A newborn
   b. A patient with cardiovascular disease
   c. An older adult with arthritis
   d. A critical care patient
10. The nurse considers the impact of shearing forces in the development of pressure injury in patients. Which patient would be most likely to develop a pressure injury from shearing forces?
    a. A patient sitting in a chair who slides down
    b. A patient who lifts himself up on his elbows
    c. A patient who lies on wrinkled sheets
    d. A patient who must remain on his back for long periods of time
11. The nurse is assessing the wounds of patients in a burn unit. Which wound would most likely heal by primary intention?
    a. A surgical incision with sutured approximated edges
    b. A large wound with considerable tissue loss allowed to heal naturally

c. A wound left open for several days to allow edema to subside

d. A wound healing naturally that becomes infected

## ALTERNATE-FORMAT QUESTIONS

### Multiple Response Questions

***Circle the letters that correspond to the best answers for each question.***

1. The nurse is assessing the wounds of patients. Which patients would the nurse place at risk for delayed wound healing? *(Select all that apply.)*

   a. An older adult who is bedridden.

   b. A patient with a peripheral vascular disorder

   c. A patient who is obese

   d. A patient who eats a diet high in vitamins A and C

   e. A patient who is taking corticosteroid drugs

   f. A 10-year-old patient with a surgical incision

2. A med-surg nurse is assessing wounds of patients. Which wound complications are accurately described below? *(Select all that apply.)*

   a. Symptoms of wound infection, which are usually apparent within 1 to 2 weeks after the injury or surgery

   b. Dehiscence, which is present when there is a partial or total disruption of wound layers

   c. Evisceration, which occurs when the viscera protrudes through the incisional area

   d. Delayed wound healing in patients who are thin and at greater risk for complications owing to a thinner layer of tissue cells

   e. A wound with an increase in the flow of serosanguineous fluid between postoperative days 4 and 5, which is a sign of an impending evisceration

   f. Postoperative fistula formation, most often the result of delayed healing, commonly manifested by drainage from an opening in the skin or surgical site

3. A nurse assessing patient wounds would document which examples of wounds as healing normally without complications? *(Select all that apply.)*

   a. The edges of a healing surgical wound appear clean and well approximated, with a crust along the edges

   b. A wound that takes approximately 2 weeks for the edges to appear normal and heal together

   c. A wound with increased swelling and drainage that may occur during the first 5 days of the wound healing process

   d. A wound that does not feel hot upon palpation

   e. A wound that forms exudate due to the inflammatory response

   f. Incisional pain during the wound healing, which is most severe for the first 3 to 5 days and then progressively diminishes

4. In which situations has the nurse used a dressing properly? *(Select all that apply.)*

   a. A nurse places a Surgipad directly over an incision.

   b. A nurse places transparent dressings over an ABD to help keep the wound dry.

   c. A nurse places OpSite over a central venous access device insertion site.

   d. A nurse uses appropriate aseptic techniques when changing a dressing.

   e. A nurse places Sof-Wick around a drain insertion site.

   f. A nurse applies Telfa to a wound to keep drainage from passing through to a secondary dressing.

5. Which interventions might a nurse be expected to perform when providing competent care for a patient with a draining wound? *(Select all that apply.)*

   a. Administer a prescribed analgesic 30 to 45 minutes before changing the dressing, if necessary.

   b. Change the dressing midway between meals.

   c. Apply a protective ointment or paste, if appropriate, to cleansed skin surrounding the draining wound.

   d. Apply another layer of protective ointment or paste on top of the previous layer when changing dressings.

   e. Apply an absorbent dressing material as the first layer of the dressing.

   f. Apply a nonabsorbent material over the first layer of absorbent material.

6. A nurse is using the RYB wound classification system to document patient wounds. Which wounds would the nurse document as a Y (yellow) wound? *(Select all that apply.)*
   a. A wound that reflects the color of normal granulation tissue
   b. A wound that is characterized by oozing from the tissue covering the wound
   c. A wound with drainage that is a beige color
   d. A wound that requires wound cleaning and irrigation
   e. A wound that is covered with thick eschar
   f. A wound that is treated by using sharp, mechanical, or chemical debridement
7. Which teaching points would the nurse use to explain the development of pressure injuries to patients and how to prevent them? *(Select all that apply.)*
   a. "Pressure injuries usually occur over bony prominences where body weight is distributed over a small area without much subcutaneous tissue."
   b. "Most pressure injuries occur over the trochanter and calcaneus."
   c. "Generally, a pressure injury will not appear within the first 2 days in a person who has not moved for an extended period of time."
   d. "The major predisposing factor for a pressure injury is internal pressure over an area, resulting in occluded blood capillaries and poor circulation to the tissues."
   e. "The skin can tolerate considerable pressure without cell death, but for short periods only."
   f. "The duration of pressure, compared to the amount of pressure, plays a larger role in pressure injury formation."
8. Which would be appropriate actions for the nurse to take when cleaning and dressing a pressure injury? *(Select all that apply.)*
   a. Clean the wound with each dressing change using aggressive motions to remove necrotic tissue.
   b. Use povidone–iodine or hydrogen peroxide to irrigate and clean the injury.
   c. Use whirlpool treatments, if ordered, until the injury is considered clean.
   d. Keep the injury tissue moist and the surrounding skin dry.
   e. Use a dressing that absorbs exudate but maintains a moist healing environment.
   f. Pack wound cavities densely with dressing material to promote tissue healing.
9. Which nursing interventions reflect the accurate use of heat or cold during wound care? *(Select all that apply.)*
   a. The nurse makes more frequent checks of the skin of an older adult using a heating pad.
   b. The nurse places a heating pad on a sprained wrist that is in the acute stage.
   c. The nurse instructs the patient to lean or lie directly on the heating device.
   d. The nurse fills an ice bag with small pieces of ice to about two thirds full.
   e. The nurse covers a cold pack with a cotton sleeve to keep it in place on an arm.
   f. The nurse applies moist cold to a patient's eye for 40 minutes every 2 hours.
10. Which actions would a nurse be expected to perform when applying a saline-moistened dressing to a patient's wound? *(Select all that apply.)*
    a. Put on clean gloves and squeeze excess fluid from the gauze dressing before packing it tightly in the wound.
    b. Position the patient so the wound cleanser or irrigation solution will flow from the clean end of the wound toward the dirtier end.
    c. Carefully and gently remove the soiled dressings; if there is resistance, use a silicone-based adhesive remover to help remove the tape.
    d. Apply one dry, sterile gauze pad over the wet gauze, and then place an ABD pad over the gauze pad.
    e. Using clean technique, open the supplies and dressings and place the fine mesh gauze into the basin, pouring the ordered solution over the mesh to saturate it.
    f. Gently press to loosely pack the moistened gauze into the wound; if necessary, use forceps or cotton-tipped applicators to press gauze into all wound surfaces.

### Prioritization Question

1. Place the following steps to collecting a wound culture in the order in which they should be performed.
   - **a.** Using aseptic technique, don sterile gloves and clean wound. Remove sterile gloves.
   - **b.** Explain the procedure to patient; gather equipment; perform hand hygiene.
   - **c.** Apply clean dressing to wound.
   - **d.** Perform hand hygiene. Remove all equipment and make patient comfortable.
   - **e.** Remove gloves from inside out, and discard them in plastic waste bag. Perform hand hygiene.
   - **f.** Twist cap to loosen swab in Culturette tube, or open separate swab and remove cap from culture tube, keeping inside uncontaminated. Don clean glove or new sterile glove, if necessary.
   - **g.** Label specimen container appropriately, attach laboratory requisition to tube with a rubber band or place tube in plastic bag with requisition attached; send to lab within 20 minutes.
   - **h.** Carefully insert swab into wound and rotate the swab several times. Use another swab if collecting specimen from another site.
   - **i.** Place swab in Culturette tube, being careful not to touch outside of container. Twist cap to secure; if using Culturette tube, crush ampule of medium at bottom of tube.
   - **j.** Don clean disposable gloves. Remove dressing and assess wound and drainage.
   - **k.** Record collection of specimen, appearance of wound, and description of drainage in chart.

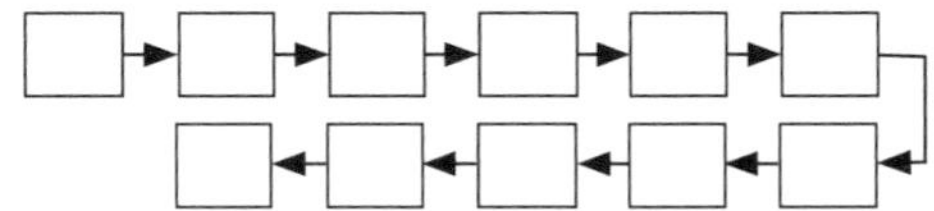

## NURSING PROCESS WORKSHEET

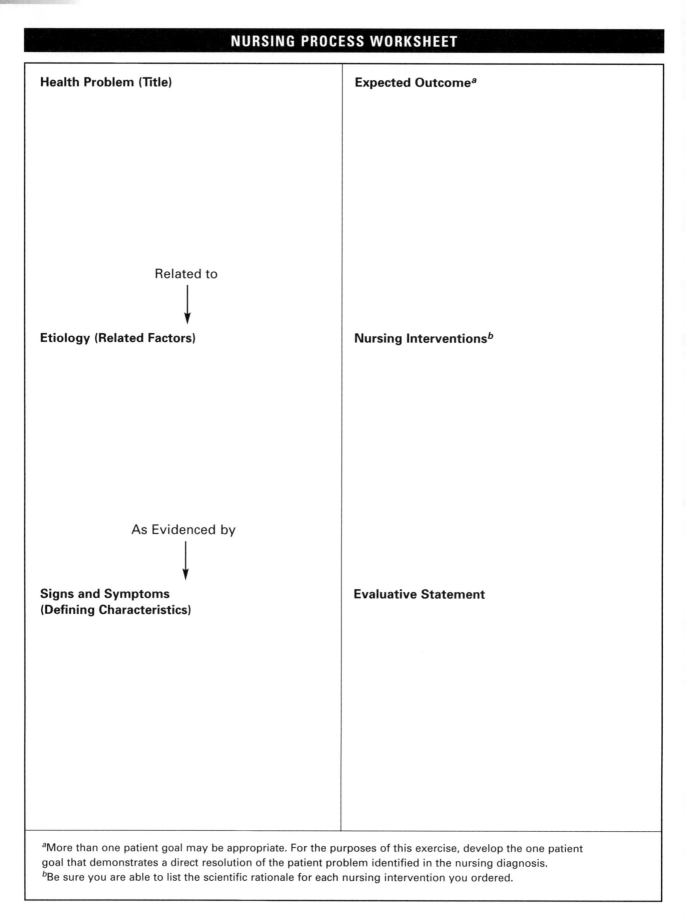

| **Health Problem (Title)** | **Expected Outcome**[a] |
|---|---|
| Related to ↓ | |
| **Etiology (Related Factors)** | **Nursing Interventions**[b] |
| As Evidenced by ↓ | |
| **Signs and Symptoms (Defining Characteristics)** | **Evaluative Statement** |

[a]More than one patient goal may be appropriate. For the purposes of this exercise, develop the one patient goal that demonstrates a direct resolution of the patient problem identified in the nursing diagnosis.
[b]Be sure you are able to list the scientific rationale for each nursing intervention you ordered.

CHAPTER 33

# Activity

## ASSESSING YOUR UNDERSTANDING

### IDENTIFICATION

1. Identify the bed-lying positions illustrated below by placing the names of the positions on the lines provided.

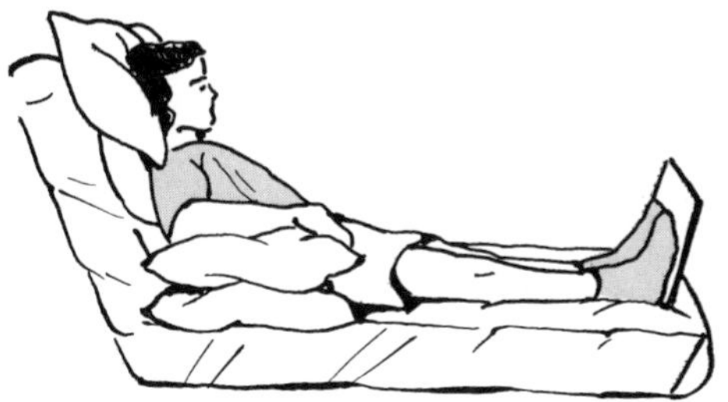

a. ______________________________

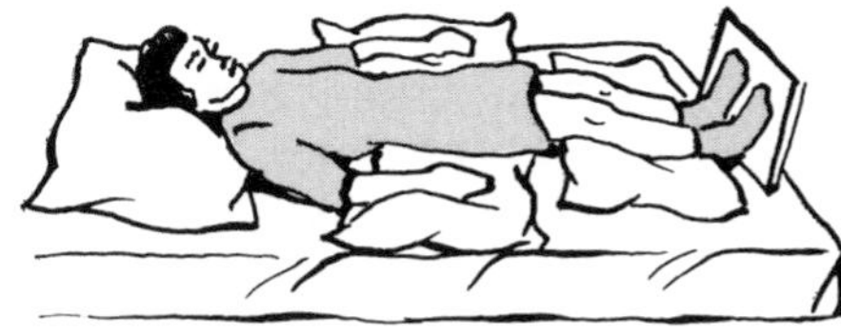

b. ______________________________

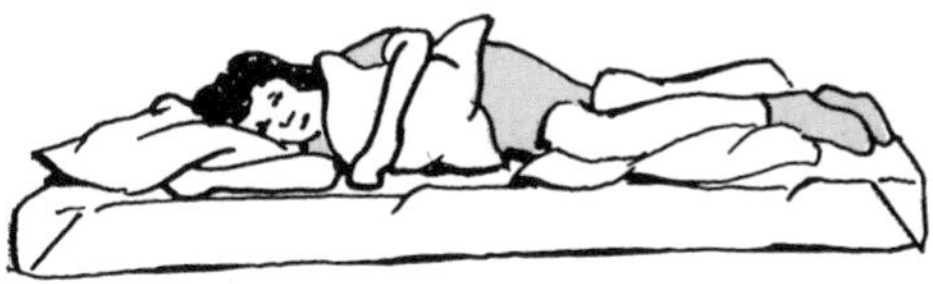

c. ______________________________

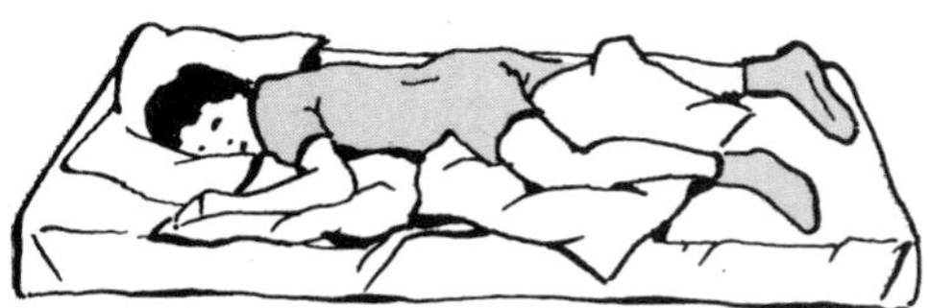

d. ______________________________

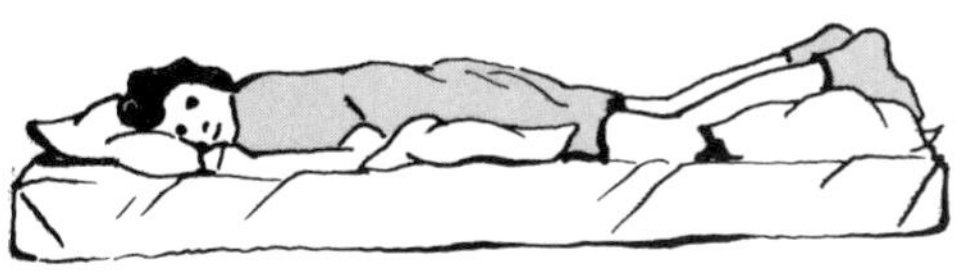

e. ______________________________

### MATCHING EXERCISES

***Match the type of joint listed in Part A with the examples listed in Part B.***

**PART A**

**a.** Ball-and-socket joint
**b.** Condyloid joint
**c.** Gliding joint
**d.** Hinge joint
**e.** Pivot joint
**f.** Saddle joint

**PART B**

____ **1.** The joints between the axis and atlas and the proximal ends of the radius and ulna

____ **2.** Carpal bones of the wrist; tarsal bones of the feet

____ 3. The joint between the trapezium and metacarpal of the thumb

____ 4. Wrist joint

____ 5. Shoulder and hip joints

***Match the term used to describe body positions and movements in Part A with its definition listed in Part B.***

**PART A**

a. Abduction
b. Adduction
c. Circumduction
d. Flexion
e. Extension
f. Hyperextension
g. Dorsiflexion
h. Plantar flexion
i. Rotation
j. Internal rotation
k. External rotation
l. Pronation
m. Supination
n. Inversion
o. Eversion

**PART B**

____ 6. The assumption of a prone position

____ 7. Lateral movement of a body part away from the midline of the body

____ 8. Backward bending of the hand or foot

____ 9. Movement of the sole or foot outward

____ 10. The state of being bent

____ 11. A body part turning on its axis away from the midline of the body

____ 12. Lateral movement of a body part toward the midline of the body

____ 13. Movement of the sole of the foot inward

____ 14. Movement of the distal part of the limb to trace a complete circle while the proximal end of the bone remains fixed

____ 15. The assumption of a supine position

____ 16. A body part turning on its axis toward the midline of the body

____ 17. Flexion of the foot

____ 18. The state of being in a straight line

____ 19. The turning point of a body part on the axis provided by its joint

***Match the condition related to muscle mass listed in Part A with its definition listed in Part B.***

**PART A**

a. Atrophy
b. Hypertrophy
c. Muscle tone
d. Flaccidity
e. Spasticity
f. Paresis
g. Hemiparesis
h. Paraplegia
i. Quadriplegia

**PART B**

____ 20. Increased muscle mass resulting from exercise or training

____ 21. Increased tone that interferes with movement

____ 22. Impaired muscle strength or weakness

____ 23. Muscle mass that is decreased through disuse or neurologic impairment

____ 24. Paralysis of the arms and legs

____ 25. The slight residual tension that remains in a normal resting muscle with an intact nerve supply

____ 26. Decreased tone that results from disuse or neurologic impairment

____ 27. Weakness of half of the body

## CORRECT THE FALSE STATEMENTS

***Circle the word "true" or "false" that follows the statement. If you circled "false," change the underlined word or words to make the statement true. Place your answer in the space provided.***

1. The bones of the jaw and spinal column are classified as <u>short bones</u>.
   a. True
   b. False ____________________

2. In a <u>gliding joint</u>, articular surfaces are flat; flexion–extension and abduction–adduction are permitted.
   a. True
   b. False ____________________

3. Ligaments are tough, fibrous bands that bind joints together and connect bones and cartilage.
   a. True
   b. False ______________________

4. It is a nerve impulse that stimulates muscles to contract.
   a. True
   b. False ______________________

5. Body dynamics are the efficient use of the body as a machine and as a means of locomotion.
   a. True
   b. False ______________________

6. Tonus is the term used to describe the state of slight contraction or the usual state of skeletal muscles.
   a. True
   b. False ______________________

7. The narrower a base of support and the lower the center of gravity, the greater the stability of the object.
   a. True
   b. False ______________________

8. The labyrinthine sense informs the brain of the location of a limb or body part as a result of joint movements stimulating special nerve endings in muscles, tendons, and fascia.
   a. True
   b. False ______________________

9. The cerebral motor cortex integrates semivoluntary movements such as walking, swimming, and laughing.
   a. True
   b. False ______________________

10. Rehabilitative exercises for knee or elbow injuries are examples of isokinetic exercises.
    a. True
    b. False ______________________

11. Atelectasis is an incomplete expansion or collapse of lung tissue.
    a. True
    b. False ______________________

12. Footdrop is a complication of immobility in which the foot cannot maintain itself in the perpendicular position, heel–toe gait is impossible, and the patient experiences extreme difficulty in walking.
    a. True
    b. False ______________________

13. Should a patient faint or begin to fall while walking, the nurse should stand with his or her feet apart to create a wide base of support and rock the pelvis out on the side opposite the patient.
    a. True
    b. False ______________________

14. When a patient stands between the back legs of a walker, the walker should extend from the floor to the patient's hip joint; the patient's elbows should be flexed about 30 degrees.
    a. True
    b. False ______________________

15. A nurse should lift an object to be moved to reduce the energy needed to overcome the pull of gravity.
    a. True
    b. False ______________________

## SHORT ANSWER

1. Briefly explain the effects of exercise and immobility on the body systems listed in the table below. Write your answers in the spaces provided in the table.

| Body System | Effects of Exercise | Effects of Immobility |
|---|---|---|
| Cardiovascular | | |
| Respiratory | | |
| Gastrointestinal | | |
| Urinary | | |
| Musculoskeletal | | |
| Metabolic | | |
| Integumentary | | |
| Psychological Well-Being | | |

2. List three functions performed by the muscles through contraction.
   a. ______
   b. ______
   c. ______

3. Describe the following points of attachment of muscle to bone.
   a. Point of origin: ______
   b. Point of insertion: ______

4. Describe the four steps the nervous system completes to stimulate muscles to contract.
   a. ______
   b. ______
   c. ______
   d. ______

5. Briefly describe the following concepts of ergonomics.
   a. Body alignment or posture: ______
   b. Balance: ______
   c. Coordinated body movement: ______

6. List four guidelines for the use of ergonomics when a person is at work.
   a. ______
   b. ______
   c. ______
   d. ______

7. Briefly describe how the following types of exercise provide health benefits to patients, and give an example of each.
   a. Aerobic exercises: ____________________
   b. Stretching exercises: ____________________
   c. Strength and endurance exercises: ____________________
   d. Activities of daily living: ____________________

8. List four psychological benefits of regular exercise.
   a. ____________________
   b. ____________________
   c. ____________________
   d. ____________________

9. Briefly describe how the following devices are used to promote correct alignment or alleviate discomfort on body parts.
   a. Pillows: ____________________
   b. Mattresses: ____________________
   c. Adjustable bed: ____________________
   d. Bed side rails: ____________________
   e. Trapeze bar: ____________________
   f. Cradle: ____________________
   g. Sandbags: ____________________
   h. Trochanter rolls: ____________________
   i. Hand/wrist splints or rolls: ____________________

10. Describe how you would teach a patient the following exercises.
   a. Quadriceps drills: ____________________
   b. Pushups: ____________________
   c. Dangling: ____________________

11. Mrs. Mulherin is a 60-year-old woman admitted to a health care facility for degenerative joint disease. Explain how you would assess, diagnose, and plan an exercise program for this patient.
   a. Physical assessment: ____________________
   b. Diagnosis: ____________________
   c. Exercise program: ____________________

12. Give two examples of normal and abnormal findings when assessing the mobility status of a patient in the following areas.
   a. General ease of movement:
      Normal: ____________________
      Abnormal: ____________________

**b.** Gait and posture:
Normal: ______________________________

______________________________

Abnormal: ______________________________

______________________________

**c.** Alignment:
Normal: ______________________________

______________________________

Abnormal: ______________________________

______________________________

**d.** Joint structure and function:
Normal: ______________________________

______________________________

Abnormal: ______________________________

______________________________

**e.** Muscle mass, tone, and strength:
Normal: ______________________________

______________________________

Abnormal: ______________________________

______________________________

**f.** Endurance:
Normal: ______________________________

______________________________

Abnormal: ______________________________

______________________________

## APPLYING YOUR KNOWLEDGE

### CRITICAL THINKING QUESTIONS

**1.** Visit a center for rehabilitative medicine and observe how the physical therapists assist patients to become mobile. Interview several patients to find out how the lack of mobility has affected their lives. See if you can help with some of the exercise routines, and try some of the exercises yourself. Develop a nursing care plan to incorporate what you learned about mobility and exercise into your own patient care routine.

**2.** Using a partner, practice putting each other into the following positions: Fowler's, supine, prone, lateral side-lying, and Sims'. What did this teach you about the experience of being positioned that will be helpful in your practice? Assess each position for health risks that may arise from the following factors: comfort level, body alignment, and pressure points. Write down the advantages and disadvantages of each position.

**3.** Try maneuvering on a busy street while on crutches or in a wheelchair. How does impaired mobility affect your ability to perform everyday chores? How did the public react to your impaired mobility? What effects might a permanent disability have on patients, and how can you promote their coping?

### REFLECTIVE PRACTICE: CULTIVATING QSEN COMPETENCIES

***Use the following expanded scenario from Chapter 33 in your textbook to answer the questions below.***

***Scenario:*** Kelsi Lester is a 10-year-old girl admitted to the pediatric unit as a result of a skiing accident. Unconscious for 2 days, she may or may not regain consciousness. She is on complete bed rest and requires frequent positioning to maintain correct body alignment and range of motion. Her parents are nearby and express concerns about the redness developing around her shoulder blades. They ask, "Is there anything we can do to make our daughter more comfortable?"

**1.** What patient teaching might the nurse incorporate into the plan of care to help Kelsi's parents minimize the complications of immobility for their daughter?

______________________________

______________________________

______________________________

**2.** What would be a successful outcome for this patient?

______________________________

______________________________

______________________________

**3.** What intellectual, technical, interpersonal, and/or ethical/legal competencies are most likely to bring about the desired outcome?

______________________________

______________________________

______________________________

4. What resources might be helpful for the Lester family?

______________________________

______________________________

______________________________

### PATIENT CARE STUDY

***Read the following patient care study and use your nursing process skills to answer the questions below.***

***Scenario:*** Robert Witherspoon, a 42-year-old university professor, presents for a checkup shortly after his father's death. His father died of complications of coronary artery disease. Mr. Witherspoon is 5 ft 9 in tall, weighs 235 lb, has a decided "paunch," and reports that until now he has made no time for exercise because he preferred to use his free time reading or listening to classical music. He enjoys French cuisine, including rich desserts, and has a total cholesterol level of 310 mg/dL (optimal is under 200 mg/dL). He admits being frightened by his father's death and is appropriately concerned about his elevated cholesterol level. "I guess I've never given much thought to my health before, but my Dad's death changed all that," he tells you. "I know that coronary artery disease runs in families, and I can tell you that I'm not ready to pack it all in yet. Tell me what I have to do to fight this thing." He admits that he used to tease a colleague—who lowered his own cholesterol from 290 to 200 mg/dL by diet and exercise alone—by accusing him of being a fitness freak. "Now, I'm recognizing the wisdom of his health behaviors and wondering if diet and exercise won't do the trick for me. Can you help me design an exercise program that will work?"

1. Identify pertinent patient data by placing a single underline beneath the objective data in the patient care study and a double underline beneath the subjective data.
2. Complete the Nursing Process Worksheet on page 215 to develop a three-part diagnostic statement and related plan of care for this patient.
3. Write down the patient and personal nursing strengths you hope to draw on as you assist this patient to better health.

   Patient strengths: ______________________________

   ______________________________

   ______________________________

   Personal strengths: ______________________________

   ______________________________

   ______________________________

4. Pretend that you are performing a nursing assessment of this patient after the plan of care has been implemented. Document your findings.

   ______________________________

   ______________________________

## PRACTICING FOR NCLEX

### MULTIPLE CHOICE QUESTIONS

***Circle the letter that corresponds to the best answer for each question.***

1. A nurse is performing range-of-motion exercises on a patient who is on bedrest. What would be the nurse's best action when the patient complains: "I'm just too tired to do these exercises today."
   a. Encourage the patient to finish the exercises and then reevaluate the nursing plan.
   b. Stop the exercises and reevaluate the nursing care plan.
   c. Finish the exercises and report the incident to the primary care provider.
   d. Modify the number of repetitions for each exercise and then modify the plan.
2. The nurse moves a person's arm from an outstretched position to a position at the side of the patient's body. What is the term used to describe this type of body movement?
   a. Adduction
   b. Abduction
   c. Circumduction
   d. Extension

**3.** Using proper ergonomics, which motions would the nurse make to move an object?

**a.** The nurse balances the head over the shoulders, leans forward, and relaxes the stomach muscles when moving an object.

**b.** The nurse uses the muscles of the back to help provide the power needed in strenuous activities.

**c.** The nurse uses the internal girdle and a long midriff to stabilize the pelvis and to protect the abdominal viscera when stooping, reaching, lifting, or pulling.

**d.** The nurse directly lifts an object rather than sliding, rolling, pushing, or pulling it to reduce the energy needed to lift the weight against the pull of gravity.

**4.** A nurse is assisting a patient from a bed to a wheelchair. Which nursing action is appropriate?

**a.** The nurse discourages the patient from helping with the transfer.

**b.** The nurse administers pain medication following the transfer.

**c.** The nurse grabs and holds the patient by his arms.

**d.** The nurse uses assistive devices when lifting more than 35 lb of patient weight.

**5.** The nurse uses gait belts when assisting patients to ambulate. Which patient would be a likely candidate for this assistive device?

**a.** A patient who has leg strength and can cooperate with the movement

**b.** A patient who has an abdominal incision

**c.** A patient with a thoracic incision

**d.** A patient who is confined to bedrest

**6.** The nurse is assessing a patient who is bedridden. For which condition would the nurse consider this patient to be at risk?

**a.** Increase in the movement of secretions in the respiratory tract

**b.** Increase in circulating fibrinolysin

**c.** Predisposition to renal calculi

**d.** Increased metabolic rate

**7.** A nurse is promoting exercise and activities for an older adult patient. Which teaching point would be appropriate for this patient?

**a.** Encourage the patient to quickly increase the repetitions for arm and leg exercises.

**b.** Encourage the patient to warm up before beginning exercises and to cool down after exercising.

**c.** Instruct the patient to continue exercise even if feeling weakness, to build up stamina.

**d.** Teach the patient to force joints to meet their natural limit and beyond prior to modifying exercises.

**8.** The nurse is assessing an ambulatory patient for gait. Which documentation describes this mobility status?

**a.** A straight line can be drawn from the ear through the shoulder and hip.

**b.** Patient displays full range of motion in arms and legs.

**c.** Arms swing freely in alternation with legs.

**d.** Adequate muscle mass, tone, and strength are available to accomplish movement.

**9.** A patient will be ambulating for the first time since his cardiac surgery. What should the nurse consider when assisting this patient?

**a.** Patients who are fearful of walking should be told to look at their feet when walking to ensure correct positioning.

**b.** Patients who can lift their legs only 1 to 2 in off the bed do not have sufficient muscle power to permit walking.

**c.** Nurses should never assist patients with ambulation without a physical therapist present.

**d.** If an ambulating patient whom a nurse is assisting begins to fall, the nurse should slide the patient down his or her own body to the floor, carefully protecting the patient's head.

**10.** Which patient would the nurse place in a protective prone position?

**a.** A patient prone to internal shoulder rotation and adduction

**b.** A patient prone to edema of the hand

**c.** A patient prone to hyperextension of the spine

**d.** A patient prone to flexion contracture of the neck

11. A nurse is logrolling a patient who has a spinal injury. Which nursing action follows the recommended guidelines for this procedure?
    a. Enlist the assistance of two or three other nurses to perform the procedure.
    b. Use a friction-reducing sheet that extends from below shoulder to above hips.
    c. Have the patient cross his or her arms on the chest and place a pillow over them.
    d. Have two nurses stand on the side of the bed in the direction the patient will be turned.
12. A nurse is recommending aerobic exercise for a patient who is overweight. Which exercise might the nurse suggest?
    a. Swimming
    b. Lifting weights
    c. Yoga
    d. Stretching exercises
13. The nurse is performing range-of-motion exercises on a patient's arm. The nurse starts by lifting the arm forward to above the head of the patient. Which action would the nurse perform next?
    a. Move the opposite arm forward to above the head of the patient.
    b. Return the arm to the starting position at the side of the body.
    c. Rotate the lower arm and hand so the palm is up.
    d. Move the arm across the body as far as possible.
14. During range-of-motion exercises, the nurse turns the sole of a patient's foot toward the midline and then turns the sole of the foot outward. Which type of movement is this nurse promoting by these actions?
    a. Internal and external rotation of the ankle
    b. Dorsiflexion and plantar flexion of the ankle
    c. Flexion and extension of the ankle
    d. Inversion and eversion of the ankle
15. A nurse assesses a patient's alignment and documents which data as a normal finding?
    a. The chest is held upward and backward.
    b. The abdominal muscles are held downward and the buttocks upward.
    c. The knees are slightly bent.
    d. The base of support is on the soles of the feet.

## ALTERNATE-FORMAT QUESTIONS

### Multiple Response Questions

***Circle the letters that correspond to the best answers for each question.***

1. Which exercises would the nurse recommend when planning isometric exercise for a patient? *(Select all that apply.)*
    a. Jogging
    b. Range-of-motion exercises
    c. Contracting the quadriceps
    d. Kegel exercises
    e. Bicycling
    f. Contracting and releasing the gluteal muscles
2. A nurse is promoting body movements for a patient during range-of-motion exercises. Which movements provide for flexion? *(Select all that apply.)*
    a. Bending the hand or foot backward and forward
    b. Turning the sole of the foot toward the midline, then turning the sole of the foot outward
    c. Bending the leg and bringing the heel toward the back of the leg and then returning the leg to the straight position
    d. Curling the toes downward and then straightening them out
    e. Moving the head from side to side, then bringing the chin toward each shoulder
    f. Extending the leg and lifting it upward, then returning the leg to the original position
3. A nurse is teaching a patient about the beneficial effects of exercise on his body. Which teaching point would the nurse include in the plan? *(Select all that apply.)*
    a. Exercise increases resting heart rate and blood pressure.
    b. Exercise increases intestinal tone.
    c. Exercise increases efficiency of metabolic system.
    d. Exercise increases blood flow to kidneys.
    e. Exercise decreases appetite.
    f. Exercise decreases rate of carbon dioxide excretion.

4. Which body system effects would the nurse state as occurring due to immobility? *(Select all that apply.)*
   a. Increased cardiac workload
   b. Increased depth of respiration
   c. Increased rate of respiration
   d. Decreased urinary stasis
   e. Increased risk for renal calculi
   f. Increased risk for electrolyte imbalance

5. A nurse is assessing a patient's mobility status. What data would the nurse document as normal findings? *(Select all that apply.)*
   a. Increased joint mobility
   b. Independent maintenance of correct alignment
   c. Scissors gait
   d. Head, shoulders, and hips aligned in bed
   e. Full range of motion
   f. Fasciculations

6. A nurse is caring for patients with alterations in mobility. Which nursing interventions are recommended for these patients? *(Select all that apply.)*
   a. For increased cardiac workload, instruct the patient to lie in the prone position.
   b. For ineffective breathing patterns, encourage shallow breathing and coughing.
   c. For orthostatic hypotension, have the patient sleep sitting up or in an elevated position.
   d. For impaired physical mobility, perform ROM exercises every 2 hours.
   e. For constipation, increase fluid intake and roughage.
   f. For impaired skin integrity, reposition the patient in correct alignment at least every 1 to 2 hours.

7. A nurse is teaching a patient how to walk with crutches. Which teaching points are recommended guidelines for this activity? *(Select all that apply.)*
   a. Keep elbows close to sides.
   b. Prevent crutches from getting closer than 3 inches to the feet.
   c. Use the four-point gait for patients who may bear weight on both feet.
   d. Use the swing-to gait for patients who may bear weight on one foot.
   e. Use the two-point gait for patients who may not bear weight on either foot.
   f. When climbing stairs, advance the unaffected leg past the crutches, then place weight on the crutches, then advance the affected leg and then the crutches.

8. Which nursing actions would the nurse perform when assisting patients with passive ROM exercises? *(Select all that apply.)*
   a. Raise the bed to the highest position.
   b. Adjust the bed to the flat position or as low as the patient can tolerate.
   c. Begin ROM exercises at the patient's head and move down one side of the body at a time.
   d. Perform each exercise 10 to 15 times.
   e. Move each joint in a smooth, rhythmic manner.
   f. Use a flat palm to support joints during ROM exercises.

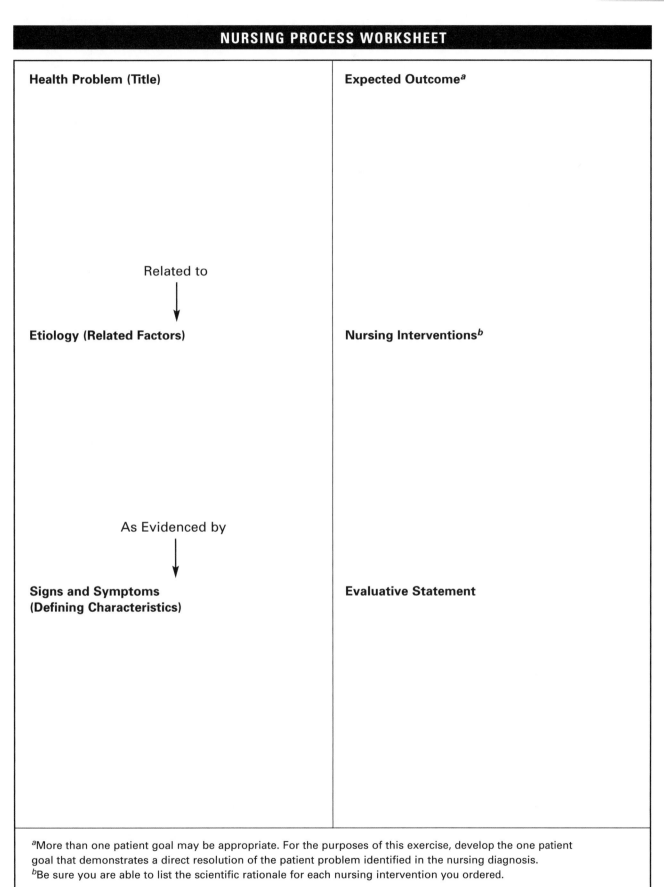

## NURSING PROCESS WORKSHEET

| Health Problem (Title) | Expected Outcome[a] |
|---|---|
| Related to ↓ | |
| **Etiology (Related Factors)** | **Nursing Interventions[b]** |
| As Evidenced by ↓ | |
| **Signs and Symptoms (Defining Characteristics)** | **Evaluative Statement** |

[a]More than one patient goal may be appropriate. For the purposes of this exercise, develop the one patient goal that demonstrates a direct resolution of the patient problem identified in the nursing diagnosis.
[b]Be sure you are able to list the scientific rationale for each nursing intervention you ordered.

CHAPTER 34

# Rest and Sleep

## ASSESSING YOUR UNDERSTANDING

### FILL IN THE BLANKS

1. The nurse explains to a patient that two systems in the brainstem known as the ___________ and the ___________ are believed to work together to control the cyclic nature of sleep.
2. When patients are in stages III and IV sleep, representing about 10% of total sleep time, they are experiencing deep-sleep states termed ___________ or slow-wave sleep.
3. A patient tells the nurse that he experiences patterns of waking behavior during his sleep at night. These types of sleep disorders are termed ___________.
4. A patient who has difficulty falling asleep, intermittent sleep, or early awakening from sleep is experiencing the sleep disorder known as ___________.
5. A patient confides to the nurse that she is sleeping more than normal during the day. This condition, characterized by excessive sleep, is termed ___________.
6. During a sleep assessment, a patient tells the nurse that she can fall asleep standing up or even in the middle of a conversation. This sleep disorder, known as ___________, is a condition characterized by an uncontrollable desire to sleep.

### MATCHING EXERCISES

***Match the sleep disorder listed in Part A with its appropriate definition listed in Part B.***

**PART A**

**a.** Insomnia
**b.** Hypersomnia
**c.** Narcolepsy
**d.** Sleep apnea
**e.** Parasomnia
**f.** Somnambulism
**g.** Enuresis
**h.** Sleep deprivation
**i.** Restless leg syndrome

**PART B**

____ **1.** Bedwetting during sleep

____ **2.** Difficulty in falling asleep, intermittent sleep, or early awakening from sleep

____ **3.** A condition characterized by an uncontrollable desire to sleep

____ **4.** A condition characterized by excessive sleep, particularly during the day

____ **5.** Periods of no breathing between snoring intervals

____ **6.** Decrease in the amount, consistency, and quality of sleep

____ **7.** Condition in which patient cannot lie still and reports unpleasant creeping, crawling, or tingling sensations in the legs

____ **8.** Sleepwalking

____ **9.** Patterns of waking behavior that appear during REM or NREM stages of sleep

***Match the stage of NREM sleep listed in Part A with the characteristics of that stage listed in Part B. Some answers may be used more than once, and some questions may have more than one answer.***

**PART A**

a. Stage I
b. Stage II
c. Stage III
d. Stage IV

**PART B**

____ 10. The depth of sleep increases, and arousal becomes increasingly difficult.

____ 11. It is a transitional stage between wakefulness and sleep.

____ 12. Involuntary muscle jerking may occur and waken the person.

____ 13. The person reaches the greatest depth of sleep, called delta sleep.

____ 14. The person falls into a deep sleep from which he or she cannot be aroused with ease.

____ 15. Constitutes about 10% of sleep.

____ 16. Constitutes 50% to 55% of sleep.

____ 17. Metabolism slows and the body temperature is low.

____ 18. Constitutes about 5% of sleep.

## CORRECT THE FALSE STATEMENTS

***Circle the word "true" or "false" that follows the statement. If you circled "false," change the underlined word or words to make the statement true. Place your answer in the space provided.***

1. During sleep, stimuli from the cortex are minimal.
   a. True
   b. False ____________________

2. Sleep stages III and IV are deep-sleep states termed delta sleep or slow-wave sleep.
   a. True
   b. False ____________________

3. If a person is awakened from sleep at any time, he or she will return to sleep again by starting at the point in the cycle where he or she was when disturbed.
   a. True
   b. False ____________________

4. Most people go through 8 to 10 cycles of sleep each night.
   a. True
   b. False ____________________

5. On average, infants require 10 to 12 total hours of sleep each day.
   a. True
   b. False ____________________

6. During times of stress, REM sleep decreases in amount, which tends to add to anxiety and stress.
   a. True
   b. False ____________________

7. A small protein snack before bedtime is recommended for patients with insomnia.
   a. True
   b. False ____________________

8. Exercise that occurs within a 2-hour interval before normal bedtime promotes sleep.
   a. True
   b. False ____________________

9. The administration of a larger midafternoon dose of asthma medication may prevent attacks that commonly occur at night during sleep.
   a. True
   b. False ____________________

10. Parasomnias are patterns of waking behavior that appear during sleep.
    a. True
    b. False ____________________

11. Narcolepsy refers to periods of no breathing between snoring intervals.
    a. True
    b. False ____________________

## SHORT ANSWER

1. List three benefits of sleep.
   a. ____________________
   b. ____________________
   c. ____________________

2. List the average amount of sleep required for the following age groups.
   a. Infants: ______
   b. Growing children: ______
   c. Adults: ______
   d. Older adults: ______

3. Briefly describe how the following factors influence sleep.
   a. Physical activity: ______
   b. Psychological stress: ______
   c. Motivation: ______
   d. Culture: ______
   e. Diet: ______
   f. Alcohol and caffeine: ______
   g. Smoking: ______
   h. Environmental factors: ______
   i. Lifestyle: ______
   j. Exercise: ______
   k. Illness: ______
   l. Medications: ______

4. List the information that should be determined in a sleep history when a sleep disturbance is noted.

5. Describe four physical findings that either confirm that a patient is getting sufficient rest to provide energy for the day's activities or validate the existence of a sleep disturbance that is decreasing the quantity or quality of sleep.
   a. ______
   b. ______
   c. ______
   d. ______

6. Describe how you would prepare a restful environment for a home health care patient who is experiencing a sleep disorder.

7. Write a sample nursing diagnosis for the following sleep problems.
   a. Mr. Smith is admitted to the hospital for surgery. He normally has no problem falling asleep, but the noise of the hospital and the need for periodic treatments keep him awake at night.
   b. Mr. Loper, a 74-year-old patient in a long-term care facility, is bored during the day and takes a nap in the afternoon and early evening. He cannot sleep at night.
   c. Dr. Harris, a resident working varying shifts in the emergency room, complains that he is sleepy all the time but cannot sleep when he lies down after work.
   d. Mrs. Maher, age 28, consumes four alcoholic drinks when watching television at night before bedtime. After eliminating the alcohol from her diet, she complains of waking after a short period and not being able to fall back to sleep.

**e.** Mrs. Eichorn, age 45, has two teenage sons who are often out late at night. She cannot get to sleep until they are both home safely, and even then she continues to worry about them.

______________________________

______________________________

**8.** Describe how each of the following is affected by REM sleep.

**a.** Eyes: ______________________________

**b.** Muscles: ______________________________

**c.** Respirations: ______________________________

**d.** Pulse: ______________________________

**e.** Blood pressure: ______________________________

**f.** Gastric secretions: ______________________________

**g.** Metabolism: ______________________________

**h.** Sleep cycle: ______________________________

**9.** List three measures a nurse can take to help alleviate a patient's sleep problem.

**a.** ______________________________

**b.** ______________________________

**c.** ______________________________

**10.** Give an example of a question you would ask a patient to assess for the following sleep factors.

**a.** Usual sleeping and waking times: ______________________________

______________________________

**b.** Number of hours of undisturbed sleep:

______________________________

______________________________

**c.** Quality of sleep: ______________________________

______________________________

**d.** Number and duration of naps: ______________________________

______________________________

**e.** Energy level: ______________________________

______________________________

**f.** Means of relaxing before bedtime:

______________________________

______________________________

**g.** Bedtime rituals: ______________________________

______________________________

**h.** Sleep environment: ______________________________

______________________________

**i.** Pharmacologic aids: ______________________________

______________________________

**j.** Nature of a sleep disturbance: ______________________________

______________________________

**k.** Onset of a disturbance: ______________________________

______________________________

**l.** Causes of a disturbance: ______________________________

______________________________

**m.** Severity of a disturbance: ______________________________

______________________________

**n.** Symptoms of a disturbance: ______________________________

______________________________

**o.** Interventions attempted and results:

______________________________

______________________________

## APPLYING YOUR KNOWLEDGE

### CRITICAL THINKING QUESTIONS

**1.** Imagine visiting a busy hospital unit at night and assessing the factors on the ward that would contribute to a patient's sleep deficit. What could be done to change the hospital environment to promote healthy sleeping patterns in the occupants?

**2.** Develop a sleep teaching tool that assesses the typical sleep patterns and requirements for patients of all ages (infants to older adults). Include common factors that disrupt sleep patterns, total amount of sleep required, and possible interventions to minimize sleep pattern disturbances. Interview people who have tried your interventions, and evaluate the likelihood that your teaching tool will resolve sleep problems.

**3.** Interview several friends or relatives to find out what they do to prepare for a restful night's sleep. Do they have any bedtime routines that are different from yours? What are some methods they use when they cannot fall asleep? Discuss the effect of lack of sleep on their work performance the following day.

## REFLECTIVE PRACTICE: CULTIVATING QSEN COMPETENCIES

***Use the following expanded scenario from Chapter 34 in your textbook to answer the questions below.***

*Scenario:* Charlie Bitner is an 86-year-old man who has recently been admitted to a long-term care facility. He tells his daughter that "even though I go to bed around 9 PM, I don't fall asleep until after midnight and then I'm up twice to go to the bathroom and have a lot of trouble falling back to sleep." His daughter has mentioned to the nurse that her father spends a lot of time napping during the day.

1. What nursing interventions might the nurse employ to help alleviate Mr. Bitner's sleep disturbances?

______________________________

______________________________

______________________________

2. What would be a successful outcome for this patient?

______________________________

______________________________

______________________________

3. What intellectual, technical, interpersonal, and/or ethical/legal competencies are most likely to bring about the desired outcome?

______________________________

______________________________

______________________________

4. What resources might be helpful for Mr. Bitner?

______________________________

______________________________

______________________________

## PATIENT CARE STUDY

***Read the following patient care study and use your nursing process skills to answer the questions below.***

*Scenario:* Gina Cioffi, a 23-year-old graduate nurse, has been in her new position as a critical care staff nurse in a large tertiary-care medical center for 3 months. "I was so excited about working three 12-hour shifts a week when I started this job, thinking I'd have lots of time for other things I want to do, but I'm not so sure anymore," she says. "I've been doing extra shifts when we're short-staffed because the money is so good, and right now it seems I'm always tired and all I think about all day long is how soon I can get back to bed. Worst of all, when I do finally get into bed, I often can't fall asleep, especially if things have been busy at work and someone 'went bad.' Does everyone else feel like me?" Looking at Gina, you notice dark circles under her eyes and are suddenly struck by the change in her appearance from when she first started working. At that time, she "bounced into work" looking fresh each morning, and her features were always animated. Now, her skin is pale, her hair and clothes look rumpled, and the "brightness" that was so characteristic of her earlier is strikingly absent. With some gentle questioning, you discover that she frequently goes out with new friends she has made at the hospital when her shift is over, and she sometimes goes for 48 hours without sleep. "I know I've gotten myself into a rut. How do I get out of it? I used to think my sleep habits were bad at school, but this is a hundred times worse because there never seems to be time to crash. I just have to keep on going."

1. Identify pertinent patient data by placing a single underline beneath the objective data in the case study and a double underline beneath the subjective data.
2. Complete the Nursing Process Worksheet on page 224 to develop a three-part diagnostic statement and related plan of care for this patient.
3. Write down the patient and personal nursing strengths you hope to draw on as you assist this patient to better health.

   Patient strengths: ______________________________

   ______________________________

   ______________________________

   Personal strengths: ______________________________

   ______________________________

   ______________________________

4. Pretend that you are performing a nursing assessment of this patient after the plan of care is implemented. Document your findings.

______________________________

______________________________

## PRACTICING FOR NCLEX

### MULTIPLE CHOICE QUESTIONS

***Circle the letter that corresponds to the best answer for each question.***

1. A nurse notes that a patient admitted to a long-term care facility sleeps for an abnormally long time. After researching sleep disorders, the nurse learns that which area of this patient's brain may have suffered damage?
   a. Cerebral cortex
   b. Hypothalamus
   c. Medulla
   d. Midbrain
2. The pediatric nurse teaches parents about normal sleep patterns in their children. Which of the following teaching points should the nurse include?
   a. Inform parents that daytime napping decreases during the preschool period, and, by the age of 5 years, most children no longer nap.
   b. Teach parents of infants to report any eye movements, groaning, or grimacing by their infant during sleep periods.
   c. Advise parents that waking from nightmares or night terrors is common during the adolescent stage.
   d. Inform parents about the preschool child's awareness of the concept of death possibly occurring and encourage parents to help alleviate the child's fears.
3. What interview question would be the best choice for the nurse to use to assess for recent changes in a patient's sleep–wakefulness pattern?
   a. In what way does the sleep you get each day affect your everyday living?
   b. How much sleep do you think you need to feel rested?
   c. What do you usually do to help yourself fall asleep?
   d. Do you usually go to bed and wake up about the same time each day?
4. A nurse attempts to wake a patient who is scheduled for tests and is able to arouse him relatively easily. Which stage of sleep is this patient most likely experiencing?
   a. Stage I
   b. Stage II
   c. Stage III
   d. Stage IV
5. A nurse on the night shift checks on a patient and suspects that the patient is in REM sleep. Which patient cue is indicative of this stage of sleep?
   a. The patient's eyes dart back and forth quickly.
   b. The patient has a slow, regular pulse.
   c. The patient's metabolism and body temperature have decreased.
   d. The patient's blood pressure decreases.
6. The nurse is implementing nursing interventions to promote sleep on a busy hospital ward. Which intervention is the best choice for these patients?
   a. Encourage the patients to take a shower prior to bedtime.
   b. Have the patients set an alarm clock so they are not worried about getting up.
   c. Create a warm, dark environment in the patients' rooms.
   d. Offer patients a small carbohydrate and protein snack before bedtime.
7. For which of the following patients would the nurse be most likely to administer a benzodiazepine-like drug?
   a. A patient who needs long-term therapy for chronic insomnia
   b. A patient who has insomnia and awakens in the middle of the night
   c. A patient who is being treated for short-term insomnia
   d. A patient who has insomnia combined with restless leg syndrome.
8. The nurse should obtain a sleep history on which patients as a protocol?
   a. Only patients who have been suffering from a sleep disorder
   b. Only patients who suffer from a sleep disorder or have been unconscious
   c. Patients who suffer from a sleep disorder or who are spending time in the CCU
   d. All patients admitted to a health care facility

9. A patient diagnosed with hypothyroidism is suffering from fatigue, lethargy, depression, and difficulty executing the tasks of everyday living. What type of sleep deprivation would the nurse suspect is affecting this patient?
   a. REM deprivation
   b. NREM deprivation
   c. Total sleep deprivation
   d. Insomnia

10. Most authorities agree that a person's sleep–wake cycle is fully developed by what age?
    a. 9 months to 1 year
    b. 1 year to 18 months
    c. 2 to 3 years
    d. 4 to 6 years

11. When caring for a patient with insomnia, the nurse would appropriately institute which intervention?
    a. Encourage the patient to nap frequently during the day to make up for the lost sleep at night.
    b. Have the patient eliminate caffeine and alcohol in the evening because both are associated with disturbances in the normal sleep cycle.
    c. Advise the patient to exercise vigorously before bedtime to promote drowsiness.
    d. Advise the patient to avoid food high in carbohydrates before bedtime.

12. A new patient in the medical–surgical unit complains of difficulty sleeping and is scheduled for an exploratory laparotomy in the morning. The nursing diagnosis is: Disturbed sleep pattern: Insomnia related to fear of impending surgery. Which step is most appropriate in planning care for this diagnosis?
    a. Help the patient maintain normal bedtime routine and time for sleep.
    b. Provide an opportunity for the patient to talk about concerns.
    c. Use tactile relaxation techniques, such as a back massage.
    d. Bring the patient a warm glass of milk at bedtime.

## ALTERNATE-FORMAT QUESTIONS

### Multiple Response Questions

***Circle the letters that correspond to the best answers for each question.***

1. The nurse is managing the environment for patients on a busy hospital ward. Which interventions would the nurse perform to facilitate a more restful environment? *(Select all that apply.)*
   a. Maintain a brighter room during daylight hours and dim lights in the evening.
   b. Keep the room warm and provide earplugs and eye masks if requested.
   c. Decrease the volume on alarms, pages, telephones, and staff conversations.
   d. Schedule procedures separately to avoid tiring out the patients.
   e. Medicate for pain if needed.
   f. Keep the doors to the patients' rooms open.

2. The nurse is teaching a patient about nonpharmacologic measures to alleviate restless leg syndrome (RLS). Which teaching points would the nurse include in her plan? *(Select all that apply.)*
   a. Drinking a cup of coffee before bed can help relieve the tingling sensations.
   b. Applying heat or cold to the extremity can help relieve the symptoms.
   c. An alcoholic drink is recommended before bed to relax the patient.
   d. Biofeedback and transcutaneous electrical nerve stimulation (TENS) can help relax the patient and relieve symptoms.
   e. Massaging the legs may relieve symptoms.
   f. A mild analgesic before bed can help relieve symptoms.

3. The nurse is providing patient teaching for the parents of an obese child diagnosed with obstructive sleep apnea. What treatment measures would the nurse explain during the teaching session? *(Select all that apply.)*
   a. A weight loss plan
   b. Treatment with intranasal antibiotics
   c. Treatment with sleeping pills
   d. Use of a continuous passive airway pressure machine
   e. Counseling for depression
   f. Use of a mandibular advancement device (MAD)

4. The nurse is teaching the practice of stimulus control to a patient who has insomnia. The nurse would include which teaching points in the teaching plan? *(Select all that apply.)*
   a. Recommend that the patient use the bedroom for sex and sleep only.
   b. Instruct the patient to leave the bedroom if he or she cannot get to sleep within 15 to 20 minutes; he or she should return to the bedroom when sleepy.
   c. Instruct the patient to get up the same time every day, no matter what time he or she fell asleep.
   d. Allow the patient to nap during the day if he or she could not sleep during the night.
   e. Instruct the patient to exercise moderately 1 hour before going to bed.
   f. Encourage the patient to consume one or two alcoholic drinks to help him or her relax before bedtime.

5. A nurse explains cognitive behavioral therapy (CBT) to a patient who is experiencing chronic insomnia. Which statements by the nurse best describe this therapy? *(Select all that apply.)*
   a. "Sedatives and hypnotics are used in conjunction with CBT."
   b. "You will meet with a therapist to work through any maladaptive sleep beliefs."
   c. "Used with other complementary therapies, CBT is very successful."
   d. "Pharmacologic approaches should be attempted prior to CBT to resolve the insomnia."
   e. "CBT may include progressive muscle relaxation measures, stimulus control, and sleep restriction therapy."
   f. "Patients undergoing CBT are asked to stay in bed during normal sleep hours even if they are unable to sleep."

6. A nurse caring for a patient with hypersomnia investigates the cause of the sleep disorder. What are possible causes to consider? *(Select all that apply.)*
   a. Another sleep disorder, such as sleep apnea
   b. Depression
   c. Malnourishment
   d. Alcohol abuse
   e. Some medications
   f. Eating disorders

**Prioritization Question**

1. Place the following stages of a sleep cycle in the order in which they would normally occur.
   a. NREM stage III
   b. NREM stage I
   c. NREM stage II
   d. Wakefulness
   e. REM
   f. NREM stage IV
   g. Second NREM stage II
   h. Second NREM stage III
   i. Third NREM stage II

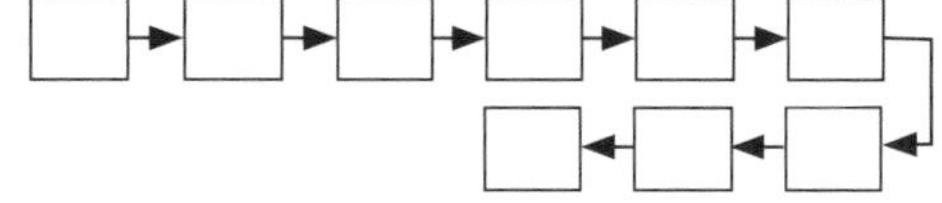

## NURSING PROCESS WORKSHEET

| Health Problem (Title) | Expected Outcome[a] |
|---|---|
| Related to ↓ | |
| **Etiology (Related Factors)** | **Nursing Interventions[b]** |
| As Evidenced by ↓ | |
| **Signs and Symptoms (Defining Characteristics)** | **Evaluative Statement** |

[a]More than one patient goal may be appropriate. For the purposes of this exercise, develop the one patient goal that demonstrates a direct resolution of the patient problem identified in the nursing diagnosis.
[b]Be sure you are able to list the scientific rationale for each nursing intervention you ordered.

CHAPTER 35

# Comfort and Pain Management

## ASSESSING YOUR UNDERSTANDING

### FILL IN THE BLANKS

1. A patient who experiences acute pain following a noxious stimulus is experiencing ___________ pain.
2. A patient who has pain related to a surgical incision is experiencing ___________ pain.
3. A patient who complains of pain that is poorly localized following abdominal surgery is most likely experiencing ___________ pain.
4. A person who experiences a "head rush" from eating ice cream too fast is experiencing ___________.
5. A patient who has sharp pains in his left arm following a myocardial infarction is experiencing ___________ pain.

### MATCHING EXERCISES

***Match the type of pain listed in Part A with its definition listed in Part B.***

#### PART A

a. Nociceptive pain
b. Cutaneous pain
c. Somatic pain
d. Visceral pain
e. Neuropathic pain
f. Allodynia
g. Psychogenic pain
h. Referred pain
i. Acute pain
j. Chronic pain
k. Intractable pain

#### PART B

____ 1. Pain that results from an injury to, or abnormal functioning of, peripheral nerves or the central nervous system

____ 2. Pain that is resistant to therapy and persists despite a variety of interventions

____ 3. Pain that occurs following a normally weak or nonpainful stimulus, such as a light touch or a cold drink

____ 4. Pain that may be limited, intermittent, or persistent but that lasts for 6 months or longer and interferes with normal functioning

____ 5. Pain that is usually acute and transmitted following normal processing of noxious stimuli

____ 6. Pain that is diffuse or scattered and originates in tendons, ligaments, bones, blood vessels, and nerves

____ 7. Pain for which no physical cause can be found

____ 8. Superficial pain that usually involves the skin or subcutaneous tissue

____ 9. Pain that is poorly localized and originates in body organs, the thorax, cranium, and abdomen

____ 10. Pain that is perceived in an area distant from its point of origin

***Match the examples in Part B with the type of pain listed in Part A. Answers may be used more than once.***

**PART A**

**a.** Cutaneous pain

**b.** Deep somatic pain

**c.** Visceral pain

**d.** Referred pain

**PART B**

____ **11.** Pain associated with cancer of the uterus

____ **12.** Pain associated with a myocardial infarction

____ **13.** Pain associated with a knee injury

____ **14.** Pain associated with burns

____ **15.** Pain associated with a brain tumor

____ **16.** Pain associated with a gash in the skin

____ **17.** Pain associated with a broken leg

____ **18.** Pain associated with stomach ulcers

***Match the term for nonpharmacologic pain relief listed in Part A with its definition listed in Part B.***

**PART A**

**a.** Imagery

**b.** Relaxation techniques

**c.** TENS

**d.** Cutaneous stimulation

**e.** Placebo

**f.** Hypnosis

**g.** Acupuncture

**h.** Biofeedback

**i.** Acupressure

**j.** Therapeutic touch

**k.** Distraction

**PART B**

____ **19.** Involves using one's hands to consciously direct an energy exchange from the health care provider to the patient

____ **20.** Reduce skeletal muscle tension and lessen anxiety; the nurse acknowledges the patient's pain and expresses a willingness to help the patient relieve the distress caused by that pain

____ **21.** Involves stimulating the skin's surface to relieve pain; can be explained by the gate control theory

____ **22.** Requires the patient to focus attention on something other than the pain

____ **23.** An example of mind–body interaction used to decrease pain that involves one or all of the senses and focusing on a mental picture

____ **24.** Involves the use of the fingertips to create gentle but firm pressure to usual acupuncture sites

____ **25.** A noninvasive alternative technique that involves electrical stimulation of large-diameter fibers to inhibit the transmission of painful impulses carried over small-diameter fibers

____ **26.** A technique that influences a subconscious condition by means of suggestion

____ **27.** A technique that uses a machine with a signal to help the patient learn by trial and error to control the supposedly involuntary body mechanisms that may cause pain

____ **28.** A technique that uses needles of various lengths to prick specific parts of the body to produce insensitivity to pain

**SHORT ANSWER**

**1.** Read each of the situations below and use the box on page 227 to describe behavioral, physiologic, and affective responses to pain that you might observe in these patients:

*Situation A:* Mrs. Novinger tells you that she frequently gets migraine headaches and feels one coming on.

*Situation B:* Ryan Goode, age 3, reached out to pet a stray cat, who hissed and scratched his forearm.

*Situation C:* Mrs. Carol Chung underwent a cesarean birth 2 days ago and is using her call light to request something for her incisional pain.

*Situation D:* Joseph Miles, age 79, has a long history of degenerative joint disease and tells you this is a "bad morning" for his joints: "I think the weather must be affecting my arthritis."

Write a three-part diagnosis statement for each of these patients using the assessment data in the box.

*Situation A:* ______________________

*Situation B:* ______________________

*Situation C:* ______________________

*Situation D:* ______________________

| Situation | Behavioral | Physiologic | Affective |
|---|---|---|---|
| A | | | |
| B | | | |
| C | | | |
| D | | | |

**2.** Briefly describe the events that occur when the threshold of pain has been reached and there is injured tissue.

______________________

______________________

______________________

**3.** Explain why referred pain can be transmitted to a cutaneous (skin) site different from its origin.

______________________

______________________

**4.** Explain the mechanics of the gate control theory and how it is believed to control pain.

______________________

______________________

______________________

______________________

**5.** Describe the following types of pain and give an example of each from your own experience with patients.

**a.** Acute pain: ______________________

**b.** Chronic pain: ______________________

**c.** Intractable pain: ______________________

**6.** Give an example of how the following factors may influence a patient's pain experience.

**a.** Culture/ethnicity: ______________________

**b.** Family, biologic sex, or age: ______________________

**c.** Religious beliefs: ______________________

**d.** Environment and support people: ______________________

**e.** Anxiety and other stressors: ______________________

f. Past pain experience: ____________________

7. List two experiences you have had with pain management for patients. Note your response to their pain and the effectiveness of your pain management techniques. Which pain control measures were most effective, and what could you have done differently to provide better pain control?
   a. ____________________
   b. ____________________

8. Describe how you would respond to a patient who tells you the following about his or her pain experience.
   a. "I know you'll know when I'm in pain and will do something to relieve it." ____________________
   b. "If I ask for something for pain, I'm afraid I may become addicted." ____________________
   c. "It's natural to have pain when you get older. It's just something I've learned to live with." ____________________

9. Give an example of an interview question you could use to assess a patient for the following characteristics of pain.
   a. Duration of pain: ____________________
   b. Quantity and intensity of pain: ____________________
   c. Quality of pain: ____________________
   d. Physiologic indicators of pain: ____________________

10. State your opinion of the use of placebos to satisfy a person's demand for a drug. Is lying to the patient ever justifiable? How could this action affect the nurse–patient relationship? What, if anything, would you say to a health care provider who prescribed a placebo for your patient?

____________________

11. How would you modify your means of assessing for pain in the following patients?
   a. A patient with a cognitive impairment: ____________________
   b. A 5-year-old patient: ____________________
   c. An older adult: ____________________

## APPLYING YOUR KNOWLEDGE

### CRITICAL THINKING QUESTIONS

1. Think back to the last time you experienced acute pain (e.g., a toothache, headache, backache). If you were at work, were you able to concentrate on anything but the pain? How did the people around you respond to your pain? What measures did you take to relieve the pain, and how successful were they? Interview several patients who are experiencing acute pain. How are they coping psychologically and physically with the pain? What comfort measures work best for them? How has medication helped to control their pain? How can you use this knowledge to improve your care?

2. Find a tool to assess pain. Be sure it includes physical assessment, pain scales, location and duration of the pain, coping measures, pain management, and the effect of pain on daily living. Use this tool to assess the pain of people with similar problems (e.g., migraine, cramps, arthritis) and look for factors to explain their different experiences.

3. You notice a young woman who is experiencing intense pain. When you ask the nurses about this patient, they tell you she is in end-stage cancer and has received all the pain medication she has been prescribed. They could not administer more medication without a doctor's order. How would you react to this patient? What would you do to provide alternative comfort measures? Would you be an advocate for this patient and attempt to have more medication prescribed? How might who you are and your competence in pain management affect this woman's last days?

## REFLECTIVE PRACTICE: CULTIVATING QSEN COMPETENCIES

***Use the following expanded scenario from Chapter 35 in your textbook to answer the questions below.***

***Scenario:*** Carla Potter is a 26-year-old White woman. She experiences "bad cramps" and periodic fatigue, anxiety, irritability, and mood swings approximately 1 week before the start of her menses. She told the nurse practitioner that her job as a computer programmer is stressful and that these monthly symptoms are affecting her job performance and relationships. She asks the nurse if there is anything available to control these symptoms.

1. What nursing interventions might the nurse use to help minimize the effects of premenstrual syndrome on Ms. Potter?

______________________________

______________________________

______________________________

2. What would be a successful outcome for this patient?

______________________________

______________________________

______________________________

3. What intellectual, technical, interpersonal, and/or ethical/legal competencies are most likely to bring about the desired outcome?

______________________________

______________________________

______________________________

4. What resources might be helpful for Ms. Potter?

______________________________

______________________________

______________________________

## PATIENT CARE STUDY

***Read the following case study and use your nursing process skills to answer the questions below.***

***Scenario:*** Tabitha Wilson is a 24-month-old infant with AIDS who is hospitalized with infectious diarrhea. She is well known to the pediatric staff, and there is real concern that she might not pull through this admission. She has suffered many of the complications of AIDS and is no stranger to pain. At present, the skin on her buttocks is raw and excoriated, and tears stream down her face whenever she is moved. Her blood pressure also shoots up when she is touched. The severity of her illness has left her extremely weak and listless, and her foster mother reports that she no longer recognizes her child. When alone in her crib, she seldom moves, and she moans softly. Several nurses have expressed great frustration caring for Tabitha because they find it hard to perform even simple nursing measures like turning, diapering, and weighing her when they see how much pain these procedures cause.

1. Identify pertinent patient data by placing a single underline beneath the objective data in the case study and a double underline beneath the subjective data.

2. Complete the Nursing Process Worksheet on page 233 to develop a three-part diagnostic statement and related plan of care for this patient.

3. Write down the patient and personal nursing strengths you hope to draw on as you assist this patient to better health.

   Patient strengths: ______________________________

   ______________________________

   ______________________________

   Personal strengths: ______________________________

   ______________________________

   ______________________________

4. Pretend that you are performing a nursing assessment of this patient after the plan of care is implemented. Document your findings.

______________________________

______________________________

## PRACTICING FOR NCLEX

### MULTIPLE CHOICE QUESTIONS

***Circle the letter that corresponds to the best answer for each question.***

1. A nurse implements cutaneous stimulation for a patient as part of a strategy for pain relief. Which nursing action exemplifies the use of this technique?
   a. The nurse plays soft music in the patient's room.
   b. The nurse assists the patient to focus on something pleasant rather than on pain.
   c. The nurse gives the patient a massage before bed.
   d. The nurse teaches the patient deep breathing techniques for relaxation.

2. The nurse is visiting a patient at home who is recovering from a bowel resection. The patient complains of constant pain and discomfort and displays signs of depression. When assessing this patient for pain, what should be the nurse's ***focal point***?
   a. Judging whether the patient is in pain or is just depressed
   b. Beginning pain medications before the pain is too severe
   c. Administering a placebo and performing a reassessment of the pain
   d. Reviewing and revising the pain management treatment

3. When performing a pain assessment on a patient, the nurse observes that the patient guards his arm, which was fractured in a car accident, and he refuses to move out of his chair. The nurse notes this reaction as what type of pain response?
   a. Behavioral
   b. Physiologic
   c. Affective
   d. Psychosomatic

4. A patient who is in pain strikes out at a nurse who is attempting to perform a bed bath. This patient is displaying what pain response?
   a. Involuntary
   b. Behavioral
   c. Physiologic
   d. Affective

5. The nurse is teaching a novice nurse about the therapeutic effects of laughter. Which example correctly identifies one of these effects?
   a. It activates the immune system.
   b. It increases the level of epinephrine.
   c. It decreases heart rate.
   d. It causes shallow breathing.

6. A patient who recently underwent amputation of a leg complains of pain in the amputated part. What would be the nurse's best response?
   a. "Your pain cannot exist because the leg has been amputated."
   b. "Your pain is a phenomenon known as 'ghost pain'."
   c. "Your pain is a real experience."
   d. "You are experiencing central pain syndrome."

7. The nurse instructs a patient to enter a hot whirlpool gradually. What is the theory that explains why a body part becomes acclimated to water temperature gradually?
   a. Threshold of pain theory
   b. Adaptation theory
   c. Gate control theory
   d. Regulation by neuromodulators

8. Which of the following means of pain control is based on the gate control theory?
   a. Biofeedback
   b. Distraction
   c. Hypnosis
   d. Acupuncture

9. The nurse is assessing a patient for the chronology of the pain she is experiencing. Which is an example of an appropriate interview question to obtain this data?
   a. How does the pain develop and progress?
   b. How would you describe your pain?
   c. How would you rate the pain on a scale of 1 to 10?
   d. What do you do to alleviate your pain and how well does it work?

**10.** A patient complains of severe pain following a mastectomy. The nurse would expect to administer what type of pain medication to this patient?

**a.** NSAIDs

**b.** Corticosteroids

**c.** Opioid analgesics

**d.** Nonopioid analgesics

**11.** A nurse administers pain medication to patients on a med-surg ward. Which patient would benefit from a PRN drug regimen as an effective method of pain control?

**a.** A patient experiencing acute pain

**b.** A patient in the early postoperative period

**c.** A patient experiencing chronic pain

**d.** A patient in the postoperative stage with occasional pain

**12.** A patient is experiencing acute pain following the amputation of a limb. What nursing interventions would be most appropriate when treating this patient?

**a.** Treat the pain only as it occurs to prevent drug addiction.

**b.** Encourage the use of nondrug complementary therapies as adjuncts to the medical regimen.

**c.** Increase and decrease the serum level of the analgesic as needed.

**d.** Do not provide analgesia if there is any doubt about the likelihood of pain occurring.

**13.** Three days after surgery, a patient continues to have moderate to severe incisional pain. Based on the gate control theory, what action should the nurse take?

**a.** Administer pain medications in smaller doses but more frequently.

**b.** Decrease external stimuli in the room during painful episodes.

**c.** Reposition the patient and gently massage the patient's back.

**d.** Advise the patient to try to sleep following administration of pain medication.

**14.** A nurse is treating a young boy who is in pain but cannot vocalize this pain. What would be the nurse's best intervention in this situation?

**a.** Ignore the boy's pain if he is not complaining about it.

**b.** Ask the boy to draw a cartoon about the color or shape of his pain.

**c.** Medicate the boy with analgesics to reduce the anxiety of experiencing pain.

**d.** Distract the boy so he does not notice his pain.

**15.** After sedating a patient, the nurse assesses that the patient is frequently drowsy and drifts off during conversations. What number on the sedation scale would the nurse document for this patient?

**a.** 1

**b.** 2

**c.** 3

**d.** 4

## ALTERNATE-FORMAT QUESTIONS

### Multiple Response Questions

***Circle the letters that correspond to the best answers for each question.***

**1.** A nurse is performing pain assessments on patients in a health care provider's office. Which patients would the nurse document as having acute pain? *(Select all that apply.)*

**a.** A patient who is having an MI

**b.** A patient who has diabetic neuropathy

**c.** A patient who presents with the signs and symptoms of appendicitis

**d.** A patient who fell and broke an ankle

**e.** A patient who has rheumatoid arthritis

**f.** A patient who has bladder cancer

**2.** The nurse is giving a back massage to a patient who is having trouble sleeping. Which nursing actions are performed appropriately? *(Select all that apply.)*

**a.** The nurse massages the patient's shoulder, entire back, areas over iliac crests, and sacrum with light vertical stroking motions.

**b.** The nurse kneads the patient's skin using continuous grasping and pinching motions.

**c.** The nurse assists the patient to a prone position and drapes the patient's body as needed with the bath blanket.

**d.** The nurse completes the massage with additional short, stroking movements that eventually become heavier in pressure.

**e.** The nurse applies warmed lotion to patient's shoulders, back, and sacral area.

f. The nurse places hands at the base of the spine and strokes upward to the shoulder and back down to the buttocks.

3. The nurse is massaging an older adult's back and notices a reddened area on the patient's sacrum. What actions would the nurse perform in response? *(Select all that apply.)*
   a. Lightly massage the area.
   b. Document the reddened area on the patient medical record.
   c. Following the massage, position the patient on the sacral area.
   d. Report the finding to the primary care provider.
   e. Institute a turning schedule.
   f. Do not massage the patient's back; immediately report the area to the health care provider.

4. The nurse recognizes common pain syndromes that cause neuropathic pain. Which patients would the nurse place at risk for this type of pain? *(Select all that apply.)*
   a. A patient who has a tooth abscess
   b. A patient with postherpetic neuralgia
   c. A patient with phantom limb pain
   d. A patient with diabetic neuropathy
   e. A patient who has lung cancer
   f. A patient with complex regional pain syndrome

5. Nurses assess patients who have physiologic responses to pain. Which examples of pain response are physiologic responses? *(Select all that apply.)*
   a. Exaggerated weeping and restlessness
   b. Protecting the painful area
   c. Increased blood pressure
   d. Muscle tension and rigidity
   e. Nausea and vomiting
   f. Grimacing and moaning

## NURSING PROCESS WORKSHEET

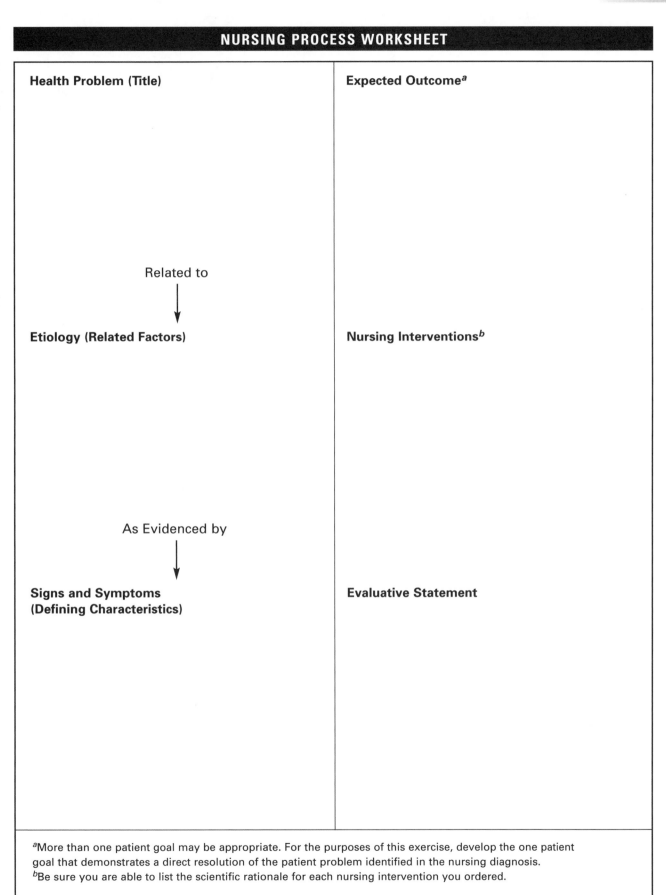

| Health Problem (Title) | Expected Outcome[a] |
| --- | --- |
| Related to ↓ | |
| Etiology (Related Factors) | Nursing Interventions[b] |
| As Evidenced by ↓ | |
| Signs and Symptoms (Defining Characteristics) | Evaluative Statement |

[a]More than one patient goal may be appropriate. For the purposes of this exercise, develop the one patient goal that demonstrates a direct resolution of the patient problem identified in the nursing diagnosis.
[b]Be sure you are able to list the scientific rationale for each nursing intervention you ordered.

CHAPTER 36

# Nutrition

## ASSESSING YOUR UNDERSTANDING

### FILL IN THE BLANKS

1. What would the nurse document as the body mass index (BMI) for a 220-lb man who is 6 ft 3 in tall? ___________

2. Following MyPlate food guidelines, what would be the daily caloric requirement for a sedentary male whose IBW is 165? ___________

3. The nurse teaches a patient that it is recommended that carbohydrates provide ___________% to ___________ % of calories for adults, focusing on complex carbohydrates, such as whole grains.

4. Most health care experts recommend that protein intake should contribute what percentage of total caloric intake? ___________

5. What percentage of an adult's total body weight is water? ___________

6. Dysphagia is associated with an increased risk for ___________, the misdirection of oropharyngeal secretions or gastric contents into the larynx and lower respiratory tract.

7. ___________ is the energy required to carry on the involuntary activities of the body at rest—the energy needed to sustain the metabolic activities of cells and tissues

### MATCHING EXERCISES

***Match the nutrient in Part A with the type of function it performs listed in Part B. Answers will be used more than once.***

**PART A**

**a.** Carbohydrates

**b.** Protein

**c.** Fat

**PART B**

____ **1.** Spares protein so it can be used for other functions

____ **2.** Insulates the body

____ **3.** Promotes tissue growth and repair

____ **4.** Prevents ketosis from inefficient fat metabolism

____ **5.** When metabolized it burdens the kidneys

____ **6.** Cushions internal organs

____ **7.** Delays glucose absorption

____ **8.** Is necessary for absorption of fat-soluble vitamins

____ **9.** Detoxifies harmful substances

____ **10.** Forms antibodies

***Match the function in Part B with the mineral listed in Part A. List one food source for each mineral on the line provided at the end of the sentence. Reference*** thePoint ***for a table summarizing these minerals.***

**PART A**

**a.** Calcium
**b.** Phosphorus
**c.** Magnesium
**d.** Sulfur
**e.** Sodium
**f.** Selenium
**g.** Chlorine
**h.** Iron
**i.** Iodine
**j.** Zinc
**k.** Copper
**l.** Manganese
**m.** Fluoride
**n.** Chromium
**o.** Molybdenum

**PART B**

____ **11.** Promotes certain enzyme reactions and detoxification reactions

____ **12.** Bone and tooth formation, blood clotting, nerve transmission, muscle contraction

____ **13.** Component of HCl in stomach; fluid balance; acid–base balance

____ **14.** Component of thyroid hormones

____ **15.** Major ion of extracellular fluid; fluid balance; acid–base balance

____ **16.** Aids in iron metabolism and activity of enzymes

____ **17.** Tooth formation and integrity; bone formation and integrity

____ **18.** Antioxidant

____ **19.** Oxidizes sulfur and products of sulfur metabolism

____ **20.** Bone and tooth formation; acid–base balance; energy metabolism

____ **21.** Oxygen transported by way of hemoglobin; constituent of enzyme systems

____ **22.** Tissue growth; sexual maturation; immune response

____ **23.** Part of enzyme system needed for protein and energy metabolism

____ **24.** Cofactor for insulin; proper glucose metabolism

***Match the terms listed in Part A with their definition listed in Part B.***

**PART A**

**a.** Nutrition
**b.** Nutrients
**c.** Macronutrients
**d.** Micronutrients
**e.** Calories
**f.** Basal metabolism
**g.** RDA
**h.** Cholesterol
**i.** MyPlate Food Guide

**PART B**

____ **25.** The measurement of energy in the diet

____ **26.** The study of nutrients and how they are handled by the body

____ **27.** The recommendation for average daily amounts that healthy population groups should consume over time

____ **28.** Specific biochemical substances used by the body for growth, development, activity, reproduction, lactation, health maintenance, and recovery from injury or illness

____ **29.** A graphic device designed to represent a total diet and provide a firm foundation for health

____ **30.** Essential nutrients that supply energy and build tissue

____ **31.** The amount of energy required to carry on the involuntary activities of the body at rest

____ **32.** Vitamins and minerals that are required in much smaller amounts to regulate and control body processes

**SHORT ANSWER**

**1.** Briefly explain the body's state of nitrogen balance.

________________________________________

________________________________________

________________________________________

**2.** Explain the difference between the following fatty acids and give an example of each. Note which of the two lowers serum cholesterol levels.

**a.** Saturated fatty acids: ____________________

____________________

____________________

**b.** Unsaturated fatty acids: ____________________

____________________

____________________

**3.** List four conditions that may predispose a person to mild or subclinical deficiencies of vitamin A, vitamin C, folate, and vitamin $B_6$.

**a.** ____________________

**b.** ____________________

**c.** ____________________

**d.** ____________________

**4.** Briefly describe the nutritional needs of the following age groups:

**a.** Infancy: ____________________

____________________

**b.** Toddlers and preschoolers: ____________________

____________________

**c.** School-aged children: ____________________

____________________

**d.** Adolescents: ____________________

____________________

**e.** Adults: ____________________

____________________

**f.** Pregnant women: ____________________

____________________

**g.** Older adults: ____________________

____________________

**5.** Complete the table below that depicts the function and recommended percentage of the diet for the energy nutrients.

| Nutrient | Function | Recommended % |
|---|---|---|
| **a.** Carbohydrates | | |
| **b.** Proteins | | |
| **c.** Fats | | |
| **d.** Vitamins | | |
| **e.** Minerals | | |
| **f.** Water | | |

6. List four interventions to increase fiber in a patient's diet.
   a. ______
   b. ______
   c. ______
   d. ______

7. Briefly describe the following eating disorders and the typical characteristics of individuals affected by them.
   a. Anorexia nervosa: ______
   b. Bulimia: ______

8. Give an example of how the following variables may affect a patient's nutritional needs.
   a. Biologic sex: ______
   b. State of health: ______
   c. Alcohol abuse: ______
   d. Medications: ______
   e. Megadoses of nutrient supplements: ______
   f. Religion: ______
   g. Economics: ______

9. Describe the following methods of collecting dietary data.
   a. Food diaries: ______
   b. Diet history: ______
   c. Food frequency record: ______

10. Describe how a nurse would assess a patient who is using home health care services for adequate nourishment.

    ______

11. List three teaching strategies a nurse may use to achieve compliance with diet instructions.
    a. ______
    b. ______
    c. ______

12. Describe the following types of diets, noting their nutritional value, and give an example of the types of food provided in each.
    a. Clear liquid diet: ______
    b. Full liquid diet: ______

13. Briefly describe the following types of enteral feedings, noting their advantages and disadvantages.
    a. Nasogastric feeding tube: ______
    b. Nasointestinal feeding tube: ______

14. List five areas that need to be evaluated for a patient at home who is receiving TPN.
    a. ______
    b. ______
    c. ______
    d. ______
    e. ______

## APPLYING YOUR KNOWLEDGE

### CRITICAL THINKING QUESTIONS

1. Develop a nutritional assessment for the following patients. What developmental factors influence their nutritional needs?
   a. An 18-month-old healthy infant
   b. A 5-year-old who is extremely active
   c. A 12-year-old who is 50 lb overweight
   d. A teenager who is concerned about body image and borders on being anorexic
   e. A middle-aged adult with high blood pressure
   f. A senior citizen who is anemic
2. Keep a diary of all the foods you eat in a week. Does your diet follow the USDA's dietary guidelines for a healthy diet? Does your diet include the recommended number of servings of foods from MyPlate? Is your diet high or low in fat? Perform a nutritional nursing assessment of your dietary habits. Develop a plan of care to improve your nutritional intake, if necessary. What personal factors might interfere with your making the necessary changes? How might this self-knowledge influence your nursing care?

### REFLECTIVE PRACTICE: DEVELOPING QSEN COMPETENCIES

***Use the following expanded scenario from Chapter 36 in your textbook to answer the questions below.***

*Scenario:* William Johnston, a 42-year-old executive, is newly diagnosed with high blood pressure and high cholesterol. He confides that his health has been the last thing on his mind and that his health habits are less than admirable. "I usually eat on the run, often fast food, or big dinners with lots of alcohol. I can't remember the last time I worked out or did any exercise, unless running from my car to the train counts! I guess it's no wonder I've gained a few pounds over the years!"

1. What patient teaching might the nurse provide to help Mr. Johnston meet his nutritional and exercise needs?

   ______________________________________
   ______________________________________
   ______________________________________

2. What would be a successful outcome for this patient?

   ______________________________________
   ______________________________________
   ______________________________________

3. What intellectual, technical, interpersonal, and/or ethical/legal competencies are most likely to bring about the desired outcome?

   ______________________________________
   ______________________________________
   ______________________________________

4. What resources might be helpful for Mr. Johnston?

   ______________________________________
   ______________________________________
   ______________________________________

### PATIENT CARE STUDY

***Read the following case study and use your nursing process skills to answer the questions below.***

*Scenario:* Mr. Church, a 74-year-old White man, is being admitted to the geriatric unit of the hospital for a diagnostic workup. He was diagnosed with Alzheimer's disease 4 years ago, and 1 year ago, he was admitted to a long-term care facility. His wife of 49 years is extremely devoted and informs the nurse taking the admission history that she instigated his admission to the hospital because she was alarmed by the amount of weight he was losing. Assessment reveals a 6-ft, 1-in tall, emaciated man who weighs 149 lb. His wife reports that he has lost 20 lb in the past 2 months. The staff at the long-term care facility report that he was eating his meals, and his wife validated that this was the case. No one seems sure, however, of the caloric content of his diet. Mrs. Church nods her head vigorously when asked if her husband had seemed more agitated and hyperactive recently. Mr. Church has dull, sparse hair; pale, dry skin; and dry mucous membranes.

1. Identify pertinent patient data by placing a single underline beneath the objective data in the case study and a double underline beneath the subjective data.

2. Complete the Nursing Process Worksheet on page 242 to develop a three-part diagnostic statement and related plan of care for this patient.
3. Write down the patient and personal nursing strengths you hope to draw on as you assist this patient to better health.

   Patient strengths: ______________________

   ______________________

   Personal strengths: ______________________

   ______________________
4. Pretend that you are performing a nursing assessment of this patient after the plan of care is implemented. Document your findings.

   ______________________

   ______________________

## PRACTICING FOR NCLEX

### MULTIPLE CHOICE QUESTIONS

***Circle the letter that corresponds to the best answer for each question.***

1. A nurse is planning a high-energy diet for a patient. What nutrient provides energy to the body and should be increased in the diet?
   a. Carbohydrates
   b. Vitamins
   c. Minerals
   d. Water
2. The nurse is assessing patients for BMR. Which patient would the nurse suspect would have an increased BMR?
   a. An older adult patient
   b. A patient who has a fever
   c. A patient who is fasting
   d. A patient who is asleep
3. The nurse is performing a nutritional assessment of an obese patient who visits a weight control clinic. What information should the nurse take into consideration when planning a weight reduction plan for this patient?
   a. To lose 1 lb/wk, the daily intake should be decreased by 200 calories.
   b. One pound of body fat equals approximately 5,000 calories.
   c. Psychological reasons for overeating should be explored, such as eating as a release for boredom.
   d. Obesity is very treatable, and 50% of obese people who lose weight maintain the weight loss for 7 years.
4. What consideration based on biologic sex would a nurse make when planning a menu for a male patient with well-defined muscle mass?
   a. Men have a lower need for carbohydrates.
   b. Men have a higher need for minerals.
   c. Men have a higher need for proteins.
   d. Men have a lower need for vitamins.
5. Which nursing action is performed according to guidelines for aspirating fluid from small-bore feeding tube?
   a. Use a small syringe and insert 10 mL of air.
   b. Inject air boluses into the tube with a large syringe and slowly apply negative pressure to withdraw fluid.
   c. Continue to instill air until fluid is aspirated.
   d. Place the patient in the Trendelenburg position to facilitate the fluid aspiration process.
6. When checking the placement of a gastrostomy or jejunostomy tube, the nurse must make regular comparisons of:
   a. Tube length
   b. Gastric fluid
   c. pH
   d. Air pressure
7. Which method of feeding would a nurse normally provide if a patient can attempt eating regular meals during the day and is prepared to ambulate and resume activities?
   a. Continuous feeding
   b. Intermittent feeding
   c. Cyclic feeding
   d. Ambulatory feeding
8. Which nursing action associated with successful tube feedings follows recommended guidelines?
   a. Check tube placement by adding food dye to the tube feed as a means of detecting aspirated fluid.
   b. Check the residual before each feeding or every 4 to 8 hours during a continuous feeding.

c. Assess for bowel sounds at least four times per shift to ensure the presence of peristalsis and a functional intestinal tract.
d. Prevent contamination during enteral feedings by using an open system.

9. A nurse is assessing the nutritional needs of patients. Which criterion indicates that a patient most likely needs TPN?
a. Serum albumin level of 2.5 g/dL or less
b. Residual of more than 100 mL
c. Absence of bowel sounds
d. Presence of dumping syndrome

## ALTERNATE-FORMAT QUESTIONS

### Multiple Response Questions

***Circle the letters that correspond to the best answers for each question.***

1. A nurse who is planning a diet for a patient who has anorexia chooses nutrients that supply energy to the body including: *(Select all that apply.)*
a. Vitamins
b. Minerals
c. Carbohydrates
d. Protein
e. Water
f. Lipids

2. Which examples of patients would the nurse expect to have an increase in BMR? *(Select all that apply.)*
a. A toddler who is having a growth spurt
b. An older adult who is in a long-term care facility
c. A teenager who has been fasting to lose weight
d. An adolescent who has a fever
e. An adult who is going through an emotional time due to divorce
f. An adult who has hypersomnia

3. As a nurse is aspirating the contents during a tube feeding, the nurse finds that the tube is clogged. What would be appropriate nursing interventions in this situation? *(Select all that apply.)*
a. Use warm water and gentle pressure to remove clog.
b. Flush with a carbonated beverage such as a cola soft drink.
c. Use a stylet to unclog the tube.
d. If necessary, replace the tube.
e. Ensure that adequate flushing is completed after each feeding.
f. Administer an antiemetic to the patient.

4. The nurse is assessing adequate nutrition for residents of a long-term care facility. Which strategies are recommended to address age-related changes affecting nutrition? *(Select all that apply.)*
a. Avoid cold liquids with decreased peristalsis in the esophagus.
b. Serve a variety of foods at each meal for loss of sense of taste and smell.
c. Avoid eating right before bedtime for gastroesophageal reflux.
d. Eat a high-fiber diet for slowed intestinal peristalsis.
e. Eat more protein for lowered glucose tolerance.
f. Offer large meals at frequent intervals for reduction in appetite and thirst sensation.

5. A home health care nurse is teaching a patient and caregivers how to administer an enteral feeding. Which teaching points are appropriate? *(Select all that apply.)*
a. When checking residuals, routinely discard residuals to prevent an acid–base imbalance.
b. When cleaning around a gastric tube insertion site, be careful not to rotate the guard after cleaning around it.
c. Check for leaking of gastric contents around the insertion site. (Is guard too loose or balloon not filled adequately?)
d. Clean around the gastric tube with soap and water, making sure it is adequately rinsed.
e. Keep the head elevated while delivering a gastric feeding and for approximately an hour after the feeding.
f. Mark gastrostomy tubes with an indelible marker and check the mark to make sure it is at the level of the abdominal wall.

6. The nurse researches factors that may alter nutrition. Which statements accurately describe factors that influence nutritional status? *(Select all that apply.)*
   - **a.** During adulthood, there is an increase in the basal metabolic rate with each decade.
   - **b.** Because of the changes related to aging, the caloric needs of the older adult increase.
   - **c.** During pregnancy and lactation, nutrient requirements increase.
   - **d.** Nutritional needs per unit of body weight are greater in infancy than at any other time in life.
   - **e.** Men and women differ in their nutrient requirements.
   - **f.** Trauma, surgery, and burns decrease nutrient requirements.

7. Which nursing actions follow guidelines for preventing complications with enteral feedings? *(Select all that apply.)*
   - **a.** Elevate the head of the bed by 30 to 45 degrees during the feeding and for at least 1 hour afterward.
   - **b.** Give large, infrequent feedings.
   - **c.** Flush the tube before and after feeding.
   - **d.** Clean and moisten the nares every 4 to 8 hours.
   - **e.** Change the delivery set every other day according to facility policy.
   - **f.** Check the residual before intermittent feedings and every 8 hours during continuous feedings.

## NURSING PROCESS WORKSHEET

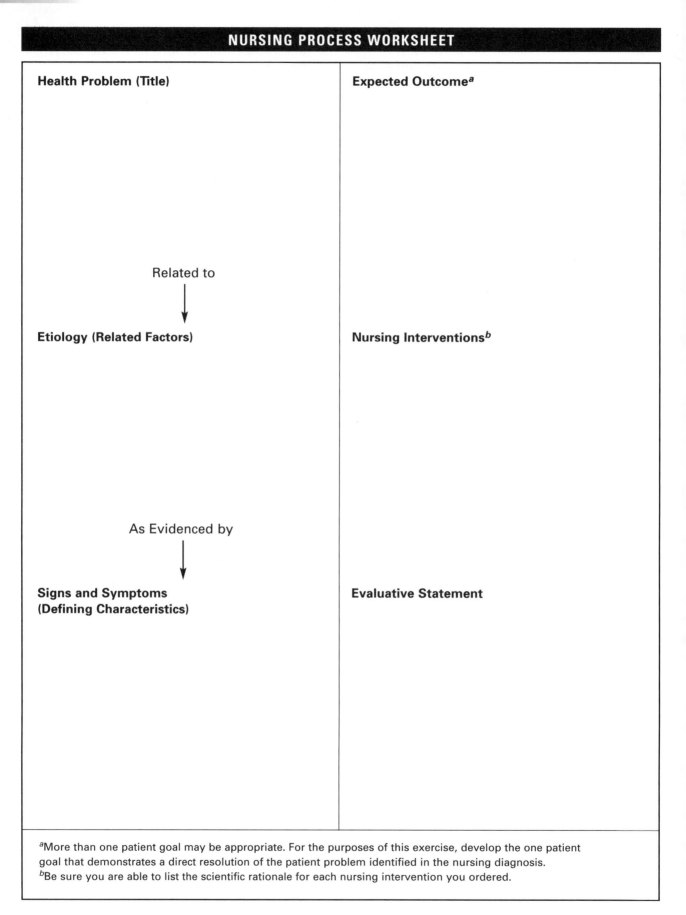

| **Health Problem (Title)** | **Expected Outcome**[a] |
|---|---|
| Related to ↓ | |
| **Etiology (Related Factors)** | **Nursing Interventions**[b] |
| As Evidenced by ↓ | |
| **Signs and Symptoms (Defining Characteristics)** | **Evaluative Statement** |

[a]More than one patient goal may be appropriate. For the purposes of this exercise, develop the one patient goal that demonstrates a direct resolution of the patient problem identified in the nursing diagnosis.
[b]Be sure you are able to list the scientific rationale for each nursing intervention you ordered.

CHAPTER 37

# Urinary Elimination

## ASSESSING YOUR UNDERSTANDING

### MATCHING EXERCISES

***Match the terms associated with micturition in Part A with their definitions listed in Part B.***

**PART A**

**a.** Micturition
**b.** Frequency
**c.** Urinary retention
**d.** Enuresis
**e.** Autonomic bladder
**f.** Hesitancy
**g.** Stress incontinence
**h.** Urge incontinence
**i.** Mixed incontinence
**j.** Overflow incontinence
**k.** Functional incontinence
**l.** Total incontinence

**PART B**

____ **1.** A delay or difficulty in initiating voiding

____ **2.** The involuntary loss of urine associated with an abrupt and strong desire to void

____ **3.** Urine loss caused by factors outside the lower urinary tract, such as chronic impairments of physical or cognitive functioning

____ **4.** The process of emptying the bladder

____ **5.** Involuntary urination that occurs after an age when continence should be present

____ **6.** Occurs when urine is produced normally but not appropriately excreted from the bladder

____ **7.** The involuntary loss of urine associated with overdistention and overflow of the bladder

____ **8.** Continuous and unpredictable loss of urine resulting from surgery, trauma, or physical malformation

____ **9.** Voiding by reflex only

____ **10.** Occurs when there is an involuntary loss of urine related to an increase in intra-abdominal pressure during coughing, sneezing, laughing, or other physical activities

____ **11.** Symptoms of urge and stress incontinence are present, although one type may predominate

***Match the color of urine listed in Part A with the medication that produces that color listed in Part B. Answers may be used more than once.***

**PART A**

**a.** Pale yellow
**b.** Orange, orange-red, or pink
**c.** Green or green-blue
**d.** Brown or black
**e.** Red

**PART B**

____ **12.** Levodopa

____ **13.** Diuretics

____ **14.** B-complex vitamins

____ **15.** Amitriptyline

____ **16.** Phenazopyridine

____ **17.** Anticoagulants

____ **18.** Injectable iron compounds

**SHORT ANSWER**

**1.** Describe how the following factors affect micturition.

**a.** Developmental considerations: ____________________

**b.** Food and fluid: ____________________

**c.** Psychological variables: ____________________

**d.** Activity and muscle tone: ____________________

**e.** Pathologic conditions: ____________________

**f.** Medications: ____________________

**2.** List three factors that indicate a child is ready for toilet training.

**a.** ____________________

**b.** ____________________

**c.** ____________________

**3.** Describe special urinary considerations that should be included in the nursing history for the following patients.

**a.** Infants and young children: ____________________

**b.** Older adults: ____________________

**c.** Patients with limited or no bladder control or urinary diversions: ____________________

**4.** Describe how you would examine the following areas of the urinary system when performing a physical assessment.

**a.** Kidneys: ____________________

**b.** Bladder: ____________________

**c.** Urethral orifice: ____________________

**d.** Skin integrity and hydration: ____________________

**e.** Urine: ____________________

**5.** List four expected outcomes that denote normal voiding in a patient.

**a.** ____________________

**b.** ____________________

**c.** ____________________

**d.** ____________________

**6.** Explain how the following factors influence a patient's voiding patterns.

**a.** Schedule: ____________________

**b.** Privacy: ____________________

**c.** Position: ____________________

**d.** Hygiene: ____________________

**7.** List three reasons for catheterization.

**a.** ____________________

**b.** ____________________

**c.** ____________________

**8.** List two expected outcomes for a patient with a urinary appliance.

**a.** ____________________

**b.** ____________________

## APPLYING YOUR KNOWLEDGE

### CRITICAL THINKING QUESTIONS

**1.** Develop a teaching plan to teach a postsurgical patient and his wife how to insert and care for a Foley catheter in a home setting. What factors are likely to influence the success of your teaching plan?

2. Keep a record of your fluid intake and output for 3 days. Note how your intake influenced urinary elimination. Write down the factors that could affect urine elimination. Are you at risk for urinary problems? If possible, perform routine tests on a sample of your urine and record the results.

## REFLECTIVE PRACTICE: CULTIVATING QSEN COMPETENCIES

***Use the following expanded scenario from Chapter 37 in your textbook to answer the questions below.***

*Scenario:* Midori Morita, age 69, is taking care of her 70-year-old husband at home. She states, "I'd like to talk with my husband's doctor about getting him a urinary catheter. Ever since he came back from the hospital this last time, he seems unable to use the urinal. He dribbles constantly and I can't keep up with the laundry. He had a catheter in the hospital, and I'm going to request that he has one at home."

1. How might the nurse respond to Mrs. Morita's remarks regarding her husband's home care?

______________________________

______________________________

______________________________

2. What would be a successful outcome for this patient?

______________________________

______________________________

______________________________

3. What intellectual, technical, interpersonal, and/or ethical/legal competencies are most likely to bring about the desired outcome?

______________________________

______________________________

______________________________

4. What resources might be helpful for the Morita family?

______________________________

______________________________

______________________________

## PATIENT CARE STUDY

***Read the following case study and use your nursing process skills to answer the questions below.***

*Scenario:* Mr. Eisenberg, age 84, was admitted to a long-term care facility when his wife of 62 years died. He has two adult children, neither of whom feels prepared to care for him the way his wife did. "We don't know how Mom did it year after year," his son says. "After he retired from his law practice, he was terribly demanding, and it just seemed nothing she did for him pleased him. His Parkinson's disease does make it a bit difficult for him to get around, but he's able to do a whole lot more than he is letting on. He's always been this way." The aides have reported to you that Mr. Eisenberg is frequently incontinent of both urine and stool during the day, as well as during the night. He is alert and appears capable of recognizing the need to void or defecate and signaling for any assistance. His son and daughter report that this was never a problem at home and that he was able to go into the bathroom with assistance. He has been depressed about his admission to the home and seldom speaks, even when directly approached. He has refused to participate in any of the floor social events since his arrival.

1. Identify pertinent patient data by placing a single underline beneath the objective data in the case study and a double underline beneath the subjective data.
2. Complete the Nursing Process Worksheet on page 250 to develop a three-part diagnostic statement and related plan of care for this patient.
3. Write down the patient and personal nursing strengths you hope to draw on as you assist this patient to better health.

   Patient strengths: ______________________________

   ______________________________

   Personal strengths: ______________________________

   ______________________________

4. Pretend that you are performing a nursing assessment of this patient after the plan of care is implemented. Document your findings.

______________________________

______________________________

## PRACTICING FOR NCLEX

### MULTIPLE CHOICE QUESTIONS

***Circle the letter that corresponds to the best answer for each question.***

1. The nurse is assessing a female patient who states that she notices an involuntary loss of urine following a coughing episode. What would be the nurse's best reply?
   a. "You are experiencing stress incontinence. Do you know how to do Kegel exercises?"
   b. "You are experiencing reflex incontinence. Have you had a spinal cord injury in the past?"
   c. "You are experiencing total incontinence. Have you had any surgeries or trauma that may be causing this?"
   d. "You are experiencing transient incontinence. Have you been administered diuretics or IV fluids lately?"
2. The nurse measures a patient's residual urine by catheterization after the patient voids. What condition would this test verify?
   a. Urinary tract infection
   b. Urinary retention
   c. Urinary incontinence
   d. Urinary suppression
3. What catheter would the nurse use to drain a patient's bladder for short periods (5 to 10 minutes)?
   a. Foley catheter
   b. Suprapubic catheter
   c. Indwelling urethral catheter
   d. Straight catheter
4. The nurse is preparing to catheterize a patient who is incontinent of urine following bladder surgery. What fact should the nurse keep in mind when performing catheterization?
   a. The bladder normally is a sterile cavity.
   b. The external opening to the urethra should always be sterilized.
   c. Pathogens introduced into the bladder remain in the bladder.
   d. A normal bladder is as susceptible to infection as an injured one.
5. The nurse is collecting a clean-catch specimen from a patient. Which nursing action is performed correctly in this procedure?
   a. Clean the area at the meatus with antiseptic solution.
   b. Collect the first 10 mL of urine voided in the sterile specimen container.
   c. Position the container near the meatus, and collect at least 10 mL of urine.
   d. Continue collecting the urine in the container until the bladder is empty.
6. The nurse is choosing a collection device to collect urine from a nonambulatory male patient? What would be the nurse's best choice?
   a. Specimen hat
   b. Large urine collection bag
   c. Bedpan
   d. Urinal
7. A male patient is being transferred to the hospital from a long-term care facility with a diagnosis of dehydration and urinary bladder infection. His skin is also excoriated from urinary incontinence. Which nursing diagnosis is most appropriate for this patient?
   a. Impaired skin integrity related to functional incontinence
   b. Stress urinary incontinence related to urinary tract infection
   c. Impaired skin integrity related to urinary bladder infection and dehydration
   d. Risk for urinary tract infection related to dehydration
8. A nurse is inserting a catheter into a female urinary bladder. Which nursing action is performed correctly?
   a. Clean the perineal area with a gauze pad and alcohol using a different corner of the gauze with each stroke.
   b. Assist the patient to a prone position with knees flexed, feet about 2 ft apart, with legs abducted.
   c. Using dominant hand, hold the catheter 12 in from the tip and insert slowly into the urethra.
   d. Use dominant hand to inflate the catheter balloon, and inject entire volume of sterile water supplied in prefilled syringe.

9. A nurse assessing an older adult finds that the patient has had four urinary tract infections in the past year. Which physiologic change of aging would the nurse suspect is the cause?
   a. Decreased bladder contractility
   b. Diminished ability to concentrate urine
   c. Decreased bladder muscle tone
   d. Neurologic weakness
10. The doctor has ordered the collection of a fresh urine sample for a particular examination. Which urine sample would the nurse discard?
    a. The sample collected immediately after lunch
    b. The bedtime voiding
    c. The voiding collected at 1600
    d. The first voiding of the day
11. The nurse is caring for a male patient who has a urinary obstruction and is not a candidate for surgery. What intervention would the nurse expect the health care provider to perform?
    a. Insertion of an indwelling urethral catheter
    b. Insertion of a suprapubic catheter
    c. Insertion of a straight catheter
    d. Insertion of a urologic stent

## ALTERNATE-FORMAT QUESTIONS

### Multiple Response Questions

***Circle the letters that correspond to the best answers for each question.***

1. The nurse is preparing a patient for an intravenous pyelogram. Which nursing actions are performed correctly? *(Select all that apply.)*
   a. Tell the patient not to void before the test.
   b. Withhold or limit foods before testing.
   c. Give an enema the day of the examination.
   d. Restrict fluids and foods immediately after the examination.
   e. Obtain patient's allergy history.
   f. Give a laxative the evening before the examination.
2. A nurse is collecting a urine specimen for urinalysis. What factors should the nurse consider when performing this procedure? *(Select all that apply.)*
   a. Sterile urine specimens may be obtained by catheterizing the patient's bladder.
   b. A sterile urine specimen is required for a routine urinalysis.
   c. If a woman is menstruating, a urine specimen cannot be obtained for urinalysis.
   d. Strict aseptic technique must be used when collecting and handling urine specimens.
   e. Urine should be left standing at room temperature for a 24-hour period before being sent to the laboratory.
   f. A clean-catch specimen of urine may be collected in midstream.
3. A nurse is assessing the freshly voided urine of a patient. What characteristics of the urine would indicate a urinary problem? *(Select all that apply.)*
   a. The urine is amber colored.
   b. The urine smells like ammonia.
   c. The urine pH is 6.0.
   d. The urine is translucent.
   e. There is pus in the urine.
   f. The urine is cloudy.
4. A nurse is performing a physical assessment of a patient's urinary system. Which nursing actions are appropriate during this assessment? *(Select all that apply.)*
   a. If using a bedside scanner, the nurse places the patient in a supine position.
   b. The nurse measures the height of the edge of the bladder below the symphysis pubis.
   c. The nurse inspects the urethral orifice for any signs of inflammation, discharge, or foul odor.
   d. The nurse places male patients in the dorsal recumbent position for good visualization of the meatus.
   e. The nurse retracts the foreskin of an uncircumcised male patient to visualize the meatus.
   f. The nurse assesses the patient's urine for color, odor, clarity, and the presence of any sediment.

5. The nurse is assessing a patient's bladder volume using an ultrasound bladder scanner. Which nursing actions are performed correctly? *(Select all that apply.)*
   a. The nurse gently palpates the patient's symphysis pubis.
   b. The nurse places a generous amount of ultrasound gel or gel pad midline on the patient's abdomen, about 1 to 1.5 in above the symphysis pubis.
   c. The nurse places the scanner head on the gel or gel pad, with the directional icon on the scanner head pointed away from the patient's head.
   d. The nurse aims the scanner head toward the bladder (points the scanner head slightly downward toward the coccyx).
   e. The nurse adjusts the scanner head to center the bladder image on the crossbars.
   f. The nurse presses and holds the END button until it beeps three times and then reads the volume measurement on the screen.
6. The nurse is catheterizing a male urinary bladder, and urine leaks out of the meatus around the catheter. What actions would the nurse perform next? *(Select all that apply.)*
   a. Increase the size of the indwelling catheter.
   b. Make sure the smallest sized catheter with a 10-mL balloon is used.
   c. Consider an evaluation for urinary tract infection.
   d. Ensure that the correct amount of solution was used to inflate the balloon.
   e. If under fill is suspected, attempt to push the catheter further into the bladder.
   f. Assess the patient for diarrhea.
7. The nurse is changing a stoma appliance on an ileal conduit. Which of the following nursing actions are recommended procedure? *(Select all that apply.)*
   a. Gently remove the appliance, starting at the top and keeping the abdominal skin taut.
   b. Remove appliance faceplate by pulling appliance from skin rather than pushing.
   c. Apply a silicone-based adhesive remover by spraying or wiping as needed.
   d. Clean skin around stoma with alcohol on a gauze pad.
   e. Make sure skin around stoma is thoroughly dry by patting it dry.
   f. Apply faceplate by using firm, even pressure for approximately 60 seconds.

### Hot Spot Questions

1. Place an X on figures A and B below to identify the female and male urethras.

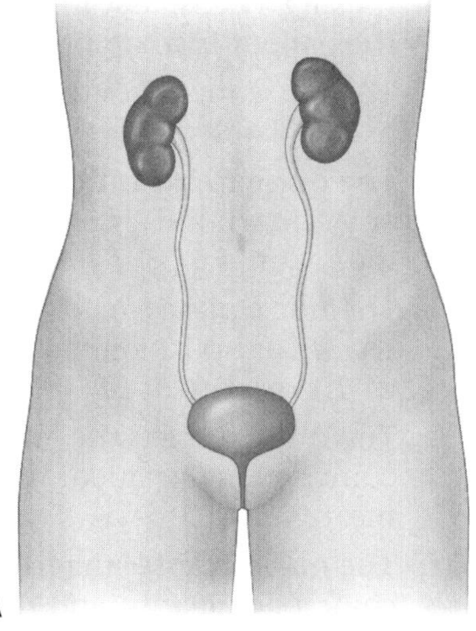


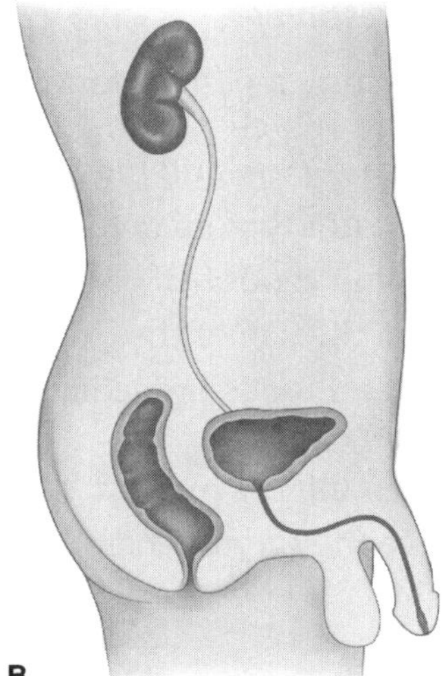

**2.** Place an X on the figure below to identify the location of the external sphincter.

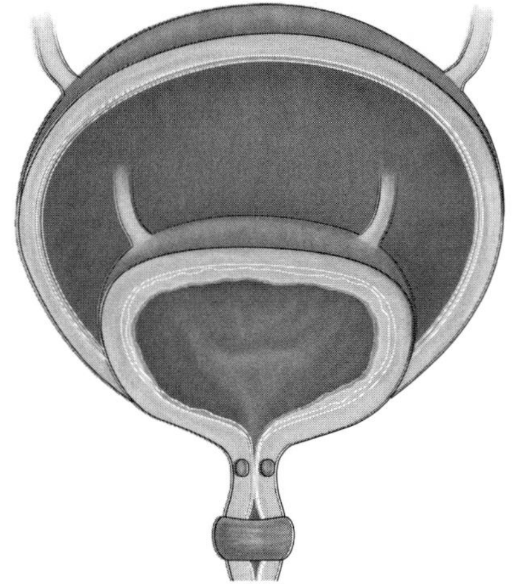

**3.** Place an X on the figure below to identify the urinary bladder.

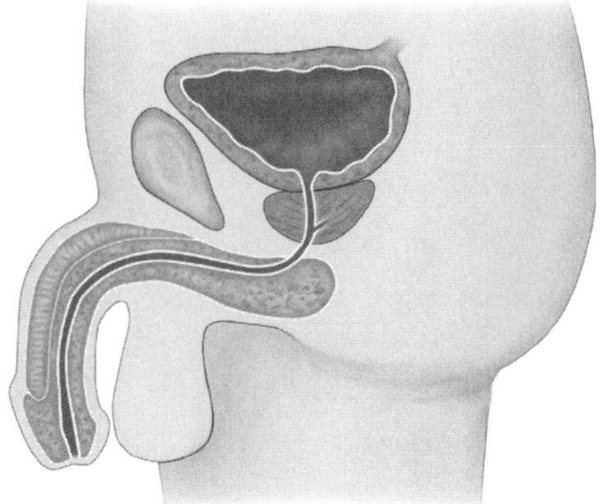

**4.** Place an X on the figure below to mark the spot where a suprapubic catheter would be inserted into the bladder.

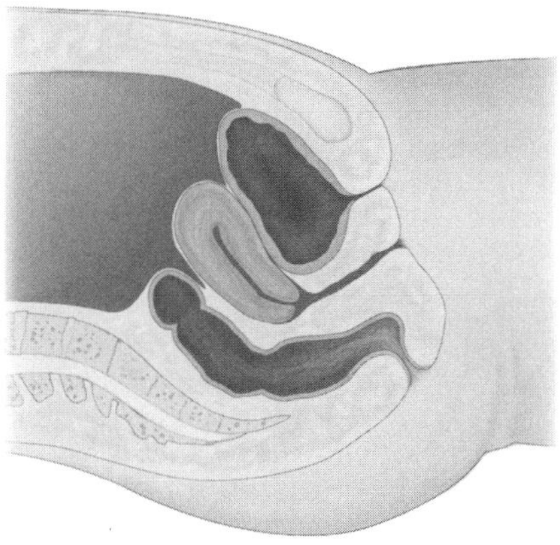

## NURSING PROCESS WORKSHEET

| **Health Problem (Title)**<br><br>Related to<br>↓ | **Expected Outcome**[a] |
| --- | --- |
| **Etiology (Related Factors)**<br><br>As Evidenced by<br>↓ | **Nursing Interventions**[b] |
| **Signs and Symptoms (Defining Characteristics)** | **Evaluative Statement** |

[a]More than one patient goal may be appropriate. For the purposes of this exercise, develop the one patient goal that demonstrates a direct resolution of the patient problem identified in the nursing diagnosis.
[b]Be sure you are able to list the scientific rationale for each nursing intervention you ordered.

CHAPTER 38

# Bowel Elimination

## ASSESSING YOUR UNDERSTANDING

### IDENTIFICATION

1. Locate the internal anal sphincter, the external anal sphincter, the anal canal, the rectum, and the anal valve on the figure below and write the appropriate body part on the lines provided.

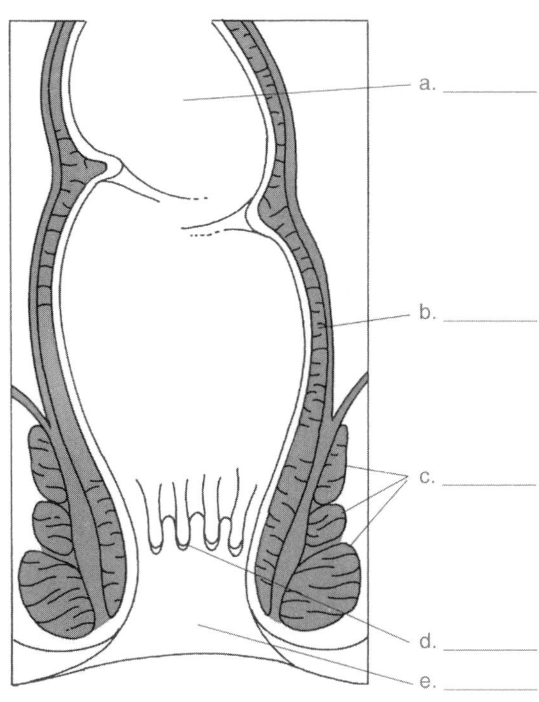

2. Name the type of ostomy depicted in the figures below by writing your answers on the lines provided. Indicate the type of stool that would be expected with each ostomy.

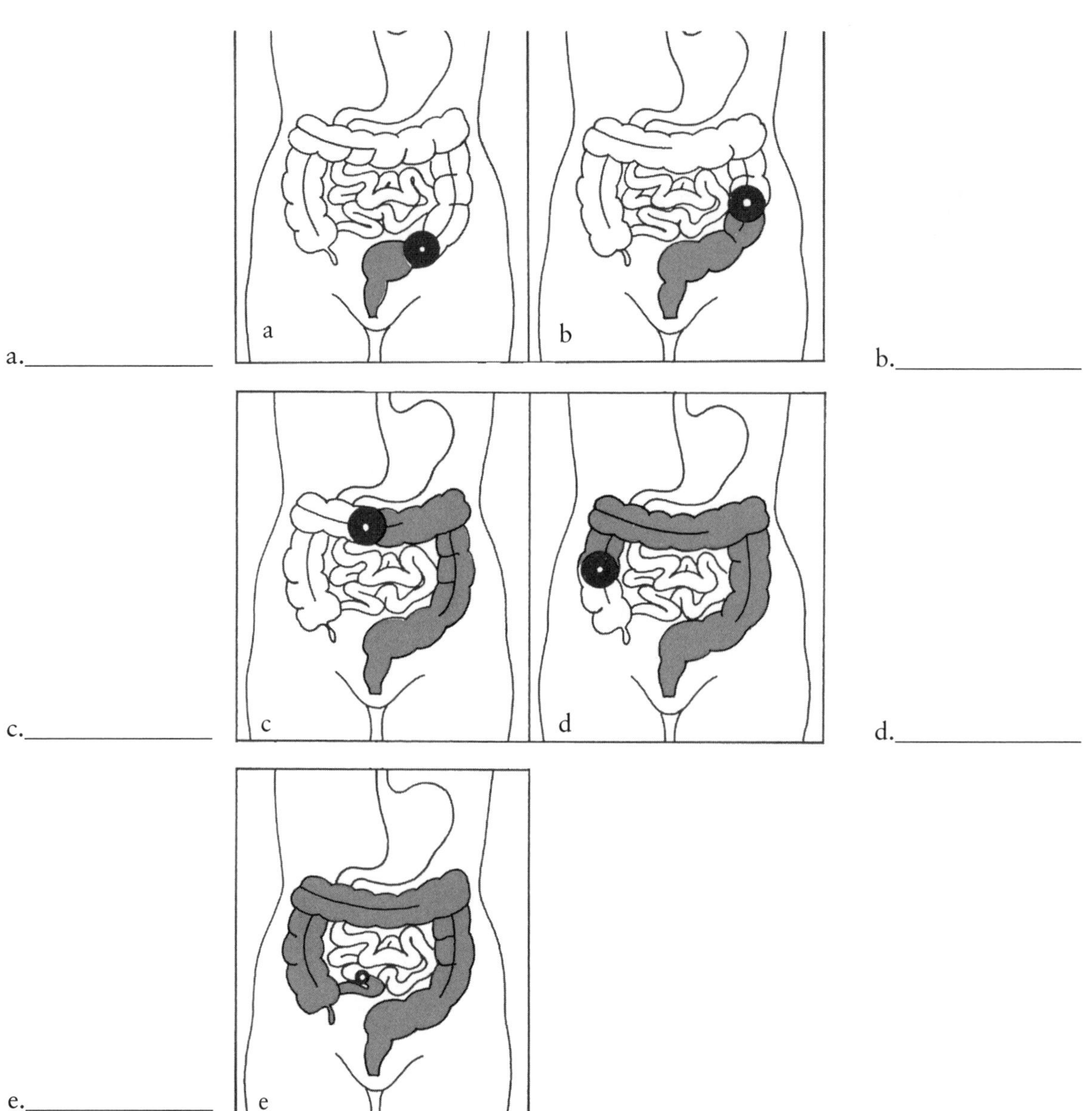


## MATCHING EXERCISES

***Match the bowel studies listed in Part A with their definition listed in Part B.***

### PART A

**a.** Endoscopy
**b.** Esophagogastroduodenoscopy
**c.** Colonoscopy
**d.** Sigmoidoscopy
**e.** Upper gastrointestinal examination
**f.** Lower gastrointestinal examination
**g.** Fecal occult blood test (FOBT)
**h.** Timed specimens
**i.** Pinworm test
**j.** Barium enema

### PART B

____ **1.** The collection of a specimen of every stool passed within a designated time period

____ **2.** The direct visualization of the lining of a hollow body organ using a long flexible tube containing glass fibers that transmit light into the organ, allowing the return of an image that can be viewed

____ **3.** The visual examination of the lining of the distal sigmoid colon, the rectum, and the anal canal using either a flexible or rigid instrument

____ **4.** Barium sulfate is instilled into the large intestine through a rectal tube inserted through the anus. Fluoroscopy projects consecutive x-ray images onto a screen for continuous observation of the flow of the barium

____ **5.** Visual examination of the lining of the large intestine with a flexible, fiber-optic endoscope

____ **6.** The patient drinks barium sulfate, which coats the esophagus, stomach, and small intestine to produce better visualization

____ **7.** Visual examination of the lining of the esophagus, the stomach, and the upper duodenum with a flexible, fiber-optic endoscope

____ **8.** Use of a commercial tape, dipstick, or solution to test for pH or blood in the stool

____ **9.** Involves a series of radiographs that examine the large intestine after rectal instillation of barium sulfate

***Match the type of enema in Part A with its use listed in Part B. Some questions may have more than one answer.***

**PART A**

**a.** Oil-retention enemas
**b.** Carminative enemas
**c.** Medicated enemas
**d.** Anthelmintic enemas

**PART B**

____ **10.** Used to lubricate the stool and intestinal mucosa, making defecation easier

____ **11.** Administered to destroy intestinal parasites

____ **12.** Used to administer medications that are absorbed through the rectal mucosa

____ **13.** Used to help expel flatus from the rectum and provide relief from gaseous distention

***Match the term in Part A with its definition listed in Part B.***

**PART A**

**a.** Chyme
**b.** Feces
**c.** Stool
**d.** Flatus
**e.** Bowel movement
**f.** Hemorrhoids
**g.** Constipation
**h.** Diarrhea
**i.** Incontinence
**j.** Valsalva maneuver
**k.** Peristalsis

**PART B**

____ **14.** The passage of dry, hard stools

____ **15.** Waste product of digestion

____ **16.** The passage of excessively liquid and unformed stools

____ **17.** Waste product that reaches the distal end of the colon

____ **18.** Intestinal gas

____ **19.** The inability of the anal sphincter to control the discharge of fecal and gaseous material

____ **20.** Excreted feces

____ **21.** The emptying of the intestines

____ **22.** The contraction of the circular and longitudinal muscles of the intestine

***Match the organs of the gastrointestinal system listed in Part A with the illustration in Part B.***

**PART A**

**a.** Splenic flexure
**b.** Sigmoid colon
**c.** Cecum
**d.** Hepatic flexure
**e.** Common bile duct
**f.** Stomach
**g.** Esophagus
**h.** Descending colon
**i.** Ileum
**j.** Hepatic duct
**k.** Gallbladder

**l.** Duodenum
**m.** Jejunum
**n.** Rectum
**o.** Ascending colon
**p.** Pancreatic duct
**q.** Ileocecal junction
**r.** Transverse colon

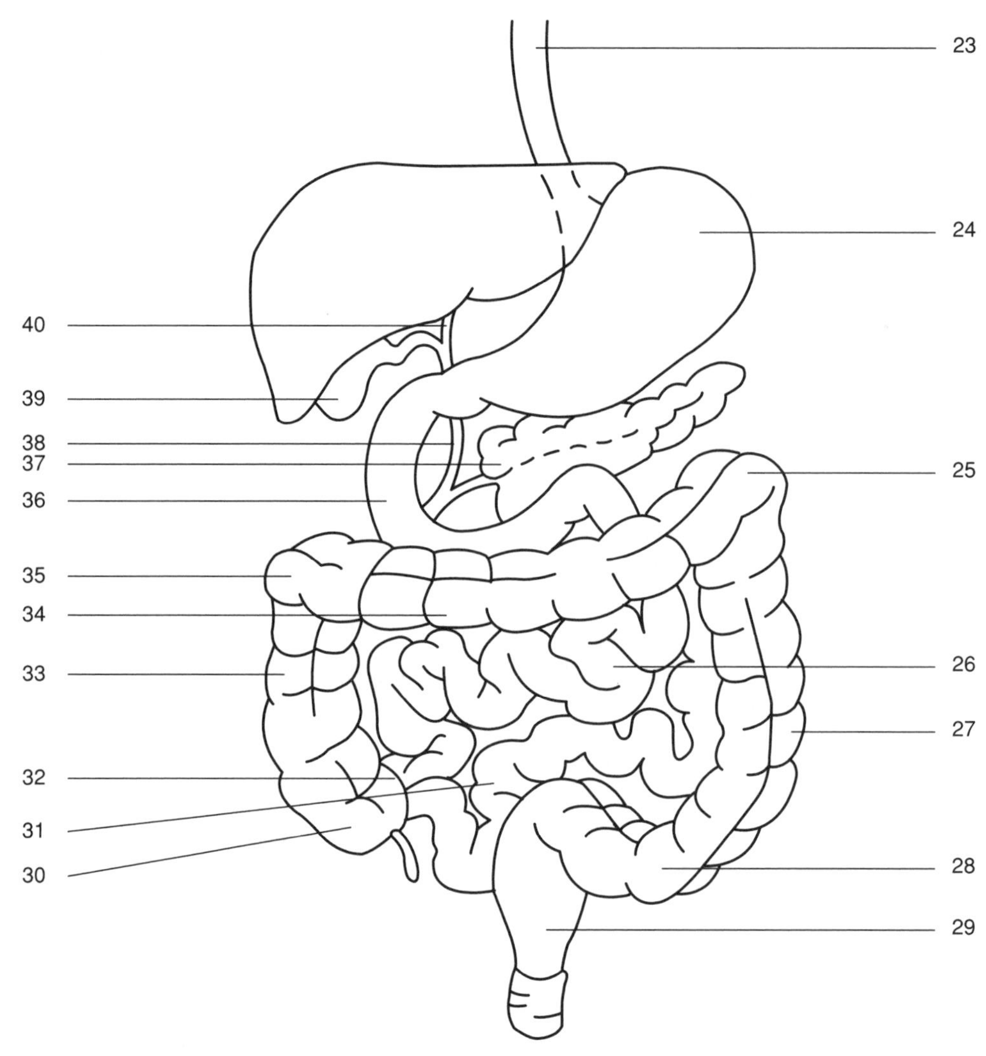


**PART B**

____ **23.**

____ **24.**

____ **25.**

____ **26.**

____ **27.**

____ **28.**

____ **29.**

____ **30.**

____ **31.**

____ **32.**

____ **33.**

____ **34.**

____ **35.**

____ **36.**

____ **37.**

____ **38.**

____ **39.**

____ **40.**

## SHORT ANSWER

1. List four functions of the large intestine.
   a. ______
   b. ______
   c. ______
   d. ______
2. List the two centers of the nervous system that govern the reflex to defecate.
   a. ______
   b. ______
3. Describe two effects the following surgical procedures may have on peristalsis.
   a. Direct manipulation of the bowel: ______
   b. Inhalation of general anesthetic agents: ______
4. List the characteristics of the abdomen the nurse would assess by the following methods.
   a. Inspection: ______
   b. Auscultation: ______
   c. Percussion: ______
   d. Palpation: ______
5. Give an example of how the following factors might affect a patient's bowel elimination.
   a. Developmental considerations: ______
   b. Daily patterns: ______
   c. Food and fluids: ______
   d. Activity and muscle tone: ______
   e. Lifestyle: ______
   f. Psychological variables: ______
   g. Medications: ______
   h. Diagnostic studies: ______
6. Mrs. Manganello is a 52-year-old patient with acute stomach pain related to diverticular disease. Prepare an interview to assess Mrs. Manganello's bowel elimination.
7. List four factors that promote healthy elimination patterns.
   a. ______
   b. ______
   c. ______
   d. ______
8. Give three examples of foods that have the following effects on elimination.
   a. Constipating: ______
   b. Laxative: ______
   c. Gas producing: ______
9. Mrs. Azhner is a 65-year-old postsurgical patient complaining of painful defecation due to hard, dry stools. List three expected outcomes for this patient.
   a. ______
   b. ______
   c. ______
10. Specify dietary measures to alleviate the following gastrointestinal problems.
    a. Constipation: ______
    b. Diarrhea: ______
    c. Flatulence: ______
    d. Ostomies: ______

**11.** Describe the following exercises designed for patients with weak abdominal and perineal muscles who are using a bedpan.

**a.** Abdominal settings: ______________________

______________________

**b.** Thigh strengthening: ______________________

______________________

**12.** List four reasons for prescribing cleansing enemas.

**a.** ______________________

**b.** ______________________

**c.** ______________________

**d.** ______________________

**13.** Briefly describe the following types of ostomies.

**a.** Ileostomy: ______________________

______________________

**b.** Colostomy: ______________________

______________________

**14.** Describe how the following factors help promote healthy bowel habits in patients.

**a.** Timing: ______________________

______________________

**b.** Positioning: ______________________

______________________

**c.** Privacy: ______________________

______________________

**d.** Nutrition: ______________________

______________________

**e.** Exercise: ______________________

______________________

## APPLYING YOUR KNOWLEDGE

### CRITICAL THINKING QUESTIONS

**1.** Develop a list of preferred foods to ensure healthy bowel elimination for the following patients.

**a.** A woman complains of constipation following a cesarean section.

**b.** A 40-year-old man who is under stress in his job complains of frequent diarrhea.

**c.** A toddler's stools are hard and dry, and he complains of frequent stomachaches.

What other factors are likely to promote healthy bowel elimination in these patients?

**2.** Perform a physical assessment and write a nursing diagnosis for a patient who has just had a colostomy performed. What changes will this patient face in his life, and what can be done to help him cope with them? How can you best learn this? Be sure to assess this patient's physical and psychological factors, body image, coping mechanisms, and support system. Develop a nursing care plan to provide postoperative care, hospital care, and follow-up care for this patient.

### REFLECTIVE PRACTICE: CULTIVATING QSEN COMPETENCIES

***Use the following expanded scenario from Chapter 38 in your textbook to answer the questions below.***

***Scenario:*** Leroy Cobbs, age 56, was recently diagnosed with prostate cancer. He is taking acetaminophen (Tylenol) with codeine for pain and is hospitalized for fecal impaction. During the physical examination, Mr. Cobbs says, "Nobody told me I would get so constipated. It's been almost a week and I'm still not moving my bowels normally. I didn't know anything could hurt so bad!" Mr. Cobbs reports that he had regular, pain-free bowel movements, once daily, before taking the pain medication. He appears frustrated and says, "I'll take my chances with the cancer pain in the future rather than take more pain medicine and have this happen again."

**1.** What nursing interventions might the nurse implement for this patient?

______________________

______________________

______________________

**2.** What would be a successful outcome for Mr. Cobbs?

______________________

______________________

______________________

3. What intellectual, technical, interpersonal, and/or ethical/legal competencies are most likely to bring about the desired outcome?

_______________

_______________

_______________

4. What resources might be helpful for Mr. Cobbs?

_______________

_______________

_______________

**PATIENT CARE STUDY**

***Read the following patient care study and use your nursing process skills to answer the questions below.***

***Scenario:*** Ms. Elgaresta, age 54, a single Hispanic woman, is being followed by a cardiologist who monitors her arrhythmia. Last month, she started taking a new heart medication. At this visit, she says to the nurse practitioner who works with the cardiologist: "Right after I started taking that medication, I got terribly constipated, and nothing seems to help. I'm desperate and about ready to try dynamite unless you can think of something else!" She reports a change in her bowel movements from one soft stool daily to one or two hard stools weekly, stools that cause much straining. The nurse practitioner realizes that regulating Ms. Elgaresta's heart is difficult and that her best cardiac response to date has been with the medication that is now causing constipation. Reluctant to suggest substituting another medication too quickly, she asks more questions and Ms. Elgaresta responds, "I've never been much of a drinker, 2 cups of coffee in the morning and maybe a glass of wine at night. Water? Almost never. And I don't drink juices or soft drinks." Analysis of her diet reveals a diet low in fiber: "I never was one much for vegetables, and they can just keep all this bran stuff that's out on the market! Coffee and a cigarette. That's for me!" Ms. Elgaresta is a workaholic computer programmer and spends what little spare time she has watching TV. She reports tiring after walking one flight of stairs and says she avoids all forms of vigorous exercise.

1. Identify pertinent patient data by placing a single underline beneath the objective data in the case study and a double underline beneath the subjective data.
2. Complete the Nursing Process Worksheet on page 261 to develop a three-part diagnostic statement and related plan of care for this patient.
3. Write down the patient and personal nursing strengths you hope to draw on as you assist this patient to better health.

   Patient strengths: _______________

   _______________

   _______________

   Personal strengths: _______________

   _______________

   _______________

4. Pretend that you are performing a nursing assessment of this patient after the plan of care is implemented. Document your findings.

   _______________

   _______________

## PRACTICING FOR NCLEX

**MULTIPLE CHOICE QUESTIONS**

***Circle the letter that corresponds to the best answer for each question.***

1. The nurse is administering a large-volume cleansing enema to a patient. Which nursing action is performed correctly?
   a. The nurse places the patient on bedpan in the supine position while receiving enema.
   b. The nurse uses cool tap water for the enema solution.
   c. The nurse elevates solution to no higher than 10 in above level of anus.
   d. The nurse gives the solution slowly over a period of 5 to 10 minutes.

2. The nurse is changing a patient's ostomy appliance and observes that the peristomal skin is excoriated. What would be the nurse's ***priority*** intervention in this situation?
   a. Notify the primary care provider.
   b. Suspect ischemia and notify the primary care provider immediately.
   c. Clean outside of bag thoroughly when emptying.
   d. Make sure that the appliance is not cut too large.
3. The nurse is inserting a rectal tube to administer a large-volume enema. Which nursing action is performed correctly in this procedure?
   a. Position the patient on his or her back and drape properly.
   b. Slowly and gently insert the enema tube 3 to 4 in (7 to 10 cm) for an adult.
   c. Introduce solution quickly over a period of 3 to 5 minutes.
   d. Encourage the patient to hold the solution for at least 20 minutes.
4. The nurse is irrigating a nasogastric tube attached to suction and finds that the flush solution is meeting a lot of force when plunger is pushed. What would be the nurse's ***first*** intervention in this situation?
   a. Inject 20 to 30 mL of free air into the abdomen in attempt to reposition the tube and enable flushing of the tube.
   b. Check the suction canister to ensure that the suction is working appropriately.
   c. Assess the abdomen for distention and ask the patient if he or she is experiencing any nausea or any abdominal discomfort.
   d. Attempt to flush the tube to ensure its patency.
5. The nurse is caring for a patient who is scheduled for an esophagogastroduodenoscopy (EGD). What action would the nurse take to prepare the patient for this procedure?
   a. Ensure that the patient ingests a gallon of bowel cleanser, such as GoLytely, in a short period of time.
   b. Inform patient that a chalky-tasting barium contrast mixture will be given to drink before the test.
   c. Provide a light meal before the test and administer two Fleet enemas.
   d. Ensure that the patient fasts 6 to 12 hours before the test as per policy.
6. The nurse is scheduling tests for a patient who is experiencing bowel alterations. What is the most logical sequence of tests to ensure an accurate diagnosis?
   a. Barium studies, endoscopic examination, fecal occult blood test
   b. Fecal occult blood test, barium studies, endoscopic examination
   c. Barium studies, fecal occult blood test, endoscopic examination
   d. Endoscopic examination, barium studies, fecal occult blood test
7. The nurse is administering psyllium to a patient with constipation. What mechanism of action would the nurse expect from this drug?
   a. Chemical stimulation of peristalsis
   b. Softening of the fecal material
   c. Increasing intestinal bulk to enhance mechanical stimulation of the intestine
   d. Drawing water into the intestines to stimulate peristalsis

## ALTERNATE-FORMAT QUESTIONS

### Multiple Response Questions

***Circle the letters that correspond to the best answers for each question.***

1. The nurse is administering an oil-retention enema to a patient. Which nursing actions in this procedure are performed correctly? *(Select all that apply.)*
   a. The nurse chooses a large rectal tube.
   b. The nurse instills the solution into the rectum by applying gentle pressure on the collapsible solution container.
   c. The nurse administers the oil-retention enema at body temperature.
   d. The nurse instructs the patient to retain the oil for at least 30 minutes.
   e. The nurse administers a cleansing enema prior to the oil-retention enema.
   f. The nurse administers a cleansing enema after the oil-retention enema.

**2.** A nurse is assessing the bowel elimination of patients in a med-surg unit. What developmental factors affecting elimination should the nurse consider? *(Select all that apply.)*

**a.** Voluntary control of defecation occurs between the ages of 12 and 18 months.

**b.** The number of stools that infants pass varies greatly.

**c.** Some children have bowel movements only every 2 or 3 days.

**d.** A child who has not had a bowel movement daily is most likely constipated.

**e.** In an infant, a liquid stool signifies diarrhea.

**f.** Constipation is often a chronic problem for older adults.

**3.** A nurse who is planning menus for a patient in a long-term care facility takes into consideration the effects of foods and fluids on bowel elimination. Which examples correctly describe these effects? *(Select all that apply.)*

**a.** Patients with lactose intolerance may experience diarrhea or gas when consuming starchy foods.

**b.** A patient who is constipated should eat eggs and pasta to relieve the condition.

**c.** Patients who are constipated should eat more fruits and vegetables.

**d.** Patients experiencing flatulence should avoid gas-producing foods such as cauliflower and onions.

**e.** Alcohol and coffee tend to have a constipating effect on patients.

**f.** Patients with food intolerances may experience altered bowel elimination.

**4.** A nurse is assessing the bowel elimination patterns of hospitalized patients. Which nursing actions related to the assessment process are performed correctly? *(Select all that apply.)*

**a.** The nurse auscultates the abdomen before inspection and palpation are performed.

**b.** The nurse places the patient in the supine position with the abdomen exposed.

**c.** The nurse drapes the patient's chest and pubic area and extends the patient's legs flat against the bed.

**d.** The nurse encourages the patient to drink fluids before the assessment so that the bladder is full and can be examined.

**e.** The nurse uses a warmed stethoscope to listen for bowel sounds in all abdominal quadrants.

**f.** The nurse notes the character of bowel sounds, which are normally high pitched, gurgling, and soft.

**5.** A nurse is collecting a stool specimen from a patient. Which measures are appropriate for this procedure? *(Select all that apply.)*

**a.** The patient should be asked to void first because the lab study may be inaccurate if the stool contains urine.

**b.** The patient should be asked to defecate into a clean bedpan or toilet bowl, depending on the nature of the study.

**c.** The patient should be instructed not to place toilet tissue in the bedpan or specimen container.

**d.** Medical aseptic techniques are always followed.

**e.** Handwashing is performed before and after glove use when handling a stool specimen.

**f.** Generally, 2 in of formed stool or 20 to 30 mL of liquid stool is sufficient for a stool specimen.

**6.** The nurse inspects the stool of patients admitted to the hospital with abdominal distress. Which statements accurately describe the normal characteristics of stool and special considerations for observation? *(Select all that apply.)*

**a.** Consistently large diarrheal stools suggest a disorder of the left colon or rectum.

**b.** The rapid rate of peristalsis in the breastfed infant causes the stool to be yellow.

**c.** The absence of bile may cause the stool to appear black.

**d.** Antacids in the diet cause the stool to be whitish.

**e.** A gastrointestinal obstruction may result in a narrow, pencil-shaped stool.

**f.** The odor of the stool is influenced by its pH value, which normally is slightly acidic.

7. The nurse is selecting antidiarrheal medications for patients with diarrhea. Which statements accurately describe the action of specific antidiarrheal medications? *(Select all that apply.)*
   a. Atropine may be used in older adults as it does not affect level of consciousness.
   b. Diphenoxylate should be used in patients taking opioids to decrease constipation.
   c. Diphenoxylate should not be used if antibiotic-associated diarrhea is suspected.
   d. Pepto-Bismol contains salicylates; a health care provider should be consulted before giving it to children or patients taking aspirin.
   e. Higher than recommended doses of loperamide may increase serious cardiac events.
   f. Loperamide has a shorter duration than diphenoxylate and atropine.

8. Which of the following commonly used enema solutions would the nurse administer to distend the intestine and increase peristalsis? *(Select all that apply.)*
   a. Tap water
   b. Soap
   c. Normal saline
   d. Mineral oil
   e. Hypertonic
   f. Olive oil

9. The nurse is performing digital removal of a fecal impaction. Which nursing actions follow guidelines for this procedure? *(Select all that apply.)*
   a. Have the patient lie on his stomach and pie-fold top linens over him.
   b. Place the patient in a side-lying position.
   c. Vigorously work the finger around and into the hardened mass to break it up.
   d. Use nonsterile gloves for the procedure because the intestinal tract is not sterile.
   e. Use a cleansing enema if necessary.
   f. Lubricate the index finger generously to reduce irritating the rectum, and insert the finger gently into the anal canal.

**Prioritization Question**

1. Place the following steps for digital removal of stool in the order in which they would normally occur:
   a. Slowly and gently work the finger around and into the hardened mass to break it up and then remove pieces of it. Instruct the patient to bear down if possible while extracting feces to ease in removal.
   b. Place the patient in a side-lying position and place a bedpan on the bed for depositing removed feces.
   c. Use an oil-retention enema if necessary.
   d. Remove the impaction at intervals if it is severe. This helps to avoid discomfort as well as irritation, which can injure intestinal mucosa.
   e. Wash and dry the patient's buttocks and anal area. Assist the patient to a comfortable position.
   f. Lubricate the forefinger generously to reduce irritation of the rectum, and insert the finger gently into the anal canal. The presence of the finger added to the mass tends to cause discomfort for the patient if the work is not done slowly and gently.
   g. Use nonsterile gloves for the procedure because the intestinal tract is not sterile.
   h. Have a second person assist with the procedure to reassure and comfort the patient while the first person breaks up the mass.

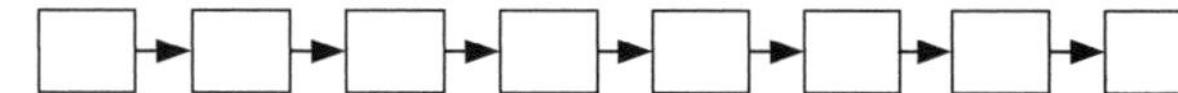

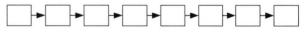

## NURSING PROCESS WORKSHEET

| **Health Problem (Title)** | **Expected Outcome**[a] |
|---|---|
| Related to ↓ | |
| **Etiology (Related Factors)** | **Nursing Interventions**[b] |
| As Evidenced by ↓ | |
| **Signs and Symptoms (Defining Characteristics)** | **Evaluative Statement** |

[a]More than one patient goal may be appropriate. For the purposes of this exercise, develop the one patient goal that demonstrates a direct resolution of the patient problem identified in the nursing diagnosis.
[b]Be sure you are able to list the scientific rationale for each nursing intervention you ordered.

CHAPTER 39

# Oxygenation and Perfusion

## ASSESSING YOUR UNDERSTANDING

### IDENTIFICATION

1. Identify the location of the organs of the respiratory tract listed here by writing the appropriate organ on the lines provided on the figure below.

Diaphragm
Epiglottis
Esophagus
Frontal sinus
Laryngeal pharynx
Larynx and vocal cords
Left lung
Mediastinum
Nasal cavity
Nasopharynx
Oropharynx
Right bronchus
Right lung
Sphenoidal sinus
Terminal bronchiole
Trachea

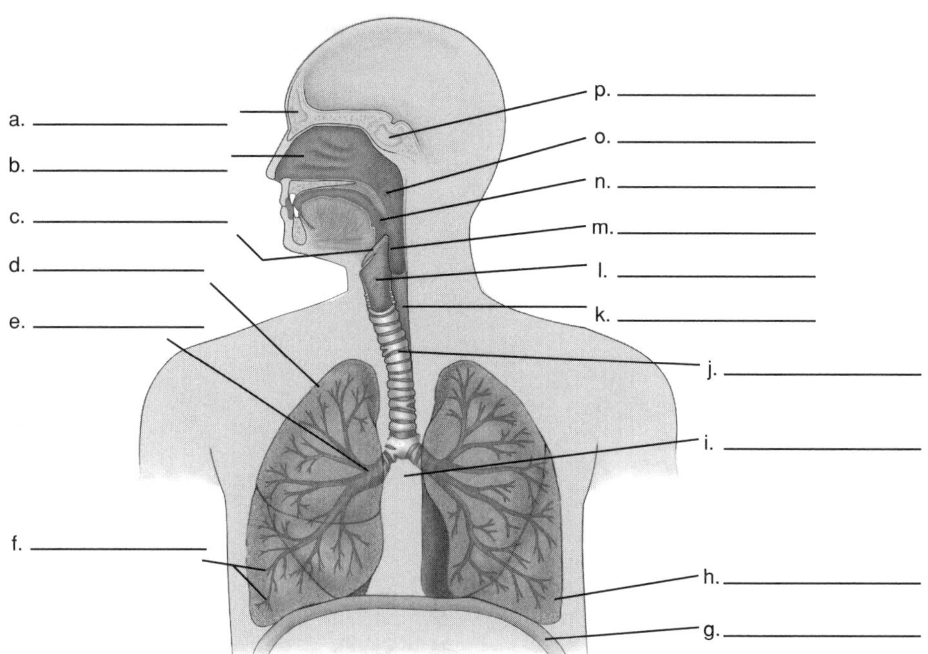

2. Identify the equipment illustrated below by placing your answer on the line provided.

_______________

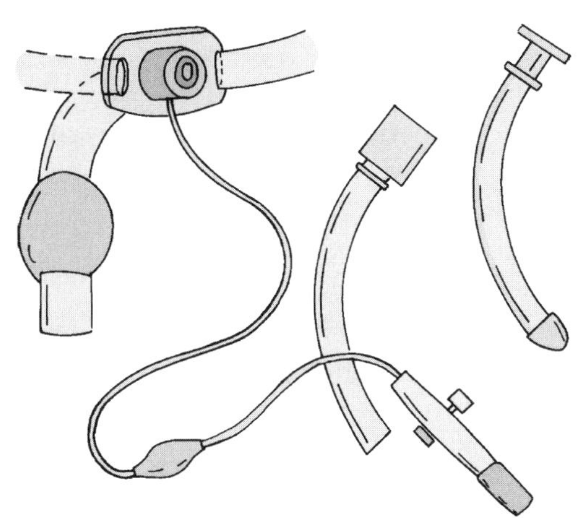

## MATCHING EXERCISES

***Match the definition in Part B with the term listed in Part A.***

**PART A**

**a.** Ventilation
**b.** Inspiration
**c.** Expiration
**d.** Lung compliance
**e.** Airway resistance
**f.** Diffusion
**g.** Perfusion
**h.** Hypoventilation
**i.** Atelectasis
**j.** Hyperventilation
**k.** Hypoxia

**PART B**

____ **1.** Movement of muscles and thorax to bring air into the lungs

____ **2.** Movement of oxygen and carbon dioxide between the air and the blood

____ **3.** Incomplete lung expansion or lung collapse

____ **4.** An inadequate amount of oxygen in the cells

____ **5.** Movement of air in and out of the lungs

____ **6.** Any impediment or obstruction that air meets as it moves through the airway

____ **7.** Stretchability of the lungs or the ease with which the lungs can be inflated

____ **8.** Process by which the oxygenated capillary blood passes through tissue

____ **9.** A decreased rate of air movement into the lungs

____ **10.** An increased rate and depth of ventilation above the body's normal metabolic requirements

***Match the type of oxygen delivery system listed in Part A with its description listed in Part B.***

**PART A**

**a.** Nasal cannula
**b.** Nasopharyngeal catheter
**c.** Simple facemask
**d.** Partial rebreather mask
**e.** Nonrebreather mask
**f.** Venturi mask
**g.** Oxygen tent
**h.** Transtracheal oxygen delivery

**PART B**

____ **11.** Connects to oxygen tubing, a humidifier, and flow meter and uses a delivery flow rate greater than 5 L/min; it should be comfortably snug over face but not tight; it has vents in sides to allow room air to leak in at many places, diluting the source oxygen.

____ **12.** Produces the highest concentration of oxygen with a mask; contains two one-way valves that prevent conservation of exhaled air, which escapes through side vents.

____ **13.** This mask delivers the most precise concentration of oxygen and has a large tube with an oxygen inlet. As the tube narrows, pressure drops, causing air to be sucked in through the side ports.

____ **14.** Probably the most commonly used respiratory aid, this consists of a disposable, plastic device with two protruding prongs for insertion into the nostrils; it is connected to an oxygen source with a humidifier and a flow meter.

____ **15.** A small catheter is inserted into the trachea under local anesthesia and the catheter is attached to the oxygen source.

____ **16.** This mask is equipped with a reservoir bag for the collection of the first part of the patient's exhaled air. The air is mixed with 100% oxygen for the next inhalation.

## SHORT ANSWER

**1.** List three factors on which normal respiratory functioning depends.

**a.** ____________________

**b.** ____________________

**c.** ____________________

**2.** Briefly describe the functions of the upper and lower airways, listing their main components.

**a.** Upper airway: ____________________

____________________

**b.** Lower airway: ____________________

____________________

**3.** List four factors that influence the diffusion of gas in the lungs.

**a.** ____________________

____________________

**b.** ____________________

____________________

**c.** ____________________

____________________

**d.** ____________________

____________________

**4.** Describe the two ways that oxygen is carried in the body.

**a.** ____________________

**b.** ____________________

**5.** Briefly describe the variations in respiration experienced by the following age groups.

**a.** Infant: ____________________

____________________

**b.** Preschool- and school-aged child: ____________________

____________________

**c.** Older adult: ____________________

____________________

**6.** Describe nursing responsibilities before, during, and after a thoracentesis.

____________________

____________________

____________________

**7.** How would you describe the effects of smoking on the lungs to a patient who smokes a pack of cigarettes a day?

____________________

____________________

**8.** Briefly describe the following techniques designed to promote proper breathing.

**a.** Deep breathing: ____________________

____________________

**b.** Incentive spirometry: ____________________

____________________

**c.** Pursed lip breathing: ____________________

____________________

**d.** Diaphragmatic breathing: ____________________

____________________

**e.** Voluntary coughing: ____________________

____________________

____________________

**9.** You are the visiting nurse for a patient with emphysema who is receiving oxygen therapy. List five precautions you would take to prevent fire and injury to this patient.

**a.** ____________________

**b.** ____________________

**c.** ____________________

**d.** ____________________

**e.** ____________________

**10.** Briefly describe the following types of airways and their uses.

**a.** Oropharyngeal/nasopharyngeal airway:

____________________

____________________

**b.** Endotracheal tube: ____________________

____________________

____________________

c. Tracheostomy tube: ______________________

______________________

______________________

11. What is the nurse's responsibility when managing a patient's chest tube?

______________________

______________________

______________________

______________________

12. Describe seven comfort measures for patients with impaired respiratory functioning.
   a. ______________________
   b. ______________________
   c. ______________________
   d. ______________________
   e. ______________________
   f. ______________________
   g. ______________________

13. Describe the nurse's role in providing tracheostomy care for a patient.

______________________

______________________

14. Briefly describe the following components in the procedure for administering cardiopulmonary resuscitation (CPR):
   a. Chest compression: ______________________

   ______________________

   b. Airway: ______________________

   ______________________

   c. Breathing: ______________________

   ______________________

   d. Defibrillation: ______________________

   ______________________

## APPLYING YOUR KNOWLEDGE

### CRITICAL THINKING QUESTIONS

1. Develop a set of nursing strategies to promote adequate respiratory functioning in the following patients.
   a. A patient with lung cancer presents with blood in his sputum.
   b. A child with cystic fibrosis is having difficulty breathing.
   c. A young woman with asthma develops pneumonia.
   d. A 48-year-old man who smokes a pack of cigarettes a day presents with emphysema.

   What is it that makes the strategies you selected appropriate/effective?

2. Interview young people who are smokers to find out their opinions about the health risks associated with smoking. See if they would be willing to quit with your help. Is the knowledge of health risk sufficient to motivate lifestyle modifications? What are the implications for your practice?

### REFLECTIVE PRACTICE: CULTIVATING QSEN COMPETENCIES

***Use the following expanded scenario from Chapter 39 in your textbook to answer the questions below.***

***Scenario:*** Joan McIntyre, age 72, is in the medical intensive care unit, diagnosed with severe COPD. Unable to breathe on her own, she has a tracheostomy and is receiving mechanical ventilation. Efforts are being made to wean her from the ventilator, but she has been unable to breathe on her own for any length of time. She has written notes asking the staff to "let me go" the next time she fails to be weaned. Her only daughter is by her side and asks that all measures to save her mother's life be initiated.

1. How might the nurse respond to Ms. McIntyre's request for a DNR order while taking into consideration the wishes of her daughter?

______________________

______________________

______________________

2. What would be a successful outcome for this patient?

______________________

______________________

______________________

3. What intellectual, technical, interpersonal, and/or ethical/legal competencies are most likely to bring about the desired outcome?

_______________

_______________

_______________

4. What resources might be helpful for Ms. McIntyre?

_______________

_______________

_______________

### PATIENT CARE STUDY

***Read the following case study and use your nursing process skills to answer the questions below.***

*Scenario:* Toni is a 14-year-old girl who is in the adolescent mental health unit following a suicide attempt. Her chart reveals that on several occasions when her mother was visiting, she began hyperventilating (respiratory rate of 42 and increased depth). Gasping for breath on these occasions, she nevertheless pushed away all who approached her to assist. Her mother confided that she and her husband are in the midst of a divorce and that it hasn't been easy for Toni at home: "I know she's been having a rough time at school, and I guess I've been too caught up in my own troubles to be there for her." When you attempt to discuss this with Toni and mention her mother's concern, she begins hyperventilating again.

1. Identify pertinent patient data by placing a single underline beneath the objective data in the case study and a double underline beneath the subjective data.
2. Complete the Nursing Process Worksheet on page 270 to develop a three-part diagnostic statement and related plan of care for this patient.
3. Write down the patient and personal nursing strengths you hope to draw on as you assist this patient to better health.

Patient strengths: _______________

_______________

_______________

Personal strengths: _______________

_______________

_______________

4. Pretend that you are performing a nursing assessment of this patient after the plan of care is implemented. Document your findings.

_______________

_______________

## PRACTICING FOR NCLEX

### MULTIPLE CHOICE QUESTIONS

***Circle the letter that corresponds to the best answer for each question.***

1. The nurse schedules a pulmonary function test to measure the amount of air left in a patient's lungs at maximal expiration. What test does the nurse order?
   a. Tidal volume (TV)
   b. Total lung capacity (TLC)
   c. Forced expiratory volume (FEV)
   d. Residual volume (RV)
2. The nurse is assessing the respiratory rates of patients in a community health care facility. Which patient exhibits an abnormal value?
   a. An infant with a respiratory rate of 20 bpm
   b. A 4-year-old with a respiratory rate of 40 bpm
   c. A 12-year-old with a respiratory rate of 20 bpm
   d. A 70-year-old with a respiratory rate of 18 bpm
3. The nurse assesses a patient and detects the following findings: difficulty breathing, increased respiratory and pulse rates, and pale skin with regions of cyanosis. What condition would the nurse suspect as causing these respiratory alterations?
   a. Hyperventilation
   b. Hypoxia
   c. Perfusion
   d. Atelectasis
4. When inspecting a patient's chest to assess respiratory status, the nurse should be aware of which normal finding?
   a. The contour of the intercostal spaces should be rounded.
   b. The skin at the thorax should be cool and moist.

**c.** The anteroposterior diameter should be greater than the transverse diameter.

**d.** The chest should be slightly convex with no sternal depression.

**5.** When percussing a normal lung, which sound would the nurse hear?

**a.** Tympany

**b.** Resonance

**c.** Dullness

**d.** Hyperresonance

**6.** The nurse is auscultating the lungs of a patient and detects normal vesicular breath sounds. What is a characteristic of vesicular breath sounds?

**a.** They are loud, high-pitched sounds heard primarily over the trachea and larynx.

**b.** They are medium-pitched blowing sounds heard over the major bronchi.

**c.** They are low-pitched, soft sounds heard over peripheral lung fields.

**d.** They are soft, high-pitched discontinuous (intermittent) popping lung sounds.

**7.** A nurse auscultates the lungs of a patient with asthma. Which lung sound is characteristic of this condition?

**a.** Crackles

**b.** Bronchial sounds

**c.** Wheezes

**d.** Vesicular sounds

**8.** What assessments would a nurse make when auscultating the lungs?

**a.** Cardiovascular function

**b.** Abnormal chest structures

**c.** Presence of edema

**d.** Volume of air exhaled or inhaled

**9.** The nurse is caring for a patient who complains of difficulty breathing. In what position would the nurse place this patient?

**a.** Prone position

**b.** Lateral position

**c.** Supine position

**d.** Fowler's position

**10.** The nurse is teaching an adolescent with asthma how to use a metered-dose inhaler. Which teaching point follows recommended guidelines?

**a.** Inhale through the nose instead of the mouth.

**b.** Be sure to shake the canister before using it.

**c.** Inhale the medication rapidly.

**d.** Inhale two sprays with one breath for faster action.

**11.** The nurse sets up an oxygen tent for a patient. Which patient is the best candidate for this oxygen delivery system?

**a.** An older adult patient who has COPD

**b.** A child who has pneumonia

**c.** An adult who is receiving oxygen at home

**d.** An adolescent who has asthma

**12.** Mr. Parks has chronic obstructive pulmonary disease. His nurse has taught him pursed lip breathing, which helps him in which of the following ways?

**a.** Increases carbon dioxide, which stimulates breathing

**b.** Teaches him to prolong inspiration and shorten expiration

**c.** Helps liquefy his secretions

**d.** Decreases the amount of air trapping and resistance

**13.** A nurse suctioning a patient through a tracheostomy tube should be careful not to occlude the Y-port when inserting the suction catheter because it would cause what condition to occur?

**a.** Trauma to the tracheal mucosa

**b.** Prevention of suctioning

**c.** Loss of sterile field

**d.** Suctioning of carbon dioxide

**14.** When caring for a patient with a tracheostomy, the nurse would perform which recommended action?

**a.** Clean the wound around the tube and inner cannula at least every 24 hours.

**b.** Assess a newly inserted tracheostomy every 3 to 4 hours.

**c.** Use gauze dressings over the tracheostomy that are filled with cotton.

**d.** Suction the tracheostomy tube using sterile technique.

15. A nurse is performing CPR on a patient who is in cardiac arrest. What action would the nurse perform second?
    a. Check the victim for a response.
    b. Begin CPR with the CAB sequence.
    c. Get an automated external defibrillator (AED) or defibrillator.
    d. Activate the emergency response system.

## ALTERNATE-FORMAT QUESTIONS

### Multiple Response Questions

***Circle the letters that correspond to the best answers for each question.***

1. The nurse is reviewing the results of a patient's arterial blood gas and pH analysis. Normal findings include: *(Select all that apply.)*
    a. pH 7.45
    b. $PCO_2$ 40 mm Hg
    c. $PO_2$ 70 mm Hg
    d. $HCO_3$ 30 mEq/L
    e. Base excess or deficit +2 mmol/L
    f. pH 8.5
2. The nurse is preparing a patient for a complete blood count test. Which actions would the nurse perform? *(Select all that apply.)*
    a. Emphasize that there is no discomfort during the venipuncture.
    b. Inform the patient that this test can assist in evaluating the body's response to illness.
    c. Inform the patient that specimen collection takes approximately 5 to 10 minutes.
    d. Administer an analgesic to the patient prior to the test.
    e. Explain that, based on results, additional testing may be performed.
    f. Ensure that no food is consumed 6 hours prior to the test.
3. When preparing a patient for a cardiac catheterization, what are the responsibilities of the nurse? *(Select all that apply.)*
    a. Verify that an informed consent was obtained.
    b. Inform the patient that bedrest is required for 24 hours after the procedure.
    c. Tell the patient to avoid heavy lifting, sports, and strenuous housework for 1 week.
    d. Make sure the patient is NPO after midnight before the procedure.
    e. Inform the patient that when dye is given, a feeling of warmth or flushing, or a metallic taste may occur.
    f. Inform the patient that bathing and showering are not allowed for 48 hours following the procedure.
4. The nurse performs assessments of cardiopulmonary functioning and oxygenation during regular physical assessments. Based on developmental variations, which findings would the nurse consider normal? *(Select all that apply.)*
    a. Blood pressure increases over time until it reaches the adult level around age 8.
    b. The power of the respiratory and abdominal muscles is reduced in older adults, and therefore the diaphragm moves less efficiently.
    c. The normal infant's chest is small and the airways are short, making aspiration a potential problem.
    d. Alterations in respiratory function due to aging in older adults increase the risk for disease, especially pneumonia and other chest infections.
    e. The respiratory rate is more rapid in infants until the alveoli increase in number and size to produce adequate oxygenation at lower respiratory rates.
    f. The chest in the older adult is unable to stretch as much, resulting in an increase in maximum inspiration and expiration.
5. Which normal conditions would a nurse expect to find when performing a physical assessment of a patient's respiratory system? *(Select all that apply.)*
    a. Slightly contoured chest with no sternal depression
    b. Anteroposterior diameter of the chest less than the transverse diameter
    c. Quiet and nonlabored respiration occurring at a rate of 18 to 30 bpm
    d. Barrel chest appearance in older adults
    e. Bronchial, vesicular, and bronchovesicular breath sounds
    f. Crackles heard on inspiration.
6. Which actions should a nurse perform when inserting an oropharyngeal airway? *(Select all that apply.)*
    a. Use an airway that reaches from the nose to the back angle of the jaw.
    b. Wash hands and put on PPE, as indicated.

c. Position patient flat on his or her back with the head turned to one side.
d. Insert the airway with the curved tip pointing down toward the base of the mouth.
e. Rotate the airway 180 degrees as it passes the uvula.
f. Remove airway for a brief period every 4 hours or according to facility policy.

7. The nurse is teaching a patient the proper use of inhaled medications. What are appropriate teaching points to include? *(Select all that apply.)*
   a. Bronchodilators are used to liquefy or loosen thick secretions or reduce inflammation in airways.
   b. Nebulizers are used to deliver a controlled dose of medication with each compression of the canister.
   c. When using an MDI, the patient must activate the device before and after inhaling.
   d. DPIs are actuated by the patient's inspiration, so there is no need to coordinate the delivery of puffs with inhalation.
   e. Metered-dose inhalers deliver a controlled dose of medications with each compression of the canister.
   f. Inhalers can be used safely without serious side effects whenever they are needed by the patient.

## Prioritization Questions

1. Place the following steps for teaching a patient to use an incentive spirometer in the order in which they should occur.
   a. Instruct the patient to exhale normally and then place lips securely around mouthpiece and not to breathe through his or her nose.
   b. Medicate with ordered pain medication if needed.
   c. Tell patient to hold breath and count to three when unable to inhale anymore. Check position of gauge to determine progress and level attained.
   d. Tell patient to complete breathing exercises about 5 to 10 times every 1 to 2 hours, if possible, and to rest between breaths as necessary.
   e. Assist patient to an upright or semi-Fowler's position if possible and remove dentures if they fit poorly.
   f. Demonstrate how to steady device with one hand and hold mouthpiece with other hand.
   g. Instruct the patient not to breathe through the nose and to inhale slowly and as deeply as possible through the mouthpiece.
   h. Instruct the patient to remove lips from mouthpiece and exhale normally.

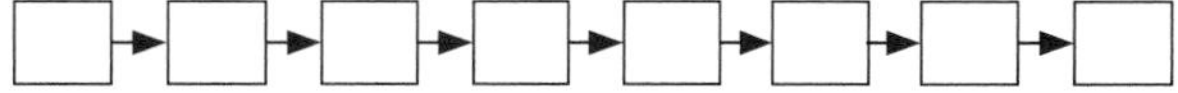

2. Place the following steps for inserting a nasopharyngeal airway in the order in which they should occur.
   a. Remove the airway, clean it, and place it in the other naris at least every 8 hours or according to facility policy. Assess for any evidence of skin breakdown.
   b. Wash your hands, put on PPE as indicated, and identify the patient.
   c. Explain what you are going to do and the reason for doing it, even though the patient does not appear to be alert.
   d. Gently insert the airway into the naris, narrow end first, pointing it down toward the back of the throat until the rim is touching the naris. If resistance is met, stop and try inserting in the other naris.
   e. Put on gloves; put on mask and goggles or face shield as indicated. Lubricate the airway with the water-soluble lubricant, covering the airway from the tip to the guard rim.
   f. Use an airway that is the correct size. Measure the nasopharyngeal airway for correct size. Measure the nasopharyngeal airway length by holding the airway on the side of the patient's face. The airway should reach from the tip of the nose to the earlobe. The airway with the largest outer diameter that fits the patient's nostril should be used.
   g. If the patient is awake and alert, position in semi-Fowler's position. If the patient is not conscious or alert, position in a side-lying position.
   h. Check placement by closing the patient's mouth and placing your fingers in front of the tube opening to check for air movement. Assess the pharynx to visualize the tip of the airway behind the uvula. Assess the nose for blanching or stretching of the skin.

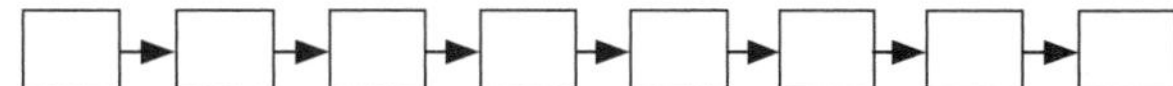

## NURSING PROCESS WORKSHEET

| **Health Problem (Title)**<br><br>Related to ↓ | **Expected Outcome**[a] |
|---|---|
| **Etiology (Related Factors)**<br><br>As Evidenced by ↓ | **Nursing Interventions**[b] |
| **Signs and Symptoms (Defining Characteristics)** | **Evaluative Statement** |

[a]More than one patient goal may be appropriate. For the purposes of this exercise, develop the one patient goal that demonstrates a direct resolution of the patient problem identified in the nursing diagnosis.
[b]Be sure you are able to list the scientific rationale for each nursing intervention you ordered.

CHAPTER 40

# Fluid, Electrolyte, and Acid–Base Balance

## ASSESSING YOUR UNDERSTANDING

### MATCHING EXERCISES

***Match the cation in Part A with its function listed in Part B. Some answers may be used more than once.***

**PART A**

**a.** Sodium
**b.** Potassium
**c.** Calcium
**d.** Magnesium

**PART B**

____ **1.** It is the chief regulator of cellular enzyme activity and cellular water content.

____ **2.** It is necessary for nerve impulse transmission and blood clotting.

____ **3.** It controls and regulates the volume of body fluids.

____ **4.** It is the primary regulator of ECF volume.

____ **5.** It is important for the metabolism of carbohydrates and proteins.

____ **6.** It is a catalyst for muscle contraction.

____ **7.** It assists in the regulation of acid–base balance by cellular exchange with $H^+$.

____ **8.** It acts on the cardiovascular system, producing vasodilation.

***Match the anion in Part A with its function listed in Part B. Some answers may be used more than once.***

**PART A**

**a.** Chloride
**b.** Bicarbonate
**c.** Phosphate

**PART B**

____ **9.** It acts with sodium to maintain the osmotic pressure of the blood.

____ **10.** It promotes energy storage; carbohydrate, protein, and fat metabolism.

____ **11.** It is a major component of interstitial and lymph fluid; gastric and pancreatic juices; sweat, bile, and saliva.

____ **12.** It is an anion that is the major chemical base buffer within the body.

____ **13.** It has a role in acid–base balance as a hydrogen buffer.

____ **14.** It combines with hydrogen ions to produce hydrochloric acid.

____ **15.** It plays a role in muscle and red blood cell function.

***Match the equations in Part B with the type of imbalance listed in Part A.***

**PART A**

**a.** Respiratory acidosis
**b.** Metabolic acidosis

c. Respiratory alkalosis
d. Metabolic alkalosis

**PART B**

____ 16. Low pH, normal $PaCO_2$, low $HCO_3$

____ 17. Low pH, high $PaCO_2$, normal $HCO_3$

____ 18. High pH, normal $PaCO_2$, high $HCO_3$

____ 19. High pH, low $PaCO_2$, normal $HCO_3$

***Match the term in Part A with its definition listed in Part B.***

**PART A**

a. Ion
b. Electrolyte
c. Cation
d. Anion
e. Solvents
f. Solutes
g. Osmolarity
h. Filtration
i. Oncotic pressure
j. Hydrostatic pressure
k. Diffusion
l. Active transport
m. Filtration pressure
n. Buffer
o. Intravascular fluid
p. Interstitial fluid

**PART B**

____ 20. Ions that develop a positive charge

____ 21. Substances that are dissolved in a solution

____ 22. Fluid that surrounds tissue cells, including lymph

____ 23. Measured in terms of their chemical combining power, or chemical activity

____ 24. The liquid constituent of blood

____ 25. A process that requires energy for the movement of substances through a cell membrane from an area of lesser concentration to an area of higher concentration

____ 26. The passage of a fluid through a permeable membrane

____ 27. An atom or molecule carrying an electric charge

____ 28. An ion with a negative charge

____ 29. Liquids that hold a substance in solution

____ 30. A force exerted by a fluid against the container wall

____ 31. The difference between colloid osmotic pressure and blood hydrostatic pressure

____ 32. A substance that prevents body fluids from becoming overly acidic or alkaline

____ 33. The concentration of particles in a solution, or its pulling power

____ 34. The tendency of solutes to move freely throughout a solvent

**CORRECT THE FALSE STATEMENTS**

***Circle the word "true" or "false" that follows the statement. If you circled "false," change the underlined word or words to make the statement true. Place your answer in the space provided.***

1. The human body is composed of <u>50% to 60%</u> water by weight.
   a. True
   b. False ____________

2. Substances capable of breaking into electrically charged ions when dissolved in a solution are called <u>solutes</u>.
   a. True
   b. False ____________

3. A <u>hypertonic solution</u> has less osmolarity than plasma.
   a. True
   b. False ____________

4. <u>Ingested liquids</u> make up the largest amount of water normally taken into the body.
   a. True
   b. False ____________

5. The acidity or alkalinity of a solution is determined by its concentration of <u>oxygen</u> ions.
   a. True
   b. False ____________

6. An <u>acid</u> is a substance that can accept or trap hydrogen ions.
   a. True
   b. False ____________

7. Normal blood plasma is slightly acidic and has a normal pH of 7.35 to 7.45.
   a. True
   b. False ______
8. The kidneys are the primary controller of the body's carbonic acid supply.
   a. True
   b. False ______
9. Excessive retention of water and sodium in ECF results in a condition termed fluid volume excess or hypervolemia.
   a. True
   b. False ______
10. Hypokalemia refers to a surplus of sodium in ECF that can result from excess water loss or an overall excess of sodium.
    a. True
    b. False ______
11. Acid–base imbalances occur when the ECF and ICF carbonic acid or bicarbonate levels become equal.
    a. True
    b. False ______
12. Arterial blood gases are most commonly used to assess and treat acid–base imbalances.
    a. True
    b. False ______

## SHORT ANSWER

1. Briefly describe how the following processes transport materials to and from intracellular compartments.
   a. Osmosis: ______
   b. Diffusion: ______
   c. Active transport: ______
2. Give an example of how water is derived from the following sources.
   a. Ingested liquids: ______
   b. Food: ______
   c. Metabolic oxidation: ______
3. List three mechanisms for water loss in the body.
   a. ______
   b. ______
   c. ______
4. Explain how the following organs/systems of the body maintain fluid homeostasis.
   a. Kidneys: ______
   b. Cardiovascular system: ______
   c. Lungs: ______
   d. Thyroid: ______
   e. Parathyroid glands: ______
   f. Gastrointestinal tract: ______
   g. Nervous system: ______
5. Give a brief description of the following conditions.
   a. Acidosis: ______
   b. Alkalosis: ______
6. Describe the following acid–base imbalances and their effect on the body.
   a. Respiratory acidosis: ______
   b. Respiratory alkalosis: ______
   c. Metabolic acidosis: ______
   d. Metabolic alkalosis: ______

7. Describe the causes of the following changes in hemoglobin and hematocrit.
   a. Increased hematocrit: ______
   b. Decreased hematocrit: ______
   c. Increased hemoglobin: ______
   d. Decreased hemoglobin: ______

8. Briefly describe the following screening tests.
   a. Urine pH and specific gravity: ______
   b. Serum electrolytes: ______
   c. Arterial blood gases: ______

9. You are the visiting nurse for an older adult patient with diabetes. List four factors you should consider to prevent fluid imbalance for this patient.
   a. ______
   b. ______
   c. ______
   d. ______

10. List the important points a home health care nurse should address when caring for a patient on home infusion therapy.

______

## APPLYING YOUR KNOWLEDGE

### CRITICAL THINKING QUESTIONS

1. Assess the following patients for fluid, electrolyte, and acid–base balance. What knowledge of the factors that influence fluid and electrolyte and acid–base balance would you draw on to develop a plan to prevent recurrence of these patient problems?
   a. A long-distance runner who is practicing on a hot day experiences dizziness and shows signs of dehydration.
   b. An older man with persistent heartburn ingests a large amount of sodium bicarbonate in 1 day.
   c. An infant is brought to the ER severely dehydrated after an extended bout of diarrhea.

2. Plan a low-salt diet for a patient who has high blood pressure. List healthy foods that are low in salt, as well as foods that are high in salt and that should be avoided. Check the sodium content of fast food in restaurants to see if any of these foods could be included on the diet.

### REFLECTIVE PRACTICE: CULTIVATING QSEN COMPETENCIES

***Use the following expanded scenario from Chapter 40 in your textbook to answer the questions below.***

***Scenario:*** Jack Soo Park, a 78-year-old man receiving intravenous (IV) therapy with antibiotics, states, "I'm having trouble breathing. It just started a little while ago." Physical examination reveals a bounding pulse; distended neck veins; shallow, rapid respirations; and crackles and wheezes in the lungs. Excess fluid volume is suspected. Further checking reveals an IV fluid administration error that has resulted in overhydration.

1. Based on the data in this scenario, what body systems are involved in Mr. Park's fluid volume excess? What interventions would be appropriate?

______

2. What would be a successful outcome for Mr. Park?

______

3. What intellectual, technical, interpersonal, and/or ethical/legal competencies are most likely to bring about the desired outcome?

_______________

_______________

_______________

4. What resources might be helpful for Mr. Park?

_______________

_______________

_______________

## PATIENT CARE STUDY

***Read the following patient care study and use your nursing process skills to answer the questions below.***

*Scenario:* Rebecca is a college freshman who had her wisdom teeth removed yesterday morning. She had a sore throat several days before the extraction but did not mention this to the oral surgeon. Because of her sore throat, she had greatly decreased her food and fluid intake. The night of the surgery, she had an oral temperature of 39.5°C (103.1°F). Friends gave her some Tylenol, which brought her temperature down, and encouraged her to drink more fluids. When they checked on her this morning, her temperature was elevated again, and she said she had felt too weak during the night to drink. They took her to the student health service, where the admitting nurse noticed her dry mucous membranes, decreased skin turgor, and rapid pulse. At 5 ft 2 in and 98 lb, Rebecca had lost 4 lb in the past week.

1. Identify pertinent patient data by placing a single underline beneath the objective data in the case study and a double underline beneath the subjective data.
2. Complete the Nursing Process Worksheet on page 281 to develop a three-part diagnostic statement and related plan of care for this patient.
3. Write down the patient and personal nursing strengths you hope to draw on as you assist this patient to better health.

   Patient strengths: _______________

   _______________

   _______________

   Personal strengths: _______________

   _______________

   _______________

4. Pretend that you are performing a nursing assessment of this patient after the plan of care has been implemented. Document your findings.

   _______________

   _______________

   _______________

# PRACTICING FOR NCLEX

## MULTIPLE CHOICE QUESTIONS

***Circle the letter that corresponds to the best answer for each question.***

1. The nurse writes a nursing diagnosis for a patient of "excess fluid volume." What risk factor would the nurse assess in this patient?
   a. Excessive use of laxatives
   b. Diaphoresis
   c. Renal failure
   d. Increased cardiac output
2. When teaching a patient about foods that affect fluid balance, the nurse would advise the patient to decrease:
   a. $Na^+$
   b. $K^+$
   c. $Ca^{++}$
   d. $Mg^{++}$
3. A healthy patient eats a regular, balanced diet and drinks 3,000 mL of liquids during a 24-hour period. In evaluating this patient's urine output for the same 24-hour period, the nurse realizes that it should total approximately how many milliliters?
   a. 3,750
   b. 3,000
   c. 1,000
   d. 500

4. The nurse is caring for a patient with "hyperkalemia related to decreased renal excretion secondary to potassium-conserving diuretic therapy." What is an appropriate expected outcome?
   a. Bowel motility will be restored within 24 hours after beginning supplemental $K^+$.
   b. ECG will show no cardiac arrhythmias within 48 hours after removing salt substitutes, coffee, tea, and other $K^+$-rich foods from diet.
   c. ECG will show no cardiac arrhythmias within 24 hours after beginning supplemental $K^+$.
   d. Bowel motility will be restored within 24 hours after eliminating salt substitutes, coffee, tea, and other $K^+$-rich foods from the diet.
5. The nurse is caring for older adults in a long-term care facility. What age-related alteration should the nurse consider when planning care for these patients?
   a. An increased sense of thirst
   b. Increase in nephrons in the kidneys
   c. Increased renal blood flow
   d. Cardiac volume intolerance
6. Which nursing diagnosis would the nurse make based on the effects of fluid and electrolyte imbalance on human functioning?
   a. Constipation related to immobility
   b. Acute pain related to surgical incision
   c. Impaired mood regulation related to cerebral edema
   d. Risk for infection related to inadequate personal hygiene
7. A nurse is measuring intake and output for a patient who has congestive heart failure. What does not need to be recorded?
   a. Fruit consumption
   b. Sips of water
   c. Parenteral fluids
   d. Frozen fluids
8. What food would the nurse provide for a patient who has hypokalemia?
   a. Canned vegetables
   b. Cheese
   c. Bread
   d. Bananas
9. A nurse is caring for a patient who has a PICC line. Which nursing action is recommended?
   a. Use clean technique when changing dressing.
   b. Flush using normal saline and/or heparin solution according to facility policy.
   c. Keep external portion of catheter coiled on top of dressing.
   d. Change catheter caps every 10 days or as per facility policy.
10. The nurse is administering 1,000-mL 0.9 normal saline over 10 hours (set delivers 60 gtt/1 mL). Using the formula below, the flow rate would be:

$$\text{gtt/min} = \frac{\text{milliliters per hour} \times \text{drop factor (gtt/mL)}}{\text{time (60 min)}}$$

   a. 60 gtt/min
   b. 100 gtt/min
   c. 160 gtt/min
   d. 600 gtt/min
11. The nurse is determining a site for an IV infusion. What guideline should the nurse consider?
   a. Scalp veins should be selected for infants because of their accessibility.
   b. Antecubital veins should be used for long-term infusions.
   c. Veins in the leg should be used to keep the arms free for the patient's use.
   d. Veins in surgical areas should be used to increase the potency of medication.
12. What blood type might be used in an emergency situation when the patient's blood type is not available?
   a. Type A
   b. Type O
   c. Type B
   d. Type AB
13. A nurse who has diagnosed a patient as having "fluid volume excess" related to compromised regulatory mechanism (kidneys) may have been alerted by what symptom?
   a. Muscle twitching
   b. Distended neck veins
   c. Fingerprinting over sternum
   d. Nausea and vomiting

## ALTERNATE-FORMAT QUESTIONS

### Multiple Response Questions

***Circle the letters that correspond to the best answers for each question.***

1. What nursing interventions would be appropriate for a patient diagnosed with deficient fluid volume? *(Select all that apply.)*
   a. Hypervolemia management
   b. Fluid restriction
   c. Intravenous therapy
   d. Electrolyte management
   e. Monitoring edema
   f. Nutrition management

2. What nursing actions would be performed when preparing an IV solution and tubing when starting an IV infusion? *(Select all that apply.)*
   a. Maintain aseptic technique when opening sterile packages and IV solution.
   b. Clamp tubing, uncap spike, and insert into entry site on bag as manufacturer directs.
   c. Squeeze drip chamber and allow it to fill one fourth full.
   d. Remove cap at end of tubing, release clamp, and allow fluid to move through tubing.
   e. Allow fluid to flow and cap at end of tubing before all air bubbles have disappeared.
   f. Apply label to tubing reflecting the day/date for next set change, per facility guidelines.

3. Following preparation of the IV solution and tubing, what nursing actions would be performed by the nurse when selecting a site and palpating a vein to start an IV infusion? *(Select all that apply.)*
   a. Place the patient in a high Fowler's position in bed.
   b. Select an appropriate site and palpate accessible veins.
   c. Apply a tourniquet 6 in above the venipuncture site to obstruct venous flow and distend the vein.
   d. Direct the ends of the tourniquet away from the site and check that the radial pulse is still present.
   e. Ask the patient to keep a tightly closed fist while observing and palpating for a suitable vein.
   f. If a vein cannot be felt, release the tourniquet and have the patient lower the arm below the level of the heart to fill the veins.

4. Which actions would a nurse perform after selecting a site and palpating accessible veins in order to start an IV infusion? *(Select all that apply.)*
   a. Clean the entry site with saline, followed by an alcohol swab according to facility policy.
   b. Place the dominant hand about 4 in below the entry site to hold the skin taut against the vein.
   c. Enter the skin gently with the catheter held by the hub in the nondominant hand, bevel side down, at a 10- to 30-degree angle.
   d. Advance the needle or catheter into the vein. A sensation of "give" can be felt when the needle enters the vein.
   e. When blood returns through the lumen of the needle or the flashback chamber of the catheter, advance device into the vein until the hub is at the venipuncture site.
   f. Release the tourniquet, quickly remove the protective cap from the IV tubing, and attach the tubing to the catheter or needle.

5. What signs of complications and their probable causes may occur when administering an IV solution to a patient? *(Select all that apply.)*
   a. Swelling, pain, coolness, or pallor at the insertion site may indicate infiltration of the IV.
   b. Redness, swelling, heat, and pain at the site may indicate phlebitis.
   c. Local or systemic manifestations may indicate an infection is present at the site.
   d. A pounding headache, fainting, rapid pulse rate, increased blood pressure, chills, back pains, and dyspnea occur when an air embolus is present.
   e. Bleeding at the site when the IV is discontinued indicates an infection is present.
   f. Engorged neck veins, increased blood pressure, and dyspnea occur when a thrombus is present.

6. The nurse is teaching a patient about the function of sodium in the body. What teaching points would the nurse make? *(Select all that apply.)*
   a. Sodium does not influence ICF volume.
   b. Sodium is the primary regulator of ECF volume.
   c. The daily value of sodium cited on nutrition facts labels is 1,200 mg.

**d.** Sodium is normally maintained in the body within a relatively narrow range, and deviations quickly result in serious health problems.

**e.** The normal extracellular concentration of sodium is 85 to 95 mEq/L.

**f.** Sodium participates in the generation and transmission of nerve impulses.

**7.** A nurse monitoring an IV infusion notes the signs and symptoms of a thrombus. What nursing interventions would the nurse perform? *(Select all that apply.)*

**a.** Stop the infusion immediately.

**b.** Apply warm compresses as ordered by the primary care provider.

**c.** Rub or massage the affected area.

**d.** Monitor vital signs and pulse oximetry.

**e.** Restart the IV at another site.

**f.** Place patient on left side in Trendelenburg position.

**8.** What IV solutions would the nurse expect to be ordered for a patient who has hypovolemia? *(Select all that apply.)*

**a.** 10% dextrose in water ($D_{10}W$)

**b.** 0.45% NaCl (½-strength normal saline)

**c.** 0.9% NaCl (normal saline)

**d.** Lactated Ringer's solution

**e.** 5% dextrose in 0.9% NaCl

**f.** 5% dextrose in water ($D_5W$)

**9.** The nurse is assisting with a patient blood transfusion. What type of reactions may occur during this procedure? *(Select all that apply.)*

**a.** Dyspnea, dry cough, and pulmonary edema may occur during a bacterial reaction.

**b.** Hives, itching, and anaphylaxis may occur during an allergic reaction.

**c.** Fever, chills, headache, and malaise may occur during a febrile reaction.

**d.** Fever; hypertension; abdominal pain; and dry, flushed skin may occur during circulatory overload.

**e.** Facial flushing, fever, chills, headache, low back pain, and shock may occur during a hemolytic transfusion reaction.

**f.** Shortness of breath and auscultated crackles bilaterally in the bases may occur during a febrile reaction.

## Chart/Exhibit Questions

***Determine the acid–base imbalance in the cases in the following questions and circle the letter that corresponds to the best answer for each scenario. Refer to the Rules of ABG Interpretation table below for your answers.***

| Rules of ABG Interpretation | | |
|---|---|---|
| **pH** | **$PaCO_2$** | **$HCO_3$** |
| <7.35 = acidosis | >45 mm Hg = respiratory acidosis | <22 mEq/L = metabolic acidosis |
| >7.45 = alkalosis | >35 mm Hg = respiratory alkalosis | >26 mEq/L = metabolic alkalosis |

- It is OK to use what you know about your patient.
- The body responds to acid–base imbalances by activating compensatory mechanisms that minimize pH changes; a metabolic disturbance is compensated by the lungs, and a respiratory system disturbance is compensated by the kidneys.
- Any pH less than 7.35 = state of acidosis. Any pH greater than 7.45 = state of alkalosis.
- $CO_2$ is an acid; $HCO_3$ is a base. Any change in $CO_2$ reflects a respiratory change. Any change in $HCO_3$ reflects a metabolic change.
- If the pH has returned to *normal,* compensation has taken place.
- If the primary event is a *fall* in pH, whether respiratory or metabolic in origin, the arterial pH stays on the *acid* side after compensation.
- If the primary event is an *increase* in pH, whether respiratory or metabolic in origin, the arterial pH stays on the *base* side after compensation.

1. Mr. W. is a 90-year-old man who had a successful cardiopulmonary resuscitation a few hours ago. He received bicarbonate during that resuscitation.

   ABGs: pH = 7.55; $PaCO_2$ = 43; $HCO_3$ = 36

   a. Respiratory acidosis
   b. Metabolic acidosis
   c. Metabolic alkalosis
   d. Respiratory alkalosis

2. Mr. F. is a 56-year-old man with a history of COPD.

   ABGs: pH = 7.36; $PaCO_2$ = 60; $HCO_3$ = 35

   a. Respiratory acidosis with renal compensation
   b. Metabolic acidosis with partial respiratory compensation
   c. Respiratory alkalosis
   d. Respiratory acidosis

3. A 55-year-old woman is admitted with chronic renal failure. She is weak and tired.

   ABGs: pH = 7.24; $PaCO_2$ = 30; $HCO_3$ = 12

   a. Respiratory acidosis
   b. Respiratory alkalosis
   c. Metabolic alkalosis with partial respiratory compensation
   d. Metabolic acidosis with partial respiratory compensation

4. Mrs. S. is a 55-year-old woman with heart failure and dyspnea. She complains of pleuritic pain.

   ABGs: pH = 7.56; $PaCO_2$ = 22; $HCO_3$ = 24

   a. Respiratory alkalosis
   b. Respiratory acidosis
   c. Metabolic acidosis
   d. Metabolic alkalosis

5. Ms. S. is a 21-year-old woman who was found by her friends on the floor of her room. She is "out of it."

   ABGs: pH = 7.18; $PaCO_2$ = 79; $HCO_3$ = 26

   a. Respiratory alkalosis
   b. Respiratory acidosis
   c. Metabolic alkalosis with partial respiratory compensation
   d. Metabolic acidosis with partial respiratory compensation

6. Indicate on the chart below the nature of the acid–base disturbance, whether compensation is present or not, and if present, whether compensation is renal or respiratory, and partial or complete.

| | | | | Comp. Present? | | IF Yes | | IF Yes | |
|---|---|---|---|---|---|---|---|---|---|
| **pH** | **$PaCO_2$** | **$HCO_3^-$** | **Nature of Disturbance** | **Yes** | **No** | **Renal** | **Respiratory** | **Partial** | **Complete** |
| 7.28 | 63 | 25 | | | | | | | |
| 7.20 | 40 | 14 | | | | | | | |
| 7.52 | 40 | 35 | | | | | | | |
| 7.16 | 82 | 30 | | | | | | | |
| 7.36 | 68 | 35 | | | | | | | |
| 7.56 | 23 | 26 | | | | | | | |
| 7.40 | 40 | 26 | | | | | | | |
| 7.56 | 23 | 26 | | | | | | | |
| 7.26 | 70 | 25 | | | | | | | |
| 7.52 | 44 | 38 | | | | | | | |
| 7.32 | 30 | 18 | | | | | | | |
| 7.49 | 34 | 26 | | | | | | | |

## Hot Spot Questions

1. Place an "X" on the figure below to indicate the spot where a peripherally inserted central catheter (PICC) would be inserted.

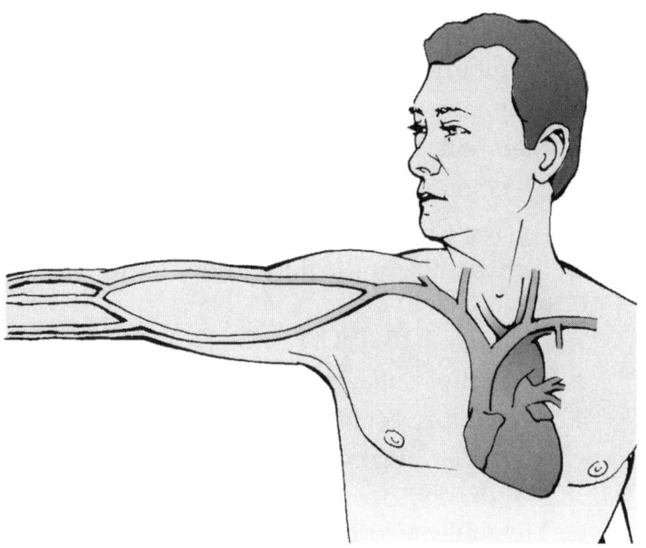

2. Indicate the proper placement of a triple-lumen nontunneled percutaneous central venous catheter by placing an "X" on the figure below where it would be inserted.

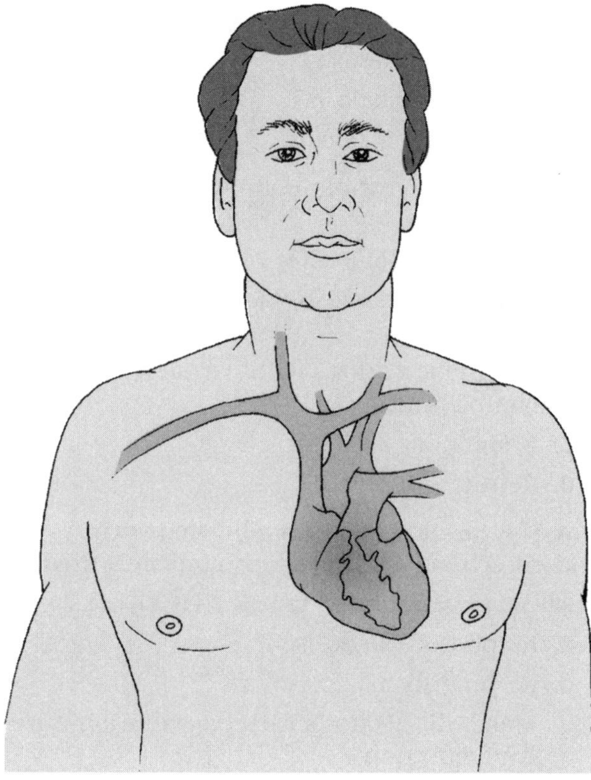

## NURSING PROCESS WORKSHEET

| **Health Problem (Title)** | **Expected Outcome**[a] |
|---|---|
| Related to ↓ | |
| **Etiology (Related Factors)** | **Nursing Interventions**[b] |
| As Evidenced by ↓ | |
| **Signs and Symptoms (Defining Characteristics)** | **Evaluative Statement** |

[a]More than one patient goal may be appropriate. For the purposes of this exercise, develop the one patient goal that demonstrates a direct resolution of the patient problem identified in the nursing diagnosis.
[b]Be sure you are able to list the scientific rationale for each nursing intervention you ordered.

CHAPTER 41

# Self-Concept

## ASSESSING YOUR UNDERSTANDING

### FILL IN THE BLANKS

1. A person who is a talented musician strives to reach full potential by constantly studying and practicing the craft. This human need is termed ____________.
2. All of the feelings, beliefs, and values associated with "I" or "me" comprise ____________.
3. The composite of all the basic facts, qualities, traits, images, and feelings one holds about oneself is known as ____________.
4. The self one wants to be that developed in childhood and was based on the image of role models is known as the ____________.
5. When a teenager attempts to please his parents by attending church although he doesn't believe in organized religion, he is displaying his ____________.
6. ____________ describes a person's conscious sense of who he or she is.

### MATCHING EXERCISES

***Match the definition in Part B with the term listed in Part A.***

**PART A**

**a.** Self-esteem
**b.** Self-actualization
**c.** Self-concept
**d.** Body image
**e.** Self-knowledge
**f.** Self-expectations
**g.** Self-evaluation
**h.** Personal identity

**PART B**

____ **1.** The need to feel good about oneself and believe others also hold one in high regard

____ **2.** The person's subjective view of his or her physical appearance

____ **3.** Describes a person's conscious sense of who he or she is

____ **4.** Includes basic facts (sex, age, race, occupation, cultural background, sexual orientation); a person's position within social groups; and qualities or traits that describe typical behaviors, feelings, moods, and other characteristics

____ **5.** These flow from the ideal self, the self one wants to be or thinks one should be.

____ **6.** The mental image or picture of self

____ **7.** The assessment of how well I like myself

***Match the examples of risk factors for self-concept disturbances in Part B with the factors listed in Part A. Some answers may be used more than once.***

**PART A**

**a.** Personal identity disturbances
**b.** Body image disturbances
**c.** Self-esteem disturbances
**d.** Altered role performance

**PART B**

____ **8.** A 55-year-old executive is laid off from his job due to cutbacks.

____ **9.** A 45-year-old woman undergoes a radical mastectomy.

____ **10.** A 30-year-old woman finds herself in a relationship with an abusive husband.

____ **11.** An exchange student from France attends high school in America to learn a new language and customs.

____ **12.** A new mother discovers she is terrified of taking care of her newborn son on her own.

____ **13.** An 11-year-old girl starts menstruating and developing earlier than her peers.

____ **14.** A 65-year-old retired lawyer regrets that he was unable to become a judge as he had always dreamed of doing.

____ **15.** An athlete loses his pitching arm to cancer.

____ **16.** A 38-year-old woman who is recently divorced is lost without her husband.

**SHORT ANSWER**

**1.** What measures could you, as a nurse, employ to promote self-esteem in older adults?

______________________________________

______________________________________

______________________________________

**2.** Reflect on your personal self-concept and how it affects the way you live your life. Keeping this in mind, answer the following questions.

**a.** Who am I? ______________________________________

______________________________________

**b.** Who or what do I want to be? ______________________________________

______________________________________

**c.** How well do I like me? ______________________________________

______________________________________

**3.** Give an example of a question you might use to assess a patient for the following concepts.

**a.** Significance: ______________________________________

______________________________________

**b.** Competence: ______________________________________

______________________________________

**c.** Virtue: ______________________________________

______________________________________

**d.** Power: ______________________________________

______________________________________

**4.** Give an example of how each of the following factors might influence a person's self-concept.

**a.** Developmental considerations: ______________________________________

______________________________________

**b.** Culture: ______________________________________

______________________________________

**c.** Internal and external resources: ______________________________________

**d.** History of success or failure: ______________________________________

______________________________________

**e.** Stressors: ______________________________________

______________________________________

**f.** Aging, illness, or trauma: ______________________________________

______________________________________

**5.** List one example from your experience as a nurse that exemplifies the use of the following strategies for developing self-esteem in your practice.

**a.** Dispel the myth that it is necessary to know all there is to know about nursing to be a good nurse: ______________________________________

______________________________________

**b.** Realistically evaluate strengths and weaknesses: ______________________________________

______________________________________

**c.** Accentuate the positive: ______________________________________

______________________________________

**d.** Develop a conscious plan for changing weaknesses into strengths: ______________________________________

______________________________________

**e.** Work to develop team self-esteem: ______________________________________

______________________________________

______________________________________

**f.** Actively demonstrate your commitment to nursing and concern about the nursing profession's public image:

______________________________________

______________________________________

6. Describe how you would record a self-concept assessment using your own personal strengths as an example. ____________________

7. Give an example of an interview question you could use to assess self-concept in the following areas.
   a. Personal identity: ____________________
   b. Patient strengths: ____________________
   c. Body image: ____________________
   d. Self-esteem: ____________________
   e. Role performance: ____________________

8. Write a sample nursing diagnosis and goal for the following disturbances in self-concept.
   a. A 42-year-old woman is anxious about disfigurement from her mastectomy.
      Diagnosis: ____________________
      Patient goal: ____________________
   b. A teen is anxious about being able to cope with pregnancy.
      Diagnosis: ____________________
      Patient goal: ____________________
   c. A 76-year-old man stops taking care of his physical needs because he doesn't want to go on with life without his recently deceased spouse.
      Diagnosis: ____________________
      Patient goal: ____________________
   d. A parent doesn't know how to teach a child who is being ridiculed by his peers in school how to establish self-esteem.
      Diagnosis: ____________________
      Patient goal: ____________________
   e. A battered woman feels her situation is hopeless and believes she deserves to be abused because she is so weak.
      Diagnosis: ____________________
      Patient goal: ____________________
   f. A woman who underwent a hysterectomy feels she can no longer have a sexual relationship with her husband.
      Diagnosis: ____________________
      Patient goal: ____________________

9. Describe three strategies nurses can use to help patients identify and use personal strengths.
   a. ____________________
   b. ____________________
   c. ____________________

10. Give three examples of how nurses can help patients maintain a sense of self-worth.
   a. ____________________
   b. ____________________
   c. ____________________

11. Describe nursing strategies to develop self-esteem that you might use to meet the needs of the following older adult patients with disturbances in self-concept.
   a. An 88-year-old woman, newly admitted to a long-term care facility, says she has lost all sense of self (Self-Identity Disturbance): ____________________

**b.** A 75-year-old man with crippling arthritis tells you he no longer recognizes himself when he looks in the mirror (Body Image Disturbance):

______________________________

______________________________

**c.** A 62-year-old man who is recovering from a stroke that has paralyzed his right side says, "I don't know if I can live like this." (Self-Esteem Disturbance):

______________________________

______________________________

______________________________

**d.** A 67-year-old woman complains that she no longer has the patience to babysit for her grandchildren whom she loves (Role Performance Disturbance):

______________________________

______________________________

______________________________

______________________________

## APPLYING YOUR KNOWLEDGE

### CRITICAL THINKING QUESTIONS

1. There are many factors that influence the self-concept of patients, including developmental considerations, culture, internal or external resources, history of success or failure, stressors, and aging, illness, or trauma. Interview several patients to find out how these factors have influenced their self-concept. Once you've identified these factors, write a nursing diagnosis for each patient and develop patient health goals where appropriate.
2. Would you describe yourself as having high or low self-concept? Ask your friends if they agree with your assessment. How might your self-concept influence the relationships you establish with patients and colleagues?

### REFLECTIVE PRACTICE: CULTIVATING QSEN COMPETENCIES

***Use the following expanded scenario from Chapter 41 in your textbook to answer the questions below.***

***Scenario:*** Anthony Santorini is a middle-aged man with a history of diabetes. He recently underwent a below-the-knee amputation due to complications resulting from poor glucose control. One morning, he states, "I feel like damaged goods. I'm not a whole man anymore." When the nurse attempts to initiate an assessment of his self-concept, he turns his back on her and states: "Just leave me alone, I don't want to talk about it."

1. What interventions might the nurse employ to try to resolve Mr. Santorini's self-image disturbance?

______________________________

______________________________

______________________________

2. What would be a successful outcome for Mr. Santorini?

______________________________

______________________________

______________________________

3. What intellectual, technical, interpersonal, and/or ethical/legal competencies are most likely to bring about the desired outcome?

______________________________

______________________________

______________________________

4. What resources might be helpful for Mr. Santorini?

______________________________

______________________________

______________________________

### PATIENT CARE STUDY

***Read the following patient care study and use your nursing process skills to answer the questions below.***

***Scenario:*** An English teacher asks you, the school nurse, to see one of her students, Julie, whose grades have recently dropped and who no longer seems to be interested in school or anything else. "She was one of my best students, and I can't figure out what's going on," the teacher says. "She seems reluctant to talk about this change." When Julie, a 16-year-old junior, walks into your office, you are immediately struck by her stooped posture, unstyled hair, and sloppy appearance. Julie is attractive, but at 5 ft 3 in and 150 lb, she is overweight. Julie is initially reluctant to talk, but she breaks down at one point and confides that for the first time in her life she feels "absolutely awful" about herself. "I've always concentrated on getting good grades and achieved this easily. But now, this doesn't seem so important. I don't have any friends. All I hear the girls talking about is boys, and I was never even asked out by a boy, which I guess isn't surprising. Look at me!" After a few questions, it becomes clear that Julie has new expectations for herself based on what she observes in her peers, and she finds herself falling far short of her new, ideal self. Julie admits that, in the past, once she set a goal for herself, she was always able to achieve it because she is strongly self-motivated. Although she has withdrawn from her parents and teachers, she admits that she does know adults she can trust who have been a big support to her in the past. She says, "If only I could become the kind of teenager other kids like and have lots of friends!"

1. Identify pertinent patient data by placing a single underline beneath the objective data in the case study and a double underline beneath the subjective data.
2. Complete the Nursing Process Worksheet on page 288 to develop a three-part diagnostic statement and related plan of care for this patient.
3. Write down the patient and personal nursing strengths you hope to draw on as you assist this patient to better health.

   Patient strengths: ______________________

   ______________________

   ______________________

   Personal strengths: ______________________

   ______________________

   ______________________

4. Pretend you are performing a nursing assessment of this patient after the plan of care has been implemented. Document your findings.

   ______________________

   ______________________

## PRACTICING FOR NCLEX

### MULTIPLE CHOICE QUESTIONS

***Circle the letter that corresponds to the best choice for each question.***

1. A child lists his favorite sports figures and tells the nurse he is going to be just like them. What human need is displayed in this example?
   a. Self-knowledge
   b. Self-expectations
   c. Self-evaluation
   d. Self-actualization
2. A nurse encourages a young female whose leg was amputated to continue to pursue her dream to become a dancer. What is the need to reach one's potential through full development of one's unique capability?
   a. Self-actualization
   b. Self-concept
   c. Self-esteem
   d. Ideal self
3. A nurse assessing children in a pediatrician's office would expect a child to achieve self-recognition at what age?
   a. At birth
   b. By 18 months
   c. By 3 years
   d. By 6 years
4. A student nurse who has not maintained healthy relationships with his or her peers would be at risk for what self-concept disturbance?
   a. Personal identity disturbance
   b. Body image disturbance
   c. Self-esteem disturbance
   d. Altered role performance
5. When a nurse asks a patient to describe her personal characteristics and traits, the nurse is most likely assessing the patient for what self-concept factors?
   a. Body image
   b. Role performance
   c. Self-esteem
   d. Personal identity

6. Which question would the nurse include on a self-concept assessment related to body image?
   a. Do you like who you are?
   b. Who influenced you the most growing up?
   c. How do you feel about any physical changes you noticed recently?
   d. Who would you most like to be?
7. Which question would the nurse ask to assess a patient's self-identity during a focused self-concept assessment?
   a. Who would you like to be?
   b. What do you like most about your body?
   c. What are your personal strengths?
   d. Do you like being a teacher?
8. Which nursing diagnosis lacks a self-concept disturbance etiology?
   a. Feeding self-care deficit related to dysfunctional grieving
   b. Noncompliance related to low self-esteem
   c. Post-trauma syndrome related to disturbance in personal identity
   d. Ineffective health maintenance related to altered role performance
9. Which question would provide the nurse with the information needed first when assessing self-concept?
   a. How would you describe yourself to others?
   b. Do you like yourself?
   c. What do you see yourself doing 5 years from now?
   d. What are some of your personal strengths?

## ALTERNATE-FORMAT QUESTIONS

### Multiple Response Questions

***Circle the letters that correspond to the best answers for each question.***

1. The nurse is preparing a focused assessment guide to assess patients for self-esteem. Which questions address personal identity? *(Select all that apply.)*
   a. Is there anything about your body that you would change?
   b. How would you describe yourself?
   c. What would you list as your strengths?
   d. How satisfied are you with yourself?
   e. What are your relationships with others like?
   f. What are your fears in life?
2. The school nurse is teaching parents how to build self-esteem in children. Which strategies would the nurse include? *(Select all that apply.)*
   a. Notice examples of your child's ability in many different circumstances and point this out to the child.
   b. Listen to what your child says about his or her behavior and try to provide a possible "fix" for the problem.
   c. Address your child's negative qualities including those that are a matter of taste, preference, or personal style.
   d. Find occasions to frequently and honestly praise your child.
   e. Ask yourself what need is being expressed by your child's negative behavior and address that behavior.
   f. Let your child know what to expect; let your child practice the necessary skills; be patient; and make it safe to fail.
3. A nurse is counseling adolescents in a group home setting. What aspect of self-esteem is developed in this age group? *(Select all that apply.)*
   a. Sense of self is consolidated.
   b. Emphasis is on sexual identity.
   c. It is important to meet role expectations well.
   d. Parental influences on self-concept are often rejected.
   e. A sense of being trusted and loved, of being competent and trustworthy develops.
   f. Differentiation of self and nonself is beginning.

## NURSING PROCESS WORKSHEET

| | |
|---|---|
| **Health Problem (Title)**<br><br>Related to<br>↓ | **Expected Outcome**[a] |
| **Etiology (Related Factors)**<br><br>As Evidenced by<br>↓ | **Nursing Interventions**[b] |
| **Signs and Symptoms (Defining Characteristics)** | **Evaluative Statement** |

[a]More than one patient goal may be appropriate. For the purposes of this exercise, develop the one patient goal that demonstrates a direct resolution of the patient problem identified in the nursing diagnosis.
[b]Be sure you are able to list the scientific rationale for each nursing intervention you ordered.

CHAPTER 42

# Stress and Adaptation

## ASSESSING YOUR UNDERSTANDING

### FILL IN THE BLANKS

1. A person who is in an automobile accident may experience __________ stressors.
2. The pain response is an example of the __________ syndrome.
3. The __________ response is a local response to injury or infection.
4. The __________ response is the body's method of preparing the body to either fight off a stressor or run away from it.
5. A person who develops diarrhea while under prolonged stress is said to be experiencing a(n) __________ disorder.
6. The most common human response to stress is __________.
7. Behaviors used to decrease stress and anxiety are called __________.
8. The prolonged stress experienced by family members caring for a loved one at home is known as __________.

### MATCHING EXERCISES

***Match the type of defense mechanism listed in Part A with its example listed in Part B.***

#### PART A

**a.** Compensation
**b.** Denial
**c.** Displacement
**d.** Introjection
**e.** Projection
**f.** Rationalization
**g.** Reaction formation
**h.** Regression
**i.** Repression
**j.** Sublimation
**k.** Suppression
**l.** Undoing
**m.** Dissociation

#### PART B

____ **1.** A patient bangs his hand on the bed tray in frustration over his rehabilitation progress.

____ **2.** A patient doesn't remember striking a nurse during a painful procedure.

____ **3.** A patient who screamed at a nurse in anger over a lack of privacy gives the nurse a box of candy.

____ **4.** A patient who continually forgets to take his medications complains, "There are too many pills to take."

____ **5.** A patient refuses to accept her diagnosis of cancer.

____ **6.** A patient who has sexual feelings for a nurse accuses her of sexual harassment.

____ **7.** A patient who cannot stop smoking becomes a fitness fanatic.

____ **8.** A patient adopts his spiritual director's philosophy of life.

____ **9.** A patient who actually admires her doctor's medical ability questions his competency.

____ 10. A long-term care facility patient who is depressed becomes incontinent.

____ 11. A wheelchair-bound patient becomes involved in wheelchair races.

____ 12. An adult cannot recall memories of a car accident occurring in his childhood, that killed his mother.

***Match the homeostatic regulators of the body listed in Part A with their action listed in Part B.***

**PART A**

**a.** Parasympathetic
**b.** Sympathetic
**c.** Pituitary
**d.** Adrenals
**e.** Thyroid
**f.** Cardiovascular
**g.** Renal
**h.** Respiratory
**i.** Gastrointestinal

**PART B**

____ 13. Secretes adrenocorticotropic hormone and thyroid-stimulating hormone

____ 14. Takes in food and fluids and eliminates waste products

____ 15. Functions under stress conditions to bring about the fight-or-flight response

____ 16. Regulates intake and output of oxygen and carbon dioxide

____ 17. Functions under normal conditions and at rest

____ 18. Secretes thyroid hormone and calcitonin

____ 19. Serves as a transport system and pump

____ 20. Filters, excretes, and reabsorbs metabolic products and water

**SHORT ANSWER**

1. Briefly describe the following adaptive responses to stress and give an example of each response.
   a. Mind–body interaction: ____________
   b. Local adaptation syndrome: ____________
   c. General adaptation syndrome: ____________

2. Describe the inflammatory response.
   a. ____________

3. List three variables affecting the length of the alarm stage.
   a. ____________
   b. ____________
   c. ____________

4. Describe the following types of anxiety. In your practice, have you experienced any of these levels of anxiety?
   a. Mild anxiety: ____________
   b. Moderate anxiety: ____________
   c. Severe anxiety: ____________
   d. Panic: ____________

5. Give an example of a situation in which you experienced the following coping mechanisms personally or witnessed them in a friend, relative, or patient.
   a. Attack behavior: ____________
   b. Withdrawal behavior: ____________
   c. Compromise behavior: ____________

6. List three examples of situations in which stress may have a positive impact on a person.
   a. ____________
   b. ____________
   c. ____________

7. Give three examples of the following sources of stress.
   a. Developmental stress: ______

   ______

   ______

   b. Situational stress: ______

   ______

   ______

8. An 18-year-old boy is admitted to your unit with a broken leg and facial lacerations from an automobile accident. List two remarks a nurse might make during the nursing history to assess this patient for anxiety.
   a. ______
   b. ______

9. You are a visiting nurse for a patient recovering from a stroke who is being taken care of by her daughter-in-law, who is also the mother of 2-year-old twins. During your visit, you notice that your patient's daughter is restless and unfocused. She tells you she has resumed her smoking habit. You suspect she is suffering from caregiver burden. How would you plan and implement care to help relieve her stress?

   ______

   ______

   ______

   ______

10. Briefly describe how the following components can help reduce stress.
    a. Exercise: ______

    ______

    b. Rest and sleep: ______

    ______

    c. Nutrition: ______

    ______

11. List the five steps of the problem-solving technique used in crisis intervention.
    a. ______
    b. ______
    c. ______
    d. ______
    e. ______

12. List four personal factors that affect stress.
    a. ______
    b. ______
    c. ______
    d. ______

13. Give three examples of how a family can help a patient manage stress.
    a. ______
    b. ______
    c. ______

## APPLYING YOUR KNOWLEDGE

### CRITICAL THINKING QUESTIONS

1. Describe the nursing interventions you would use to relieve the stress of the following patients:
   a. A 42-year-old man with a wife and three children is being treated for an ulcer. He recently lost his job and is having a hard time finding a new one. He doesn't know if he can make his mortgage and school payments.
   b. A 16-year-old boy is admitted to a unit for drug rehabilitation. He put pressure on himself to be "the best" in sports and schoolwork and says he couldn't handle the stress without getting high.

   How would you use your knowledge of the patients to individualize the plan of care?

2. Think of a period in your life when you were under a considerable amount of stress, such as during exams, following a death, or during an illness. How did the stress affect you physically? Did it alter your health state? What did you do to compensate for the effects of stress on your body? How can you use this information in caring for patients?

### REFLECTIVE PRACTICE: CULTIVATING QSEN COMPETENCIES

***Use the following expanded scenario from Chapter 42 in your textbook to answer the questions below.***

***Scenario:*** Joan Rogerrio is a middle-aged woman with a history of inflammatory bowel disease. She comes to the outpatient clinic with complaints of increasing episodes of diarrhea. She says, "I think my bowel disease is flaring up again." Further assessment reveals that she started a new job 1 month ago after being out of the workforce for the past 15 years. She tells the nurse, "Since the children are in school most of the day, my husband and I decided it was time for me to go back to work to help out financially." She says her skills are rusty, and she is having a difficult time adapting to her new work schedule.

1. What might be the cause of the flare-up of Ms. Rogerrios's inflammatory bowel disease? What nursing interventions would be beneficial for this patient?

_______________

_______________

_______________

2. What would be a successful outcome for this patient?

_______________

_______________

_______________

3. What intellectual, technical, interpersonal, and/or ethical/legal competencies are most likely to bring about the desired outcome?

_______________

_______________

_______________

4. What resources might be helpful for Ms. Rogerrio?

_______________

_______________

_______________

**PATIENT CARE STUDY**

***Read the following patient care study and use your nursing process skills to answer the questions below.***

***Scenario:*** Tisha Brent, age 52, comes to the clinic complaining of feelings of nervousness and an inability to sleep. During the health history, she says, "This past year has been almost more than I could stand." She tells you that in 1 year, her grandmother and father died, her husband was diagnosed with cancer, her daughter got a divorce, and her son became depressed and unable to work. She believes herself to be "the strong person in the family; the one who always takes care of everyone else."

Mrs. Brent works full time as a social worker but is finding it more and more difficult to help others because of her own worries. She tells you that she rarely sees her friends anymore because she must care for her husband. She also says that she has no appetite, cries often, and sometimes has trouble catching her breath. Findings from the physical assessment included a weight loss of 10 lb in the past 3 months (with weight 5% below normal for height), tachycardia, slightly elevated blood pressure, and hand tremors.

1. What additional questions might you ask to complete the health history?

_______________

_______________

_______________

2. What physical manifestations of stress might be elicited during the health history and physical assessment?

_______________

_______________

_______________

3. List the nursing diagnoses obtained from your data.

_______________

_______________

_______________

4. List the expected outcomes for Mrs. Brent.

_______________

_______________

_______________

5. Mrs. Brent is diagnosed as being in crisis. What does this mean?

_______________

_______________

_______________

6. What are the steps of crisis intervention that may be used with Mrs. Brent?

_______________

_______________

_______________

**7.** What would you teach Mrs. Brent about reducing stress through healthy activities of daily living?

**a.** Exercise

**b.** Rest and sleep

**c.** Nutrition

**8.** How would you know if Mrs. Brent had decreased her level of stress and increased her ability to cope with stressors?

______________________________________

______________________________________

______________________________________

## PRACTICING FOR NCLEX

### MULTIPLE CHOICE QUESTIONS

***Circle the letter that corresponds to the best answer for each question.***

**1.** A nurse assesses patients in a long-term care facility for diseases that are exacerbated by stressors. What is an autoimmune disease that is related to stress?

**a.** Graves' disease

**b.** Asthma

**c.** Hypertension

**d.** Esophageal reflux

**2.** Which patient is handling stress by using the defense mechanism termed displacement?

**a.** An athlete who doesn't make the team concentrates on body building instead.

**b.** A man with symptoms of prostate cancer refuses to see a doctor.

**c.** A mother who is angry at her husband shouts at the kids to "keep quiet."

**d.** A man who forgets his medication blames his wife for putting it away.

**3.** The nurse is assessing a patient who was involved in a neighborhood shooting. The patient's vital signs show that his body is attempting to adapt to the stressor. What stage of the general adaptation syndrome is this patient experiencing?

**a.** Alarm reaction

**b.** Resistance

**c.** Exhaustion

**d.** Homeostasis

**4.** A patient who responds to bad news concerning his lab reports by crying uncontrollably is handling stress by using:

**a.** Adaptation technique

**b.** Coping mechanism

**c.** Withdrawal behavior

**d.** Defense mechanism

**5.** Which statement correctly explains a person's interactions with basic human needs?

**a.** As a person strives to meet basic human needs at each level, stress can serve as either a stimulus or barrier.

**b.** Basic human needs and responses to stress are generalized.

**c.** Basic human needs and responses to stress are unaffected by sociocultural backgrounds, priorities, and past experiences.

**d.** Stress affects all people in their attainment of basic human needs in the same manner.

**6.** A withdrawn and isolated patient is most likely suffering from what type of stressors on basic human needs?

**a.** Physiologic needs

**b.** Safety and security needs

**c.** Self-esteem needs

**d.** Love and belonging needs

**7.** Which patent reaction is indicative of a person experiencing anxiety due to a psychological response?

**a.** Tremors

**b.** Sleep disturbances

**c.** Expressions of anger

**d.** Withdrawal from interactions with others

**8.** A patient's body uses physiologic mechanisms from within to respond to internal changes and maintain an essential balance. This process is known as:

**a.** Stress

**b.** Self-regulation

**c.** Homeostasis

**d.** Fight-or-flight response

**9.** A patient responds to an approaching diagnostic test with a rapidly beating heart and shaking hands. This is the result of what type of response?

**a.** Coping mechanism

**b.** Stress adaptation

c. Defense mechanism
d. Withdrawal behavior

10. Which patient is experiencing the panic level of anxiety?
    a. A patient loses control and expresses irrational thinking.
    b. A patient experiences increased alertness and motivated learning.
    c. A patient focuses narrowly on specific detail.
    d. A patient displays a narrow perception field.

11. When nurses become overwhelmed in their jobs and develop symptoms of anxiety and stress, they are experiencing what condition?
    a. Culture shock
    b. Adaptation syndrome
    c. Ineffective coping
    d. Burnout

12. What is a general task for a patient adapting to acute and chronic illness?
    a. Maintain self-esteem
    b. Handle pain
    c. Carry out medical treatment
    d. Confront family problems

13. Which of the following conditions most likely occur when a patient is experiencing stress related to scheduled surgery?
    a. Anger
    b. Anxiety
    c. Despair
    d. Depression

## ALTERNATE-FORMAT QUESTIONS

### Multiple Response Questions

***Circle the letters that correspond to the best answers for each question.***

1. Which examples describe the four levels of anxiety that occur in people's lives? *(Select all that apply.)*
   a. Moderate anxiety is present in day-to-day living, and it increases alertness and perceptual fields.
   b. Although mild anxiety may interfere with sleep, it also facilitates problem solving.
   c. Mild anxiety is manifested by a quivering voice, tremors, increased muscle tension, and a slight increase in respirations and pulse.
   d. Severe anxiety creates a very narrow focus on specific detail, causing all behavior to be geared toward getting relief.
   e. Severe anxiety causes a person to lose control and experience dread and terror.
   f. During the panic stage, the person cannot learn, concentrates only on the present situation, and often experiences feelings of impending doom.

2. Which statements accurately describe the body's defense mechanisms against stressors? *(Select all that apply.)*
   a. Withdrawal behavior involves physical withdrawal from the threat or emotional reactions such as admitting defeat, becoming apathetic, or feeling guilty and isolated.
   b. Defense mechanisms are conscious reactions to stressors.
   c. Displacement occurs when a person refuses to acknowledge the presence of a condition that is disturbing.
   d. Projection occurs when a person's thoughts or impulses are attributed to another person.
   e. Repression occurs when a person voluntarily excludes an anxiety-producing event from conscious awareness.
   f. Reaction formation occurs when a person tries to give questionable behavior a logical or socially acceptable explanation.

3. The nurse is describing the effect of stress on the body to a group of health practitioners. Which statements accurately describe the role of stress on the health and illness of patients? *(Select all that apply.)*
   a. Stress has a negative impact on a person as he or she strives to meet basic human needs at each level.
   b. People react to stress in a consistent and predictable manner.
   c. The health–illness continuum is affected by stress.
   d. The effects of stress on a sick or injured person are usually positive.
   e. As the duration, intensity, or number of stressors increases, a person's ability to adapt is lessened.

f. Recovery from illness and return to normal function are compromised by prolonged stress.

4. What are examples of situational stress? *(Select all that apply.)*
   a. A toddler learning to control elimination
   b. A school-aged child attending her first party
   c. A man getting married to his high school sweetheart
   d. A woman recovering from a car accident
   e. A teenager being offered a cigarette by a friend
   f. A high school graduate enrolling in the armed services

5. What are examples of psychosocial stressors? *(Select all that apply.)*
   a. News reports on television about a war
   b. Being caught in a blizzard
   c. Acquiring a nosocomial infection
   d. Being diagnosed with HIV
   e. Fearing a terrorist attack
   f. Being involved in an accident

**Prioritization Question**

1. Place the following steps of the general adaptation syndrome (GAS) in the order in which they would normally occur:
   a. Rest and recovery or death occur.
   b. Alarm reaction begins.
   c. Fight-or-flight response occurs.
   d. Neuroendocrine activity increases vital signs.
   e. Stage of resistance begins.
   f. Panic, crisis, and exhaustion occur.
   g. Neuroendocrine activity returns to normal.
   h. Stage of exhaustion begins.
   i. Threat occurs.

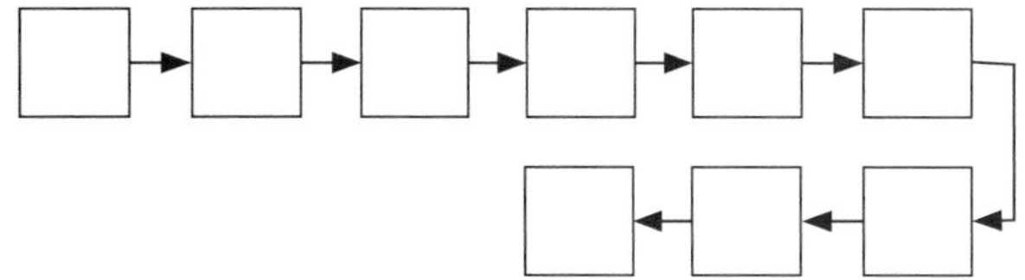

CHAPTER 43

# Loss, Grief, and Dying

## ASSESSING YOUR UNDERSTANDING

### FILL IN THE BLANKS

1. When an older man grieves for the loss of his youth, this type of loss is known as ___________ loss.
2. ___________ is a state of grieving due to loss of a loved one.
3. According to Engel, ___________ is the final resolution of the grief process.
4. Abnormal or distorted grief that may be unresolved or inhibited is known as ___________ grief.
5. According to the Uniform Definition of Death Act (1981), death is defined as present when a person has sustained either irreversible cessation of circulation and respiratory functions or ___________.
6. The goal of ___________ care is to give patients with life-threatening illnesses the best quality of life they can have by the aggressive management of symptoms. It involves taking care of the whole person—body, mind, and spirit, heart and soul.

### MATCHING EXERCISES

***Match the term in Part A with the appropriate definition listed in Part B.***

**PART A**

**a.** Actual loss
**b.** Perceived loss
**c.** Physical loss
**d.** Psychological loss
**e.** Anticipatory loss
**f.** Grief
**g.** Bereavement
**h.** Mourning

**PART B**

____ **1.** Actions and expressions of grief, including the symbols and ceremonies (e.g., a funeral or final celebration of life) that make up the outward expressions of grief

____ **2.** A type of loss in which a person displays loss and grief behaviors for a loss that has yet to take place

____ **3.** A type of loss that can be recognized by others as well as by the person sustaining the loss

____ **4.** The state of grieving due to loss of a loved one

____ **5.** A type of loss that is felt by the person but is intangible to others, such as loss of youth or financial independence

____ **6.** A type of loss that may be caused by an altered self-image and inability to return to work

____ **7.** A type of loss that is tangible, such as the loss of a limb or organ

***Match Engel's six stages of grief listed in Part A with the appropriate conversation that may occur during each stage listed in Part B.***

**PART A**

**a.** Shock and disbelief
**b.** Developing awareness

**c.** Restitution

**d.** Resolving the loss

**e.** Idealization

**f.** Outcome

**PART B**

____ **8.** "I know I won't be having Sunday dinner with my mother anymore. Maybe my husband and I can eat out this Sunday."

____ **9.** "I can't believe my mother died of breast cancer! She was never seriously ill in her life."

____ **10.** "My mother was the perfect parent. I wish I could be more like her with my kids."

____ **11.** "Every time I think of my mother, I can't help but cry."

____ **12.** "I've been attending Mass every morning to pray for my mother's soul and to help me get over her death."

____ **13.** "I miss my mother, but at least now I can accept her death and try to get on with my life."

## CORRECT THE FALSE STATEMENTS

***Circle the word "true" or "false" that follows the statement. If you circled "false," change the underlined word or words to make the statement true. Place your answer in the space provided.***

**1.** A person experiencing <u>abbreviated grief</u> may have trouble expressing feelings of loss or may deny them.

**a.** True

**b.** False ____________________

**2.** In the <u>denial and isolation</u> stage of dying, the patient expresses rage and hostility and adopts a "why me?" attitude.

**a.** True

**b.** False ____________________

**3.** In the case of a terminal illness, the <u>health care provider</u> is usually responsible for deciding what and how much the patient should be told.

**a.** True

**b.** False ____________________

**4.** In a <u>living will</u>, the patient appoints an agent he or she trusts to make decisions if he or she becomes incapacitated.

**a.** True

**b.** False ____________________

**5.** The <u>Patient Self-Determination Act of 1990</u> requires all hospitals to inform their patients of advance directives.

**a.** True

**b.** False ____________________

**6.** A <u>slow-code</u> order may be written on the chart of a terminally ill patient if the patient or family has expressed a wish that there be no attempts to resuscitate the patient in the event of cardiopulmonary failure.

**a.** True

**b.** False ____________________

**7.** <u>Terminal weaning</u> is the gradual withdrawal of mechanical ventilation from a patient with a terminal illness or an irreversible condition with a poor prognosis.

**a.** True

**b.** False ____________________

**8.** The <u>nurse</u> assumes responsibility for handling and filing the death certificate with proper authorities.

**a.** True

**b.** False ____________________

**9.** After the patient has been pronounced dead, the <u>health care provider</u> is responsible for preparing the body for discharge.

**a.** True

**b.** False ____________________

## SHORT ANSWER

**1.** List two nursing responsibilities that should be carried out after the death of a patient in each of the following areas.

**a.** Care of the body: ____________________

____________________

**b.** Care of the family: ____________________

____________________

**c.** Discharging legal responsibilities: ____________________

____________________

2. Briefly describe the following stages of dying, according to Kübler-Ross.
   a. Denial and isolation: ______
   b. Anger: ______
   c. Bargaining: ______
   d. Depression: ______
   e. Acceptance: ______
3. Your patient is a 50-year-old woman newly diagnosed with terminal uterine cancer. What information should be provided to her regarding her condition?
4. How would you respond to a patient dying of AIDS who says: "Nurse, please help me die"?
5. Describe the role of the nurse in terminal weaning.
6. List three goals for nurses who wish to become effective in caring for patients experiencing loss, grief, or dying and death.
   a. ______
   b. ______
   c. ______
7. Your patient is a 62-year-old man dying of liver cancer at home with his family. List three patient goals or outcomes for this patient and his family.
   a. ______
   b. ______
   c. ______
8. List three arguments in favor of and against assisted suicide and direct voluntary euthanasia.
   a. In favor of: ______
   b. Against: ______
9. What is the role of the nurse during the following code situations?
   a. No-code: ______
   b. Comfort measures only: ______
   c. Do-not-hospitalize order: ______
   d. Terminal weaning: ______
10. Explain the role of the nurse in obtaining the following advance directives for a patient.
   a. Durable power of attorney: ______
   b. Living will: ______

## APPLYING YOUR KNOWLEDGE

### CRITICAL THINKING QUESTIONS

1. Develop nursing plans to help the following patients deal with their grief.
   a. A 22-year-old male athlete has his left leg amputated after it was crushed in a car accident.
   b. You find a 30-year-old woman crying softly in her bed after undergoing a hysterectomy.
   c. A 50-year-old woman has just been told she has an inoperable brain tumor.

What knowledge and skills would you need to meet their needs?

2. Think of a time when you lost someone dear to you. How did you cope with your loss? Were you aware of going through Engel's six stages of grief? How long did it take you to resolve the loss and get back to normal life activities? Interview some friends about coping with losing a loved one and compare their experiences to yours. How can you use this knowledge in your care of patients?

## REFLECTIVE PRACTICE: CULTIVATING QSEN COMPETENCIES

***Use the following expanded scenario from Chapter 43 in your textbook to answer the questions below.***

***Scenario:*** Yvonne Malic, age 20, is admitted to the hospital after her water broke, and labor begins 7 weeks early. She delivers a female infant who is immediately transported to the neonatal intensive care unit. Yvonne is single and desperately wants to be a mother. She had a normal pregnancy up to this point and was expecting a healthy baby girl. The nurse informs Ms. Malic that her baby has less than a 50% chance of surviving the next 24 hours. Ms. Malic tearfully tells the nurse, "Leave me alone!" and turns her body to face the wall.

1. How might the nurse react to Ms. Malic in a manner that respects her right to privacy while at the same time helping her through the grief process?

______________________________________

______________________________________

______________________________________

2. What would be a successful outcome for this patient?

______________________________________

______________________________________

______________________________________

3. What intellectual, technical, interpersonal, and/or ethical/legal competencies are most likely to bring about the desired outcome?

______________________________________

______________________________________

______________________________________

4. What resources might be helpful for Ms. Malic?

______________________________________

______________________________________

______________________________________

## PATIENT CARE STUDY

***Read the following patient care study and use your nursing process skills to answer the questions below.***

***Scenario:*** LeRoy is a 40-year-old architect whose life partner, Michael, is dying of AIDS. Although both LeRoy and Michael "did the bathhouse scene" in the early 1980s and had multiple unprotected sexual encounters, they have been in a monogamous relationship for the past 14 years. Michael has been in and out of the hospital during the past 3 years and is now dying of end-stage AIDS at home. He is enrolled in a hospice program. LeRoy has been very supportive of Michael throughout the different phases of his illness but at present seems to be "losing it." Michael noticed that LeRoy is sleeping at odd times and seems to be losing weight. He suspects that LeRoy may be drinking more than usual and using recreational drugs. He also says that LeRoy is "acting strangely"; he seems emotionally withdrawn and unusually uncommunicative. "I don't think he's able to deal with the fact that I'm dying," Michael tells you. "He won't let me talk about it at all." The hospice nurse notes that LeRoy is now rarely home when he comes to visit. When the hospice nurse calls to arrange a meeting with LeRoy, LeRoy informs him that he is "managing quite well, thank you" and that he has no concerns or problems to discuss.

1. Identify pertinent patient data by placing a single underline beneath the objective data in the patient care study and a double underline beneath the subjective data.

2. Complete the Nursing Process Worksheet on page 303 to develop a three-part diagnostic statement and related plan of care for this patient.

3. Write down the patient and personal nursing strengths you hope to draw on as you assist this patient to better health.

   Patient strengths: ______________________

   ______________________

   ______________________

   Personal strengths: ______________________

   ______________________

   ______________________

4. Pretend that you are performing a nursing assessment of LeRoy after the plan of care is implemented. Document your findings.

   ______________________

   ______________________

## PRACTICING FOR NCLEX

### MULTIPLE CHOICE QUESTIONS

***Circle the letter that corresponds to the best answer for each question.***

1. With the help of the nurse, the parents of an infant who died shortly after birth arrange for a funeral service. What stage of grief, according to Engel, involves the rituals surrounding loss, including funeral services?
   a. Shock and disbelief
   b. Developing awareness
   c. Restitution
   d. Resolving the loss

2. The husband of a patient who has died cannot express his feelings of loss and at times denies them. His bereavement has extended over a lengthy period. What type of grief is the husband experiencing?
   a. Anticipatory grief
   b. Inhibited grief
   c. Normal grief
   d. Unresolved grief

3. A patient who was brought to the emergency room for gunshot wounds dies in intensive care 15 hours later. Which statement concerning the need for an autopsy would apply to this patient?
   a. The closest surviving family member should be consulted to determine whether an autopsy should be performed.
   b. The coroner must be notified to determine the need for an autopsy.
   c. The health care provider should be present to prepare the patient for an autopsy.
   d. An autopsy should not be performed because the nature of death has been established.

4. Mr. Cooney, age 85, is in advanced stages of pneumonia with a no-code order in his chart. Which of the following nursing care actions will help establish a trusting nurse–patient relationship?
   a. The nurse discusses the patient's fears and doubts openly and serves as a nonjudgmental listener.
   b. The nurse reduces verbal and nonverbal contact with the patient to avoid confusing him.
   c. The nurse avoids providing counseling and death education because it is not within the scope of professional nursing practice.
   d. The nurse arranges a visit from a spiritual advisor for dying patients, regardless of the patient's wishes, to provide hope in the face of death.

5. A nurse informs a woman that there is nothing more that can be done medically for her premature infant who is expected to die. The mother suppresses her grief and tells the nurse she is experiencing heart palpitations. What type of grief might the mother be experiencing?
   a. Anticipatory grief
   b. Inhibited grief
   c. Unresolved grief
   d. Dysfunctional grief

6. The wife of a man who is dying tells the nurse: "Harold was so good to me. He was like a saint with his patience. I will miss him terribly." Which stage of grief is this woman experiencing, according to Engel?
   a. Restitution
   b. Awareness
   c. Outcome
   d. Idealization

7. Before the death of her husband, Mrs. Sardi complained of frequent headaches and loss of appetite. No medical cause was found. Mrs. Sardi probably was experiencing which type of grief?

a. Abbreviated grief
b. Anticipatory grief
c. Unresolved grief
d. Inhibited grief

8. Which diagnosis specifically addresses human response to loss and impending death in the problem statement?
 a. Complicated grieving related to loss of partner
 b. Anxiety related to unknown reaction to stages of death
 c. Dressing self-care deficit related to weakness
 d. Impaired comfort related to complications of chemotherapy for end-stage liver cancer

## ALTERNATE-FORMAT QUESTIONS

### Multiple Response Questions

***Circle the letters that correspond to the best answers for each question.***

1. A nurse is assessing a dying patient for realism of expectations and perception of condition. Which interview questions address this concern? *(Select all that apply.)*
 a. Have you had any previous experience with this condition before?
 b. Do you know how to contact your doctor and get answers to your questions?
 c. How do you see the next few weeks playing out?
 d. What have you been told about your condition?
 e. How well do you think those around you are coping?
 f. What do you think may be happening in the midst of all of this?

2. Which signs assessed in a dying patient would the nurse recognize as signs of death? *(Select all that apply.)*
 a. Increased body temperature
 b. Nausea, flatus, abdominal distention
 c. Racing pulse
 d. Cheyne–Stokes respirations
 e. Loss of movement, sensation, and reflexes
 f. Increased blood pressure

3. A nurse is conducting grief resolution for a patient who lost his wife in a motor vehicle accident in which he was the driver. Which interventions best accomplish this goal? *(Select all that apply.)*
 a. Encourage the patient's desire to keep silent about the event.
 b. Avoid making emphatic statements about the patient's grief.
 c. Avoid identification of fears regarding the loss.
 d. Listen to expressions of grief.
 e. Include significant others in discussions and decisions as appropriate.
 f. Communicate acceptance of discussing loss.

4. The nurse is discussing end-of-life decisions with a patient who has terminal cancer. Which statements describe the patient's options? *(Select all that apply.)*
 a. Living wills provide specific instructions about the kinds of health care that should be provided or foregone in particular situations.
 b. In a living will, a patient appoints an agent that he or she trusts to make decisions if he or she becomes incapacitated.
 c. The Patient Self-Determination Act of 1990 requires all hospitals to inform their patients about advance directives.
 d. The status of advance directives varies from state to state.
 e. Nurses are legally responsible for arranging for a durable power of attorney for all terminal patients.
 f. Legally, all attempts must be made by the health care team to resuscitate a terminal patient.

5. A nurse is explaining the preparation of a death certificate to a student nurse. Which statements accurately describe this process? *(Select all that apply.)*
 a. U.S. law requires that a death certificate be prepared for each person who dies.
 b. Death certificates are sent to a national health department, which compiles many statistics from the information.
 c. The nurse assumes responsibility for handling and filing the death certificate with the proper authorities.

d. A health care provider's signature is required on a death certificate.
e. It is the nurse's responsibility to ensure that the health care provider has signed a death certificate.
f. A death certificate is signed by the pathologist, the coroner, and others in special cases.

6. Which actions are performed by the nurse when a patient dies? *(Select all that apply.)*
   a. Washing the patient's body
   b. Removing all tubes according to facility policy, unless an autopsy is to be performed
   c. Placing identification on the shroud or garment and wrist
   d. Placing identification tags on the patient's dentures or other prostheses
   e. Arranging for family members to view the body before it is discharged to the mortician
   f. Attending the funeral of a deceased patient and making follow-up visits to the family

## NURSING PROCESS WORKSHEET

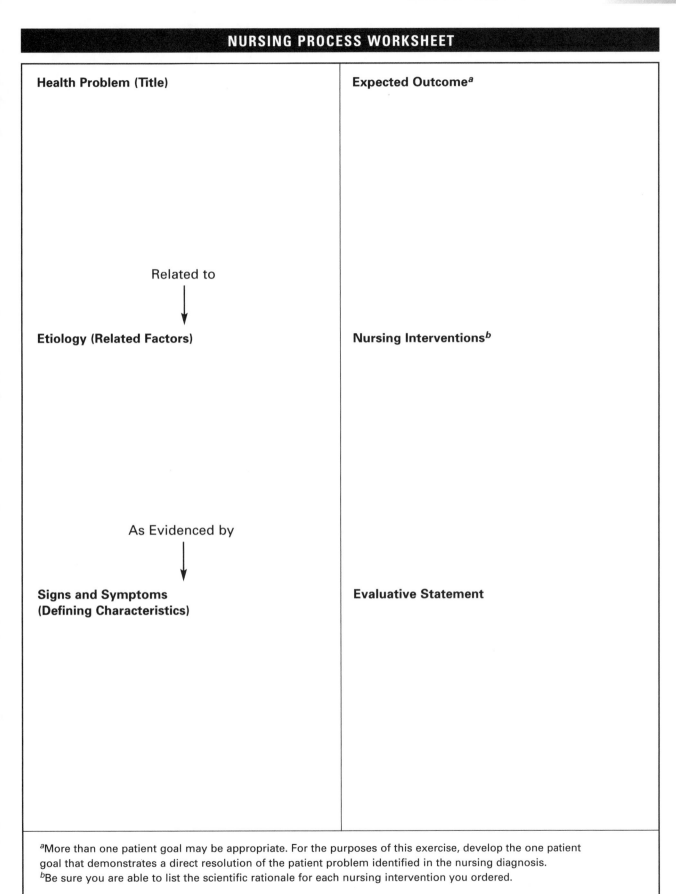

| **Health Problem (Title)**<br><br>Related to<br>↓ | **Expected Outcome**[a] |
|---|---|
| **Etiology (Related Factors)**<br><br>As Evidenced by<br>↓ | **Nursing Interventions**[b] |
| **Signs and Symptoms (Defining Characteristics)** | **Evaluative Statement** |

[a]More than one patient goal may be appropriate. For the purposes of this exercise, develop the one patient goal that demonstrates a direct resolution of the patient problem identified in the nursing diagnosis.
[b]Be sure you are able to list the scientific rationale for each nursing intervention you ordered.

CHAPTER 44

# Sensory Functioning

## ASSESSING YOUR UNDERSTANDING

### FILL IN THE BLANKS

1. ____________ is the process of receiving data about the internal or external environment through the senses.
2. ____________ refers to awareness of positioning of body parts and body movement.
3. ____________ is the sense that perceives the solidity of objects and their size, shape, and texture.
4. The state in which a person cannot remember bits of information or behavior skills is known as ____________ and is attributed to pathophysiologic or situational causes that are either temporary or permanent.
5. Impaired or absent functioning in one or more senses is termed ____________.

### MATCHING EXERCISES

***Match the senses in Part A with their definition in Part B.***

**PART A**

**a.** Visual
**b.** Auditory
**c.** Olfactory
**d.** Gustatory
**e.** Tactile
**f.** Kinesthesia
**g.** Visceral
**h.** Stereognosis

**PART B**

____ **1.** The sense that perceives the solidity of objects and their size, shape, and texture
____ **2.** The sense of taste
____ **3.** The sense of sight
____ **4.** The sense of smell
____ **5.** The sense of hearing
____ **6.** The awareness of positioning of body parts and body movement
____ **7.** The sense of touch

***Match the examples in Part B with the appropriate stimulation listed in Part A. Some answers may be used more than once.***

**PART A**

**a.** Visual stimulation
**b.** Auditory stimulation
**c.** Gustatory/olfactory stimulation
**d.** Tactile stimulation

**PART B**

____ **8.** A nurse wears a brightly colored top when caring for patients confined to bed.
____ **9.** A nurse collaborates with the hospital nutritionist to prepare meals with varied seasonings and textures.
____ **10.** A patient confined to bed is given daily massages.
____ **11.** Soft music is played in the room of a patient who has eye patches following his surgery.

____ **12.** In a long-term care facility, a nurse checks a patient for properly fitting dentures.

____ **13.** A nurse hugs a depressed patient who has made the effort to bathe and dress herself.

____ **14.** A nurse explains a procedure to a comatose patient.

____ **15.** A nurse arranges a patient's cards in a heart shape on her wall.

## SHORT ANSWER

**1.** List four conditions that must be present for a person to receive data necessary to experience the world.

**a.** ____

**b.** ____

**c.** ____

**d.** ____

**2.** Give an example of how the following factors may place a patient at high risk for sensory deprivation.

**a.** Environment: ____

**b.** Impaired ability to receive environmental stimuli: ____

**c.** Inability to process environmental stimuli: ____

**3.** Briefly describe the following effects of sensory deprivation:

**a.** Perceptual responses: ____

**b.** Cognitive responses: ____

**c.** Emotional responses: ____

**4.** List three examples of sensory overload you have observed when caring for patients on your nursing unit.

**a.** ____

**b.** ____

**c.** ____

**5.** Describe the concept of cultural care deprivation and list an example from your own experience of a patient who has experienced this alteration.

____

**6.** Give an example of sensory stimulation that could be provided for each of the following age groups.

**a.** Infant: ____

**b.** Adult: ____

**c.** Older adult: ____

**7.** Give an example of two goals for patients with impaired sensory functioning.

**a.** ____

**b.** ____

**8.** You have been assigned to visit a home health care patient, a 75-year-old woman with diabetes living at home with her husband. When you arrive at their home, you notice the drapes are shut; the room is dark and bleak; and there are no pictures, flowers, or the like to visually stimulate the patient. The patient appears in good physical health but slightly disoriented and confused about the date and time of day. Develop a nursing care plan for this patient with emphasis on the need for sensory stimulation.

____

**9.** List four precautions you could teach a patient to avoid eye injury in the home.

**a.** ____

**b.** ____

**c.** ____

**d.** ____

**10.** Give two suggestions for increasing environmental stimulation and role model appropriate interactional behaviors for children in the following areas.

**a.** Visual: ____________________

**b.** Auditory: ____________________

**c.** Olfactory: ____________________

**d.** Gustatory: ____________________

**e.** Tactile: ____________________

**11.** Give an example of how each of the following factors may influence the amount and quality of stimuli needed to maintain cortical arousal.

**a.** Developmental considerations: ____________________

**b.** Culture and lifestyle: ____________________

**c.** Personality: ____________________

**d.** Stress: ____________________

**e.** Illness and medication: ____________________

**12.** Explain how you might assess a patient for the following sensory experiences.

**a.** Stimulation: ____________________

**b.** Reception: ____________________

**c.** Transmission–perception–reaction: ____________________

**13.** Give three examples of how a nurse might communicate with the following patients.

**a.** Visually impaired patients: ____________________

**b.** Hearing-impaired patients: ____________________

**c.** Unconscious patients: ____________________

## APPLYING YOUR KNOWLEDGE

### CRITICAL THINKING QUESTIONS

**1.** Test your friends' senses by trying out these tactile, gustatory, and olfactory exercises.

**a.** Gather several items from your home/work area and place them in a paper bag. These items could include things such as a key, a cotton ball, a toothpick, a tongue depressor, etc. Have your friends take turns feeling the objects in the bag and guessing what they are without looking at them. As an item is identified, remove it from the bag. Discuss the importance of tactile experiences to the vision-impaired patient.

**b.** Gather several foods for your friends to taste and identify. You could use pudding, gelatin, mints, chocolate, etc. Blindfold your friends and give them a taste of each food. See how many they can identify correctly.

**c.** Gather items with a pungent odor for your friends to smell and identify. You could use alcohol, lemon juice, pickle juice, cinnamon, mint, etc. See how many odors they can identify correctly.

Reflect on the role different senses play. Do you believe using only one sense at a time heightens the awareness of that sense? Relate the exercises above to the special needs of hearing-impaired and vision-impaired patients.

**2.** Walk down a busy street in a city and try to pick out individual noises. How many noises were you able to identify? How many noises became indistinct due to sensory overload? Relate this experience to a patient in a critical care unit.

## REFLECTIVE PRACTICE: CULTIVATING QSEN COMPETENCIES

***Use the following expanded scenario from Chapter 44 in your textbook to answer the questions below.***

***Scenario:*** Dolores Pirolla, age 74, comes to the older adult clinic with her 77-year-old husband who was diagnosed with macular degeneration and progressive vision loss. She says, "Now I've noticed he's also having difficulty hearing me. I'm worried because he doesn't want to leave the house. We hardly see any of our friends anymore. We used to go out to the movies or dinner at least once a week, and lately if we get out once a month, that's a lot!" Mrs. Pirolla also expresses concerns about her husband's safety when moving about the house and neighborhood.

1. What nursing interventions might be appropriate for Mr. Pirolla?

 ______________________________________

 ______________________________________

 ______________________________________

2. What would be a successful outcome for this patient?

 ______________________________________

 ______________________________________

 ______________________________________

3. What intellectual, technical, interpersonal, and/or ethical/legal competencies are most likely to bring about the desired outcome?

 ______________________________________

 ______________________________________

 ______________________________________

4. What resources might be helpful for Mr. Pirolla?

 ______________________________________

 ______________________________________

 ______________________________________

## PATIENT CARE STUDY

***Read the following patient care study and use your nursing process skills to answer the questions below.***

***Scenario:*** George Gibson, an 81-year-old, married, African-American man, reluctantly reports, after much prodding from his wife, that he is not hearing as well as he used to be. "I don't know what the trouble is," he tells you. "I'm in perfect health, always have been. More and more, people just seem to be mumbling instead of talking." You notice he is seated on the edge of his chair and bends toward you when you speak to him. His wife reports that he has stopped going out and pretty much stays in his room whenever people come to visit because he is embarrassed by his inability to hear. "This is really a shame, because George was always the life of the party," she says. You ask Mr. Gibson if he has ever had his hearing evaluated, and he tells you no, until now, he's been trying to convince himself that nothing's wrong with his hearing.

1. Identify pertinent patient data by placing a single underline beneath the objective data in the patient care study and a double underline beneath the subjective data.
2. Complete the Nursing Process Worksheet on page 310 to develop a three-part diagnostic statement and related plan of care for this patient.
3. Write down the patient and personal nursing strengths you hope to draw on as you assist this patient to better health.

 Patient strengths: ______________________

 ______________________________________

 ______________________________________

 Personal strengths: ______________________

 ______________________________________

 ______________________________________

4. Pretend that you are performing a nursing assessment of this patient after the plan of care is implemented. Document your findings.

 ______________________________________

 ______________________________________

## PRACTICING FOR NCLEX

### MULTIPLE CHOICE QUESTIONS

***Circle the letter that corresponds to the best answer for each question.***

1. A patient who has been living in a long-term care facility for the past 5 years no longer responds to the everyday noises outside his room. This ability to ignore continuing noise is known as:
   a. Sensoristasis
   b. Sensory overload
   c. Adaptation
   d. Stereognosis
2. The nurse takes into consideration factors that affect sensory stimulation in hospitalized patients when planning patient care. Which statement is true?
   a. Different personality types demand the same level of stimulation.
   b. Decreased sensory stimulation may be sought during periods of low stress.
   c. Illness does not affect the reception of sensory stimuli.
   d. A person's culture may dictate the amount of sensory stimulation considered normal.
3. A nurse admitting an unconscious person to the unit considers which guideline when performing care for this patient?
   a. Hearing is the first sense lost in an unconscious patient; therefore, verbal communication is unnecessary.
   b. Assume the patient can hear you, and talk with him or her in a normal tone of voice.
   c. Do not touch the unconscious patient unnecessarily because it may confuse him or her.
   d. Keep the environmental noise level high in the patient's room to help stimulate the patient.
4. Which patient would the nurse consider most at risk for sensory deprivation?
   a. A patient in an isolation room
   b. A patient who visits a health care provider's office
   c. A patient in the emergency department
   d. A patient in a long-term care facility
5. A patient who hallucinates simply to maintain an optimal level of arousal is experiencing what condition?
   a. Sensory overload
   b. Sensory deprivation
   c. Cultural care deprivation
   d. Sleep deprivation
6. A patient in a long-term care facility cannot control the direction of thought content, has a decreased attention span, and cannot concentrate. Which effects of sensory deprivation might the patient be experiencing?
   a. Perceptual response
   b. Emotional response
   c. Physical response
   d. Cognitive response
7. What condition is a patient who is blind said to be experiencing?
   a. Sensory overload
   b. Sensory deficit
   c. Sensory deprivation
   d. Sensory overstimulation

### ALTERNATE-FORMAT QUESTIONS

#### Multiple Response Questions

***Circle the letters that correspond to the best answers for each question.***

1. For which conditions would the nurse assess a patient to determine if he or she is able to adequately receive the data necessary to experience the world? *(Select all that apply.)*
   a. A response
   b. A stimulus
   c. A receptor or sense organ
   d. An arousal mechanism
   e. An intact nerve pathway
   f. A functioning brain
2. A nurse is assessing patients in a burn unit for sensory alterations. Which factors contribute to severe sensory alterations? *(Select all that apply.)*
   a. Sensory saturation
   b. Sensory discrepancies
   c. Sensory overload
   d. Sensory deprivation
   e. Sleep deprivation
   f. Cultural overload

3. What conditions occur in patients who are experiencing the effects of sensory deprivation? *(Select all that apply.)*
   - a. Inaccurate perception of sights, sounds, tastes, and smells
   - b. Increased coordination and equilibrium
   - c. Inability to control direction of thought content
   - d. Increased attention span and ability to concentrate
   - e. Difficulty with memory, problem solving, and task performance
   - f. Emotionally caring attitude and stable moods
4. The nurse is planning strategies to increase sensory stimulation for patients in isolation. Which considerations should the nurse keep in mind? *(Select all that apply.)*
   - a. The amount of stimuli different people consider optimal is constant.
   - b. Sensory functioning is established at birth and is independent of stimulation received during childhood.
   - c. It is recommended that medically fragile infants have greater light and visual and vestibular stimulation.
   - d. Sensory functioning tends to decline progressively throughout adulthood.
   - e. A person's culture may dictate the amount of sensory stimulation considered normal.
   - f. Different personality types demand different levels of stimulation.
5. For which conditions would the nurse assess to determine if a patient is suffering from sensory deprivation or overload? *(Select all that apply.)*
   - a. Boredom
   - b. Decreased sleeping
   - c. Quickness of thought
   - d. Anxiety
   - e. Dreamless sleep
   - f. Thought disorganization
6. Which actions are performed according to guidelines for caring for visually impaired patients? *(Select all that apply.)*
   - a. Wait for the person to sense your presence in the room before identifying yourself.
   - b. Speak in a normal tone of voice.
   - c. Explain the reason for touching the person after doing so.
   - d. Orient the person to the arrangement of the room and its furnishings.
   - e. Assist with ambulation by walking slightly behind the person.
   - f. Sit in the person's field of vision if he or she has partial or reduced peripheral vision.
7. Which actions are performed according to guidelines for caring for patients with hearing impairments? *(Select all that apply.)*
   - a. Increase the noise level in the room.
   - b. Clean ears on a daily basis.
   - c. Position yourself so that the light is on your face when you speak.
   - d. Talk to the person from a distance so that he or she may read your lips.
   - e. Demonstrate or pantomime ideas you wish to express.
   - f. Write down any ideas that you cannot convey to the person in another manner.

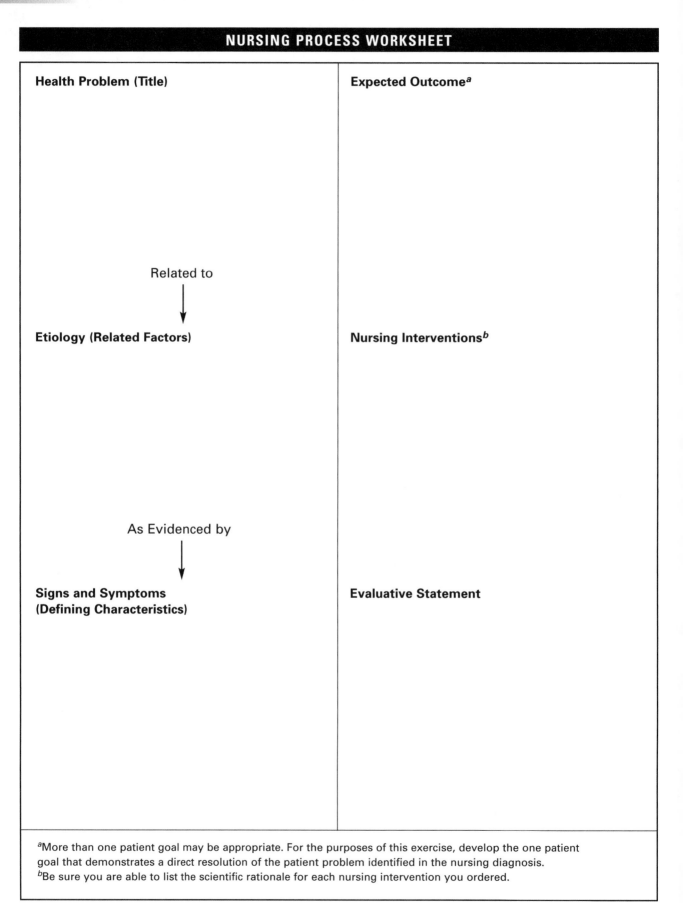

## NURSING PROCESS WORKSHEET

| Health Problem (Title)<br><br>Related to<br>↓ | Expected Outcome[a] |
|---|---|
| **Etiology (Related Factors)**<br><br>As Evidenced by<br>↓ | **Nursing Interventions[b]** |
| **Signs and Symptoms (Defining Characteristics)** | **Evaluative Statement** |

[a]More than one patient goal may be appropriate. For the purposes of this exercise, develop the one patient goal that demonstrates a direct resolution of the patient problem identified in the nursing diagnosis.
[b]Be sure you are able to list the scientific rationale for each nursing intervention you ordered.

CHAPTER 45

# Sexuality

## ASSESSING YOUR UNDERSTANDING

### FILL IN THE BLANKS

1. ____________ is the degree to which a person exhibits and experiences maleness or femaleness physically, emotionally, and mentally.
2. ____________ refers to romantic, emotional, affectionate, or sexual attraction to other people.
3. ____________ refers to the preferred biologic sex of the partner of an individual.
4. A woman who experiences menstrual cycle–related distress is said to have ____________.
5. Areas that when stimulated cause sexual arousal and desire are called ____________.
6. The ____________ system of contraception is a reversible, 5-year, low-dose progestin-only contraceptive consisting of six capsules placed under the skin of the woman's upper arm.
7. The ____________ patch supplies continuous daily circulating levels of ethinyl estradiol and norelgestromin to prevent conception.

### MATCHING EXERCISES

***Match the terms listed in Part A with their definition listed in Part B.***

**PART A**

a. Biologic sex
b. Gender role
c. Gender identity
d. Sexual orientation
e. Heterosexual
f. Gay or lesbian
g. Bisexual
h. Transsexual
i. Transvestite

**PART B**

____ 1. Refers to the preferred biologic sex of an individual's sexual partner

____ 2. Term used to denote chromosomal sexual development

____ 3. People who live full-time as members of a biologic sex that differs from the sex and gender they were assigned at birth

____ 4. The behavior a person exhibits in relation to being male or female, which may or may not be the same as biologic sex or gender identity

____ 5. Refers to a person who is attracted to both men and women

____ 6. One who experiences sexual fulfillment with a person of the opposite biologic sex

____ 7. The inner sense a person has of being male or female

____ 8. One who experiences sexual fulfillment with a person of the same biologic sex

### SHORT ANSWER

1. Give an example of an intervention that could improve their sexual relations for patients with the following health problems.
   a. Chronic pain: ____________________
   ____________________
   b. Diabetes: ____________________
   ____________________

c. Cardiovascular disease: ______

d. Loss of body part: ______

e. Spinal cord injury: ______

f. Mental illness: ______

g. Sexually transmitted infections: ______

2. Briefly describe the four phases of the menstrual cycle.
   a. Follicular phase: ______
   b. Proliferation phase: ______
   c. Luteal phase: ______
   d. Secretory phase: ______

3. Briefly describe the male and female responses in the following phases of the sexual response cycle.
   a. Excitement phase—Female: ______
      Male: ______
   b. Plateau—Female: ______
      Male: ______
   c. Orgasm—Female: ______
      Male: ______
   d. Resolution—Female: ______
      Male: ______

4. List three general categories of patients who should have a sexual history recorded by the nurse.
   a. ______
   b. ______
   c. ______

5. List three interview questions a nurse may use during a sexual history when assessing a male for impotence.
   a. ______
   b. ______
   c. ______

6. List three major goals of patient teaching about sexuality and wellness.
   a. ______
   b. ______
   c. ______

7. Complete the following table, listing the advantages and disadvantages associated with contraceptive methods.

| Method | Advantages | Disadvantages |
|---|---|---|
| **a.** Behavioral | | |
| **b.** Barrier methods | | |
| **c.** Intrauterine devices | | |
| **d.** Hormonal methods | | |
| **e.** Sterilization | | |

## APPLYING YOUR KNOWLEDGE

### CRITICAL THINKING QUESTIONS

1. Write down the interview questions you would use to obtain a sexual history from the following patients.
   a. An 18-year-old female victim of date rape who is brought to the emergency room for testing and treatment
   b. A 48-year-old man diagnosed with prostate cancer who is seeking a prescription for Viagra
   c. An HIV-positive woman who has had multiple sexual partners and admits she probably infected other people through unsafe practices
   d. A 5-year-old girl who presents with soreness and redness in the genital area

   How comfortable would you be asking these patients the necessary questions, and how might you develop the skills necessary to perform the interview?
2. Describe the knowledge and skills you would need to care for patients experiencing the following sexual dysfunctions.
   a. A man undergoing radiation treatment for colon cancer complains of impotence.
   b. A menopausal woman complains of vaginal dryness and pain during intercourse.
   c. A sexually active teenager complains of a burning sensation during urination.

### REFLECTIVE PRACTICE: CULTIVATING QSEN COMPETENCIES

***Use the following expanded scenario from Chapter 45 in your textbook to answer the questions below.***

***Scenario:*** Jefferson Smith is a middle-aged man who was recently married after the death of his first wife 10 years ago. He has a history of diabetes and hypertension and is receiving numerous medications as treatment. During a routine visit to his primary care physician, Mr. Smith confides that he has been having problems "in the bedroom." He reports difficulty attaining and maintaining an erection. He asks, "What about all those new drugs they keep advertising on TV? Would they work for me?"

1. What issues might the nurse address in the plan of care for Mr. Smith? What patient teaching should be incorporated into the plan of care?

   ______________________________

   ______________________________

   ______________________________

2. What would be a successful outcome for this patient?

   ______________________________

   ______________________________

   ______________________________

3. What intellectual, technical, interpersonal, and/or ethical/legal competencies are most likely to bring about the desired outcome?

   ______________________________

   ______________________________

   ______________________________

4. What resources might be helpful for Mr. Smith?

   ______________________________

   ______________________________

   ______________________________

### PATIENT CARE STUDY

***Read the following patient care study and use your nursing process skills to answer the questions below.***

***Scenario:*** Anthony Piscatelli, a 6-ft tall, muscular, healthy 19-year-old college freshman in the School of Nursing, confides to his nursing advisor that "everything is great" about college life, with one exception: "All of a sudden, I find myself questioning the values I learned at home about sex and marriage. My mom was really insistent that each of her sons should respect women and that intercourse was something you saved until you were ready to get married. If she told us once, she told us a hundred times, that we'd save ourselves, the girls in our lives, and her and dad a lot of heartache if we could just learn to control ourselves sexually. Problem is that no one here seems to subscribe to this philosophy. I feel like I'm abnormal in some way to even think like this. There's a lot of sexual activity in the dorms, and no one even thinks you're serious if you talk about virginity positively. What do you think? Did my mom sell me a bill of goods? Is it true that if you take the proper precautions, no one gets hurt and everyone has a good time?" Tony reports that he is a virgin and that he really misses his close family back home: "I do get lonely at times and would love to just cuddle with someone or even give and get a big hug, but no one seems to understand this."

1. Identify pertinent patient data by placing a single underline beneath the objective data in the patient care study and a double underline beneath the subjective data.
2. Complete the Nursing Process Worksheet on page 318 to develop a three-part diagnostic statement and related plan of care for this patient.
3. Write down the patient and personal nursing strengths you hope to draw on as you assist this patient to better health.

   Patient strengths: ______________________

   ______________________

   ______________________

   Personal strengths: ______________________

   ______________________

   ______________________

4. Pretend that you are performing a nursing assessment of this patient after the plan of care is implemented. Document your findings.

   ______________________

   ______________________

## PRACTICING FOR NCLEX

### MULTIPLE CHOICE QUESTIONS

***Circle the letter that corresponds to the best answer for each question.***

1. The nurse is teaching patients about sexually transmitted infections (STIs). What would the nurse include as a teaching point?
   a. Most of the time, STIs cause no symptoms.
   b. Health problems from STIs tend to be more severe in males.
   c. Reported STIs are at an all-time low due to targeted education about STIs.
   d. STIs are most prevalent among the adult population.
2. The nurse is preparing a talk on health issues in the LGBT population. Which statistics would the nurse include?
   a. Lesbians and bisexual females are more likely to be underweight or anorexic.
   b. LGBT populations have lower rates of tobacco, alcohol, and other drug use.
   c. LGBT youth are two to three times more likely to attempt suicide.
   d. Lesbians are more likely to get preventive services for cancer.
3. In which of these situations does the nursing action not advocate for patient sexual needs?
   a. The nurse anticipates potentially shaming situations for the patient.
   b. The nurse interfaces with the primary care provider to obtain information for the patient.
   c. The nurse ensures the patient wears a hospital gown to protect personal clothing.
   d. The nurse refers to the patient as Mr., Mrs., Miss, or Ms., according to the patient's preference.
4. The nurse caring for patients in a health care provider's office takes into consideration developmental stage when assessing sexuality. Which is an example of a developmentally appropriate intervention?
   a. The nurse teaches parents of an 18-month-old to discourage self-manipulation of genitals.
   b. The nurse teaches parents of a 4-year-old that they may cause anxiety in the child by intolerance of inconsistency of sex-role behavior.
   c. The nurse warns parents of 2-year-old that toilet training should be initiated immediately to prevent compulsive behaviors later on.
   d. The nurse states that same-sex preference for relationships in the school-aged child may be related to heterosexual or homosexual tendencies.

5. The nurse is caring for a patient diagnosed with human papillomavirus (HPV). What is a symptom of this STI?
   a. Foul-smelling, thin, grayish white vaginal discharge
   b. Possible vaginal bleeding or spotting
   c. Single painless genital lesion 10 days to 3 months after exposure
   d. Profuse watery vaginal discharge

6. A patient visits a community clinic with complaints of foul-smelling vaginal discharge that is thin, foamy, and green in color; itching of vulva and vagina; and burning on urination. What STI would the nurse suspect?
   a. Acquired immunodeficiency syndrome (AIDS)
   b. *Chlamydia trachomatis*
   c. *Trichomonas vaginalis*
   d. *Neisseria gonorrhoeae*

7. The nurse recommends a barrier method of contraception for a patient who is concerned about the side effects of hormonal contraception. What method might the nurse suggest?
   a. Abstinence
   b. Cervical cap
   c. Norplant system
   d. Sterilization

8. The nurse is discussing contraception with an adolescent patient who asks the nurse: "What if I can't have an orgasm?" What is the nurse's best response?
   a. "Women who have multiple orgasms are promiscuous."
   b. "A mature sexual relationship does not require a man and woman to achieve simultaneous orgasm."
   c. "The larger the penis, the greater the potential for achieving orgasm."
   d. "The ability to achieve orgasm is the only indicator of a person's sexual responsiveness."

9. Which example best supports the diagnosis of Sexual dysfunction, related to dyspareunia?
   a. A patient with a colostomy believes she cannot have a sexual relationship with her husband because he will be repulsed by her stoma.
   b. A 50-year-old woman with a history of stroke is afraid to have sex with her partner for fear it will elevate her blood pressure.
   c. A 50-year-old woman in the process of menopause has pain and burning during intercourse.
   d. A 39-year-old alcoholic woman is no longer interested in having sex with her partner.

## ALTERNATE-FORMAT QUESTIONS

### Multiple Response Questions

***Circle the letters that correspond to the best answers for each question.***

1. The nurse is discussing the use of hormonal contraception with a woman who just delivered twins and is not ready to get pregnant in the near future. Which methods might the nurse recommend? *(Select all that apply.)*
   a. Oral contraceptives
   b. Norplant system
   c. Depo-Provera
   d. Vaginal sponge
   e. Vaginal ring
   f. Intrauterine device

2. The nurse is counseling a young rape victim in the emergency department and recommends emergency contraception. Which statements describe this process? *(Select all that apply.)*
   a. A vaginal sponge will be prescribed to be worn daily for 7 days.
   b. The health care provider will prescribe increased doses of oral contraceptives.
   c. The health care provider will order a copper IUD within 5 to 7 days of the unprotected sex.
   d. An emergency DNC will be performed within 24 hours of unprotected sex.
   e. A vaginal ring will be inserted within 36 hours of unprotected sex.
   f. Plan B One-Step may be obtained without a prescription at a drugstore or family planning clinic.

3. The nurse is teaching a male adolescent how to use a condom. Which teaching points would the nurse include? *(Select all that apply.)*
   a. "Roll the condom onto the penis before it becomes erect."
   b. "If the condom does not have a nipple receptacle, leave a small space at the end for semen to collect."
   c. "Use a condom with every act of intercourse."
   d. "Immediately after ejaculation remove the condom and discard it."
   e. "Do not use a spermicide with the condom."
   f. "If using a lambskin condom, the condom may be reused a second time."
4. The nurse is advising an adolescent male about sexual myths that have him concerned. Which statements describe ***accurate*** patient teaching regarding these concerns? *(Select all that apply.)*
   a. A larger penis allows for a more satisfying sexual experience.
   b. Nocturnal emissions indicate the existence of a sexual disorder.
   c. Nocturnal emissions are signs of a sexually transmitted infection.
   d. Masturbation or self-stimulation is a natural and healthy outlet for sexual urges.
   e. No male or female should feel pressured into sexual activity at any age.
   f. Nocturnal emissions are normal in men of all ages.
5. Which patients would be more likely to meet the criteria for the NANDA diagnosis: Sexual dysfunction? *(Select all that apply.)*
   a. A 25-year-old male patient in traction
   b. A 52-year-old male with a history of hypertension
   c. A 19-year-old male who is still a virgin
   d. A postmenopausal female patient
   e. A 49-year-old male diagnosed with an enlarged prostate (BPH)
   f. A 30-year-old female experiencing PMS
6. A nurse is planning strategies to address factors that affect sexual dysfunction in older adults. Which interventions would be appropriate? *(Select all that apply.)*
   a. Teach the patient that sexual intercourse and similar forms of sexual expression are considered dangerous for older adults with cardiovascular disease.
   b. Actively seek a new partner for older adult patients who have lost a spouse and are not sexually active.
   c. Educate older adult patients, intimate partners, and family about the sexual side effects of specific medications.
   d. Assist in attitude and value clarification about substance use, sexuality, and sexual behavior.
   e. Encourage older adult patients to have a thorough physical evaluation by a health care provider.
   f. Provide an open, nonjudgmental response when older adult patients display a need for warmth, close contact, and companionship.
7. Which statements describe sexual dysfunction in males or females? *(Select all that apply.)*
   a. Premature ejaculation is a condition in which a man consistently reaches ejaculation or orgasm before or soon after entering the vagina.
   b. Delayed ejaculation refers to the man's inability to ejaculate into the vagina or delayed intravaginal ejaculation.
   c. Vaginismus is painful intercourse.
   d. Dyspareunia is a condition in which the vaginal opening closes tightly and prevents penile penetration.
   e. Vulvodynia is a chronic vulvar discomfort or pain characterized by burning, stinging, irritation, or rawness of the female genitalia that interferes with sexual activity.
   f. Inhibited sexual desire refers to the inability of a woman to reach orgasm.

### Prioritization Questions

1. Place the following series of reactions that control the menstrual cycle in the order in which they occur.
   a. The leftover empty follicle fills up with a yellow pigment and is then called the corpus luteum.
   b. A number of follicles mature, but only one produces a mature ovum.
   c. Ovulation occurs.
   d. If fertilization does not occur, the body sheds the lining of the uterus.
   e. Menstrual flow begins.

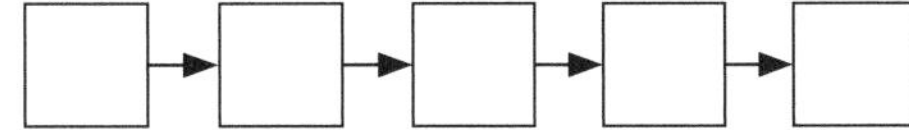

2. Place the following events in the order in which they occur in the sexual response cycle.
   a. The climax occurs.
   b. There is a heightened feeling of physical pleasure followed by overwhelming release and involuntary contraction of the genitals.
   c. The excitement phase is initiated by erotic stimulation and arousal.
   d. The women's breasts swell, and the nipples become erect. The penis becomes erect in the man.
   e. The intensity of the plateau phase builds and intensifies; the woman's clitoris retracts and disappears under the clitoral hood and secretions from Cowper's glands may appear at the glans of the penis.
   f. The body returns to normal functioning; the man experiences a refractory period.

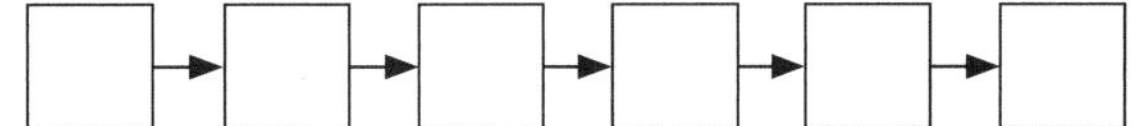

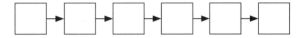

## NURSING PROCESS WORKSHEET

| Health Problem (Title) | Expected Outcome[a] |
| --- | --- |
| Related to ↓ | |
| Etiology (Related Factors) | Nursing Interventions[b] |
| As Evidenced by ↓ | |
| Signs and Symptoms (Defining Characteristics) | Evaluative Statement |

[a]More than one patient goal may be appropriate. For the purposes of this exercise, develop the one patient goal that demonstrates a direct resolution of the patient problem identified in the nursing diagnosis.
[b]Be sure you are able to list the scientific rationale for each nursing intervention you ordered.

CHAPTER 46

# Spirituality

## ASSESSING YOUR UNDERSTANDING

### FILL IN THE BLANKS

1. A patient recently diagnosed with prostate cancer tells the nurse that he believes God is far away and could care less about his condition. This patient may be suffering from spiritual __________.
2. __________ is the impaired ability to experience and integrate meaning and purpose in life through one's connectedness with self, others, art, music, literature, nature, or a power greater than one's self.
3. A nurse who asks a patient how his religious beliefs help or hinder him to feel at peace is assessing the patient for the spiritual need for __________.
4. A patient who tells a nurse that she no longer goes to church on Sunday may be experiencing what form of spiritual distress? __________
5. A mother who refuses to sign a consent form for a blood transfusion for her daughter due to religious reasons is most likely practicing what faith? __________

### MATCHING EXERCISES

***Match the type of spiritual distress listed in Part A with the appropriate example listed in Part B.***

**PART A**

**a.** Spiritual pain
**b.** Spiritual alienation
**c.** Spiritual anxiety
**d.** Spiritual guilt
**e.** Spiritual anger
**f.** Spiritual loss
**g.** Spiritual despair

**PART B**

____ **1.** A Roman Catholic college student stops going to Mass on Sundays and moves in with her boyfriend; she tells you, "I really want to do this, but it still feels wrong."

____ **2.** A woman cannot accept the death of her newborn and says, "How long will it hurt this bad?"

____ **3.** A man with a terminal illness cannot accept his eventual death and asks, "What kind of God are you?"

____ **4.** An older adult with a hip replacement is confined to home and cannot get to usual daily religious services.

____ **5.** A man dying of AIDS has no friends or support system and believes that God and humanity have abandoned him.

____ **6.** A young man challenges his faith and his own belief in God.

***Match the examples of a nurse's supportive presence listed in Part B with the appropriate measure listed in Part A. Answers may be used more than once.***

**PART A**

**a.** Facilitating the practice of religion
**b.** Promoting meaning and purpose
**c.** Promoting love and relatedness
**d.** Promoting forgiveness

**PART B**

____ **7.** A nurse attempts to meet a patient's religious dietary restrictions.

____ **8.** A nurse explores with a patient the importance of learning to accept himself, even with his faults.

____ **9.** A nurse treats her patient with respect, empathy, and genuine caring.

____ **10.** A nurse explores with a patient spiritual practices from which he might derive strength and hope.

____ **11.** A nurse respects a patient's need for privacy during prayer.

____ **12.** A nurse helps a patient explore his self-expectations and determine how realistic they are.

____ **13.** A nurse encourages a patient to explore her relationship with her family and identify the origin of negative beliefs about people.

**SHORT ANSWER**

**1.** List three spiritual needs underlying all religious traditions that are common to all people.

**a.** ____________________

**b.** ____________________

**c.** ____________________

**2.** List four methods nurses can use to assist patients in meeting their spiritual needs.

**a.** ____________________

**b.** ____________________

**c.** ____________________

**d.** ____________________

**3.** Explain how the following religious influences may affect a person.

**a.** Life-affirming influences: ____________________

**b.** Life-denying influences: ____________________

**4.** Give two examples of practices associated with health care that may have religious significance to a patient.

**a.** ____________________

**b.** ____________________

**5.** Briefly describe how religious faith may affect a patient in the following areas.

**a.** As a guide to daily living: ____________________

**b.** As a source of support: ____________________

**c.** As a source of strength and healing: ____________________

**d.** As a source of conflict: ____________________

**6.** Give an example of how the following factors may influence a person's spirituality.

**a.** Developmental considerations: ____________________

**b.** Family: ____________________

**c.** Ethnic background: ____________________

**d.** Formal religion: ____________________

**e.** Life events: ____________________

**7.** Describe how you would handle the following cases.

**a.** A family who insists on care deemed medically futile for a terminally ill patient because they believe that God is going to work a miracle.

____________________

**b.** Christian scientist parents of a child needing an appendectomy who refuse to sign a consent form for surgery.

____________________

**8.** List six characteristics the religions discussed in this chapter have in common.

**a.** ______________________

**b.** ______________________

**c.** ______________________

**d.** ______________________

**e.** ______________________

**f.** ______________________

**9.** Give an example of an interview question or statement you might use to assess a patient for the following types of spiritual distress.

**a.** Spiritual pain: ______________________

**b.** Spiritual alienation: ______________________

**c.** Spiritual anxiety: ______________________

**d.** Spiritual anger: ______________________

**e.** Spiritual loss: ______________________

**f.** Spiritual despair: ______________________

**10.** You are visiting a patient at home who was paralyzed in a car accident. She tells you she believes God has abandoned her and her family, which includes two small children. Suggest a nursing diagnosis for this patient and develop a nursing care plan that includes at least two interventions to help her with her spiritual needs.

Diagnosis: ______________________

Nursing care plan: ______________________

**11.** Develop a prayer expressing a patient's needs that could be used for a patient facing surgery.

______________________

**12.** List four guidelines for preparing a patient's room to receive a spiritual counselor.

**a.** ______________________

**b.** ______________________

**c.** ______________________

**d.** ______________________

**13.** List three interventions to assist a patient with the following deficits.

**a.** Deficit: Meaning and purpose: ______________________

**b.** Deficit: Love and relatedness: ______________________

**c.** Deficit: Forgiveness: ______________________

## APPLYING YOUR KNOWLEDGE

### CRITICAL THINKING QUESTIONS

**1.** How would you respond to parents who ask you to pray with them for their child's recovery from surgery? Would you feel comfortable praying with them? Do you believe nurses should pray aloud with patients and families? Write down a prayer for the sick that you can use in these situations.

**2.** Identify your own spiritual beliefs. How do these beliefs influence the way you carry on your daily routine in life? Do these beliefs affect the way you relate to others? In what ways might they affect the way you react to patients of different faiths?

### REFLECTIVE PRACTICE: CULTIVATING QSEN COMPETENCIES

***Use the following expanded scenario from Chapter 46 in your textbook to answer the questions below.***

***Scenario:*** Margot Zeuner, a 75-year-old woman, is taking care of her 80-year-old husband with advanced Alzheimer's disease who was just discharged from the hospital and requires constant supervision. When visited at home, she says, "I really miss going to church and seeing everyone. They're so supportive. That was the one thing that helped to keep me going." She further states that she no longer feels connected to her church or community.

**1.** How might the nurse use blended nursing skills to provide holistic, competent nursing care for Mrs. Zeuner?

______________________

2. What would be a successful outcome for this patient?

___

___

___

3. What intellectual, technical, interpersonal, and/or ethical/legal competencies are most likely to bring about the desired outcome?

___

___

___

4. What resources might be helpful for Mrs. Zeuner?

___

___

___

**PATIENT CARE STUDY**

***Read the following patient care study and use your nursing process skills to answer the questions below.***

***Scenario:*** Jeffrey Stein, a 31-year-old attorney, is in a step-down unit following his transfer from the cardiac care unit where he was treated for a massive heart attack. "Bad hearts run in my family, but I never thought it would happen to me," he says. "I jog several times a week and work out at the gym, eat a low-fat diet, and I don't smoke." Jeffrey is 5 ft 7 in tall, weighs about 150 lb, and is well built. During his second night in the step-down unit, he is unable to sleep and tells the nurse, "I've really got a lot on my mind tonight. I can't stop thinking about how close I was to death. If I wasn't with someone who knew how to do CPR when I keeled over, I probably wouldn't be here today." Gentle questioning reveals that Mr. Stein is worried about what would have happened had he died. "I don't think I've ever thought seriously about my mortality, and I sure don't think much about God. My parents were semiobservant Jews, but I don't go to synagogue myself. I celebrate the holidays, but that's about all. If there is a God, I wonder what He thinks about me." He asks if there is a rabbi or anyone he can talk with in the morning who could answer some questions for him and perhaps help him get himself back on track. "For the last couple of years, all I've been concerned about is paying off my school debts and making money. I guess there's a whole lot more to life, and maybe this was my invitation to sort out my priorities."

1. Identify pertinent patient data by placing a single underline beneath the objective data in the patient care study and a double underline beneath the subjective data.

2. Complete the Nursing Process Worksheet on page 325 to develop a three-part diagnostic statement and related plan of care for this patient.

3. Write down the patient and personal nursing strengths you hope to draw on as you assist this patient to better health.

   Patient strengths: ___

   ___

   ___

   Personal strengths: ___

   ___

   ___

4. Pretend that you are performing a nursing assessment of this patient after the care plan is implemented. Document your findings.

___

___

## PRACTICING FOR NCLEX

**MULTIPLE CHOICE QUESTIONS**

***Circle the letter that corresponds to the best answer for each question.***

1. The nurse is assessing a patient for spirituality using the HOPE acronym. Which statement describes an element of this tool?
   a. H = sources of help
   b. O = organized religion
   c. P = people important in the person's life
   d. E = external stressors affecting spirituality

**2.** A terminally ill patient tells the nurse that he does not belong to an organized religion. What patient knowledge would the nurse gain from this statement?
   **a.** The patient is an atheist.
   **b.** The patient has no belief system.
   **c.** The patient is an agnostic.
   **d.** The patient may still be deeply spiritual.

**3.** The nurse is differentiating beliefs of atheists from agnostics. Which statement is accurate?
   **a.** Both deny the existence of God.
   **b.** Nurses offer religious counseling to change the beliefs of both groups.
   **c.** Both are guided by a philosophy of living that does not include a religious faith.
   **d.** Both have religious influences that are life denying.

**4.** Based on religious practices, which patient would be most likely to defer to her husband when making health care decisions?
   **a.** An Islamic woman
   **b.** A Jewish woman
   **c.** A Roman Catholic woman
   **d.** A Protestant woman

**5.** In which religion are members encouraged to obtain health care provided by members of the Black community?
   **a.** Baha'i International Community
   **b.** American Muslim Mission
   **c.** Native American religion
   **d.** Islam

**6.** According to Shelly and Fish, which of the following is a spiritual need underlying all religious traditions?
   **a.** Need for formal ceremony
   **b.** Need for power in relationship with God
   **c.** Need for justice
   **d.** Need for meaning and purpose

**7.** When assessing a child's spiritual dimension, a nurse should be aware of which basic tenet?
   **a.** Children do not have a definite perception of God.
   **b.** Children attribute to God tremendous and expansive power.
   **c.** Children do not experience spiritual distress.
   **d.** Children view God as a person with divine powers.

**8.** Based on religious customs, for which patient would the nurse administering medicines avoid touching the patient's lips?
   **a.** A Hindu patient
   **b.** An Islamic patient
   **c.** A patient who is a member of the Baha'i International Community
   **d.** A Roman Catholic patient

## ALTERNATE-FORMAT QUESTIONS

### Multiple Response Questions

***Circle the letters that correspond to the best answers for each question.***

**1.** A nurse assessing children for spirituality keeps in mind which central themes in children's descriptions of God, based on David Heller's study? *(Select all that apply.)*
   **a.** Children have a notion of a God who works through human intimacy.
   **b.** Children believe in the interconnectedness of human lives.
   **c.** Children believe that God is a constant deity that limits self-change and transformation.
   **d.** Children believe that God's power is limited and has little effect on their lives.
   **e.** Children show considerable anxiety in the face of God's power.
   **f.** An image of darkness surrounds the spiritual world of the child.

**2.** A nurse determining the effects of religion on the lifestyle of patients considers that which religions prohibit the use of alcohol? *(Select all that apply.)*
   **a.** Christian Science
   **b.** Church of Jesus Christ of Latter-Day Saints
   **c.** Roman Catholicism
   **d.** American Muslim Mission
   **e.** Hinduism
   **f.** Judaism

3. A nurse is caring for a patient who practices Daoism. Which religious beliefs would the nurse keep in mind when planning care for this patient? *(Select all that apply.)*
   a. Allah, who is all-seeing, all-hearing, all-speaking, all-knowing, all-willing, and all-powerful, is their one God.
   b. They oppose the "false teachings" of other sects.
   c. They worship one God revealed to the world through Jesus Christ.
   d. They believe that health is a manifestation of the harmony of the universe, obtained through the proper balancing of internal and external forces.
   e. The universal principle is the mysterious biologic and spiritual life rhythm or order of nature.
   f. Inherent in Daoism is the appreciation of life and the desire to keep the body from untimely or unnecessary death.

4. Which nursing actions are appropriate when caring for a patient who participates in the Hindu religion? *(Select all that apply.)*
   a. Accommodate the practice of obligatory prayers and fasting on holy days.
   b. Consider the patient to be open to new ideas in health care practices.
   c. Accept that women are not allowed to make independent decisions.
   d. Anticipate many dietary restrictions, conforming to individual sect doctrine.
   e. Accommodate certain rites to be practiced following death.
   f. Learn rituals marking life changes, birth, puberty, initiation rites, and death.

5. Which religious groups would the nurse anticipate to regard Saturday as the Sabbath? *(Select all that apply.)*
   a. Roman Catholicism
   b. Buddhism
   c. Adventist
   d. Judaism
   e. Islam
   f. Hinduism

## NURSING PROCESS WORKSHEET

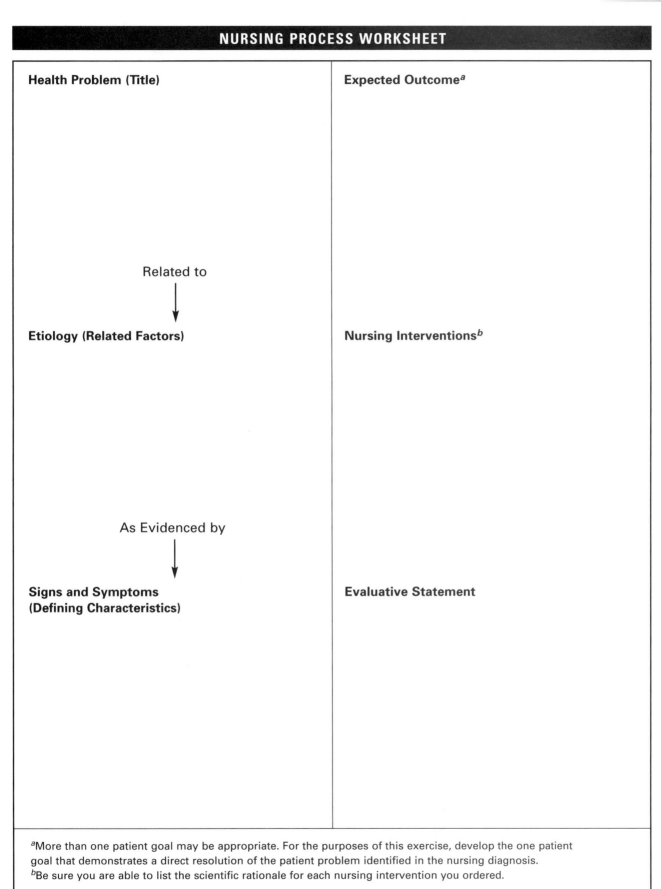

| **Health Problem (Title)** | **Expected Outcome**[a] |
|---|---|
| Related to ↓ | |
| **Etiology (Related Factors)** | **Nursing Interventions**[b] |
| As Evidenced by ↓ | |
| **Signs and Symptoms (Defining Characteristics)** | **Evaluative Statement** |

[a]More than one patient goal may be appropriate. For the purposes of this exercise, develop the one patient goal that demonstrates a direct resolution of the patient problem identified in the nursing diagnosis.
[b]Be sure you are able to list the scientific rationale for each nursing intervention you ordered.

# Answer Key

## CHAPTER 1

### ASSESSING YOUR UNDERSTANDING

#### FILL IN THE BLANKS

1. International Council of Nurses (ICN)
2. American Nurses Association (ANA)
3. Nursing: Scope and Standards of Practice
4. Nurse Practice Acts
5. Nursing Process

#### CORRECT THE FALSE STATEMENTS

1. False—patient-centered care
2. True
3. False—licensure
4. False—registered nurse
5. False—distinct and separate
6. True
7. False—the patient
8. True
9. False—the nurse facilitates coping with disability or death
10. False—person-centered process

#### SHORT ANSWER

1. Nursing is the demonstration of nonpossessive caring for and about others.
2. Nursing is sharing self with patients, other health team members, and other nurses.
3. Nursing is touching to provide comfort and give care.
4. Nursing is feeling with patients the human feelings of sorrow, joy, frustration, and satisfaction.
5. Nursing is listening attentively to the verbal and nonverbal communication signals of others.
6. Nursing is accepting self in order to accept others.
7. Nursing is respecting individual differences through unconditional acceptance, ensuring confidence and privacy, and individualizing care.
8. Sample answers:
   a. Promoting health: The nurse prepares the patient for tests, explaining each test thoroughly to the patient and focusing on any questions the patient may have. The nurse also identifies the patient's strengths (e.g., healthy diet, daily exercise routine) and weaknesses (e.g., inability to quit smoking).
   b. Preventing illness: The nurse refers the patient to a smoking cessation program and, if necessary, educates the patient about the nature and treatment of lung cancer.
   c. Restoring health: The nurse provides direct care for the patient, administers medications, and carries out procedures and treatments for the patient.
   d. Facilitating coping: The nurse facilitates patient and family coping by helping the patient to live with altered functioning or prepare for death.
9. a. Profession: A well-defined body of knowledge, strong service orientation, recognized authority as a professional group, code of ethics, professional organization that sets standards, ongoing research, and autonomy and self-regulation.
   b. Discipline: Nursing uses existing and new knowledge to solve problems creatively and meet human needs within ever-changing boundaries.
10. a. Changing demographics and increasing diversity: Greater life expectancy of people with chronic and acute conditions will challenge the health care system's ability to provide efficient and effective continuing care. Increases in diversity will affect the nature and prevalence of illness and disease requiring changes in practice that reflect and respect diverse values and beliefs.
    b. Technologic explosion: Dramatic improvements in the accessibility of clinical data across settings and time have improved both outcomes and care management. Nurses in the 21st century need to be skilled in the use of computer technology.
    c. Globalization of the world's economy and society: Nursing science needs to address health care issues, such as emerging and reemerging infections, that result from globalization. Nursing education and research must become more internationally focused to disseminate information and benefit from the multicultural experience.
    d. The era of the educated consumer, alternative therapies and genomics, and palliative care: Despite some information gaps, today's patient

is a well-informed consumer who expects to participate in decisions affecting personal and family health care. Nursing education and practice must expand to include the implications of the emerging therapies from both genetic research and alternative medicine while managing ethical conflicts and questions. A significant gap in the body of scientific knowledge and clinical education with regard to palliative and end-of-life care remains, and nursing education must prepare graduates for a significant role in these areas.

**e.** Shift to population-based care and the increasing complexity of patient care: Providing services for defined groups "covered" by managed care will demand skills and knowledge in clinical epidemiology, biostatistics, behavioral science, and their application to specific populations.

**f.** The cost of health care and the challenge of managed care: Nursing education programs must prepare students at all levels for roles in case management and employment in the managed care environment.

**g.** Impact of health policy and regulation: Nursing schools, scholars, executives, and professional nursing organizations must more actively contribute to the development of health policy and regulation.

**h.** The growing need for interdisciplinary education for collaborative practice: Teaching methods that incorporate opportunities for interdisciplinary education and collaborative practice are required to prepare nurses for their unique professional role and to understand the role of other disciplines in the care of patients.

**i.** The current nursing shortage and opportunities for lifelong learning and workforce development: Nursing shortages have a negative impact on patient care and are costly to the health care industry. Rapidly evolving technology, increasing clinical complexity in many patient care settings, advances in treatment, and the emergence of new diseases are all factors contributing to the increased need for a strong emphasis on critical thinking and lifelong learning among professional nurses.

**j.** Significant advances in nursing science and research: Nursing research is an integral part of the scientific enterprise of improving the nation's health. The growing body of nursing research provides a scientific basis for patient care and should be regularly used by the nation's nurses.

**11.** Sample answers:

**a.** Cognitive skills: A nurse selects nursing interventions to promote wound healing.

**b.** Technical skills: A nurse correctly administers medication to a patient via an IV infusion.

**c.** Interpersonal skills: A nurse displays a caring attitude when interacting with a patient.

**d.** Ethical/legal skills: A nurse explains an advance directives form to a patient.

**12.** See table below.

| Title | Education/ Preparation | Role Description |
|---|---|---|
| *Example* Nurse Researcher | Advanced degree | Conducts research relevant to nursing practice and education |
| Clinical Nurse Specialist | Advanced degree | Expert in a specialized area of nursing; carries out direct patient care; consultation; teaching of patients, families, and staff; and research |
| Nurse Midwife | Certificate or advanced degree | Provides pre/postnatal care; delivers babies in uncomplicated pregnancies |
| Nurse Practitioner | Advanced degree, certification | Works in a variety of settings, providing health assessment and primary care |
| Nurse Anesthetist | Advanced degree | Administers and monitors anesthesia |
| Nurse Administrator | Advanced degree | Functions at various levels of management in health care settings |
| Nurse Entrepreneur | Advanced degree | Manages a clinic or health-related business, conducts research, provides education, or serves as an advisor or consultant to institutions, political agencies, or businesses |
| Nurse Educator | Advanced degree (usually) | Teaches in educational or clinical settings; teaches theoretical knowledge and clinical skills; conducts research |

## APPLYING YOUR KNOWLEDGE

### REFLECTIVE PRACTICE: CULTIVATING QSEN COMPETENCIES

#### Sample Answers

1. What basic human needs should be addressed by the nurse to provide individualized, holistic care for the Pecorini family?
   When providing holistic nursing care for the Pecorini family, the nurse should address the physiologic needs related to Mr. Pecorini's health condition and his wife's inability to care for him; safety and security needs for a safe environment for a patient with weakness from radiation and chemotherapy and the development of pressure injuries; and self-actualization needs for acceptance of himself and his current situation.
2. What would be a successful outcome for this patient?
   Mr. Pecorini experiences relief from symptoms of chemotherapy and radiation and responds to wound care for his pressure injuries. Mrs. Pecorini lists community resources available to help with child care and resources to help provide nursing and/or hospice care for her husband upon discharge.
3. What intellectual, technical, interpersonal, and/or ethical/legal competencies are most likely to bring about the desired outcome?
   Intellectual: knowledge of nursing actions to alleviate symptoms of chemotherapy and radiation, and properly care for a colostomy
   Technical: ability to properly administer medications via a central venous catheter, provide wound care for pressure injuries, and care for a colostomy
   Interpersonal: ability to establish a trusting relationship with Mr. Pecorini and his wife that demonstrates respect for their human dignity throughout the patient care plan
   Ethical/Legal: empathy for the patient with commitment to getting him the help he needs to achieve health goals
4. What resources might be helpful for the Mr. Pecorini family?
   Print or audiovisual teaching aids, social services, support groups

## PRACTICING FOR NCLEX

### MULTIPLE CHOICE QUESTIONS

| | | | | |
|---|---|---|---|---|
| **1.** b | **2.** d | **3.** c | **4.** b | **5.** a |
| **6.** b | **7.** c | **8.** b | **9.** d | |

### ALTERNATE-FORMAT QUESTIONS

#### Multiple Response Questions

1. a, c, e
2. c, d, f
3. a, c, d, f
4. a, c, d
5. a, c, e, f
6. a, c, d

#### Prioritization Questions

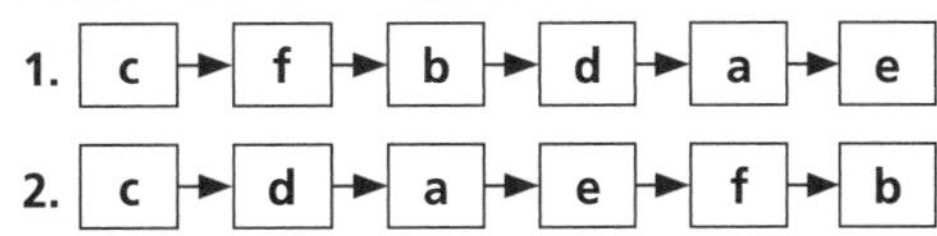
1. c → f → b → d → a → e
2. c → d → a → e → f → b

# CHAPTER 2

## ASSESSING YOUR UNDERSTANDING

### FILL IN THE BLANKS

1. Quantitative
2. Concepts
3. Adaptation
4. Informed consent
5. Evidence-based practice

### MATCHING EXERCISES

| | | | | |
|---|---|---|---|---|
| **1.** f | **2.** c | **3.** i | **4.** h | **5.** d |
| **6.** e | **7.** b | **8.** a | **9.** g | |

### SHORT ANSWER

1. **a.** General systems theory: This theory explains breaking whole things into parts and then learning how these parts work together in systems. It includes the relationship between the whole and the parts and defines concepts about how the parts will function and behave.
   **b.** Adaptation theory: This theory defines adaptation as the adjustment of living matter to other living things and to environmental conditions. Adaptation is a dynamic or continuously changing process that effects change and involves interaction and response. Human adaptation occurs on three levels—internal, social, and physical.
   **c.** Developmental theory: Outlines the process of growth and development of humans as orderly and predictable, beginning with conception and ending with death. The growth and development of a person are influenced by heredity, temperament, emotional and physical environment, life experiences, and health status.
2. **a.** Nursing theories identify and define interrelated concepts specific to nursing and clearly state the relation between these concepts.
   **b.** Nursing theories must be logical and use orderly reasoning and identify relations that are developed using a logical sequence.
   **c.** Nursing theories must be consistent with the basic assumptions used in their development. They should be simple and general.
   **d.** Nursing theories should increase the nursing profession's body of knowledge by generating research and should guide and improve practice.
3. **a.** Cultural influences on nursing: Until the past two decades, nursing essentially had been considered "women's work," and women were considered inferior to men. After Nightingale established an acceptable occupation for

educated women and facilitated improved attitudes toward nursing, the role of the woman as nurse became more favorably accepted.

**b.** Educational influences on nursing: The service orientation of nursing was the strongest influence on nursing practice until the 1950s. After World War II, women increasingly entered the workforce, became more independent, and sought higher education. Nursing education began to focus more on education instead of just training. In the 1960s, college- and university-based baccalaureate programs in nursing increased in number and enrollment, and master's and doctoral programs in nursing were established.

**c.** Research and publishing in nursing: Beginning in the 1950s, great advances were made in technology and medical research; nursing leaders realized that research about the practice of nursing was necessary to meet the health needs of modern society.

**d.** Improved communication in nursing: Nursing is based on communication with others—patients, other health care team members, community members, as well as with nurses practicing in a variety of specialty settings. Nurses need a knowledge base and common terminology to use in communicating with other professionals.

**e.** Improved autonomy of nursing: Nursing is in the process of defining its own independent functions and contributions to health care. The development and use of nursing theory provide autonomy in the practice of nursing.

**4. a.** Build the scientific foundation for clinical practice
**b.** Prevent disease and disability
**c.** Manage and eliminate symptoms caused by illness
**d.** Enhance end-of-life and palliative care

**5.** Answers will vary with student experiences.

## APPLYING YOUR KNOWLEDGE

### REFLECTIVE PRACTICE: CULTIVATING QSEN COMPETENCIES

### Sample Answers

1. How might the nurse respond to Ms. Horn's concerns regarding the care of her mother?
   The nurse should provide Ms. Horn with information and practical tips for inserting a nasogastric tube and checking its patency. After demonstrating the procedure, the nurse could ask for a return demonstration from Ms. Horn. The nurse should also reassure Ms. Horn that assistance will be available if any problems occur and provide her with the appropriate resources for help and information.
2. What would be a successful outcome for this patient?
   Ms. Horn accurately demonstrates the procedure for nasogastric tube feedings and states confidence in her ability to take care of her mother.
3. What intellectual, technical, interpersonal, and/or ethical/legal competencies are most likely to bring about the desired outcome?
   Intellectual: knowledge of nasogastric tube feedings and associated care
   Technical: ability to provide technical nursing assistance based on sound scientific rationales to meet the learning needs of Ms. Horn
   Interpersonal: ability to demonstrate empathy and respect for Ms. Horn and her situation
   Ethical/Legal: ability to provide patient education consistent with the nursing code of ethics and within the scope of legal practice
4. What resources might be helpful for Ms. Horn?
   Reference materials for teaching the procedure for nasogastric tube feedings, home health care services if applicable.

## PRACTICING FOR NCLEX

### MULTIPLE CHOICE QUESTIONS

**1.** a **2.** a **3.** c **4.** b **5.** a
**6.** d **7.** c **8.** b

### ALTERNATE-FORMAT QUESTIONS

### Multiple Response Questions

1. b, c, d
2. a, c
3. a, b, e
4. b, c, d, f

### Prioritization Question

**1.** 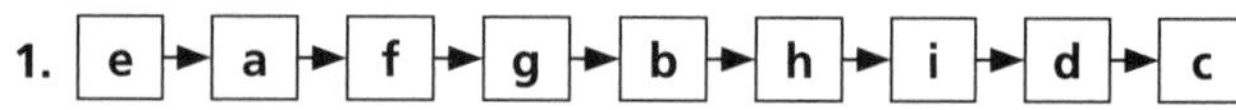


# CHAPTER 3

## ASSESSING YOUR UNDERSTANDING

### FILL IN THE BLANKS

1. Disease
2. chronic
3. acute
4. exacerbation
5. environmental

### MATCHING EXERCISES

**1.** f **2.** a **3.** e **4.** b **5.** c
**6.** d **7.** b **8.** d **9.** a **10.** c
**11.** b **12.** a **13.** c **14.** d **15.** a
**16.** b **17.** e

### SHORT ANSWER

**1.** Answers will vary with student experiences.

**2. a.** Acute illness: A temporary condition of illness in which patient goes through four stages: (1) symptoms, (2) assuming sick role, (3) dependent role; accepting diagnosis and following the treatment plan, and (4) recovery and rehabilitation; person gives up dependent role and resumes normal activities and responsibilities.

   b. Chronic illness: A permanent change caused by irreversible alterations in normal anatomy and physiology; requires patient education for rehabilitation; requires long period of care or support. Characteristics: slow onset, periods of remission.
3. Answers will vary with student experiences.
4. Sample answers:
   a. Primary health promotion: Giving immunizations, providing dental care teaching
   b. Secondary health promotion: Providing physical therapy, giving medications
   c. Tertiary health promotion: Facilitating a support system, doing diabetic teaching
5. a. Being: recognizing self as separate and individual
   b. Belonging: being part of a whole
   c. Becoming: growing and developing
   d. Befitting: making personal choices to benefit oneself for the future

## APPLYING YOUR KNOWLEDGE

### REFLECTIVE PRACTICE: CULTIVATING QSEN COMPETENCIES

#### Sample Answers

1. How might the nurse respond to Ms. Jacobi's stated desire for a higher level of wellness?
   This is the perfect opportunity for patient teaching provided throughout Ms. Jacobi's hospital stay and incorporated into the discharge plan. The nurse should present information regarding a "heart healthy diet," the need for exercise, and reinforcement for smoking cessation.
2. What would be a successful outcome for this patient?
   Ms. Jacobi describes her condition and identifies three factors in her lifestyle (smoking, diet, exercise) that can be modified for stroke prevention.
3. What intellectual, technical, interpersonal, and/or ethical/legal competencies are most likely to bring about the desired outcome?
   Intellectual: ability to integrate knowledge of preventive measures into the patient care plan
   Interpersonal: ability to assess health-related beliefs, goals, and practices
   Ethical/Legal: ability to participate as a trusted and effective patient advocate, including a commitment to securing the best possible care for Ms. Jacobi
4. What resources might be helpful for Ms. Jacobi?
   Smoking cessation materials, menu plans, support groups

## PRACTICING FOR NCLEX

### MULTIPLE CHOICE QUESTIONS

| | | | | |
|---|---|---|---|---|
| 1. a | 2. c | 3. c | 4. d | 5. a |
| 6. b | | | | |

### ALTERNATE-FORMAT QUESTIONS

#### Multiple Response Questions

1. b, c, e
2. a, d, e
3. a, c, f
4. d, e, f

#### Chart/Exhibit Questions

1. Physical dimension
2. Emotional dimension
3. Intellectual and spiritual dimension
4. Environmental dimension
5. Sociocultural dimension
6. Intellectual and spiritual dimension
7. Intellectual and spiritual dimension
8. Physical dimension

# CHAPTER 4

## ASSESSING YOUR UNDERSTANDING

### FILL IN THE BLANKS

1. oxygen
2. physiologic
3. extended
4. affective and coping
5. community

### MATCHING EXERCISES

| | | | | |
|---|---|---|---|---|
| 1. e | 2. a | 3. b | 4. b | 5. d |
| 6. b | 7. c | 8. a | 9. d | 10. c |
| 11. e | 12. b | 13. c | 14. e | |

### SHORT ANSWER

1. Sample answers:
   a. Physical: A family lives in a comfortable home located in a safe neighborhood. This meets the family needs of safety and comfort and enhances growth and development of the children.
   b. Economic: A family is able to afford adequate housing, food, clothing, and community demands. This meets the family's need for nourishment, shelter, and acceptance in society.
   c. Reproductive: A family seeks family planning to limit their offspring to three children. This meets society's need for more members without putting too heavy a demand on the family to care for their children.
   d. Affective and coping: Parents counsel their children to avoid drinking alcohol, smoking cigarettes, and using drugs. This meets the children's needs to be productive members of society and to avoid the pitfalls surrounding adolescence.
   e. Socialization: Parents seek expert counseling for a kindergarten child who is having difficulty adjusting to school and relating to other children. This meets the child's need to fit in with other schoolmates and helps correct a problem before it gets out of hand.
2. Sample answers:
   a. Physiologic needs: The nurse helps to prepare the mother for her cesarean birth and administers any medications prescribed.

b. Safety and security needs: The nurse monitors the blood pressure of the mother and baby during the procedure.
c. Love and belonging needs: The nurse helps the husband to cope with his fears and gets him ready to participate in the birth of his child.
d. Self-esteem needs: The nurse reassures the mother that having a cesarean birth is a common procedure and that she should not feel guilty for not being able to have the baby vaginally.
e. Self-actualization needs: The nurse helps the mother after surgery to continue with her original plan to breastfeed her infant.

3. Answers will vary with student experiences.
4. What is the family structure? What is the family's socioeconomic status? What are the ethnic background and religious affiliation of family members? Who cares for children if both parents work? What health practices are common (e.g., types of foods eaten, meal times, immunizations, bedtime, exercise)? What habits are common (e.g., do any family members smoke, drink to excess, or use drugs)? How does the family cope with stress? Do close friends or family members live nearby, and can they help if necessary?
5. Signed in March 2010, the Patient Protection and Affordable Care Act (PPACA) aims to provide improved health security and access to health care for all Americans. In addition to the major provisions that provide a right to coverage for Americans with pre-existing conditions, allow young adults up to 26 years of age to continue to be covered under their parents' plan, and end lifetime limits on coverage, this law expands Medicaid coverage to millions of low-income Americans and makes numerous improvements to the Children's Health Insurance Program (CHIP) (Affordable Care Act, 2012).

## APPLYING YOUR KNOWLEDGE

### REFLECTIVE PRACTICE: CULTIVATING QSEN COMPETENCIES

#### Sample Answers

1. What basic human needs should be addressed by the nurse to provide individualized, holistic care for Mr. Kaplan?
When providing holistic nursing care, the nurse should consider all the dimensions that affect how the patient's basic human needs are met in health and in illness. For Mr. Kaplan, these needs include physiologic needs related to his and his wife's health condition; safety and security needs for a safe environment for a patient with Alzheimer's disease; love and belonging needs related to his desire to remain with and care for his wife; self-esteem needs based on his pride in taking care of himself and his wife; and self-actualization needs or acceptance of himself and his current situation.
2. What would a successful outcome be for this patient?
Mr. Kaplan verbalizes the reasons he is unable to care for his wife in his home and acknowledges a plan to provide a safe environment for himself and his wife.
3. What intellectual, technical, interpersonal, and/or ethical/legal competencies are most likely to bring about the desired outcome?
Intellectual: knowledge of Alzheimer's disease and its effect on the family
Interpersonal: using strong interpersonal skills to establish a trusting relationship with Mr. Kaplan that demonstrates respect for his human dignity and autonomy
Ethical/Legal: skill in working collaboratively with colleagues and community members to advocate for the health care needs of Mr. Kaplan and his wife
4. What resources might be helpful for Mr. Kaplan?
Teaching aids for patients with Alzheimer's disease, counseling services, community services, skilled nursing care

## PRACTICING FOR NCLEX

### MULTIPLE CHOICE QUESTIONS

1. d 2. a 3. d 4. c

### ALTERNATE-FORMAT QUESTIONS

#### Multiple Response Questions

1. d, f
2. a, c, f
3. b, d, e
4. b, c

#### Prioritization Question

1. 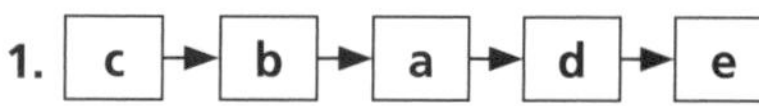


# CHAPTER 5

## ASSESSING YOUR UNDERSTANDING

### FILL IN THE BLANKS

1. subculture
2. ethnicity
3. ethnocentrism
4. Cultural blindness
5. shock
6. stereotyping

### MATCHING EXERCISES

1. b 2. c 3. e 4. f 5. a
6. e 7. b 8. f 9. f 10. c

### SHORT ANSWER

1. Sample answers:
a. Investigate bus routes from patient's home; check if medical services are available within walking distance; see if insurance will cover transportation to and from medical services.
b. Boil water before using it; check with social services to see if they can provide any necessary services for patient.

c. Research the community for free or low cost medical clinics and services and make appropriate referrals.
2. Answers will vary with student experiences.
3. Sample answers:
   a. The number of female-headed households is increasing as a result of divorce, abandonment, unmarried motherhood, and changes in abortion laws. Many households depend on two incomes for economic survival, and a single woman supporting a household is at a financial disadvantage.
   b. Most older adults live on fixed incomes, which often do not keep up with inflation. Many, particularly widows, are on the borderline of poverty or have already slipped into poverty.
   c. In some cases, poverty is passed from generation to generation. This is true in groups such as migrant farm workers, families living on welfare, and people who live in isolated areas such as Appalachia.
4. a. Feelings of despair, resignation, and fatalism
   b. "Day-to-day" attitude toward life, with no hope for the future
   c. Unemployment and need for financial or government aid
   d. Unstable family structure, possibly characterized by abusiveness and abandonment
   e. Decline in self-respect and retreat from community involvement

## APPLYING YOUR KNOWLEDGE

### REFLECTIVE PRACTICE: CULTIVATING QSEN COMPETENCIES

#### Sample Answers

1. How might the nurse respond to Ms. Dorvall's request for a Haitian folk healer?
   In order to provide culturally competent care, the nurse honors Ms. Dorvall's request and arranges a meeting with the folk healer. Prior to the meeting, the nurse researches the Haitian culture in order to properly prepare the room and patient for the visit. The nurse reassesses the patient following the visit and documents the findings in the patient record.
2. What would be a successful outcome for this patient?
   Ms. Dorvall verbalizes that the folk healer relieved her anxiety regarding the healing of her leg and states her desire to continue with the nursing care plan.
3. What intellectual, technical, interpersonal, and/or ethical/legal competencies are most likely to bring about the desired outcome?
   Intellectual: knowledge of Haitian cultural health care practices gained from research
   Interpersonal: formation of a caring relationship with the patient that encompasses the patient's beliefs and values
   Ethical/Legal: careful documentation of patient goals and outcomes
4. What resources might be helpful for Ms. Dorvall's case?
   Research materials on the Haitian culture, community services

## PRACTICING FOR NCLEX

### MULTIPLE CHOICE QUESTIONS

1. d 2. a 3. b 4. d

### ALTERNATE-FORMAT QUESTIONS

#### Multiple Response Questions

1. a, d, e
2. a, d, f

# CHAPTER 6

## ASSESSING YOUR UNDERSTANDING

### FILL IN THE BLANKS

1. Laissez-faire
2. responsible choice
3. values clarification
4. prizing
5. value system
6. advocacy

### MATCHING EXERCISES

| | | | | |
|---|---|---|---|---|
| 1. g | 2. d | 3. a | 4. f | 5. i |
| 6. b | 7. e | 8. c | 9. d | 10. e |
| 11. a | 12. c | 13. b | 14. e | 15. d |
| 16. a | 17. c | | | |

### SHORT ANSWER

1. Sample answers:
   a. Values clarification: Have the mother state the three most important things in her life. Explore her answers with her and find out why she chose them and how her choices may affect her situation.
   b. Choosing: After exploring the mother's values, have her choose her key values freely. She may choose her child or profession.
   c. Prizing: Reinforce the mother's choices and, if possible, involve the husband and child in decision making.
   d. Acting: Assist the mother to plan new behaviors consistent with the values she has chosen and incorporate them into her life. For example, if she values her child, she may reduce the number of classes she takes at night and spend more time with her.
2. Sample answers:
   a. Cost-effectiveness and allocation
   b. Issues of cultural and/or religious variation
   c. Consideration of power
   d. The relationship between health care providers and patients

3. a. Autonomy: Respect the decision-making capacity of autonomous persons (e.g., patients have the right to refuse treatment they do not feel would be helpful to their condition).
   b. Nonmaleficence: Avoid causing harm (e.g., be sure you are fully knowledgeable about a procedure before performing it).
   c. Beneficence: Provide benefits and balance these benefits against risks and harms (e.g., securing a patient with restraints who is at high risk for falls).
   d. Justice: Distribute benefits, risks, and costs fairly (e.g., give service to all patients regardless of their life circumstances).
   e. Fidelity: Be faithful to promises you made to the public to be competent, and be willing to use your competence to benefit patients entrusted to your care (e.g., not abandoning a patient entrusted to your care without first seeing to his or her needs).
4. Answers will vary with student experiences.
5. Answers will vary with student experiences.
6. Sample answers:
   a. Gather as much data as possible to support your diagnosis.
   b. Identify the ethical problem and explore solutions to the problem.
   c. Plan a course of action you can justify (e.g., seeking assistance for the patient at a higher level).
   d. Implement your decision by speaking to your superiors and presenting your case in a competent manner.
   e. Evaluate your decision: What was the outcome? How does this make me feel? Did I make the right decision?
7. Sample answers:
   a. Breach of confidentiality, incompetent practice
   b. Covering for another nurse who is not performing her job competently, short-staffing
   c. Health care provider incompetence, conflicts concerning the role of the nurse in certain situations
   d. Cost-containment versus hospitalization, health care rationing

## APPLYING YOUR KNOWLEDGE

### REFLECTIVE PRACTICE: CULTIVATING QSEN COMPETENCIES

#### Sample Answers

1. How might the nurse react to Mr. Raines's response to filling his prescriptions?
   The nurse should protect and support Mr. Raines's rights by being a strong patient advocate. This could be accomplished by investigating available social services and community services for Mr. Raines. The nurse could also check with the drug manufacturer to see if the company has a discount for needy patients.
2. What would be a successful outcome for this patient?
   Mr. Raines vocalizes the health benefits of taking his blood pressure medication and lists three reasons for seeking social services and other available assistance.
3. What intellectual, technical, interpersonal, and/or ethical/legal competencies are most likely to bring about the desired outcome?
   Intellectual: ability to integrate ethical principles and use an ethical framework and decision-making process to resolve ethical problems
   Technical: ability to integrate moral facility to provide the technical nursing assistance necessary to meet the needs of Mr. Raines
   Interpersonal: ability to advocate for patients whose values may be different from personal ones
   Ethical/Legal: ability to identify and develop the essential elements of moral facility, cultivate the virtues of nursing, and understand ethical theories that dictate and justify professional conduct
4. What resources might be helpful for Mr. Raines?
   Social services, counseling services, government assistance, community services, drug-assistance programs

## PRACTICING FOR NCLEX

### MULTIPLE CHOICE QUESTIONS

| | | |
|---|---|---|
| 1. b | 2. a | 3. b |
| 4. c | 5. a | 6. b |

### ALTERNATE-FORMAT QUESTIONS

#### Multiple Response Questions

1. c, f
2. d, e
3. a, b, e
4. c, e, f
5. b, d, e
6. a, b

# CHAPTER 7

## ASSESSING YOUR UNDERSTANDING

### FILL IN THE BLANKS

1. public
2. Nurse Practice Act
3. Licensure
4. expert witness
5. collective bargaining
6. incident
7. sentinel event

### MATCHING EXERCISES

| | | | | |
|---|---|---|---|---|
| 1. g | 2. e | 3. a | 4. c | 5. h |
| 6. f | 7. b | 8. i | 9. i | 10. h |
| 11. a | 12. l | 13. c | 14. d | 15. k |
| 16. b | 17. f | 18. g | 19. j | 20. c |
| 21. g | 22. a | 23. b | 24. d | 25. e |

## SHORT ANSWER

1. Sample answers:
   a. Failure to ensure patient safety: Update knowledge on patient safety and new interventions to prevent and reduce injury.
   b. Improper treatment or performance of treatment: Use proper techniques when performing procedures and follow facility procedures.
   c. Failure to monitor and report: Follow health care provider orders regarding monitoring of patient unless changes in the patient's condition necessitate a change in the frequency of monitoring; report need for change to health care provider.
   d. Medication errors and reactions: Listen to patient's objections regarding medication and investigate patient concerns before administering the medication.
   e. Failure to follow facility procedure: Advise the appropriate person of procedures that need to be revised.
   f. Equipment misuse: Learn how to operate equipment in a safe and appropriate manner. Never operate equipment with which you are unfamiliar.
   g. Adverse incidents: Do not assume, voice, or record any blame for an incident.
   h. Improper use of infection control techniques: Know and follow facility policies and procedures for the care of patients with infectious disease.
2. a. Voluntary standards: Developed and implemented by the nursing profession itself; not mandatory; used for peer review. Example: professional nursing organizations.
   b. Legal standards: Developed by legislative action; implemented by authority granted by the state (or province) to determine minimum standards for the education of nurses, set requirements for licensure or registration, and decide when to revoke or suspend nurse's licenses. Example: licensure.
3. a. For each specialized diagnostic procedure
   b. For experimentation involving patients
   c. On admission for routine treatment
   d. For medical or surgical treatment
4. Sample answers:
   a. Talking with patients in rooms that are not soundproof
   b. Pressing the patient for information not necessary for care planning
   c. Using tape recorders, dictating machines, computer banks, etc. without taking precautions to ensure patient confidentiality
5. a. Solid educational background
   b. Understanding of the legal aspects of nursing and malpractice liability
   c. Knowledge of the state (or provincial) Nurse Practice Act and standard of nursing care where the incident occurred
6. A contract must contain real consent of the parties, a valid consideration, a lawful purpose, competent parties, and the format required by law.
7. Sample answer:
   Limit telephone orders to true emergency situations; repeat a telephone order back to the health care provider; document the order, its time and date, situation necessitating order, health care provider prescribing, reconfirming the order as it is read back, and signing name; and VO or TO. If possible, two nurses should listen to a questionable telephone order, with both nurses countersigning the order.
8. a. Contraindicated by normal practice
   b. Contraindicated by patient's present condition
9. Sample answers:
   a. The nurse is liable for her actions and should file an incident report.
   b. The incident report should contain the name of the patient; all witnesses; a complete factual account of the incident; the date, time, and place of the incident; pertinent characteristics of the person involved (e.g., alert, ambulatory, asleep) and of any equipment or resources being used; and other relevant variables believed important to the incident.
   c. Answers will vary with student experiences.

## APPLYING YOUR KNOWLEDGE

### REFLECTIVE PRACTICE: CULTIVATING QSEN COMPETENCIES

#### Sample Answers

1. How might the nurses involved in this scenario respond to Ms. Bedford's disclosure that she will be pressing charges against the hospital?
   The nurse speaking to Ms. Bedford should not volunteer any information regarding the case and should refer her to the legal department of the hospital. It would also be appropriate for the nurse to seek advice from legal counsel. The nurses providing the care may be named as defendants and will need to work closely with an attorney while preparing the defense. Either the defense or the prosecuting attorney may call the first nurse to testify as a fact witness if he or she has knowledge of the actual incident prompting the legal case. This nurse must base testimony on only firsthand knowledge of the incident and not on assumptions. When in doubt about facts, the nurses should simply testify, "I do not remember that."
2. What intellectual, technical, interpersonal, and/or ethical/legal competencies are most likely to be used in this situation?
   Intellectual: knowledge of law and sources of law and ability to identify potential areas of liability in nursing
   Technical: ability to provide technical nursing assistance in a competent, legally appropriate manner
   Interpersonal: ability to work collaboratively with other members of the health care team and legal department
   Ethical/Legal: ability to identify errors in personal action

3. What resources might be helpful for the nurses in this case?
   Hospital legal department, liability insurance, risk management programs, malpractice arbitration panel

## PRACTICING FOR NCLEX

### MULTIPLE CHOICE QUESTIONS

| | | | |
|---|---|---|---|
| **1.** b | **2.** b | **3.** a | **4.** c |
| **5.** d | **6.** d | **7.** a | **8.** d |

### ALTERNATE-FORMAT QUESTIONS

#### Multiple Response Questions

1. a, b, d
2. b, e, f
3. c, d, e
4. a, c, e
5. c, d, e, f
6. a, c, d
7. a, c, e

#### Prioritization Question

1. 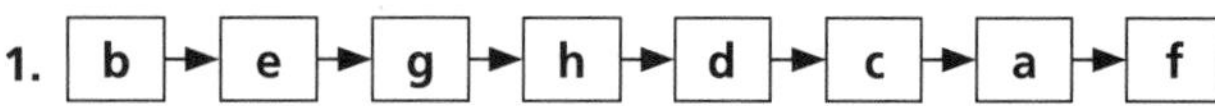


# CHAPTER 8

## ASSESSING YOUR UNDERSTANDING

### FILL IN THE BLANKS

1. stimulus
2. channel
3. feedback
4. nonverbal
5. helping
6. orientation
7. validating
8. horizontal violence

### MATCHING EXERCISES

| | | | | |
|---|---|---|---|---|
| **1.** b | **2.** d | **3.** g | **4.** a | **5.** c |
| **6.** e | **7.** b | **8.** c | **9.** a | **10.** a |
| **11.** c | **12.** b | **13.** c | **14.** a | **15.** b |
| **16.** b | **17.** c | **18.** a | **19.** e | **20.** d |
| **21.** c | | | | |

### SHORT ANSWER

1. Sample answers:
   - **a.** Touch: The nurse gently squeezes a patient's hand before surgery. The patient's response to this touch may express fear, gratitude, acceptance, etc.
   - **b.** Eye contact: A patient avoids eye contact. The patient may be expressing defenselessness or avoidance of communication.
   - **c.** Facial expressions: A patient grimaces when looking at his surgical incision. The patient may be experiencing anxiety over the alteration in his or her physical appearance.
   - **d.** Posture: A patient stands erect with good body alignment. The patient may be experiencing good health.
   - **e.** Gait: A patient walks slightly bent over. The patient may be accommodating an illness.
   - **f.** Gestures: A patient gives you a thumbs-up sign after receiving test results. The patient is most likely happy with the results.
   - **g.** General physical appearance: A patient is sweating and having difficulty breathing. The patient may be experiencing a life-threatening condition.
   - **h.** Mode of dress and grooming: A patient who has been bedridden for a week asks to take a shower and get dressed. The patient is probably feeling better.
   - **i.** Sounds: A patient sighs whenever you mention his or her significant other. The patient may be experiencing difficulty with this relationship.
   - **j.** Silence: A patient who has undergone a mastectomy remains silent when asked how she is feeling. The patient may be overwhelmed with emotion and unable to express her feelings.
2. Sample answers:
   - **a.** An 8-year-old boy: An 8-year-old boy has limited understanding of surgical procedures. Therefore, the nurse must explain the procedure in simple terms so that the child will cooperate without being frightened.
   - **b.** A 16-year-old girl: Adolescents are developing their ability to think abstractly and can understand fairly detailed descriptions of clinical procedures.
   - **c.** A 65-year-old man with a hearing impairment: The nurse should talk directly to the patient while facing him. When necessary, nonverbal communication should be used (e.g., sign language or finger spelling, or by writing any ideas that cannot be conveyed in another manner).
3. Occupation may reveal a person's abilities, talents, interests, and economic status.
4. **a.** Assessing: Verbal and nonverbal communication are essential nursing tools because the major focus of patient assessment is information gathering. Written words, patient records, spoken words, and observational skills are employed.
   - **b.** Diagnosing: Once a nurse formulates a diagnosis, it must be communicated through the spoken and written word to other nurses as well as to the patient.
   - **c.** Planning: The patient, nurse, and other health care team members must communicate with each other as patient goals and outcomes are developed and interventions selected.
   - **d.** Implementing: Verbal and nonverbal communication allows nurses to enhance basic caregiving measures and to teach, counsel, and support patients and their families.

   e. Evaluating: Nurses often rely on the verbal and nonverbal clues they receive from their patients to determine whether patient objectives or goals have been achieved.
   f. Documenting: The documentation of data promotes the continuity of care given by nurses and other health care providers.
5. a. Having specific objectives: Having a purpose for an interaction guides the nurse toward achieving a meaningful encounter with the patient.
   b. Providing a comfortable environment: A comfortable environment in which the patient and nurse are at ease helps to promote meaningful interactions. Relationships are enhanced when the atmosphere is relaxed and unhurried.
   c. Providing privacy: Every effort should be made to provide privacy during nurse–patient conversations.
   d. Maintaining confidentiality: The patient should know his or her right to specify who may have access to clinical or personal information.
   e. Maintaining patient focus: Communication in the nurse–patient relationship should focus on the patient and the patient's needs, not on the nurse or an activity in which the nurse is engaged.
   f. Using nursing observations: Observation is especially valuable in validating information and helping the nurse become aware of the patient's nonverbal communication. It also demonstrates the nurse's caring and interest in the patient.
   g. Using optimal pacing: The nurse must consider the pace of any conversation or encounter with a patient and let the patient set the pace.
   h. Providing personal space: Nurses must try to determine each patient's perception of personal space; invasion of this zone can evoke uncomfortable feelings.
   i. Developing therapeutic communication skills: Nurses must train and practice using therapeutic skills by controlling the tone of their voices, being knowledgeable about the topic, being flexible, being clear and concise, avoiding words that may be interpreted differently, being truthful and open minded, and taking advantage of opportunities for communicating.
   j. Developing listening skills: Nurses should sit when communicating with a patient, be alert and relaxed, keep the conversation natural, maintain eye contact if culturally correct, indicate that they are paying attention, think before responding to the patient, and listen for themes in the patient's comments.
   k. Using silence as a tool: The nurse can use silence appropriately by taking the time to wait for the patient to initiate or continue speaking. Nurses should be aware of the different possible meanings of silence (the patient is comfortable with the nurse, the patient is demonstrating stoicism or exploring inner thoughts, the patient may be fearful, etc.).
6. Sample answers:
   a. "Tell me about the night you had."
   b. "Let's try walking on that foot now."
   c. "What things prompted you to stop taking your insulin?"
   d. "Tell me what makes you afraid of taking the test."
   e. "Your procedure has been performed successfully every time here."
   f. Should not be said at all
7. Mrs. Clarke, age 42, underwent a mastectomy. She has a husband and two children, ages 10 and 5. When the nurse enters Mrs. Clarke's room, she finds her patient's <u>eyes are teary and there is a worried expression on her face</u>. When asked how she is feeling, Mrs. Clarke replies "fine," although <u>her face is rigid and her mouth is drawn in a firm line</u>. She is <u>moving her foot back and forth under the covers</u>. On further investigation, the nurse finds out Mrs. Clarke is worried about her children and her own ability to be a healthy, functioning wife and mother again. After prompting, Mrs. Clarke says, "I don't know if my husband will still love me like this." She <u>sighs and falls silent</u>, reflecting upon her recovery. The nurse tries to make Mrs. Clarke comfortable and <u>puts her hand over Mrs. Clarke's hand</u>. She <u>establishes eye contact</u> with Mrs. Clarke and reassures her that things have a way of working out and suggests that she give her situation some time.
8. Sample answers:
   a. Orientation phase:
      1. By 8/6/20, Mr. Uhl will call Nurse Parish by her name.
      2. By 8/6/20, Mr. Uhl will describe his freedoms/responsibilities within the institute.
   b. Working phase:
      1. By 8/10/20, Mr. Uhl will list various classes/activities available to patients.
      2. By 8/10/20, Mr. Uhl will express any anxieties he may have in his new environment to the nurse.
   c. Termination phase:
      1. By 8/25/20, Mr. Uhl will be introduced to the new nurse in charge of his case by Nurse Parish, who will continue to oversee the new relationship until her departure.
      2. By 8/27/20, Mr. Uhl will report feeling good about his past care and look forward to his new relationship.
9. Sample answers:
   a. Warmth and friendliness: A nurse who greets a patient with a pleasant smile.
   b. Openness: A nurse who provides an honest explanation of a procedure.
   c. Empathy: A nurse who listens to a woman's lament over her miscarriage while helping her bathe.
   d. Competence: A nurse who competently and smoothly inserts a Hep-Lock into a patient's vein.

e. Consideration of patient variables: A nurse who finds another nurse who speaks Spanish for her Hispanic patient.

10. Sample answers:
    a. Failure to perceive the patient as a human being: The nurse should focus on the whole person, not simply the illness or dysfunction.
    b. Failure to listen: Nurses should be open to opportunities for communication by keeping an open mind and focusing on the patient's needs instead of their own needs.
    c. Use of inappropriate comments or questions: The nurse should avoid certain types of comments and questions (clichés, questions that probe for information, leading questions, comments that give advice, judgmental comments) that tend to impede communication.
    d. Changing the subject: The nurse should avoid changing the subject; the patient may be ready to discuss something and may be frustrated if put off by a change in topic.
    e. Giving false assurance: The nurse should not try to convince the patient that things are going to turn out well when knowing the chances are not good. False assurance may give patients the impression the nurse is not interested in their problems.
11. a. Bullying: Anger and aggressive behavior between nurses, or nurse-to-nurse hostility, has been labeled horizontal violence. This negative behavior is also referred to as bullying, lateral violence, and professional incivility. According to a recent survey of new RNs in the United States, 60% quit a job after 6 months of employment as a result of being bullied. Bullying also affects patient safety because teamwork is negatively influenced, and there is deterioration in the quality of care and a greater potential for an error. It creates a toxic work environment and generates considerable emotional and physical consequences on those being bullied.
    b. Organizational response: Tactics against bullying include education for the staff, holding staff accountable, zero tolerance policies toward disruptive behaviors, protection for those who report the behaviors, training leaders to role model professional standards of behavior, surveillance and reporting systems put in place to identify unprofessional behaviors, and emphasis placed on the importance of documenting bullying behaviors.

## APPLYING YOUR KNOWLEDGE

### REFLECTIVE PRACTICE: CULTIVATING QSEN COMPETENCIES

#### Sample Answers

1. What communication skills might the nurse use to complete an assessment of Mrs. Russellinski?
   The nurse should orient Mrs. Russellinski to his or her presence before initiating conversation and talk directly to her while facing her. Important information should be communicated in a quiet environment where there is little to distract Mrs. Russellinski's attention, and conversation should be kept simple and concrete. The nurse must be patient and give Mrs. Russellinski time to respond. An interpreter should be called if the language barrier is too great, and attempts should be made to contact Mrs. Russellinski's daughter for information since she is listed as the contact person.
2. What would be a successful outcome for this patient?
   Mrs. Russellinski provides information to the nurse for the assessment and agrees to her daughter's participation in the interview.
3. What intellectual, technical, interpersonal, and/or ethical/legal competencies are most likely to bring about the desired outcome?
   Intellectual: ability to incorporate knowledge of the goals and phases of helping relationships as a component of the patient's care plan
   Interpersonal: strong people skills including the ability to communicate and interact effectively with patients who have hearing or cognitive deficits
   Ethical/Legal: ability to advocate for patients like Mrs. Russellinski who are unable to do so themselves due to language and hearing problems
4. What resources might be helpful for Mrs. Russellinski?
   An interpreter, other family members, consultation with an audiologist

## PRACTICING FOR NCLEX

### MULTIPLE CHOICE QUESTIONS

| | | | | |
|---|---|---|---|---|
| 1. d | 2. a | 3. b | 4. a | 5. c |
| 6. c | 7. d | 8. d | 9. c | 10. c |

### ALTERNATE-FORMAT QUESTIONS

#### Multiple Response Questions

1. a, b, d
2. b, c, f
3. b, d, f
4. a, c, d, f
5. c, e, f
6. a, c, f
7. c, d, e

# CHAPTER 9

## ASSESSING YOUR UNDERSTANDING

### FILL IN THE BLANKS

1. promote health
2. helping
3. Cognitive
4. affective
5. patients

6. Motivation
7. evidence based
8. counselor
9. coach

## MATCHING EXERCISES

| | | | | |
|---|---|---|---|---|
| 1. b | 2. a | 3. d | 4. h | 5. f |
| 6. g | 7. e | 8. g | 9. d | 10. c |
| 11. c | 12. b | 13. a | 14. d | 15. b |
| 16. a | 17. d | 18. c | 19. b | 20. d |
| 21. b | 22. a | 23. b | 24. c | 25. c |
| 26. a | | | | |

## SHORT ANSWER

1. Sample answers:
   a. Promoting health: Nurses can teach/counsel patients concerning health practices that lead to a higher level of wellness.
   b. Preventing illness: Nurses can teach patients health practices that help prevent specific illnesses or dangerous situations.
   c. Restoring health: Nurses can teach patients self-care practices that will facilitate recovery.
   d. Facilitating coping: Nurses can teach patients and their families to come to terms with the patient's illness and necessary lifestyle modifications.
2. Sample answers:
   a. The sensitivity and concern of the nurse in the helping relationship are the foundation for a nonthreatening learning environment for the adult patient.
   b. Honest and open communication can provide the adult learner with a realistic preview of what will be involved and allow him or her to retain some control over what is taught.
   c. New information must be presented clearly and in amounts that patients can comprehend to prevent them from becoming discouraged or overwhelmed.
3. Sample answers:
   a. Demonstration: Take Mr. Lang through the exercises and have him demonstrate them in return.
   b. Print material: Give Mr. Lang a brochure that explicitly describes and diagrams the exercises you wish him to learn.
   c. Discussion: Have a conversation with Mr. Lang about the exercises and his desire and ability to perform them.
4. a. Content must be prioritized such that essential information is taught thoroughly and promptly, and less important content is saved for last or for another time.
   b. Teamwork and cooperation allow nurses to meet deadlines for teaching. If teaching continues beyond hospitalization, the nurse can schedule additional learning opportunities through outpatient programs or referrals to community-based programs.
5. a. Formal: Planned teaching that is provided to fulfill learner objectives (e.g., viewing a film on diabetes)
   b. Informal: Unplanned teaching that represents the majority of nurse–patient interactions (e.g., a nurse showing a mother the proper way to hold an infant)
6. a. Cognitive domain: Oral questioning
   b. Affective domain: Patient's response
   c. Psychomotor domain: Return demonstration
7. A summary of the learning need, plan, implementation of the plan, and evaluated results should be documented in the patient chart. The evaluative statement should indicate whether the patient has displayed concrete evidence of learning how to bathe her infant.
8. a. Short-term counseling: Situational crisis (e.g., a nurse counsels a housebound patient after a fire destroys her bedroom)
   b. Long-term counseling: Developmental crisis (e.g., a nurse counsels an adolescent about the dangers of drugs and alcohol)
   c. Motivational counseling: Discussion of feelings and incentives with the patient (e.g., a nurse counsels a woman in a shelter about leaving her abusive spouse)
9. a. Identifying the new knowledge, attitudes, or skills that are necessary for patients and family members to manage their health care
   b. Assessing learning readiness
   c. Assessing the patient's ability to learn
   d. Identifying patient strengths and personal resources the nurse can tap
10. Answers will vary with student experiences.
11. a. Be certain that health care instructions are understandable and designed to support patient goals.
    b. Include patient and family as partners in the teaching–learning process.
    c. Use interactive teaching strategies.
    d. Remember that teaching and learning are processes that rely on strong interpersonal relationships with patients and their families.
12. a. Ignoring the restrictions of the patient's environment
    b. Failing to accept that patients have the right to change their mind
    c. Using medical jargon
    d. Failing to negotiate goals
    e. Duplicating teaching that other team members have done

## APPLYING YOUR KNOWLEDGE

### REFLECTIVE PRACTICE: CULTIVATING QSEN COMPETENCIES

#### Sample Answers

1. What should be the focus of patient teaching for this couple?
   Patient teaching should focus on health maintenance and promotion for the mother and fetus.

Teaching topics might include proper nutrition including the benefits of folic acid supplements and prenatal vitamins, substances to avoid when pregnant (tobacco, alcohol, cat litter, x-rays, etc.), methods of childbirth, and parenting skills. The nurse should encourage the couple's choice of childbirth planning and provide as much information as possible on home births.

2. What would be a successful outcome for Mr. and Mrs. Ramirez?
   By next visit, Mrs. Ramirez lists the benefits of home childbirth and signs up for a parenting class.
3. What intellectual, technical, interpersonal, and/or ethical/legal competencies are most likely to bring about the desired outcome?
   Intellectual: knowledge of how to design an appropriate teaching program for childbirth and parenting
   Interpersonal: ability to establish trusting relationships with patients to foster teaching and learning
   Ethical/Legal: strong sense of accountability for the health and well-being of patients that translates into a commitment to getting patients the information they need
4. What resources might be helpful for this couple?
   Parenting classes, prenatal classes, printed and AV materials on pregnancy, childbirth, and parenting

## PRACTICING FOR NCLEX

### MULTIPLE CHOICE QUESTIONS

| | | | | |
|---|---|---|---|---|
| **1.** a | **2.** c | **3.** b | **4.** d | **5.** a |
| **6.** c | **7.** b | **8.** d | **9.** c | **10.** c |

### ALTERNATE-FORMAT QUESTIONS

#### Multiple Response Questions

1. a, c, d
2. b, e, f
3. c, d, f
4. a, e, f
5. a, c, d, f
6. b, c, d

# CHAPTER 10

## ASSESSING YOUR UNDERSTANDING

### FILL IN THE BLANKS

1. explicit
2. autocratic
3. democratic
4. quantum
5. power
6. mentorship

### MATCHING EXERCISES

| | | | |
|---|---|---|---|
| **1.** d | **2.** b | **3.** a | **4.** d |
| **5.** e | **6.** c | **7.** b | **8.** c |
| **9.** a | **10.** a | **11.** f | **12.** g |

### SHORT ANSWER

1. Answers will vary with student experiences.
2. Sample answers:
   a. Communication skills: The nurse explains to Mr. Eng that she realizes he is in a lot of pain, and she will be available to administer medication if he feels he needs more pain relief.
   b. Problem-solving skills: When the nurse learns that Mr. Eng's pain is not being relieved by the medication prescribed by his doctor, she calls the doctor to have it adjusted. She also teaches Mr. Eng some visualization exercises to help take his mind off the pain.
   c. Management skills: The nurse meets with Mr. Eng's family to involve them in his care. She also instructs the staff to monitor Mr. Eng for signs of stress due to pain.
   d. Self-evaluation skills: The nurse realizes she is being effective in relieving Mr. Eng's suffering and vows to research techniques for pain management.
3. Sample answer:
   Step 1. Recognize symptoms that indicate a change is needed and collect data.
   Step 2. Identify a problem to be solved through change, in this case, changing record keeping to a computerized method. Analyze the symptoms and reach a conclusion. Note resistance or barriers to change and factors that promote the desired change.
   Step 3. Determine and analyze alternative solutions to the problem. Consider the advantages, disadvantages, and consequences of each alternative. An analysis of various proposed solutions to a problem may result in using a combination of alternatives.
   Step 4. Select a course of action from possible alternatives. Avoid initiating too many courses of action and thereby dissipating resources and energy.
   Step 5. Plan for making the change. This step is crucial to effect change successfully. Start by stating specific objectives, designing a plan for change, developing timetables, selecting people to assist with making the change, and anticipating how to stabilize change and deal with resistance to change. Unless a plan is clearly designed, effecting change is likely to be a chaotic experience.
   Step 6. Implement the selected course of action to effect change. Put the plan for change into effect. During this period, flexibility is important to adapt to unforeseen problems.
   Step 7. Evaluate the effects of change by comparing them with objectives stated in the plan for change. Adjustments can be made in the plan as necessary after evaluation. If the results of evaluation indicate that the course of action selected to solve a problem has been unsuccessful, an adjustment should be made or another course of action selected.

Step 8. Stabilize the change. When a solution has been found, take measures to make the change permanent. Continue follow-up until the change is firmly established.

Resistance to change: The nurse manager/leader must identify if any resistance is present in order to determine which techniques are needed to overcome it. Change alters the balance of a group, and resistance is an expected accompaniment to change.

4. a. Threat to self: Loss of self-esteem: Belief that more work will be required and that social relationships will be disrupted. Explain the proposed change to everyone affected in simple, concise language so they know how they will be affected by it.
   b. Lack of understanding: The people who will be affected by the change should be involved in the change process. When they understand the reason for and benefits of the change, they are more likely to accept it.
   c. Limited tolerance for change: Some people do not like to function in a state of flux or disequilibrium. Expedite the change so there is only a short period of confusion, and explain this tactic to the employees involved.
   d. Disagreements about the benefits of the change: Resistance may occur when the information available to the change agent is different from that received by people resisting the change. If the information available to the resisters is more accurate and relevant than the information available to the change agent, then resistance may be beneficial.
   e. Fear of increased responsibility: People often worry about having more complex responsibilities placed on them, particularly if they are unprepared for them. Since communication is the key to understanding, opportunities should be provided for open communication and feedback. Incentives may be helpful in obtaining a commitment to change.
5. Nurses can change negative portrayals of nursing in the media by organizing, monitoring the media, reacting to the media, and fostering an improved image.
6. Sample answers:
   a. Planning: Identifying problems and developing goals, objectives, and related strategies to meet the demands of the clinical arena
   b. Organizing: Acquiring, managing, and mobilizing resources to meet both clinical and financial objectives
   c. Staffing: Hiring, orienting, scheduling to facilitate team building; also includes staff development
   d. Directing: Leading others in achieving goals within the constraints of the current fiscal and workforce shortage scenarios, a demanding task for managers and staff alike
   e. Controlling: Implementing mechanisms for ongoing evaluation, particularly in areas of clinical quality and financial accountability
7. Answers will vary with students' experiences.
8. a. Identifying strengths: A nurse manager might accomplish this through feedback analysis that supports a focus on continually improving those things that he or she does best; discovering intellectual arrogance—being bright is no substitute for knowledge; initiating work on acquiring the skills and knowledge he or she needs to fully realize strengths; remedying bad habits.
   b. Evaluating work accomplishment: The manager should ask: Am I a visual or auditory learner? Do I learn best by reading or writing? Do I work more productively in teams or alone? Am I more productive as a decision maker or as an advisor?
   c. Clarifying values: Working in an organization or on a particular unit whose value system is unacceptable or incompatible condemns a person to frustration and poor performance. The nurse manager should identify his or her own values and seek a work environment that is complementary, not adversarial.
   d. Determining where he or she belongs and what he or she can contribute: In small or large organizations, the nurse manager should prepare for opportunities that emerge in response to these queries; in this dynamic industry, he or she should set reasonable short-to-medium range goals.
   e. Assuming responsibility for relationships: The nurse manager should cultivate them, nurture them, and respect the differences they might have.
9. a. What is amenable to change?
   b. How does the group function as a unit?
   c. Is the person or group ready for change and, if so, at what rate can that change be expected to be accepted?
   d. Are the changes major or minor?
10. a. The stability of the patient's condition
    b. The complexity of the activity to be delegated
    c. The potential for harm
    d. The predictability of the outcome
    e. The overall context of other patient needs
    f. The qualifications and capabilities of the UAP

## APPLYING YOUR KNOWLEDGE

### REFLECTIVE PRACTICE: CULTIVATING QSEN COMPETENCIES

#### Sample Answers

1. How might the nurse empower Ms. Kohls with the knowledge and ability to be a leader of her peers? The nurse could help Ms. Kohls identify her strengths, evaluate how she accomplishes work, clarify her values, and determine how she can

contribute to the community by being a leader in her school. The nurse can also empower Ms. Kohls by teaching her how to find the resources necessary to be knowledgeable about STIs and feel confident in her role as a leader.

2. What would be a successful outcome for Ms. Kohls?
By next visit, Ms. Kohls describes the incidence of STIs and lists interventions to prevent spreading these diseases.
By next visit, Ms. Kohls states that she feels confident in her ability to lead fellow students in a group discussion on STIs.
3. What intellectual, technical, interpersonal, and/or ethical/legal competencies are most likely to bring about the desired outcome?
Intellectual: Ability to identify leadership skills appropriately and apply personal leadership skills to a variety of patient situations; knowledge of the incidence and prevention of STIs
Interpersonal: Strong people skills; ability to communicate with and instill confidence in patients
Ethical/Legal: Ability to advocate for patients and provide them with legally sound counsel
4. What resources might be helpful for Ms. Kohls?
Information on STIs, information on leadership styles and how to propose and overcome resistance to change

## PRACTICING FOR NCLEX

### MULTIPLE CHOICE QUESTIONS

| | | | | |
|---|---|---|---|---|
| **1.** a | **2.** c | **3.** b | **4.** c | **5.** a |

### ALTERNATE-FORMAT QUESTIONS

#### Multiple Response Questions

1. c, e, f
2. a, c, f
3. b, c, d
4. b, d, f
5. c, d, f

# CHAPTER 11

## ASSESSING YOUR UNDERSTANDING

### FILL IN THE BLANKS

1. inpatient
2. Ambulatory care
3. Respite
4. Hospice
5. voluntary
6. respiratory therapist

### MATCHING EXERCISES

| | | | | |
|---|---|---|---|---|
| **1.** f | **2.** d | **3.** g | **4.** b | **5.** e |
| **6.** j | **7.** h | **8.** l | **9.** c | **10.** i |
| **11.** m | **12.** q | **13.** a | **14.** n | **15.** p |
| **16.** h | **17.** f | **18.** a | **19.** j | **20.** g |
| **21.** e | **22.** b | **23.** c | **24.** i | **25.** d |

### SHORT ANSWER

1. a. DRGs encourage early discharge from the hospital and have created a new acutely ill population who need skilled care at home.
   b. There are increasing numbers of older adults living longer with multiple chronic illnesses who are not institutionalized.
   c. With more sophisticated technology, people can be kept alive and comfortable in their own homes.
   d. Health care consumers demand that services be humane and provisions be made for a dignified death at home.
2. a. Primary care offices: Make health assessments, assist health care provider, and provide health education.
   b. Ambulatory care centers and clinics: A nurse practitioner may run these centers, which usually provide walk-in services and are open at times other than traditional office hours.
   c. Mental health centers: Nurses who work in crisis intervention centers must have strong communication and counseling skills and must be thoroughly familiar with community resources specific to the needs of patients being served.
   d. Rehabilitation centers: These centers use a health care team composed of health care providers, nurses, physical therapists, occupational therapists, and counselors.
   e. Long-term care centers: Help patients maintain function and independence with concern for the living environment, as well as for the health care provided. Provide direct care, supervise others, serve as an administrator, and teach.
3. With the trend toward discharging patients earlier, hospitals more often focus on the acute care needs of the patient. Along with this focus has come an abundance of services offered by the hospital aimed at the outpatient.
4. a. Surgical procedures
   b. Diagnostic tests
   c. Medications
   d. Physical therapy
   e. Counseling
   f. Health education
5. DRGs: Diagnosis-related groups: This plan pays the hospital a predetermined, fixed amount defined by the medical diagnosis or specific procedure rather than by the actual cost of hospitalization and care. DRGs were implemented by the federal government in an effort to control rising health care costs. If the cost of hospitalization is greater than that assigned, the hospital must absorb the additional cost. However, if cost is less than that assigned, the hospital makes a profit.
6. When patients come in contact with many different health care providers (e.g., registered nurses, licensed practical nurses, nursing assistants, nurse

specialists, physical therapists, dietitians, and students) and are frequently seen by other specialists called in on consultation or to do surgery, the patient may become confused about care and treatment. This fragmentation of care may result in the loss of continuity of care, resulting in conflicting plans of care, too much or too little medication, and higher health care costs.

## APPLYING YOUR KNOWLEDGE

### REFLECTIVE PRACTICE: CULTIVATING QSEN COMPETENCIES

#### Sample Answers

1. What nursing interventions might the nurse employ to assist Mrs. Ritchie with her caregiver duties?
   The nurse can provide Mrs. Ritchie with information about how to access respite care and make referrals for her. However, since Medicaid and most insurance providers do not cover the costs of respite care, the nurse should also check community services that may provide respite care for free. Mrs. Ritchie's husband may qualify for hospice care, and the nurse can arrange for this service.
2. What would be a successful outcome for this patient?
   Mrs. Ritchie vocalizes the benefits of respite care and hospice care programs and states that she will sign up for any services available to her.
3. What intellectual, technical, interpersonal, and/or ethical/legal competencies are most likely to bring about the desired outcome?
   Intellectual: knowledge of the various types of health care services and settings available to meet the needs of families caring for dying patients
   Technical: ability to provide technical assistance to meet the needs of families of patients on hospice
   Interpersonal: ability to work with different available resources to ensure everyone's access to safe, quality health care
   Ethical/Legal: knowledge of ethical and legal principles related to patients with terminal illnesses
4. What resources might be helpful for Mrs. Ritchie?
   Respite care, hospice services, community services

## PRACTICING FOR NCLEX

### MULTIPLE CHOICE QUESTIONS

| | | | | |
|---|---|---|---|---|
| **1.** a | **2.** b | **3.** a | **4.** d | **5.** c |
| **6.** c | **7.** d | **8.** b | **9.** d | **10.** a |

### ALTERNATE-FORMAT QUESTIONS

#### Multiple Response Questions

1. a, b, e
2. c, d, f
3. a, c, d, e
4. b, c, d, f

# CHAPTER 12

## ASSESSING YOUR UNDERSTANDING

### FILL IN THE BLANKS

1. community-based
2. Health Insurance Portability and Accountability Act (HIPAA)
3. against medical advice (AMA)
4. discharge planning

### CORRECT THE FALSE STATEMENTS

1. False—nurse
2. False—Continuity of care
3. True
4. True
5. False—patient's name, admitting provider's name, ID number, and any other information required by the particular institution
6. False—decreasing
7. False—is indicated
8. True
9. False—remains at the hospital
10. False—health care provider's order

### SHORT ANSWER

1. Sample answers:
   a. With patient's permission, check with relatives, neighbors, or fellow church or club members who could help; if necessary, employ interprofessional collaboration by checking with social agencies and community services.
   b. Describe the procedure to the patient in detail so he or she will know what to expect.
   c. Check the patient's insurance status, Medicare, or Medicaid; see if procedures are covered and what amount the patient will be responsible for. Refer to the appropriate agencies if necessary.
   d. With patient's permission, check with family; if necessary, provide interprofessional collaboration by checking into home health care possibilities, hospice, or extended care facilities.
2. a. Medications: Drug name, dosage, purpose, effect, and times taken, stated verbally and in writing.
   b. Procedures and treatments: Demonstrate all steps, practice, and put in writing. Patient and/or caregivers will be able to demonstrate procedure.
   c. Diet: Explain diet and purpose; give examples of meals and provide written plans.
   d. Referrals: Instruct patient and family how to make follow-up visits and whom to call with problems.
   e. Health promotion: All aspects of the illness or effects of treatment should be described verbally, and written materials should be supplied.
3. a. Discharge planning: Exchanges information among the patient, caregivers, and those

responsible for home care while the patient is in the institution and after the patient returns home.

**b.** Collaboration with other members of the health care team: Meets the patient's and family's physical, psychological, sociocultural, and spiritual needs in all settings and at all levels of health.

**c.** Involving patient and family in planning: Ensures that patient and family needs are consistently met as the patient moves from one level of care to another.

**4. a.** Assess the patient's need for nursing care related to admission.

**b.** Include consideration of biophysical, psychosocial, environmental, self-care, educational, and discharge planning factors in each patient's assessment.

**c.** Involve the patient and family in care as appropriate.

**d.** Nursing staff members should collaborate, as appropriate, with health care providers and members of other clinical disciplines to make decisions regarding the patient's need for nursing care.

**e.** Assess need for continuing care in preparation for discharge, and document referrals for such care in the patient's medical record.

**5. a.** Establish the health database: Age; sex; height; weight; medical history, including any prior miscarriages; and current medical treatment, follow-up treatment.

**b.** Assess for personal data: Personal feelings about her miscarriage, effectiveness of personal coping methods, strength of marital relationship.

**c.** Explore the emotional needs of the husband and his ability to cope with the situation as well as to provide emotional support to his wife.

**d.** Check if there are any support services (e.g., support groups, fertility clinics) that would be available to this couple.

**6. a.** Transfer within the hospital setting: Patient's belongings and/or furniture are moved; patient's records are moved or made available electronically, medications must be correctly labeled for the new room; and other departments must be notified as appropriate. Other hospital departments must be notified of the transfer. If transfer is to a new floor, the nurse at the original area gives a verbal report about the patient to the nurse at the new area. The report should include the patient's name, age, providers, admitting diagnosis, surgical procedure (if applicable), current condition and manifestations, allergies, medications and treatments, laboratory data, and any special equipment that will be needed to provide care. Patient goals and nursing care priorities are identified, and the existence of advance directives is noted. Accurate, concise, and complete verbal communication is essential.

**b.** Transfer to a long-term facility: All the patient's belongings are carefully packed and sent to the facility; prescriptions and appointment cards for return visits to the health care provider's office may be sent; patient is discharged from hospital setting, but a copy of the chart may be sent to long-term care facility along with a detailed assessment and care plan.

**c.** Discharge from a health care setting: Check patient discharge order, instructions, equipment and supplies, and financial arrangements. Assist patient to dress and pack belongings; check for written order for future services; transport patient to car and assist as necessary; make necessary recordings on records and complete discharge summary.

**7.** A form must be signed that releases the provider and health care institution from any legal responsibility for the patient's health status; the patient is informed of any possible risk before signing the form; the signature of the patient must be witnessed; and the form becomes part of the patient's record.

**8.** Position the bed in its highest position; arrange the furniture in the room to allow easy access to the bed. Open the bed by folding back the top bed linens. Assemble necessary equipment and supplies. Assemble special equipment and supplies (e.g., oxygen therapy equipment) and make sure it is working properly. Adjust the physical environment of the room.

**9.** Sample Answers:

**a.** Knowledgeable and skilled: A nurse knows the proper procedure for administering IV fluids and competently administers them.

**b.** Independent in making decisions: A home health care nurse encounters a situation in which caregiver burden is suspected and schedules respite care for the caregiver.

**c.** Accountable: A home health care nurse learns how to perform advanced procedures when caring for acutely ill patients in the home.

**10. a.** I: Introduction: The nurses involved in the handoff identify themselves, their roles, and their jobs.

**b.** S: Situation: The nurse performing the handoff describes the chief complaint, diagnosis, treatment plan, and patient wants and needs.

**c.** B: Background: The nurse performing the handoff lists the vital signs, mental and code status, medications, and lab results.

**d.** A: Assessment: The nurse performing the handoff gives the current patient provider's assessment of the patient.

**e.** R: Recommendation: The nurse performing the handoff identifies pending lab results and what needs to occur over the next few hours and any other recommendations for care that are appropriate.

**f.** Q: Question and answer: The nurses provide time for questions and answers regarding the patient situation.

## APPLYING YOUR KNOWLEDGE

### REFLECTIVE PRACTICE: CULTIVATING QSEN COMPETENCIES

#### Sample Answers

1. How might the admitting nurse respond to the grandmother's anxiety regarding her grandson's admission and condition?
   The nurse should explain the admission process to the grandmother and the power of attorney that is in place to admit Jeff to the hospital. The nurse should also describe the care that will be provided for her grandson to resolve his medical problems.
2. What would be a successful outcome for this patient?
   Jeff's grandmother acknowledges the policy in place to admit her grandson and states the objectives of the treatment plan.
3. What intellectual, technical, interpersonal, and/or ethical/legal competencies are most likely to bring about the desired outcome?
   Intellectual: knowledge of intellectual disability and the settings available to meet the needs of a patient with profound intellectual disability
   Interpersonal: ability to establish trusting professional relationships with patients, family caregivers, and health care professionals in different practice settings to ensure continuity of care
   Ethical/Legal: knowledge of the nurse's legal and ethical obligations as patients are transferred between home and different practice settings
4. What resources might be helpful for the nurse working with this family?
   Information on communicating with patients with intellectual disability, other health care professionals who have worked with Jeff

## PRACTICING FOR NCLEX

### MULTIPLE CHOICE QUESTIONS

**1.** c **2.** a **3.** d
**4.** a **5.** b **6.** c

### ALTERNATE-FORMAT QUESTIONS

#### Multiple Response Questions

1. a, c, e, f
2. b, c, f
3. c, d, e, f
4. b, e, f
5. a, d, f

# CHAPTER 13

## ASSESSING YOUR UNDERSTANDING

### FILL IN THE BLANKS

1. patient-centered
2. implementing
3. Quality and Safety Education for Nurses (QSEN)
4. thoughtful
5. evaluation

### MATCHING EXERCISES

| | | | | |
|---|---|---|---|---|
| **1.** a | **2.** d | **3.** e | **4.** b | **5.** c |
| **6.** a | **7.** e | **8.** b | **9.** c | **10.** e |
| **11.** d | **12.** a | **13.** c | **14.** b | **15.** d |
| **16.** a | **17.** d | **18.** b | **19.** a | **20.** c |
| **21.** b | **22.** d | | | |

### SHORT ANSWER

1. Patient:
   a. Scientifically based, holistic, individualized care
   b. The opportunity to work collaboratively with nurses
   c. Continuity of care
   Nursing:
   a. Achievement of a clear and efficient plan of action by which the entire nursing team can achieve results for patients through collaboration and communication
   b. Satisfaction that the nurse is making an important difference in the lives of patients
   c. Opportunity to grow professionally when evaluating the effectiveness of interventions and variables that contribute positively or negatively to the patient's goal achievement
2. a. Determining the need for nursing care: The nursing process provides a framework that enables the nurse to systematically collect patient data and clearly identify patient strengths and problems.
   b. Planning and implementing the care: The nursing process helps the nurse and patient develop a holistic plan of individualized care that specifies mutually agreed upon goals and the nursing actions most likely to assist the patient to meet those goals and execute the care plan.
   c. Evaluating the results of the nursing care: The nursing process provides for evaluation of the care plan in terms of patient goal achievement.
3. Defining the nursing process: The nursing process is a systematic method that directs the nurse, with the patient's participation, to accomplish the following: (1) assess the patient to determine the need for nursing care, (2) determine nursing diagnoses for actual and potential health problems, (3) identify expected outcomes and plan care, (4) implement the care, and (5) evaluate the results.
   Primary goals of the nursing process: The goals of the nursing process are to help the nurse manage each patient's care scientifically, holistically, and creatively to promote wellness, prevent disease or illness, restore health, and facilitate coping with altered functioning.
   Skills necessary for successful use of the nursing process: The skills necessary to use the nursing process successfully include intellectual, technical, interpersonal, and ethical/legal skills, as well as the willingness to use these skills creatively when working with patients.

4. Sample answers:
   a. Systematic: Each nursing task is a part of an ordered sequence of activities, and each activity depends on the accuracy of the activity that precedes it and influences the actions that follow it.
   b. Dynamic: There is great interaction and overlapping among the five steps; no one step in the process is a one-time phenomenon; each step is fluid and flows into the next step.
   c. Interpersonal: The human being is always at the heart of nursing. The nursing process ensures that nurses are patient centered rather than task centered.
   d. Outcome oriented: The nursing process offers a means for nurses and patients to work together to identify specific goals related to wellness promotion, disease and illness prevention, health restoration, and coping with altered functioning that are most important to the patient and match them with appropriate nursing actions.
   e. Universally applicable in nursing situations: Once nurses have a working knowledge of the nursing process, they can apply it to well or ill patients, young or old patients, in any type of practice setting.
5. a. Purpose of thinking: This helps to discipline thinking by keeping all thoughts directed to the goal.
   b. Adequacy of knowledge: It is important to judge whether the knowledge available to you is accurate, complete, and relevant. If you reason with false information or lack important data, it is impossible to draw a sound conclusion.
   c. Potential problems: As you become more skilled in critical thinking, you will learn to "flag" or remedy pitfalls to sound reasoning.
   d. Helpful resources: Wise professionals are quick to recognize their limits and seek help in remedying their deficiencies.
   e. Critique of judgment/decision: Ultimately, you must identify alternative judgments or decisions, weigh their merits, and reach a conclusion.
6. Sample answers:
   a. Practice a necessary skill until you feel confident in its execution before performing it on a patient.
   b. Take time to familiarize yourself with new equipment before using it in a clinical procedure.
   c. Identify nurses who are technical experts and ask them to share their secrets.
   d. Never be ashamed to seek assistance if you feel unsure of how to perform a procedure or manage equipment.
7. Answers will vary with student experiences.
8. Answers will vary with student experiences.
9. Sample answers:
   a. "I'm Nurse Brown and I'll be your nurse this week. What would you like to accomplish with this time, and how can I help you get through this period?"
   b. "What family members do you expect to see while you are here? Would you trust them to make decisions about your care if you were unable to do so yourself?"
   c. "What are your goals, hopes, and dreams in life? How do you hope to accomplish them? How will your hospitalization affect these goals?"
   d. "Tell me about your life at home/school/work. Is there anyone or anything in particular that you will miss during your recuperation?"
10. a. Do I know the legal boundaries of my practice?
    b. Do I own my personal strengths and weaknesses and seek assistance as needed?
    c. Am I knowledgeable about, and respectful of, patient rights?
    d. Does my documentation provide a legally defensible account of my practice?
11. a. Open-mindedness: A nurse is open to learning new ideas from a patient.
    b. Profound sense of the value of the person: A nurse goes to bat for a homeless woman who needs medical care.
    c. Self-awareness and knowledge of own beliefs and values: A nurse examines her own beliefs to see how they affect her practice.
    d. Sense of personal responsibility for actions: A nurse is committed to using expertise to provide health care to those who need it.
    e. Caring about well-being of patients and acting accordingly: A nurse is committed to learning new techniques to be the best nurse possible for patients.
    f. Leadership skills: A nurse uses leadership skills to persuade nurses to join professional nursing organizations.
    g. Bravery to question the "system": A nurse questions the staffing choices of a superior after working several shifts short-staffed.

## APPLYING YOUR KNOWLEDGE

### REFLECTIVE PRACTICE: CULTIVATING QSEN COMPETENCIES

#### Sample Answers

1. How might the nurse use blended nursing skills to respond to this patient situation?
   The nurse should investigate the reasons Ms. Horvath is not cooperating with the teaching session on wound care for her child. Possible reasons include fear, fatigue, lack of knowledge of possible consequences if the wound is not kept clean (i.e., infection), and being overwhelmed with family responsibilities. The nurse should use blended skills to advocate for this family and seek out possible resources (such as help from relatives or the community) to help remedy this situation.

2. What would be a successful outcome for this patient and her family?
   Ms. Horvath states the consequences of improper wound care and demonstrates changing the dressings on her daughter's wound.
3. What intellectual, technical, interpersonal, and/or ethical/legal competencies are most likely to bring about the desired outcome?
   Intellectual: knowledge of the science of nursing care related to wound care
   Technical: ability to competently change dressings on a wound and teach this skill to the caretaker
   Interpersonal: ability to counsel Ms. Horvath who is finding it difficult to respond to the challenge of caring for her daughter at home
   Ethical/Legal: commitment to patient safety and quality care, including the ability to report problem situations immediately
4. What resources might be helpful for Ms. Horvath?
   Counseling services, community services, help from relatives, printed materials on wound care

## PRACTICING FOR NCLEX

### MULTIPLE CHOICE QUESTIONS

| | | | |
|---|---|---|---|
| **1.** c | **2.** a | **3.** b | **4.** c |
| **5.** d | **6.** c | **7.** d | |

### ALTERNATE-FORMAT QUESTIONS

#### Multiple Response Questions

1. a, b, c
2. c, e, f
3. a, c, d, e
4. b, e, f
5. b, d, e

#### Prioritization Questions

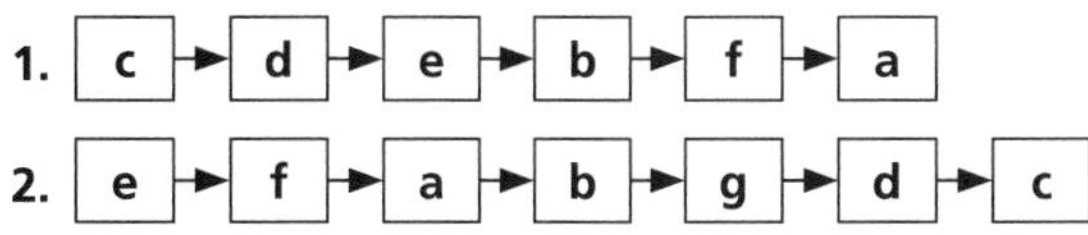


# CHAPTER 14

## ASSESSING YOUR UNDERSTANDING

### FILL IN THE BLANKS

1. patient support people, patient record
2. initial assessment
3. validation
4. Patient Centered Assessment Method (PCAM)
5. focused
6. time-lapsed
7. minimum data set

### MATCHING EXERCISES

| | | | |
|---|---|---|---|
| **1.** f | **2.** j | **3.** e | **4.** c |
| **5.** g | **6.** i | **7.** k | **8.** a |
| **9.** b | **10.** d | **11.** a | **12.** b |
| **13.** a | **14.** a | **15.** b | **16.** b |

### SHORT ANSWER

1. **a.** Make a judgment about a person's health status.
   **b.** Make a judgment about a patient's ability to manage his or her own health care.
   **c.** Make a judgment about a patient's need for nursing.
   **d.** Refer the patient to a health care provider or other health care professional.
   **e.** Plan and deliver thoughtful, person-centered, holistic nursing care that draws on the patient's strengths and promotes optimum functioning, independence, and well-being.
2. **a.** Patient: Most patients are willing to share information when they know it is helpful in planning their care.
   **b.** Support people: Family members, friends, and caregivers are helpful sources of data when a patient is a child or has a limited capacity to share information with the nurse.
   **c.** Patient record: A review of the records prepared by different members of the health care team provides information essential to comprehensive nursing care.
   **d.** Medical history, physical examination, and progress notes: Sources that record the findings of health care providers as they assess and treat the patient.
   **e.** Reports of laboratory and other diagnostic studies: These sources (e.g., x-rays and diagnostic tests) can either confirm or conflict with data collected during the nursing history or examination.
   **f.** Reports of therapies by other health care professionals: Other health care professionals record their findings and note progress in specific areas (e.g., nutrition, physical therapy, or speech therapy).
   **g.** Other health care professionals: Other nurses, health care providers, social workers, etc. can provide information about a patient's normal health habits and patterns and response to illness.
   **h.** Nursing and other health care literature: If a nurse is unfamiliar with a disease, it is important for him/her to read about the clinical manifestations of the disease and its usual progression to know what to look for when assessing the patient.
3. **a.** Purposeful: The nurse identifies the purpose of the nursing assessment (comprehensive, focused, emergency, time-lapsed) and then gathers the appropriate data.
   **b.** Prioritized: The nurse gets the most important information first.
   **c.** Complete: The nurse identifies all patient data to understand a patient's health problem and develop a care plan to maximize health promotion.
   **d.** Systematic: The nurse gathers the information in an organized manner.

e. Accurate: The nurse continually verifies what is heard with what is observed and uses other senses to validate all questionable data.
f. Relevant: The nurse determines what type of data and how much data to collect for each patient.
g. Recorded in a standard manner: The nurse records the data according to facility policy so that all caregivers can easily access the data.

4. Sample answers:
   a. What are the patient's current responses to his or her situation?
   b. What is the patient's current ability to manage his or her care?
   c. What factors are relevant in the immediate environment and in the larger environment (hospital/community)?
5. Sample answers:
   a. How will you modify your diet now that you have been diagnosed with diabetes?
   b. What do you know about insulin injections?
6. a. Patient's health orientation: Patients must identify potential and actual health risks and explore habits, behaviors, beliefs, attitudes, and values that influence levels of health.
   b. Patient's developmental stage: Nursing assessments are modified according to the patient's developmental stage.
   c. Patient's culture: When assessing patients from different cultural backgrounds (e.g., racial, ethnic, religious, socioeconomic), nurses must remember all the influences of cultural factors. Consideration of the patient's culture begins with how the nurse approaches the patient and whether or not the nurse makes direct eye contact or shakes the person's hand.
   d. Patient's need for nursing: Whether the nurse will interact with the patient for a short or long period and the nature of nursing care needs influence the type of data the nurse collects.
7. Sample answers:
   a. When there are discrepancies (e.g., a patient claims he has no pain but grimaces when you touch his chest)
   b. When the data lack objectivity (e.g., when a patient claims to have 20/20 vision but holds his reading material far away from his face)
8. Immediate communication of data is indicated whenever assessment findings reveal a critical change in the patient's health status that necessitates the involvement of other nurses or health care professionals.

## APPLYING YOUR KNOWLEDGE

### REFLECTIVE PRACTICE: CULTIVATING QSEN COMPETENCIES

#### Sample Answers

1. How might the nurse facilitate Ms. Morgan's ability to cope with disability?
   The nurse should assess the patient's body image and self-esteem needs. Working collaboratively with other members of the health care team, the nurse could then prepare a nursing care plan that specifically addresses these needs.
2. What would be a successful outcome for this patient?
   By discharge, Ms. Morgan will verbalize acceptance of her diagnosis of MS and state methods to keep herself as physically active as possible.
3. What intellectual, technical, interpersonal, and/or ethical/legal competencies are most likely to bring about the desired outcome?
   Intellectual: knowledge of the signs and symptoms of MS and supportive services for patients with MS
   Interpersonal: demonstration of strong people skills for dealing with people experiencing alterations in health
   Ethical/Legal: strong advocacy skills and a willingness to use them for patients needing assistance
4. What resources might be helpful for Ms. Morgan?
   Family counseling, printed materials on MS, support groups

## PRACTICING FOR NCLEX

### MULTIPLE CHOICE QUESTIONS

| | | | |
|---|---|---|---|
| 1. d | 2. d | 3. c | 4. a |
| 5. c | 6. b | 7. d | 8. d |

### ALTERNATE-FORMAT QUESTIONS

#### Multiple Response Questions

1. c, d, f
2. b, c, f
3. c, d, f

#### Prioritization Question

1. 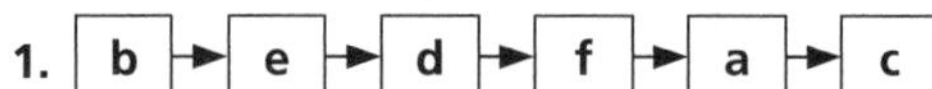


# CHAPTER 15

## ASSESSING YOUR UNDERSTANDING

### FILL IN THE BLANKS

1. collaborative
2. cues
3. standard or norm
4. data cluster
5. nursing diagnosis
6. Inability to accept the death of newborn child
7. desire for a higher level of wellness, an effective present status or function
8. syndrome

### MATCHING EXERCISES

| | | | |
|---|---|---|---|
| 1. c | 2. a | 3. b | 4. d |
| 5. a | 6. c | 7. d | |

### CORRECT THE FALSE STATEMENTS

1. False—nursing diagnoses
2. False—Nursing diagnoses

3. False—standard or norm
4. True
5. False—cluster of significant data
6. True
7. False—etiology
8. True
9. True
10. True
11. False—analyzes patient data
12. False—risk diagnosis

## SHORT ANSWER

1. a. Using legally inadvisable language
   b. X
   c. Identifying responses not necessarily unhealthy
   d. X
   e. Both clauses say the same thing.
   f. X
   g. Including value judgment
   h. Identifying responses not necessarily unhealthy
   i. X
   j. Including medical diagnosis
   k. Identifying problems as signs and symptoms
   l. Reversing clauses
   m. X
   n. Both clauses say the same thing.
   o. Identifying problems/etiologies that cannot be altered
   p. Both clauses say the same thing.
   q. X
   r. Writing diagnosis in terms of needs
2. Sample answers:
   a. Were you able to pass urine this morning? Did you drink the fluids we brought you?
   b. Do you feel like talking to other patients who are undergoing the same treatment? Would you like to see your family today?
   c. Do you feel helpless to put your life back in order? Are you overwhelmed by the changes in your life?
   d. Were you able to get some sleep last night? Did the noise on the unit keep you awake?
3. a. No problem: Reinforce patient's health habits and patterns; initiate health promotion activities to prevent disease or illness or promote higher level of wellness.
   b. Possible problem: Collect more data to confirm or rule out suspected problem.
   c. Actual or potential nursing diagnosis: Unable to treat because patient denies problem or refuses treatment; begin planning, implementing, and evaluating care designed to prevent, reduce, or resolve problem.
   d. Clinical problem other than nursing diagnosis: Consult with appropriate health care professional and work collaboratively on problem; refer to medicine.
4. Sample answers:
   a. An infant who is below the normal growth standards for his age group may be experiencing "failure to thrive."
   b. A mother who has a history of mental illness shows little or no interest in her baby.
   c. A patient placed in a long-term care facility by her son becomes incontinent without a physical cause.
5. a. Are my data accurate and complete?
   b. Have I correctly distinguished normal from abnormal findings and decided if abnormal data may be signs and symptoms of a specific health problem?
   c. Have I made and validated deductions or opinions that follow logically from patient cues?
   d. Has the patient or the patient's surrogates (if able to do so) validated that these are important problems?
   e. Have I given the patient or the patient's surrogate an opportunity to identify problems that I have missed?
   f. Is each diagnosis supported by evidence? Might these cues signify a different problem or diagnosis?
   g. Have I tried to identify what is causing the actual or potential problem and what strengths/resources the patient might use to avoid or resolve the problem?
   h. Have I followed facility guidelines to correctly document diagnostic statements in a way that clearly communicates patient problems to other health care professionals?
   i. Is this a problem that falls within nursing's independent domain or does it signify a medical diagnosis or collaborative problem?
6. a. In the presence of known problems, nurses must predict the most common and most dangerous complications and take immediate action to prevent them or manage them in case they cannot be prevented.
   b. Whether problems are present or not, nurses must look for evidence of risk factors and, if identified, aim to reduce or control them, thereby preventing the problems themselves.
   c. In all situations, nurses must ensure that safety and learning needs are met and promote optimum function and independence.
7. a. Mr. Klinetob, aged 86, has been seriously depressed since the death of his wife of 52 years, 6 months ago. Although he suffers from <u>degenerative joint disease</u> and has talked for years about having "just a touch of arthritis," this never kept him from being up and about. Recently, however, he spends all day sitting in a chair and seems to have no desire to engage in self-care activities. He tells the visiting nurse that <u>he doesn't get washed up anymore because he's "too stiff" in the morning to bathe and "I just don't seem to have the energy."</u> The visiting nurse notices that <u>his hair is matted and uncombed, his face has traces of previous meals, and he has a strong body odor</u>. His adult children have complained that their normally

fastidious father seems not to care about personal hygiene any longer.
Nursing Diagnosis: Bathing/hygiene self-care deficit, related to decreased strength and endurance, discomfort, and depression, as evidenced by matted and uncombed hair, new beard, food particles on face, and strong body odor

**b.** Ms. Adams sustained a right-sided cerebral infarct that resulted in left hemiparesis (paralysis on left side of body) and left "neglect." She ignores the left side of her body and actually denies its existence. When asked about her left leg, she stated that it belonged to the woman in the next bed—this while she was in a private room. This patient was previously quite active: she walked for 45 to 60 minutes four or five times a week and was an avid swimmer. At present, she cannot move either her left arm or leg.
Nursing Diagnosis: Disturbed body image, related to left hemiparesis (paralysis), as evidenced by her ignoring the left side of her body following her inability to move it

**c.** After trying to conceive a child for 11 years, Ted and Rosemary Hines sought the assistance of a fertility specialist who was highly recommended by a friend. It was determined that Ted's sperm was inadequate, and Rosemary was inseminated with sperm from an anonymous donor. The couple was told that the donor was healthy and that he was selected because he resembled Ted. Rosemary became pregnant after the second in vitro fertilization attempt and delivered a healthy baby girl named Sarah. Sarah is now 7 years old, and Ted and Rosemary have learned from blood tests that their fertility specialist is the biologic father of their child. It seems that he lied to some couples about using sperm from anonymous donors and deceived others into thinking the wives had become pregnant when he had simply injected them with hormones. Ted and Rosemary have joined other couples in pressing charges against this health care provider. Rosemary tells the nurse in her pediatrician's office that she is concerned about how all this is affecting her family. "Ted and I both love Sarah and would do nothing to hurt her, but I'm so angry about this whole situation that I'm afraid I may be taking it out on her," she says. Questioning reveals that Rosemary has found herself yelling at Sarah for minor disobediences and spanking her, something she rarely did before. Both Ted and Rosemary had commented before about Sarah's striking physical resemblance to the fertility specialist but attributed this to coincidence. Rosemary says, "Whenever I see her now I can't help but see Dr. Clowser and everything inside me clenches up and I want to scream." Both Ted and Rosemary express great remorse that Sarah, who is innocent, is bearing the brunt of something that is in no way her fault.
Nursing Diagnosis: Parental role conflict related to unexpected discovery about their daughter's biologic father, as evidenced by parental concern about increased incidence of parental yelling and spanking and the anger the child evokes in her parents because of her physical resemblance to the fertility specialist who deceived them.

## APPLYING YOUR KNOWLEDGE

### REFLECTIVE PRACTICE: CULTIVATING QSEN COMPETENCIES

#### Sample Answers

1. What nursing diagnosis would be appropriate for Mr. Prescott? How might the nurse advocate for Mr. Prescott to ensure that he gets tested for colon cancer?
Nursing Diagnosis: Anxiety related to constipation and possible bowel alterations
Mr. Prescott would benefit from patient teaching/counseling regarding the need for stool testing. After checking with the primary care provider, the nurse could schedule a colonoscopy if ordered to check for colon cancer. The nurse should address the patient's constipation and check with the primary care provider about scheduling a consult with a gastroenterologist.
2. What would be a successful outcome for this patient?
Mr. Prescott states the warning signs of colon cancer and agrees to schedule a colonoscopy.
3. What intellectual, technical, interpersonal, and/or ethical/legal competencies are most likely to bring about the desired outcome?
Intellectual: knowledge of gastrointestinal elimination, including hemorrhoids and risk factors for possible colon cancer
Interpersonal: ability to work collaboratively with other members of the health care team to meet the needs of patients
Ethical/Legal: ability to serve as a trusted and effective patient advocate to counsel patients with bowel alterations
4. What resources might be helpful for Mr. Prescott?
Consults with other health care professionals, educational materials on colon cancer, diet plans to prevent constipation

## PRACTICING FOR NCLEX

### MULTIPLE CHOICE QUESTIONS

**1.** c **2.** a **3.** d **4.** c **5.** d

### ALTERNATE-FORMAT QUESTIONS

#### Multiple Response Questions

1. b, c, e, f
2. c, d, f
3. a, b, d
4. a, d, e
5. a, b, c, d, e

# CHAPTER 16

## ASSESSING YOUR UNDERSTANDING

### FILL IN THE BLANKS

1. patient outcome
2. informal
3. initial, ongoing, discharge
4. Pain/the problem statement
5. Nursing Outcomes Classification (NOC)
6. evaluative
7. nursing intervention
8. nurse-initiated
9. health care provider–initiated
10. algorithm
11. nursing care plan

### MATCHING EXERCISES

| | | | | |
|---|---|---|---|---|
| **1.** a | **2.** e | **3.** b | **4.** d | **5.** c |
| **6.** g | **7.** b | **8.** h | **9.** b | **10.** a |
| **11.** b | **12.** c | **13.** a | **14.** c | **15.** b |
| **16.** a | **17.** b | **18.** c | **19.** c | **20.** a |

### SHORT ANSWER

1. **a.** Teach patient the proper technique and application for an inhaler.
   **b.** Walk with patient the length of the hallway every 5 hours, encouraging her to rely on the walker for support.
   **c.** Teach patient the importance of a well-balanced diet and daily exercise; have patient monitor daily caloric intake.
   **d.** Help patient sit up and dangle legs over side of bed; gradually help patient to stand and take several steps around the room.
2. **a.** Setting priorities: Before developing or modifying the care plan, the prioritized list of nursing diagnoses should be reviewed to determine whether they are correctly ranked as high priority, medium priority, or low priority.
   **b.** Writing goals/outcomes that determine the evaluative strategy: For each nursing diagnosis in the care plan, at least one goal must be written that, if achieved, demonstrates a direct resolution of the problem statement.
   **c.** Selecting appropriate evidence-based nursing interventions: Nursing interventions should be consistent with standards of care; realistic; compatible with patient's values, beliefs, and psychosocial background; valued by patient and family; and compatible with other planned therapies.
   **d.** Communicating the nursing care plan: Nursing orders are in writing and thus communicate to the entire nursing staff and health care team the specific nursing care to be implemented for the patient.
3. Sample answers:
   Informal planning: A postpartum nurse learns that a patient is complaining of soreness related to unsuccessful attempts to breastfeed her infant and plans to spend more time with her. A home health care nurse quickly assesses safety in the home of a patient prone to accidents.
4. A formal care plan allows the nurse to individualize care; set priorities; facilitate communication among nursing personnel; promote continuity of high-quality, cost-effective care; coordinate care; evaluate patient's response to nursing care; and promote the nurse's professional development.
5. **a.** Assess effectiveness of pain medication for patient every 4 hours.
   **b.** Speak to parents of patient to assess their ability to support patient.
   **c.** Assess patient's room for variety of colors, textures, visual stimulation.
   **d.** Teach patient to perform daily exercises and learn to ambulate with a walker.
6. **a.** Basic human needs: The nursing care plan should concisely communicate to caregivers data about the patient's usual health habits and patterns obtained during the nursing history that are needed to direct daily care (e.g., requires assistance setting up food tray).
   **b.** Nursing diagnoses: The plan should contain goals/outcomes and nursing interventions for every nursing diagnosis, as well as a place to note patient responses to the care plan; for instance, if the nursing diagnosis is Impaired skin integrity related to mobility deficit, a goal should be written to turn patient frequently and assess for skin breakdown.
   **c.** Medical and interdisciplinary care plan: The care plan should record current medical orders for diagnostic studies and specified related nursing care; for instance, if a diagnostic test is scheduled for the morning, appropriate fasting measures should be included in the care plan.
7. **a.** Have changes in the patient's health status influenced the priority of nursing diagnoses?
   **b.** Have changes in the way the patient is responding to health and illness or the care plan affected those nursing diagnoses that can be realistically addressed?
   **c.** Are there relationships among diagnoses that require that one be worked on before another can be resolved?
   **d.** Can several patient problems be dealt with together?
8. **a.** Mrs. Myers learns one lesson on nutrition per day, beginning 2/16/20.
   **b.** After viewing film on smoking, Mrs. Gray identifies three dangers of smoking.
   **c.** X
   **d.** X
   **e.** By next visit, patient will list three benefits of psychotherapy.
   **f.** X
9. Sample answers:
   **a.** By 11/12/20, patient will reestablish fluid balance as evidenced by (1) an approximate balance between fluid intake and fluid output, to average

approximately 2,500 mL; (2) urine specific gravity within the normal range (1.010–1.025).

**b.** By next visit, patient will report a resumption of usual level of sexual activity following her acceptance of her new body image.

**c.** By 6/4/20, patient will report a decrease in the number of stress incontinent episodes (less than one per day) following her use of Kegel exercises.

**d.** By 8/10/20, patient reports he has sufficient energy to carry out the priority activities identified 8/2/20.

**e.** By end of shift, patient reports better pain management (pain decreased to less than 3 on a scale of 10) related to new administration schedule.

**10. a.** Be familiar with standards and facility policies for setting priorities, identifying and recording expected patient outcomes, selecting evidence-based nursing interventions, and recording the care plan.

**b.** Remember that the goal of patient-centered care is to keep the patient and the patient's interests and preferences central in every aspect of planning.

**c.** Keep the "big picture" in focus. What are the discharge goals for this patient, and how should this direct each shift's interventions?

**d.** Trust clinical experience and judgment but be willing to ask for help when the situation demands more than your qualifications and experience can provide; value collaborative practice.

**e.** Respect your clinical intuition, but before establishing priorities, identifying outcomes, and selecting nursing interventions, be sure that research supports your plan.

**f.** Recognize personal biases and keep an open mind.

**11. a.** What problems need immediate attention, and what could happen if I wait to attend to them?

**b.** Which problems are my responsibility, and which do I need to refer to someone else?

**c.** Which problems can be dealt with by using standard plans (e.g., critical paths, standards of care)?

**d.** Which problems are not covered by protocols or standard plans but must be addressed to ensure a safe hospital stay and timely discharge?

## APPLYING YOUR KNOWLEDGE

### REFLECTIVE PRACTICE: CULTIVATING QSEN COMPETENCIES

#### Sample Answers

**1.** How might the nurse respond to Ms. Kronk's questions regarding fitness?
The nurse can teach Ms. Kronk about low-salt, low-fat diets and encourage her to begin an exercise program, such as walking each day or joining a gym. The nurse could also refer Ms. Kronk to a dietitian to explain the types of diets and diet supplements that are available, including diets that are healthy and foods to avoid with high blood pressure.

**2.** What would be a successful outcome for this patient?
Ms. Kronk lists three benefits of following a heart healthy diet and starting an exercise program to lose weight.

**3.** What intellectual, technical, interpersonal, and/or ethical/legal competencies are most likely to bring about the desired outcome?
Intellectual: knowledge of what information is needed to develop a care plan that meets the nursing needs of a woman who wants to improve her fitness level
Technical: ability to use the Internet to research literature to obtain knowledge to develop a care plan for Ms. Kronk
Interpersonal: ability to empathize with patients, sharing their struggles and celebrating their achievement of valued goals
Ethical/Legal: ability to serve as a trusted and effective patient advocate

**4.** What resources might be helpful for Ms. Kronk?
Printed materials on healthy diets, exercise plans, referrals to other health care professionals (such as fitness trainers)

## PRACTICING FOR NCLEX

### MULTIPLE CHOICE QUESTIONS

| | | | |
|---|---|---|---|
| **1.** d | **2.** a | **3.** c | **4.** b |
| **5.** c | **6.** b | **7.** c | |

### ALTERNATE-FORMAT QUESTIONS

#### Multiple Response Questions

**1.** a, c, d, f
**2.** a, c
**3.** b, d
**4.** a, d, f
**5.** a, d, e, f
**6.** c, d, f
**7.** b, c, e

# CHAPTER 17

## ASSESSING YOUR UNDERSTANDING

### FILL IN THE BLANKS

**1.** health care provider–initiated
**2.** Protocols
**3.** Community (or public health) interventions
**4.** indirect care
**5.** Nursing Interventions Classification
**6.** collaborative interventions

### MATCHING EXERCISES

| | | |
|---|---|---|
| **1.** a | **2.** b | **3.** a |
| **4.** c | **5.** b | **6.** c |

### CORRECT THE FALSE STATEMENTS

**1.** False—nurse
**2.** True
**3.** False—Protocols

4. False—nurse
5. True
6. False—nothing about the care plan is fixed
7. True
8. False—not sufficient
9. False—reassess the strategy
10. True
11. True

**SHORT ANSWER**

1. a. Interpret the specialists' findings for patients and family members.
   b. Prepare patients to participate maximally in the care plan before and after discharge.
   c. Serve as a liaison among the members of the health care team.
2. Sample answers:
   a. Nurse variable: A nurse with overwhelming outside concerns.
   b. Patient variable: A patient who gives up.
   c. Health care variable: Understaffing causes overworked nurses.
3. a. If patients and their families want to participate actively in seeking health, preventing disease and illness, recovering health, and learning to cope with altered functioning, they must possess effective self-care behavior.
   b. The nursing actions planned to promote patient goal/outcome achievement and the resolution of health problems should be carefully executed. It is important that the nurse use time wisely to maximize each patient encounter to help the patient achieve his or her goals/outcomes.
4. Sample answer:
   Mr. Franks may need a psychological evaluation to assess his adjustment to his new environment. Efforts should be made to get Mr. Franks involved in his new life so he shows interest in himself and others.
5. Sample answer:
   Along with receiving care for pregnancy, this patient should receive counseling on planning economical, nutritious meals and should be alerted to any social services in her community that could provide some relief in this area.
6. Sample answers:
   a. Administering a prescribed medication to a patient.
   b. A nurse lobbies for a new recreational facility in a long-term care facility.
   c. A nurse participates in a free blood pressure screening at a local mall.

## APPLYING YOUR KNOWLEDGE

### REFLECTIVE PRACTICE: CULTIVATING QSEN COMPETENCIES

**Sample Answers**

1. What might be the nurse's response when advocating for Antoinette and her family?
   The nurse's first responsibility is to her patient.
   In this case, the nurse must investigate the circumstances surrounding Antoinette's family life that are causing her failure to thrive. A referral to social services may be in order to help the family with child care and the necessities of life. The nurse should also investigate any community services available to help this family.
2. What would be a successful outcome for this patient?
   By next visit, Antoinette is in the normal range of growth for her age and reaches the appropriate developmental milestones.
   Antoinette's grandmother states that she is less overwhelmed with her role as caregiver and is receiving help from community services
3. What intellectual, technical, interpersonal, and/or ethical/legal competencies are most likely to bring about the desired outcome?
   Intellectual: knowledge of appropriate information necessary to implement the nursing interventions that effectively meet the nursing needs of a toddler with physical and developmental delays
   Technical: ability to competently adapt procedures and equipment to meet the needs of patients across the life span
   Interpersonal: ability to work collaboratively with members of the health care team to implement the interdisciplinary care plan
   Ethical/Legal: ability to participate as a trusted and effective patient advocate
4. What resources might be helpful for this family?
   Social services, community services, counseling services

## PRACTICING FOR NCLEX

### MULTIPLE CHOICE QUESTIONS

**1.** b **2.** c **3.** d **4.** c **5.** b

### ALTERNATE-FORMAT QUESTIONS

**Multiple Response Questions**

1. a, b
2. a, e, f
3. b, c, e, f
4. d, e, f

# CHAPTER 18

## ASSESSING YOUR UNDERSTANDING

### FILL IN THE BLANKS

1. terminate, modify, continue
2. patient
3. outcome achievement
4. criteria
5. Standards
6. Clinical practice guidelines (CPGs)
7. quality assurance
8. structure
9. retrospective

## MATCHING EXERCISES

| | | | | |
|---|---|---|---|---|
| **1.** e | **2.** c | **3.** a | **4.** d | **5.** b |
| **6.** a | **7.** b | **8.** b | **9.** a | **10.** a |

## SHORT ANSWER

**1.** Sample answers:
   **a.** Cognitive outcomes: Ask the patient to repeat the information or ask the patient to apply the new knowledge to his or her everyday situations.
   **b.** Psychomotor outcomes: Ask the patient to demonstrate the new skill.
   **c.** Affective outcomes: Observe the patient's behavior and conversation for signs that the outcomes are achieved.

**2. a** Identifying evaluative criteria: Evaluative criteria are the patient goals/outcomes developed during the planning step and must be identified to determine whether they can be met by the patient.
   **b.** Determining whether these criteria and standards are met: Because evaluative criteria reflect desired changes or outcomes in patient behavior, and because nursing actions are directed toward these outcomes, they become the core of evaluation to determine whether the plan has been effective.
   **c.** Terminating, continuing, or modifying the plan: Reviewing each step of the nursing process helps to determine whether goals have been met and whether the plan should be terminated, continued, or modified.

**3.** Sample answers:
   **a.** Patient: Is the patient motivated to learn new health behaviors?
   **b.** Nurse: Do the nurses come to work well rested and ready to help their patients?
   **c.** Health care system: Is a healthy nurse-to-patient ratio important to the institution?

**4.** The nurse should reevaluate each preceding step of the nursing process for accuracy. After this is done, it may become necessary to collect new assessment data, add or revise diagnoses, modify or rewrite patient goals/outcomes, and change the nursing orders. In addition, patient evaluations may have to be targeted more frequently.

**5. a.** Structure: An audit focused on the environment in which care is provided. Evaluation is based on physical facilities and equipment, organizational characteristics, policies and procedures, fiscal resources, and personnel resources.
   **b.** Process: An audit that focuses on the nature and sequence of activities carried out by the nurse implementing the nursing process. Evaluation is based on acceptable levels of performance of nursing actions related to patient assessment, diagnosis, planning, implementation, and evaluation.
   **c.** Outcome: Outcome evaluations focus on measurable and demonstrable changes in the health status of the patient or the results of nursing care.

**6. a.** Delete or modify the nursing diagnosis: After evaluating the data, the nurse may decide the nursing diagnosis is inadequate and delete or change the diagnosis.
   **b.** Make the goal statement more realistic: The nurse should determine the effectiveness of the goal and adjust the goal to meet the patient's needs.
   **c.** Adjust time criteria in the goal statement: If the time period was too short to accomplish the goal, it may need to be extended.
   **d.** Change nursing interventions: Reevaluate the nursing interventions and change the ones that were ineffective; tailor the interventions to the patient's needs.

**7.** *Quality by inspection* focuses on finding deficient workers and removing them. Nurses and others working in a setting using this approach may be afraid to admit a mistake or error and wrongly attempt to hide a problem. Such behavior is never acceptable and may result in serious harm to patients. *Quality as opportunity,* on the other hand, focuses on finding opportunities for improvement and fosters an environment that thrives on teamwork, with people sharing the skills and lessons they have learned.

**8. a.** Nurses measure patient outcome achievement.
   **b.** Nurses measure how effectively nurses help targeted groups of patients to achieve their specific goals.
   **c.** Nurses measure the competence of individual nurses.
   **d.** Nurses measure the degree to which external factors, such as different types of health care services, specialized equipment or procedures, or socioeconomic factors, influence health and wellness.

---

## APPLYING YOUR KNOWLEDGE

### REFLECTIVE PRACTICE: CULTIVATING QSEN COMPETENCIES

#### Sample Answers

**1.** What should be the focus of an evaluation of Mrs. Otsuki's nursing care plan conducted by the home health care nurse?
The nurse should evaluate Mrs. Otsuki's understanding of, and compliance with, the medication regime, since she admits to taking a double dose of diuretics related to confusion with brand/generic prescriptions. A secondary concern would be if Mrs. Otsuki is capable of living by herself with only a daily visit from her daughter.

**2.** What would be a successful outcome for this patient?
By next visit, Mrs. Otsuki states the dosages and frequency of administration of the drugs she is taking. By next visit, Mrs. Otsuki verbalizes that she feels comfortable with the medication administration

and is receiving help with home management from her daughter/social services.

3. What intellectual, technical, interpersonal, and/or ethical/legal competencies are most likely to bring about the desired outcome?
Intellectual: ability to incorporate knowledge of assessment, diagnosing, planning, and implementing nursing care when evaluating care for an older adult patient taking too much prescribed medication
Technical: ability to use a documentation system competently to record the patient's progress toward outcome achievement
Interpersonal: ability to identify and respond to the changing needs of a patient experiencing different alterations in health status
Ethical/Legal: commitment to evaluating patient achievement of outcomes in a timely fashion and to addressing whatever is interfering with outcome achievement within the scope of nursing practice
4. What resources might be helpful for Mrs. Otsuki?
Social services, community services, printed materials on the drugs she is taking, compartmentalized pill boxes

## PRACTICING FOR NCLEX

### MULTIPLE CHOICE QUESTIONS

| | | | | |
|---|---|---|---|---|
| **1.** a | **2.** c | **3.** b | **4.** d | **5.** b |
| **6.** d | **7.** d | **8.** d | | |

### ALTERNATE-FORMAT QUESTIONS

#### Multiple Response Questions

1. a, d, e
2. a, b, c
3. c, e, f
4. a, b, d

# CHAPTER 19

## ASSESSING YOUR UNDERSTANDING

### FILL IN THE BLANKS

1. patient record
2. variance or occurrence
3. minimum data sets
4. outcome and assessment information set (OASIS)
5. resident assessment instrument (RAI)
6. change-of-shift or hand-off report
7. incident report (variance or occurrence)
8. nursing care conference

### MATCHING EXERCISES

| | | | | |
|---|---|---|---|---|
| **1.** c | **2.** f | **3.** i | **4.** e | **5.** a |
| **6.** g | **7.** b | **8.** j | **9.** k | |

### SHORT ANSWER

1. **a.** Nursing care data related to patient assessments
   **b.** Nursing diagnoses or patient needs
   **c.** Nursing interventions
   **d.** Patient outcomes
2. **a.** Change-of-shift/hand-off reports: Given by a primary nurse to the nurse replacing him or her or by the charge nurse to the nurse who assumes responsibility for continuing care of the patient. Can be written, oral, or audiotaped.
   **b.** Telephone/telemedicine reports: Telephones can link health care professionals immediately and enable nurses to receive and give critical information about patients in a timely fashion.
   **c.** Telephone orders: Policy must be followed regarding telephone orders; they must be transcribed on an order sheet and co-signed by the health care provider within a set time.
   **d.** Transfer and discharge reports: Nurses report a summary of a patient's condition and care when transferring or discharging patients.
   **e.** Reports to family members and significant others: Nurses must keep the patient's family and significant others updated about the patient's condition and progress toward goal achievement.
   **f.** Incident reports: A tool used by health care agencies to document the occurrence of anything out of the ordinary that results in or has the potential to result in harm to a patient, employee, or visitor.
   **g.** Conferring about care: To consult with someone to exchange ideas or to seek information, advice, or instructions.
   **h.** Consultations and referrals: When nurses detect problems they cannot resolve because the problems lie outside the scope of independent nursing practice, they consult with, or make referrals to other professionals.
   **i.** Nursing and interdisciplinary team care conference: Nurses and other health care professionals frequently confer in groups to plan and coordinate patient care.
   **j.** Nursing care rounds: Procedures in which a group of nurses visit selected patients individually at each patient's bedside to gather information, evaluate nursing care, and provide the patient with an opportunity to discuss his or her care.
3. **a.** Communication: The patient record helps health care professionals from different disciplines who interact with the same patient at different times to communicate with one another.
   **b.** Care planning: Each professional working with the patient has access to the patient's baseline and updated data and can see how he or she is responding to the treatment plan from day to day. Modifications of the plan are based on these data.
   **c.** Quality process and performance improvement: Charts may be reviewed to evaluate the quality of nursing care and the competence of the nurses providing that care.
   **d.** Research: The record may be studied by researchers to determine the most effective way to recognize or treat specific health problems. The aim is to promote evidence-based practice in nursing and quality health care.

**e.** Decision analysis: Information from records review often provides the data needed by strategic planners to identify needs and the means and strategies most likely to address these needs.

**f.** Education: Health care professionals and students reading a patient's chart can learn a great deal about the clinical manifestations of health problems, effective treatment modalities, and factors that affect patient goal achievement.

**g.** Credentialing, regulation, and legislation: Documentation allows reviewers to monitor health care providers' and the health care facility's compliance with standards governing the profession and provision of care.

**h.** Legal documentation: Patient records are legal documents that may be entered into court proceedings as evidence and play an important role in implicating or absolving health providers charged with improper care.

**i.** Reimbursement: Patient records are used to demonstrate to payers that patients received the intensity and quality of care for which reimbursement is being sought.

**j.** Historical document: Because the notations in patient records are dated, they provide a chronologic account of services provided.

**4. a.** Nurses should identify themselves and the patient and state their relationship to the patient.

**b.** Nurses should report concisely and accurately the change in the patient's condition and what has already been done in response to this change.

**c.** Nurses should report the patient's current vital signs and clinical manifestations.

**d.** Nurses should have the patient record at hand so that knowledgeable responses can be made to the health care provider's inquiries.

**e.** Nurses should record concisely the time and date of the call, what was said to the health care provider, and the health care provider's response and read back any changes to the orders.

**5. a.** Residents respond to individualized care.

**b.** Staff communication becomes more effective.

**c.** Resident and family involvement increases.

**d.** Documentation becomes clearer.

**6.** See table below.

| Documentation Method | Description/Advantages/Disadvantages |
|---|---|
| ***SOURCE-ORIENTED RECORD*** | Each health care group keeps data on its own separate form. Notations are entered chronologically, with most recent entry being nearest the front of the record.<br>**Advantages:** Each discipline can easily find and chart pertinent data.<br>**Disadvantages:** Data are fragmented, making it difficult to track problems chronologically with input from different groups of professionals. |
| ***PROBLEM-ORIENTED MEDICAL RECORDS*** | Organized around a patient's problems; contributes collaboratively to care plan. SOAP is used to organize data entries in the progress notes.<br>**Advantages:** Entire health care team works together in identifying a master list of patient problems and contributes collaboratively to care plan.<br>**Disadvantages:** Some nurses believe that the SOAP method focuses too narrowly on problems and advocate a return to the traditional narrative format. |
| ***PIE—PROBLEM, INTERVENTION, EVALUATION*** | Unique in that it does not develop a care plan; the care plan is incorporated into the progress notes in which problems are identified by a number. A complete assessment is performed and documented at the beginning of each shift.<br>**Advantages:** It promotes continuity of care and saves time since there is no separate care plan.<br>**Disadvantages:** Nurses need to read all the nursing notes to determine problems and planned interventions before initiating care. |
| ***FOCUS CHARTING*** | Its purpose is to bring the focus of care back to the patient and the patient's concerns. A focus column is used that incorporates many aspects of a patient and patient care. The focus may be a patient strength, problem, or need.<br>**Advantages:** Holistic emphasis on the patient and patient's priorities; ease of charting.<br>**Disadvantages:** Some nurses report that DAR categories (Data, Action, Response) are artificial and not helpful when documenting care. |

| Documentation Method | Description/Advantages/Disadvantages |
|---|---|
| ***CHARTING BY EXCEPTION*** | Shorthand documentation method that makes use of well-defined standards of practice; only significant findings or "exceptions" to these standards are documented in the narrative notes.<br>**Advantages:** Decreased charting time, greater emphasis on significant data, easy retrieval of significant data, timely bedside charting, standardized assessment, greater communication, better tracking of important responses, and lower costs.<br>**Disadvantages:** None noted. |
| ***CASE MANAGEMENT MODEL*** | Interdisciplinary documentation tools clearly identify those outcomes that select groups of patients are expected to achieve on each day of care. Collaborative pathway is part of a computerized system that integrates the collaborative pathway and documentation flowsheets designed to match each day's expected outcomes.<br>**Advantages:** Reduced charting time by 40% and increased staff satisfaction with the amount of paperwork from 0% to 85%.<br>**Disadvantages:** Works best for "typical" patients with few individualized needs. |
| ***OCCURRENCE OR VARIANCE CHARTING*** | Variances from the plan are documented; for example, when a patient fails to meet an expected outcome or a planned intervention is not implemented in the case management model.<br>**Advantages:** Decreased charting time; only variances are charted.<br>**Disadvantages:** Loss of individualized care. |
| ***ELECTRONIC HEALTH RECORDS*** | Comprehensive computer systems have revolutionized nursing documentation in the patient record.<br>**Advantages:** The nurse can call up the admission assessment tool and key in the patient data, develop the care plan using computerized care plans, add new data to the patient data base, receive a work list showing treatments, procedures, and medications, and document care immediately.<br>**Disadvantages:** Policies should specify what type of patient information can be retrieved, by whom, and for what purpose (privacy). |

## APPLYING YOUR KNOWLEDGE

### REFLECTIVE PRACTICE: CULTIVATING QSEN COMPETENCIES

#### Sample Answers

1. What should be the focus of discharge teaching for Mr. Baron and his wife?
   The nurse should provide a report of Mr. Baron's condition and care that concisely summarizes all the patient data that his wife will need to provide immediate care. In this case, Mr. Baron's medication administration and any follow-up appointments should be discussed and written in the discharge summary.
2. What would be a successful outcome for this patient?
   Mr. Baron and his wife describe the medication dosage and frequency and state the date and time of a follow-up appointment.
3. What intellectual, technical, interpersonal, and/or ethical/legal competencies are most likely to bring about the desired outcome?
   Intellectual: knowledge of colonoscopy as a diagnostic measure and need for follow-up
   Interpersonal: ability to demonstrate that what matters is communicating the care plan so that coordination of care is achieved
   Ethical/Legal: ability to incorporate ethical and legal principles that guide decision making related to a patient needing discharge teaching
4. What resources might be helpful for Mr. Baron?
   Discharge teaching including medication administration and follow-up appointments

## PRACTICING FOR NCLEX

### MULTIPLE CHOICE QUESTIONS

| | | | | |
|---|---|---|---|---|
| **1.** d | **2.** d | **3.** c | **4.** a | **5.** b |
| **6.** b | **7.** c | **8.** a | **9.** c | **10.** c |

### ALTERNATE-FORMAT QUESTIONS

#### Multiple Response Questions

1. a, d, f
2. a, b, e, f
3. c, d, f
4. b, d, e
5. b, e, f

# CHAPTER 20

## ASSESSING YOUR UNDERSTANDING

### FILL IN THE BLANKS

1. clinical information system
2. electronic health record
3. informatics
4. superuser
5. usability
6. portal
7. data visualization
8. Big data

### MATCHING EXERCISES

| | | | | |
|---|---|---|---|---|
| **1.** p | **2.** j | **3.** a | **4.** d | **5.** o |
| **6.** b | **7.** l | **8.** c | **9.** g | **10.** k |
| **11.** n | **12.** e | **13.** m | **14.** f | **15.** h |
| **16.** i | | | | |

### SHORT ANSWER

1. **a.** Improve quality, safety, efficiency, and reduce health disparities.
   **b.** Engage patients and family.
   **c.** Improve care coordination and population and public health.
   **d.** Maintain privacy and security of patient health information.
2. **a.** Better clinical outcomes
   **b.** Improved population health outcomes
   **c.** Increased transparency and efficiency
   **d.** Empowered people
   **e.** More robust research data on health systems
3. **a.** Data: Discrete entities that are described without interpretation
   **b.** Information: Data that have been interpreted, organized, or structured
   **c.** Knowledge: Information that is synthesized so that relationships are identified
   **d.** Wisdom: Appropriate use of knowledge to manage and solve human problems
4. Sample Answers
   **a.** Analyze and plan: The nurse questions the advantages and disadvantages of switching to an electric health record and how it will affect the current workflow of the nurse. The nurse then analyzes the data and strategizes with colleagues to help implement the change.
   **b.** Design: The nurse helps to design a new work area that incorporates the use of new computers to create and access electronic health records.
   **c.** Test: The nurse collaborates with co-workers to create a testing plan that includes the use of testing scripts to ensure all components of the system are working as designed.
   **d.** Train: The head nurse schedules an in-service to train all employees involved in the use of EHRs. The nurse incorporates the five steps of ADDIE (analysis, design, development, implementation, and evaluation), in the training development process.
   **e.** Implement: The nurse ensures all testing and training has been completed, end users have been educated, and support resources are ready for any questions that arise prior to "flipping the switch." Nurse superusers are available to assist if help is needed.
   **f.** Maintain: The nurse oversees the new technology and keeps the system up and running through the allocation of resources and attention to detail.
   **g.** Evaluate: The nurse takes steps to evaluate the effectiveness of the EHR and how it has improved the practice. (Refer to Table 20-3.)
5. **a.** Usability: The extent to which a product can be used by specified users to achieve specified goals with effectiveness, efficiency, and satisfaction in a specified context of use. Making clinical systems easy to use, intuitive, and supportive of nurses' workflow is what usability is all about. Comprehensive tools for usability evaluation can be found through a number of sources both internal and external to the health care IT industry. (Refer to Box 20-2.)
   **b.** Optimization: Strategies to improve processes, maximize effective use, reduce errors, reduce costs, eliminate workflow inefficiencies, improve clinical decision support, and improve end-user skills and satisfaction with the system. Nurses in all settings can participate in organization-wide committees that discuss and make recommendations for improvements to the system.
   **c.** Standard terminologies: Nursing terminologies identify, define, and code care delivery concepts in an organized structure to represent nursing knowledge. Without the ability to aggregate and analyze data entered into the EHR, it is a challenge to represent nursing's contribution to patient outcomes and to the organization's bottom line. (Refer to Table 20-5 for a list of terminologies recognized by the ANA.)
   **d.** Interoperability: The ability of a system to exchange electronic health information with, and use electronic health information from other systems without special effort on the part of the user. This means that all people, their families, and health care providers should be able to send, receive, find, and use electronic health information in a manner that is appropriate, secure, timely, and reliable to support the health and wellness of people through informed, shared decision making. With the right information available at the right time, people and caregivers can be active partners and participants in their health and care.
   **e.** Security and privacy: Nurses are responsible to minimize the risk of harm to patients and providers through both system effectiveness and individual performance. Ensuring secure and

appropriate access to clinical systems starts with good management of passwords. Guidelines for keeping electronic systems secure with strong passwords can be found in Box 20-3.

**6.** **a.** Better health outcomes
**b.** Chronic condition management
**c.** Timely access to care
**d.** Patient retention
**e.** Patient-centered medical home recognition

**7.** **a.** Telehealth: continuing medical education, provider training
**b.** Telecare: exercise tracking tool, medication reminder systems
**c.** Telemedicine: conducting diagnostic tests, accessing specialists not from the patient's geographical area

## APPLYING YOUR KNOWLEDGE

### REFLECTIVE PRACTICE: CULTIVATING QSEN COMPETENCIES

1. What should be the focus of an evaluation of Frank's nursing care plan. How can informatics be of help in this case?
   The nurse should focus on the fact that Frank is not receiving the home care he needs to manage his condition. Frank would be identified as high risk based on population health analytic tools and appropriate referrals could be made.
2. What would be a successful outcome for this patient?
   After receiving home health care visits, Frank states that he is taking his medicine daily, is eating regular meals, and his activity level has increased.
3. What intellectual, technical, interpersonal, and/or ethical/legal competencies are most likely to bring about the desired outcome?
   Intellectual: knowledge of the effects of COPD on the body and methods to alleviate the symptoms of COPD
   Technical: ability to use informatics technology to identify Frank as a high-risk patient
   Interpersonal: ability to work with Frank in a trusting relationship to help him receive the care and services he needs
4. What resources might be helpful for Frank?
   Home health care services, social services, respiratory therapist visits

## PRACTICING FOR NCLEX

### MULTIPLE CHOICE QUESTIONS

| | | |
|---|---|---|
| **1.** d | **2.** c | **3.** b |
| **4.** b | **5.** a | **6.** a |

### Multiple Response Questions

1. a, b, e
2. b, e

### Prioritization Questions

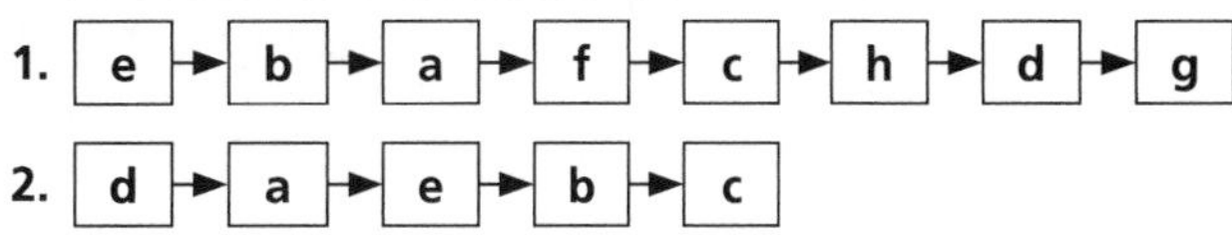


# CHAPTER 21

## ASSESSING YOUR UNDERSTANDING

### FILL IN THE BLANKS

1. proximodistal development
2. genital
3. stage 1, Intuitive-Projective Faith
4. middle adult years
5. libido
6. assimilation
7. formal operational
8. self; roles

### MATCHING EXERCISES

| | | | | |
|---|---|---|---|---|
| **1.** d | **2.** a | **3.** f | **4.** e | **5.** h |
| **6.** e | **7.** g | **8.** c | **9.** b | **10.** g |
| **11.** e | **12.** c | **13.** f | **14.** a | **15.** d |
| **16.** b | | | | |

### CORRECT THE FALSE STATEMENTS

1. True
2. False—regular and predictable
3. False—different
4. True
5. False—id
6. True
7. True
8. False—preconventional level, stage 1, punishment and obedience orientation
9. False—29 to 34

### SHORT ANSWER

1. See table below.

| Theorist and Theory | Basic Concepts of Theory | Stages of Development |
|---|---|---|
| ***EXAMPLE***<br>**Sigmund Freud**<br>Psychoanalytic theory | Stressed the impact of instinctual drives on determining behavior: unconscious mind, the id, the ego, the superego, stages of development based on sexual motivation. | Oral stage<br>Anal stage<br>Phallic stage<br>Latent stage<br>Genital stage |

*(Continued)*

| Theorist and Theory | Basic Concepts of Theory | Stages of Development |
|---|---|---|
| **Erik Erikson**<br>Psychosocial theory | Based on Freud, expanded to include cultural and social influences in addition to biologic processes:<br>(1) stages of development,<br>(2) developmental goals or tasks,<br>(3) psychosocial crises,<br>(4) process of coping. | Trust vs. mistrust<br>Autonomy vs. shame/doubt<br>Initiative vs. guilt<br>Industry vs. inferiority<br>Identity vs. role confusion<br>Intimacy vs. isolation<br>Generativity vs. stagnation<br>Ego integrity vs. despair |
| **Robert J. Havighurst**<br>Developmental tasks | Living and growing are based on learning; person must continually learn to adjust to changing social conditions, developmental tasks. | Infancy and early childhood<br>Middle childhood<br>Adolescence<br>Young adulthood<br>Middle adulthood<br>Later maturity |
| **Roger Gould**<br>Psychosocial development | Gould studied men and women between the ages of 16 and 60 years, labeling the central theme for the adult years as "transformation," with specific beliefs and developmental phases. | Ages 18 to 22<br>Ages 22 to 28<br>Ages 29 to 34<br>Ages 35 to 43<br>Ages 43 to 50<br>Ages 50 to 60 |
| **Daniel Levinson**<br>Moral development | Levinson and associates (1978) based their theory on the organizing concept of "individual life structure." The theory centered on the belief that the pattern of life at any point in time is formed by the interaction of three components: the self (values, motives), the social and cultural aspects of one's life (family, career, religion, ethnic background), and the particular set of roles in which one participates (husband, father, friend, student). | Early adult transition<br>Entering the adult world<br>Settling down<br>Midlife transition<br>The pay-off years |
| **Jean Piaget**<br>Cognitive development | Learning occurs as result of internal organization of an event, which forms a mental schemata and serves as a base for further schemata as one grows and develops. | Sensorimotor stage<br>Preoperational stage<br>Concrete operational stage<br>Formal operational stage |
| **Lawrence Kohlberg**<br>Moral development | Levels closely follow Piaget's; preconventional level, conventional level, postconventional level; moral development influenced by cultural effects on perceptions of justice or interpersonal relationships. | Preconventional level<br>Stage 1: punishment and obedience orientation<br>Stage 2: instrumental relativist orientation conventional level<br>Stage 3: "good boy–good girl" orientation<br>Stage 4: "law and order" orientation<br>Postconventional level<br>Stage 5: social contract, utilitarian orientation<br>Stage 6: universal ethical principle orientation |
| **Carol Gilligan**<br>Moral development | Conception of morality from female point of view (ethic of care); selfishness, goodness, nonviolence; female: morality of response and care; male: morality of justice. | Level 1—selfishness<br>Level 2—goodness<br>Level 3—nonviolence |
| **James Fowler**<br>Faith development | Theory of spiritual identity of humans; faith is reason one finds life worth living; six stages of faith. | Intuitive–projective faith<br>Mythical–literal faith<br>Synthetic–conventional faith<br>Individuative–reflective faith<br>Conjunctive faith<br>Universalizing faith |

2. a. Preconventional level: Follows intuitive thought and is based on external control as child learns to conform to rules imposed by authority figures. Example: Child learns that he will be sent to his room if he writes on the walls.
   b. Conventional level: This level is obtained when a person becomes concerned with identifying with significant others and shows conformity to their expectations. Example: A college student gets all A's in college so his parents will think he is a good son.
   c. Postconventional level: This level is associated with moral judgment that is rational and internalized into one's standards or values. Example: A bank teller resists the urge to steal money from a customer's account because it is against the law.
3. Sample answers:
   a. Freud: The 6-year-old is between the phallic and latency stage and will be experiencing increased interest in biologic sex differences and conflict and resolution of that conflict with parent of same sex.
   b. Erikson: The 6-year-old is becoming achievement oriented, and the acceptance of parents and peers is paramount.
   c. Havighurst: The 6-year-old is ready to learn the developmental tasks of developing physical skills, wholesome attitudes toward self, getting along with peers, sexual roles, conscience, morality, personal independence, etc. An illness could stall these processes.
   d. Piaget: The 6-year-old is in the preoperational stage, including increased language skills and play activities allowing child to better understand life events and relationships.
   e. Kohlberg: Moral development is influenced by cultural effects on perceptions of justice in interpersonal relationships. Moral development begins in early childhood and could be affected by a traumatic illness.
   f. Gilligan: Females develop a morality of response and care, level one being selfishness: a woman may tend to isolate herself to avoid getting hurt.
   g. Fowler: The 6-year-old is in stage 1—intuitive–projective faith. Children imitate the religious gestures and behaviors of others, primarily their parents, without a thorough understanding of them.
4. a. Superego
   b. Identity versus role confusion
   c. Formal operations stage
   d. Synthetic–conventional faith
5. Sample answer:
   The family plays a vital role in wellness promotion and illness prevention. Family values and cultural heritage influence interpretation of illness. A health problem of any family member can affect the remainder of the unit. Many health practices are shared by the family. Sometimes, the family may be the cause of illness.

## APPLYING YOUR KNOWLEDGE

### REFLECTIVE PRACTICE: CULTIVATING QSEN COMPETENCIES

#### Sample Answers

1. What developmental considerations may affect care planning for Mr. Logan?
   According to Havighurst, the developmental tasks of later adulthood include adjusting to decreasing physical strength and health, adjusting to retirement and reduced income, and establishing physical living arrangements. The nurse should assess Mr. Logan's self-esteem needs related to his feelings of dependency on health care providers and his family. The nurse could then base the nursing care plan on interventions to foster feelings of personal dignity and worth.
2. What would be a successful outcome for this patient?
   Mr. Logan states that he is willing to participate in his care plan and do everything in his power to adjust to his situation by accepting the assistance of others when necessary.
3. What intellectual, technical, interpersonal, and/or ethical/legal competencies are most likely to bring about the desired outcome?
   Intellectual: ability to apply knowledge of developmental theories to nurse care planning
   Technical: ability to provide technical nursing assistance to Mr. Logan as needed
   Interpersonal: ability to use therapeutic communication to meet the emotional and spiritual needs of Mr. Logan
   Ethical/Legal: ability to advocate for the unmet developmental needs of Mr. Logan
4. What resources might be helpful for Mr. Logan and his family?
   Home health care services, community services, support groups

## PRACTICING FOR NCLEX

### MULTIPLE CHOICE QUESTIONS

| | | | | |
|---|---|---|---|---|
| 1. a | 2. b | 3. a | 4. c | 5. b |
| 6. c | 7. c | 8. d | 9. a | |

### ALTERNATE-FORMAT QUESTIONS

#### Multiple Response Questions

1. b, d, e
2. a, c, d
3. b, d, e
4. a, c, f

#### Prioritization Questions

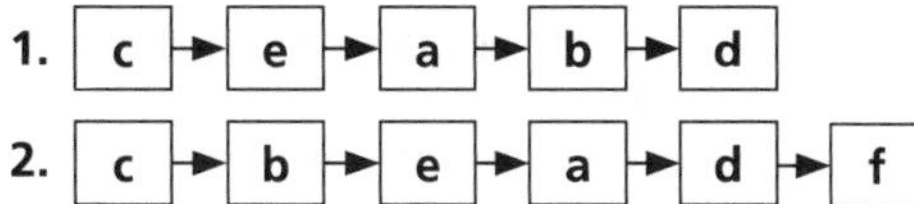

# CHAPTER 22

## ASSESSING YOUR UNDERSTANDING

### FILL IN THE BLANKS

1. endoderm
2. embryonic
3. Apgar
4. bonding
5. failure to thrive (FTT)
6. sudden infant death syndrome (SIDS)
7. Denver Developmental Screening Test (DDST)

### MATCHING EXERCISES

| | | | |
|---|---|---|---|
| **1.** f | **2.** d | **3.** d | **4.** f |
| **5.** a | **6.** c | **7.** b | **8.** e |

### SHORT ANSWER

1. Age group—Physiologic characteristics and behaviors
   P—Motor abilities include skipping, throwing and catching, copying figures, and printing letters and numbers.
   A—Puberty begins.
   I—Brain grows to about half the adult size.
   N—Reflexes include sucking, swallowing, blinking, sneezing, and yawning.
   N—Temperature control responds quickly to environmental temperatures.
   T—Walks forward and backward, runs, kicks, climbs, and rides tricycle.
   T—Drinks from a cup and uses a spoon.
   A—Sebaceous and axillary sweat glands become active.
   S—Height increases 2 to 3 in, weight increases 3 to 6 lb a year.
   A—The feet, hands, and long bones grow rapidly; muscle mass increases.
   N—Alert to environment, sees color and form, hears and turns to sound.
   I—Birth weight usually triples.
   P—Full set of 20 deciduous teeth; baby teeth fall out and are replaced.
   P—Body is less chubby and becomes leaner and more coordinated.
   A—Primary and secondary development occurs with maturation of genitals.
   T—Typically four times the birth weight and 23 to 37 in in height.
   I—Body temperature stabilizes.
   P—Average weight is 45 lb.
   S—Brain reaches 90% to 95% of adult size; nervous system almost mature.
   P—Head is close to adult size.
   I—Motor abilities develop, allowing feeding self, crawling, and walking.
   N—Can smell and taste and is sensitive to touch and pain.
   N—Begins to eliminate stool and urine.
   I—Deciduous teeth begin to erupt.
   S—All permanent teeth present except for second and third molars.
   T—Attains bladder control during the day and sometimes during the night.
   S—Holds a pencil and eventually writes in script and sentences.
   A—Full adult size is reached.
   N—Drinks breast milk, glucose water, and plain water.
   I—Eyes begin to focus and fixate.
   T—Turns pages in a book and by age 3 draws stick people.
   I—Heart doubles in weight, heart rate slows, blood pressure rises.
   T—Rapid brain growth; increase in length of long bones of the arms and legs.
   T—Uses fingers to pick up small objects.
   S—Sexual organs grow but are dormant until late in this period.
2. Age group—Psychosocial characteristics and behaviors
   I—Is in oral stage (Freud); strives for immediate gratification of needs; strong sucking need.
   S—Developmental task of learning appropriate sex's social role.
   A—In Freud's genital stage, libido reemerges in mature form.
   T—Is in anal stage (Freud); focus on pleasure of sphincter control.
   A—Self-concept is being stabilized, with peer group as greatest influence.
   I—Develops trust (Erikson) if caregiver is dependable to meet needs.
   S—Achieves personal independence; develops conscience, morality, and scale of values.
   A—Tries out different roles, personal choices, and beliefs (identity versus role confusion).
   I—Meets developmental tasks (Havighurst) by learning to eat, walk, and talk.
   S—Develops skill in reading, writing, and calculating, as well as concepts for everyday living.
   A—More mature relationships with both males and females of same age.
   T—Enters Erikson's stage of autonomy versus shame and doubt.
   P—Is in Erikson's stage of initiative versus guilt.
   A—Inner turmoil/examination of propriety of actions by rigid conscience.
   P—Getting ready to read and learning to distinguish right from wrong.
   A—One's personal appearance accepted; set of values internalized.
   S—Freud's latency stage—strong identification with own sex.
   T—Developmental tasks of learning to control elimination; begins to learn sex differences, concepts, learn language, learn right from wrong.
   P—Focus on learning useful skills with an emphasis on doing, succeeding, and accomplishing.
   P—Developmental tasks of describing social and physical reality through concept formation and language development.

P—Is in phallic stage (Freud) with biologic focus on genitals.
A—Superego and conscience begin to develop.
P—Developmental tasks of learning sex differences and modesty.
S—Developmental task of learning physical game skills.
S—Is in Erikson's industry versus inferiority stage.

3. **a.** Pre-embryonic stage: Lasts about 3 weeks; zygote implants in the uterine wall and has three distinct cell layers: ectoderm, endoderm, and mesoderm.
   **b.** Embryonic stage: fourth to eighth week; rapid growth and differentiation of the germ cell layers, all basic organs established, bones ossify, and human features are recognizable.
   **c.** Fetal stage: 9 weeks to birth; continued growth and development of all body organs and systems take place.
4. **a.** Gross motor behavior and skills
   **b.** Fine motor behavior and skills
   **c.** Language acquisition
   **d.** Personal and social interaction
5. Sample answers:
   **a.** Infant sleeps, eats, and eliminates easily; smiles spontaneously; cries in response to significant needs.
   **b.** Infant is more passive and distant than the "easy" infant.
   **c.** Infant has volatile and labile responses, often is restless sleeper, is highly sensitive to noises and eats poorly.
6. **a.** Colic is inconsolable crying or fussing in an infant that lasts more than 3 hours, occurs more than 3 days per week, and lasts for more than 3 weeks, although the more-than-3-weeks pattern is not always considered in the determination of colic. Colic durations tend to be high across the first 6 weeks of life (17% to 25%) and then decrease between 6 and 12 weeks of life (11%), then down to 0.6% at 10 to 12 weeks. The nurse should educate the parents about colic and teach them measures to help relieve the symptoms.
   **b.** Failure to thrive is a condition of inadequate growth in height and weight resulting from the infant's inability to obtain or use calories needed for growth. Collection of serial height, weight, and head circumference measurements on a reference scale such as a growth chart are helpful in determining this clinical finding. Underlying physical causes should be ruled out first; if the cause is psychosocial, specialized health interventions are warranted.
   **c.** Sudden infant death syndrome (SIDS) refers to the sudden death of an infant under the age of 1 year when consideration of the infant's history, a postmortem examination, and investigation of the scene where the death occurred fails to reveal a cause of death. Sudden unexpected infant death syndrome (SUID) is an all-encompassing term used for sudden, unexplained infant deaths where the cause of death cannot readily be identified prior to an investigation The rate of infant deaths attributed to SIDS has declined significantly since the early 1990s when the Safe to Sleep campaign promoted placing infants on their back to sleep rather than in the prone position.
   **d.** Child abuse and neglect is any recent act or failure to act on the part of a parent or caretaker which results in death, serious physical or emotional harm, sexual abuse or exploitation; or an act or failure to act which presents an imminent risk of serious harm. Health care professionals must recognize and report abuse of children and provide interventions for high-risk families.
7. Sample answers:
   **a.** Toddler: A toddler begins to understand object permanence, following simple commands and anticipating events. The perception of body image begins, and the toddler uses short sentences. The nurse should be aware that the toddler may experience separation anxiety; parents should be included in the preparation; language should be clear and simple.
   **b.** Preschooler: A preschooler may have fear of pain and body mutilation, as well as separation anxiety that must be recognized by the nurse. The child needs much reassurance and parental support. A preprocedure visit should be scheduled if possible; allowing the child to practice on a doll may be helpful.
   **c.** School-aged child: Body image, self-concept, and sexuality are interrelated. The school-aged child has well-developed language skills and ability to store information in long-term memory. The procedure should be explained clearly and thoroughly to child and caregivers.
   **d.** Adolescent and young adult: The adolescent tries out different roles, personal choices, and beliefs in the stage called identity versus role confusion. Self-concept is being stabilized, with the peer group acting as the influential body. The nurse should be aware of the adolescent's need to understand the procedure and its benefits/risks.
8. Sample answers:
   **a.** Infant: The most important role of the nurse is the prevention of illness and promotion of wellness through teaching family members. Teaching may range from scheduling immunizations to counseling parents who have a baby born with AIDS.
   **b.** Toddler: The role of the nurse is in wellness promotion, helping caregivers find the means of helping toddlers through encouraging independence while setting firm limits. Safety measures for parents of active toddlers should be taught.
   **c.** Preschooler: Promoting wellness continues for the preschooler, with emphasis on teaching accident prevention and safety, infection control, dental hygiene, and play habits and encouraging self-esteem.

d. School-aged child: Areas of concern for school-aged children are traffic, bicycle, and water safety. Substance abuse teaching should be included, and communicable conditions should be discussed. Nurses should work with parents and teachers to recognize mental health disorders and to encourage physical fitness and positive self-identity.
e. Adolescent and young adult: Nurses should educate adolescents and family members about substance abuse, motor vehicle accidents, nutrition, and sex. Nurses and parents should be aware of the adolescent's need to belong to a peer group, be like everyone else, and try on different roles.

9. a. Prepubescence: Secondary sex characteristics begin to develop, but the reproductive organs do not yet function.
b. Pubescence: Secondary sex characteristics continue to develop, and ova and sperm begin to be produced by the reproductive organs.
c. Postpubescence: Reproductive functioning and secondary sex characteristics reach adult maturity.

## APPLYING YOUR KNOWLEDGE

### REFLECTIVE PRACTICE: CULTIVATING QSEN COMPETENCIES

#### Sample Answers

1. What should be the focus of the nursing care plan developed for Ms. Jenkins?
The immediate focus should be the health habits of the mother and their effect on the fetus.
Ms. Jenkin's nursing care plan should include patient teaching regarding the detrimental effects of smoking and drinking alcohol on the fetus and the necessity to control nausea and eat a proper diet.
Ms. Jenkins could benefit from a referral to counseling and/or social services.
2. What would be a successful outcome for this patient?
By end of visit, Ms. Jenkins states that she values her health and the health of her fetus enough to stop smoking and drinking alcohol.
By next visit, Ms. Jenkins reports that her nausea is under control and she is able to eat three healthy meals a day.
3. What intellectual, technical, interpersonal, and/or ethical/legal competencies are most likely to bring about the desired outcome?
Intellectual: knowledge of the developmental needs of fetuses and the effects of maternal behaviors, such as smoking and alcohol consumption on the fetus
Technical: ability to provide the technical nursing assistance necessary to assess and meet the needs of a pregnant woman and her fetus
Interpersonal: ability to demonstrate nonjudgmental attitude when interacting in potentially emotionally charged situations, such as a high-risk pregnancy
Ethical/Legal: knowledge of the nurse's legal and ethical obligations in cases of maternal–fetal conflict
4. What resources might be helpful for Ms. Jenkins?
Counseling services, social services, community services, support groups, printed materials on healthy pregnancy behaviors

## PRACTICING FOR NCLEX

### MULTIPLE CHOICE QUESTIONS

| | | | | |
|---|---|---|---|---|
| 1. c | 2. b | 3. a | 4. b | 5. c |
| 6. b | 7. b | 8. a | 9. c | 10. b |
| 11. d | | | | |

### ALTERNATE-FORMAT QUESTIONS

#### Multiple Response Questions

1. a, d, e, f
2. b, c, e
3. b, d, e
4. a, b, e
5. a, c, e, f
6. a, b, f

#### Chart/Exhibit Questions

1. 7
2. 3
3. 10

# CHAPTER 23

## ASSESSING YOUR UNDERSTANDING

### FILL IN THE BLANKS

1. cross-linkage; cross links
2. middle
3. generation sandwich
4. 60 to 74, 75 to 84, 85 and older
5. ageism
6. identity-continuity
7. life review, reminiscence
8. Alzheimer's disease
9. Gerontology

### SHORT ANSWER

1. a. Middle adulthood:
Physiologic development: The early years are marked by maximum physical development and functioning. As time passes, gradual internal and external changes occur.
Psychosocial development: Usually a time of increased personal freedom, economic stability, social relationships, increased responsibility, and awareness of one's own mortality.
Cognitive, moral, and spiritual development: Intellectual abilities change from those of the young adult. There is increased motivation to learn. Problem-solving abilities remain, although response time may be slightly longer.

b. Older adulthood:
   Physiologic development: The process of aging becomes more rapid. All organ systems undergo some degree of decline, and the body becomes less efficient.
   Psychosocial development: Most continue their activities from middle adulthood and adapt intuitively to gradual limitations of aging.
   Cognitive, moral, and spiritual development: Cognition does not change appreciably with aging; an older adult continues to learn and solve problems, and intelligence and personality remain consistent.

2. Sample answers:
   a. Physical examination every year
   b. Pelvic examination with Pap test every 5 years for women
   c. Eye examination with test for glaucoma every 1 to 2 years
   d. Maintenance of current immunizations
   e. Cancer screening for men and women
3. a. Genetic theory: Explains that lifespan depends to a great extent on genetic factors.
   b. Immunity theory: Focuses on the functions of the immune system, which declines steadily after young adulthood.
   c. Cross-linkage theory: As one ages, cross-links accumulate, leading to essential molecules in the cell binding together and interfering with normal cell function.
   d. Free radical theory: The free radical theory is based on oxidative stress. Free radicals, formed during cellular metabolism, are molecules with unpaired, high-energy electrons that seek to combine with another molecule. This electron pairing disrupts cell membranes and affects DNA and protein synthesis. Over time, irreversible damage results from the accumulated effects of this damage. Antioxidants are thought to protect against this type of free radical damage.
   e. Disengagement theory: Maintains that an older adult withdraws from societal interactions because it is mutually desired and satisfying for both the person and society.
   f. Activity theory: Successful aging involves the ability to maintain high levels of activity and functioning.
   g. Identity-continuity theory: Assumes that healthy aging is related to the ability of the older adult to continue similar patterns of behavior that existed in young to middle adulthood.
4. Alzheimer's disease affects brain cells and is characterized by the formation of amyloid plaques and tangles of tau proteins, which have an impact on the brain structure and function in older adults with AD. It is a progressively serious and ultimately fatal disorder. In mild or early AD, forgetfulness and impaired judgment may be evident. Over a period of several years, the person progresses to moderate or middle AD, and becomes progressively more confused, forgetting family and becoming disoriented in familiar surroundings. When the ability to perform simple activities of daily living is lost, and the older adult enters the severe or late stage of AD, the person requires constant supervision and care, often in a long-term care facility.
5. a. Integumentary: Wrinkling and sagging of skin occur with decreased skin elasticity; dryness and scaling are common.
   b. Musculoskeletal: Muscle mass and strength decrease.
   c. Neurologic: Temperature regulation and pain perception become less efficient.
   d. Cardiopulmonary: The body is less able to increase heart rate and cardiac output with activity.
   e. Gastrointestinal: Malnutrition and anemia become more common.
   f. Genitourinary: Blood flow to the kidneys decreases with diminished cardiac output.

## APPLYING YOUR KNOWLEDGE

### REFLECTIVE PRACTICE: CULTIVATING QSEN COMPETENCIES

#### Sample Answers

1. How might the nurse use blended nursing skills to provide holistic, developmentally sensitive care for Mr. and Mrs. Jenkins?
   The nurse should aim to facilitate the Jenkins' achievement of the developmental tasks of older adulthood, such as adjusting to the changes of older adulthood and retirement, relating to one's age group, maintaining social roles, and continuing moral and spiritual development. The Jenkins would benefit from a referral to community services, such as physical fitness programs and social clubs designed for older adults.
2. What would be a successful outcome for this patient?
   By next visit, Mr. Jenkins will report being involved in social and physical activities and drinking less.
3. What intellectual, technical, interpersonal, and/or ethical/legal competencies are most likely to bring about the desired outcome?
   Intellectual: knowledge of the theories of aging as they relate to the changes faced by the aging adult
   Technical: ability to adapt necessary skills and techniques to address the changes associated with the aging adult
   Interpersonal: ability to establish trusting professional relationships with adult patients of different ages, respecting their developmental needs
   Ethical/Legal: ability to practice in an ethically and legally defensible manner, maintaining the rights of the aging adult
4. What resources might be helpful for Mr. and Mrs. Jenkins?
   Community services, social networks, physical fitness programs, nutrition classes

## PRACTICING FOR NCLEX

### MULTIPLE CHOICE QUESTIONS

| | | | | |
|---|---|---|---|---|
| **1.** c | **2.** a | **3.** d | **4.** b | **5.** c |
| **6.** a | **7.** d | **8.** b | **9.** b | |

### ALTERNATE-FORMAT QUESTIONS

#### Multiple Response Questions

**1.** c, e, f
**2.** a, c, d
**3.** c, d, e
**4.** a, c, f

# CHAPTER 24

## ASSESSING YOUR UNDERSTANDING

### FILL IN THE BLANKS

1. Quality and Safety Education for Nurses (QSEN)
2. bacteria
3. aerobic; anaerobic
4. fungi
5. normal flora
6. reservoirs
7. portal of entry
8. antibody
9. health care–associated infection
10. iatrogenic

### MATCHING EXERCISES

| | | | | |
|---|---|---|---|---|
| **1.** k | **2.** f | **3.** a | **4.** b | **5.** j |
| **6.** i | **7.** m | **8.** c | **9.** e | **10.** g |
| **11.** d | **12.** n | **13.** d | **14.** a | **15.** c |
| **16.** b | | | | |

### CORRECT THE FALSE STATEMENTS

1. True
2. True
3. False—Hand hygiene
4. False—Transient bacteria
5. True
6. True
7. True
8. False—surgical asepsis
9. True

### SHORT ANSWER

1. **a.** Number of organisms
   **b.** Virulence of the organism
   **c.** Competence of a person's immune system
   **d.** Length and intimacy (extent) of the contact between a person and the microorganism
2. Sample answers:
   **a.** Other humans: Tuberculosis
   **b.** Animals: Rabies
   **c.** Soil: Gas gangrene
3. **a.** Gastrointestinal
   **b.** Genitourinary tracts
   **c.** Blood and tissue
4. Sample answers:
   **a.** Direct contact: transmission of disease through touching, kissing, or sexual contact
   **b.** Indirect contact: personal contact with contaminated blood, food, water, etc.
   **c.** Vectors: mosquitoes, ticks, and lice transmit organisms from one host to another
   **d.** Fomite: an inanimate object, such as equipment or countertops
   **e.** Airborne: spread of droplet nuclei through coughing, sneezing, or talking
5. **a.** Inflammatory response: A protective mechanism that eliminates the invading pathogen and allows tissue repair to occur.
   **b.** Immune response: Involves specific reactions in the body as it responds to an invading foreign protein such as bacteria or, in some cases, the body's own proteins. The body responds to an antigen by producing an antibody.
6. **a.** Intact skin and mucous membranes protect the body against microbial invasion.
   **b.** The normal pH levels of gastric secretions and of the genitourinary tract help to ward off microbial invasion.
   **c.** The body's white blood cells influence resistance to certain pathogens.
   **d.** Age, sex, race, and hereditary factors influence susceptibility.
7. **a.** Assessing: Early detection and surveillance techniques are critical. The nurse should inquire about immunization status and previous or recurring infections, observe nonverbal cues, and obtain the history of the current disease.
   **b.** Diagnosing: The direction or focus of nursing care depends on a nursing diagnosis that accurately reflects the patient's condition.
   **c.** Planning: Effective nursing interventions can control or prevent infection. Nurses should review assessment data and consider the cycle of events that results in infection control as patient goals are formulated.
   **d.** Implementing: The nurse uses principles of aseptic technique to halt the spread of microorganisms and minimize the threat of infection.
   **e.** Evaluating: The nurse can intervene in, and improve, a patient's outcome by assessing the person at risk, selecting appropriate nursing diagnoses, planning and intervening to maintain a safe environment, and evaluating the care plan to determine whether it is working.
8. Sample answers:
   **a.** Patient's home: Wash hands before preparing food and before eating; use individual personal care items such as washcloths, towels, and toothbrushes.
   **b.** Public facilities: Wash hands after using any public bathroom; use individually wrapped drinking straws.

c. Community: Use sterilized combs and brushes in beauty and barber shops; examine food handlers for evidence of disease.
d. Health care facility: Use standard aseptic techniques to prevent further spread of a present organism and prevent nosocomial infections.

9. a. Instituting constant surveillance by infection control committees and nurse epidemiologists
b. Having written infection prevention practices for all facility personnel
c. Using practices that help promote the best possible physical condition in patients

10. a. Nature of organisms present: Some organisms are easily destroyed, whereas others can withstand certain commonly used sterilization and disinfection methods.
b. Number of organisms present: The more organisms present on an item, the longer it takes to destroy them.
c. Type of equipment: Equipment with narrow lumens, crevices, or joints requires special care. Certain items may be damaged by sterilization methods.
d. Intended use of equipment: The need for medical or surgical asepsis influences the methods used in the preparation and cleaning of equipment.
e. Available means for sterilization and disinfection: The choice of chemical or physical means of sterilization and disinfection takes into consideration the availability and practicality of the means.
f. Time: Time is a key factor. Failure to observe recommended time periods for disinfection and sterilization significantly increases the risk for infection and is grossly negligent.

11. a. Hospital: The infection control nurse is responsible for educating patients and staff about effective infection control techniques and for collecting statistics about infections.
b. Home care setting: The infection control nurse's duties include surveillance for facility-associated infections, as well as education, consultation, performance of epidemiologic investigations and quality improvement activities, and policy and procedure development.

12. a. Risk for Infection related to altered skin integrity/burns.
b. Effective nursing interventions can control or prevent infection. The nurse should review patient data, consider the cycle of events that result in the development of an infection, and incorporate infection control as a patient goal.

13. Use standard precautions for the care of all patients in the ER. The additional concern with TB necessitates using airborne precautions in addition to standard precautions. According to CDC guidelines, either a high-efficiency particulate air (HEPA) filter respirator or N95 respirator certified by NIOSH must be worn when entering the room of a patient with known or suspected tuberculosis.

## APPLYING YOUR KNOWLEDGE

### REFLECTIVE PRACTICE: CULTIVATING QSEN COMPETENCIES

#### Sample Answers

1. How might the nurse respond to Ms. Turheis in a holistic manner that respects her human dignity, while at the same time maintaining a safe environment for her?
Patients in isolation may suffer from sensory deprivation, and loss of self-esteem may occur. The nurse can reinforce Ms. Turheis's self-identity by using looks, speech, and judicious touch to communicate worth, speaking to her respectfully, spending time in conversations with her about her life experiences, and allowing her to express negative feelings. The nurse can then help Ms. Turheis to recognize her strengths and explore other options to fulfill her self-esteem needs.
2. What would be a successful outcome for Ms. Turheis?
By next visit, Ms. Turheis will report feeling better about her situation and will state three positive experiences that occurred in the last week.
3. What intellectual, technical, interpersonal, and/or ethical/legal competencies are most likely to bring about the desired outcome?
Intellectual: knowledge of the effects of isolation on the self-esteem of patients and interventions to minimize these effects
Technical: ability to use appropriate infection control precautions and barrier techniques for infection prevention
Interpersonal: ability to communicate care and compassion to patients requiring infection control precautions
Ethical/Legal: demonstration of a commitment to safety and quality; strong advocacy abilities
4. What resources might be helpful for Ms. Turheis?
Referral to counseling services, home health care visits

## PRACTICING FOR NCLEX

### MULTIPLE CHOICE QUESTIONS

**1.** b **2.** d **3.** c **4.** b **5.** a
**6.** c **7.** a

### ALTERNATE-FORMAT QUESTIONS

#### Multiple Response Questions

1. a, c, e
2. a, c, d
3. b, d, e
4. a, b, c, f
5. b, d, e
6. a, d, f

**Prioritization Questions**

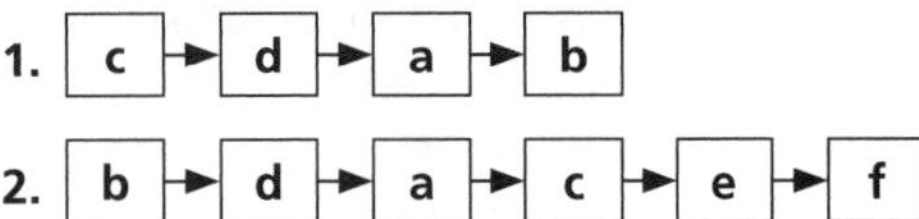


# CHAPTER 25

## ASSESSING YOUR UNDERSTANDING

### FILL IN THE BLANKS

1. heart rate
2. width 9 cm, length 18 cm
3. +1
4. 100°F
5. 102.2°F
6. 37.5°C

## DEVELOPING YOUR KNOWLEDGE BASE

### IDENTIFICATION

1. a. Temporal
   b. Carotid
   c. Brachial
   d. Radial
   e. Femoral
   f. Popliteal
   g. Posterior tibial
   h. Dorsalis pedis

### MATCHING EXERCISES

| | | | | |
|---|---|---|---|---|
| **1.** b | **2.** i | **3.** d | **4.** g | **5.** a |
| **6.** h | **7.** e | **8.** j | **9.** c | **10.** f |
| **11.** l | **12.** h | **13.** d | **14.** a | **15.** f |
| **16.** i | **17.** g | **18.** e | **19.** c | **20.** j |
| **21.** e | **22.** g | **23.** f | **24.** a | **25.** c |
| **26.** d | | | | |

### SHORT ANSWER

1. a. Circadian rhythms: Predictable fluctuations in measurements of body temperature and blood pressure exhibit a circadian rhythm. The blood pressure is usually lowest on arising in the morning. Blood pressure has been noted to rise as much as 5 to 10 mm Hg by late afternoon, and gradually falls again during sleep.
   b. Age: Body temperatures of infants and children respond more rapidly to heat and cold air temperatures than do adults. The older adult loses some thermoregulatory control and is at risk for harm from extremes in temperature.
   c. Biologic sex: Body temperature tends to fluctuate more in women than in men, probably as a result of normal, cyclic fluctuations in the release of their sex hormones.
   d. Stress: The body responds to both physical and emotional stress by increasing the production of epinephrine. As a result, the metabolic rate increases, raising the body temperature.
   e. Environmental temperature: Exposure to extreme cold without adequate protective clothing can result in heat loss severe enough to cause hypothermia. Exposure to extreme heat may result in hyperthermia.
2. See table below.

| Type of Thermometer | Brief Description | Uses/Contraindication | Normal Reading |
|---|---|---|---|
| ***A. ELECTRONIC AND DIGITAL*** | Two nonbreakable probes, disposable probe covers | Measure oral, rectal, or axillary body temperature over a time period from 1 to 60 seconds, depending on the site and product used | Site dependent |
| ***B. TYMPANIC MEMBRANE*** | Infrared sensors detect heat given off by tympanic membrane | Not used for infants to 3 months due to possible tympanic membrane damage | 36.8–37.8°C (98.2–100°F) |
| ***C. DISPOSABLE SINGLE-USE*** | Nonbreakable temperature sensitive tape or patch applied to forehead or abdomen; registers temperature within seconds | Used to screen temperature of toddler or young child | Color changes at different temperature ranges |
| ***D. TEMPORAL ARTERY*** | Forehead or abdomen; changes color at different temperatures | Newborns | 37.1–38.1°C (98.7–100.5°F) |
| ***E. AUTOMATED MONITORING DEVICE*** | Measure body temperature, pulse, and blood pressure automatically | Used in various health care settings to measure body temperature, pulse, respirations, and blood pressure simultaneously | Site dependent |

3. a. The middle three fingers may be used to palpate all peripheral pulse sites.
   b. A stethoscope may be used to auscultate the apical pulse.
   c. Doppler ultrasound may be used to assess pulses that are difficult to palpate or auscultate.
4. a. Pumping action of the heart: When the amount of blood pumped into the arteries increases, the pressure of blood against arterial walls also increases.
   b. Blood volume: When blood volume is low, blood pressure is also low because there is less fluid within the arteries.
   c. Viscosity of blood: The more viscous the blood, the higher the blood pressure.
   d. Elasticity of vessel walls: The elasticity of the walls, in addition to the resistance of the arterioles, helps to maintain normal blood pressure.
5. a. Impaired gas exchange: Excess or deficit in oxygenation and/or carbon dioxide elimination at the alveolar–capillary membrane
   b. Ineffective airway clearance: Inability to clear secretions or obstructions from the respiratory tract to maintain a clear airway
   c. Ineffective breathing pattern: Inspiration and/or expiration that does not provide adequate ventilation
   d. Impaired spontaneous ventilation: A state in which the response pattern of decreased energy reserves results in a person's inability to maintain breathing adequate to support life
6. a. Ineffective peripheral tissue perfusion: A decrease in oxygen, resulting in the failure to nourish the tissues at the capillary level
   b. Risk for deficient fluid volume: A risk for a decrease, increase, or rapid shift from one to the other of intravascular, interstitial, or intracellular fluid
   c. Excess fluid volume: The state in which a person experiences increased isotonic fluid retention
   d. Deficient fluid volume: The state in which a person experiences decreased intravascular, interstitial, or intracellular fluid
   e. Decreased cardiac output: A state in which the blood pumped by the heart is inadequate to meet the metabolic demands of the body
7. a. Stethoscope: Used to auscultate and assess body sounds, including the apical pulse and blood pressure. The acoustical stethoscope has an amplifying mechanism connected to earpieces by tubing.
   b. Sphygmomanometer: Consists of a cuff and the manometer. The cuff contains an airtight, flat, rubber bladder covered with cloth, which is closed around the limb with contact closures. Two tubes are attached to the bladder within the cuff; one is connected to a manometer, the other to a bulb used to inflate the bladder.

## APPLYING YOUR KNOWLEDGE

### REFLECTIVE PRACTICE: CULTIVATING QSEN COMPETENCIES

#### Sample Answers

1. What might be causing Noah's reaction to the nurse's attempt to assess a tympanic temperature?
   Noah may be reacting out of fear of strange people and situations. Noah may also have an earache and, in that case, a tympanic temperature is contraindicated because the movement of the tragus may cause severe discomfort.
2. What would be a successful outcome for Noah?
   Noah exhibits calmness upon examination and allows the nurse to perform necessary assessments.
3. What intellectual, technical, interpersonal, and/or ethical/legal competencies are most likely to bring about the desired outcome?
   Intellectual: knowledge of how to tailor vital signs technology to meet the needs of a 2-year-old
   Technical: ability to correctly use the equipment necessary to assess and document vital signs
   Interpersonal: ability to establish a trusting relationship with children and their families
4. What resources might be helpful for the nurse caring for Noah?
   Stuffed animal to demonstrate the procedures for taking vital signs, knowledge of distraction techniques to use when performing procedures on children

## PRACTICING FOR NCLEX

### MULTIPLE CHOICE QUESTIONS

| | | | | |
|---|---|---|---|---|
| 1. d | 2. c | 3. c | 4. d | 5. b |
| 6. a | 7. d | 8. b | 9. b | |

### ALTERNATE-FORMAT QUESTIONS

#### Multiple Response Questions

1. a, b, e
2. a, e, f
3. b, c, e
4. c, d, f
5. a, d, e
6. a, b, c, d

# CHAPTER 26

## ASSESSING YOUR UNDERSTANDING

### IDENTIFICATION

1. a. Liver
   b. Stomach
   c. Spleen
   d. Transverse colon
   e. Descending colon
   f. Small intestine
   g. Sigmoid colon
   h. Bladder
   i. Appendix

j. Cecum
k. Ascending colon
2. a. Malleus
b. Incus
c. Semicircular canals
d. Facial nerve
e. Cochlear and vestibular branch
f. Cochlea
g. Oval window
h. Round window
i. Eustachian tube
j. Stapes and footplate
k. Tympanic membrane

## MATCHING EXERCISES

| | | | | |
|---|---|---|---|---|
| 1. a | 2. b | 3. a | 4. d | 5. c |
| 6. b | 7. e | 8. d | 9. c | 10. a |
| 11. b | 12. d | 13. c | 14. a | 15. b |
| 16. e | 17. g | 18. d | 19. h | 20. f |
| 21. f | 22. b | 23. d | 24. i | 25. a |
| 26. c | 27. e | 28. g | 29. h | 30. g |
| 31. d | 32. f | 33. a | 34. c | 35. b |
| 36. e | | | | |

## SHORT ANSWER

1. a. Establish a nurse–patient relationship.
b. Gather data about the patient's general health status, integrating physiologic, psychological, cognitive, sociocultural, developmental, and spiritual dimensions.
c. Identify patient strengths.
d. Identify existing and potential health problems.
e. Establish a base for the nursing process.
2. a. Ophthalmoscope: Lighted instrument used for visualization of interior structures of the eye
b. Otoscope: Lighted instrument used for examining external ear canal and tympanic membrane
c. Snellen chart: Screening test for vision
d. Nasal speculum: Instrument that allows visualization of lower and middle turbinates of the nose
e. Vaginal speculum: Two-bladed instrument used to examine vaginal canal and cervix
f. Tuning fork: Two-pronged metal instrument used for testing auditory function and vibratory perception
g. Percussion hammer: Instrument with a rubber head, used to test reflexes and determine tissue density
h. Thermometer and sphygmomanometer: Measure temperature and blood pressure
i. Scale: Weighs and measures patient height
j. Flashlight or penlight: Assists in viewing inside of mouth and nose
k. Stethoscope: Measures blood pressure and auscultates heart, lung, abdomen, and cardiovascular sounds
l. Tape measure and ruler: A tape measure measures waist circumference in adults and head circumference in infants and children. A ruler measures abnormal findings on the skin.
3. a. patient's age
b. patient's cognitive and physical condition and energy level
c. need for privacy
d. time constraints
4. a. Patient: Consider physiologic and psychological needs of the patient. Explain that a physical assessment will be performed by the nurse, that body structures will be examined, and that such assessments are painless. Have patient put on a gown and empty bladder.
b. Environment: The time of the assessment should be mutually agreed on and should not interfere with meals or daily routines. The patient should be as free of pain as possible, and the room should be quiet and private.
5. See table below.

| Technique | Definition | Assessment/Observation |
|---|---|---|
| **a.** Inspection: | Process of deliberate, purposeful observations performed in a systematic manner | Body size, color, shape, position, symmetry, norms, and deviations from norm |
| **b.** Palpation: | Technique that uses sense of touch | Temperature, turgor, texture, moisture, vibrations, shape |
| **c.** Percussion: | The act of striking an object against another object to produce a sound | Location, shape, size, and density of tissues |
| **d.** Auscultation: | The act of listening to sound produced in the body, using stethoscope | Lung and bowel sounds; heart and vascular sounds |

6. a. Pitch—ranging from high to low
b. Loudness—ranging from soft to loud
c. Quality—for example, swishing or gurgling
d. Duration—short, medium, or long
7. a. Edema: Palpate edematous area with the fingers; an indentation may remain after the pressure is released.
b. Dehydration: Pick up the skin in a fold; when dehydration exists, normal elasticity and fullness are decreased, and skin fold returns to normal slowly.
8. a. Pupillary reaction: Ask patient to look straight ahead, bring the penlight from side of patient's face, and shine the light on one of the pupils.

Observe pupil's reaction; normally it will constrict. Repeat procedure in the same eye and observe the other eye—normally it too will constrict. Repeat the entire procedure with the other eye.

**b.** Accommodation: Hold the forefinger about 10 to 15 cm in front of the bridge of the patient's nose. Ask the patient to first look at the forefinger, then at a distant object, then the forefinger again. Normally, the pupil constricts when the patient looks at the finger and dilates when he or she looks at a distant object.

**c.** Convergence: Hold a finger about 6 to 8 in from the bridge of the patient's nose and move finger toward eyes. Normally, the patient's eyes converge (assume cross-eyed appearance).

**9.** Equipment: Vials of aromatic substances, visual acuity chart, penlight, sharp object, cotton balls, vials of solution to test taste, tuning fork, tongue depressor, reflex hammer, and familiar objects. Position: sitting.

**10.** Sample answers:
- **a.** Orientation: What is today's date?
- **b.** Immediate memory: What did you eat for lunch today?
- **c.** Past memory: When is your wedding anniversary?
- **d.** Abstract reasoning: Explain the proverb "a stitch in time, saves nine."
- **e.** Language: Would you read this passage from this book?

**11.** **a.** lub; **b.** mitral; **c.** tricuspid; **d.** ventricular; **e.** S1; **f.** apical; **g.** S2; **h.** systole; **i.** aortic; **j.** pulmonic; **k.** dub; **l.** one

**12.**
- **a.** Biographical data: "What is your birth date?"
- **b.** Reason for seeking health care: "Why are you visiting the clinic today?"
- **c.** Present health history: "When did you notice these symptoms?"
- **d.** Past health history: "When did you have your last mammogram?"
- **e.** Family history: "Do you have any close relatives who have diabetes?"
- **f.** Functional health: "Are you able to prepare your own meals?"
- **g.** Psychosocial and lifestyle factors: "How do you manage stress in your life?"
- **h.** Review of systems: "Are you experiencing any abdominal distress?"

## APPLYING YOUR KNOWLEDGE

### REFLECTIVE PRACTICE: CULTIVATING QSEN COMPETENCIES

#### Sample Answers

**1.** What type of health assessments would the nurse caring for Billy conduct?
In the emergency room, the nurse should perform an emergency assessment to determine the effects of the bee sting and the allergic reaction that occurred. Once Billy is stabilized, the nurse should perform a focused assessment of Billy's allergies and answer the parent's questions at this time.

**2.** What would be a successful outcome for Billy and his family?
Billy demonstrates the proper method for self-injecting epinephrine.
Billy and his family state methods to avoid bee stings in the future and emergency interventions in the event a bee sting occurs.

**3.** What intellectual, technical, interpersonal, and/or ethical/legal competencies are most likely to bring about the desired outcome?
Intellectual: knowledge of the typical assessment findings associated with an allergic reaction
Interpersonal: ability to communicate and interact effectively with patients and their families during times of stress
Ethical/Legal: knowledge of special regulations and legislation detailing nursing responsibilities when providing first aid in camp situations

**4.** What resources might be helpful for this family?
Printed or AV materials on allergic reactions to insect bites and how to treat them

## PRACTICING FOR NCLEX

### MULTIPLE CHOICE QUESTIONS

| | | | | |
|---|---|---|---|---|
| **1.** b | **2.** c | **3.** a | **4.** c | **5.** d |
| **6.** b | **7.** d | **8.** a | **9.** a | **10.** b |
| **11.** a | **12.** c | **13.** a | **14.** b | |

## ALTERNATE-FORMAT QUESTIONS

### Multiple Response Questions

**1.** c, d, e
**2.** b, d, e
**3.** a, d, f
**4.** c, d, e

### Hot Spot Question

**1.** See figure below.

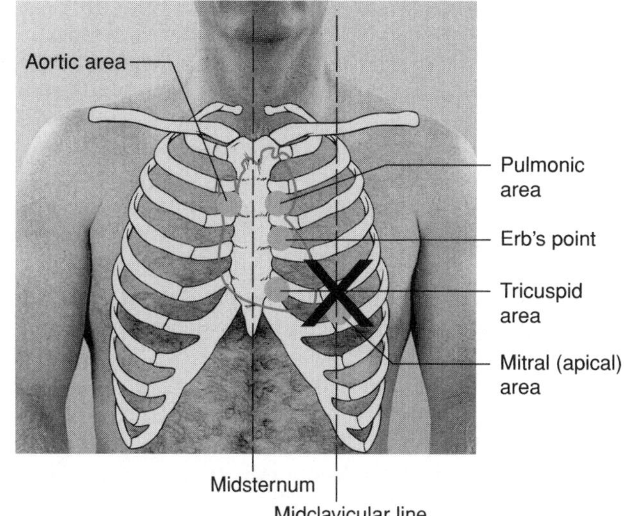

# CHAPTER 27

## ASSESSING YOUR UNDERSTANDING

### MATCHING EXERCISES

| | | | | |
|---|---|---|---|---|
| **1.** d | **2.** i | **3.** e | **4.** a | **5.** c |
| **6.** b | **7.** h | **8.** g | **9.** f | **10.** d |
| **11.** g | **12.** e | **13.** a | **14.** f | **15.** c |
| **16.** b | | | | |

### CORRECT THE FALSE STATEMENTS

1. True
2. True
3. True
4. False—home
5. False—children
6. True
7. True
8. False—preschooler
9. False—falls
10. False—unjustified
11. False—14 or younger
12. True
13. False—increase

### SHORT ANSWER

1. a. Neonates and infants: mother who smokes; mother who drinks alcohol
   b. Toddler and preschooler: child abuse; expanded environment
   c. School-aged child: accidents, fire
   d. Adolescent: drug and alcohol consumption; motor vehicle crashes
   e. Adult: spousal abuse; using alcohol to relieve stress
   f. Older adult: motor impairment; elder abuse
2. Sample answers:
   a. Developmental considerations: A teenager who drinks and drives is at risk for accidents; an adult who is under stress at work is at risk for drug or alcohol abuse.
   b. Lifestyle: A person who lives in a high-crime neighborhood is at risk for violence; a person who has a dangerous job is at risk for accidents.
   c. Limitation in mobility: An older adult with an unsteady gait is at risk for falls; recent surgery or prolonged illness can temporarily affect mobility.
   d. Limitation in sensory perception: Visual changes may cause a person to stumble, lose balance, and fall; a hearing deficit interferes with normal communication and may result in a patient who is insensitive to alarms, horns, sirens, etc.
   e. Limitation in knowledge: A mother who does not know how to childproof her home puts her toddler at risk for accidents; an older adult person who does not know how to use her walker is at risk for falls.
   f. Limitation in ability to communicate: Fatigue or stress, certain medications, aphasia, and language barriers are factors that can affect personal interchange and compromise the patient's ability to express urgent safety concerns.
   g. Limitation in health status: A patient recovering from a stroke may have muscle impairment; many patients who fall also have a primary or secondary diagnosis of cardiovascular disease.
   h. Limitation in psychosocial state: Depression may result in confusion and disorientation, accompanied by reduced awareness of environmental hazards; social isolation may be responsible for a reduced level of concentration.
3. a. Nursing history: The nurse must be alert for any history of falls because a person with a history of falling is likely to fall again. Assistive devices should be noted. A history of drug or alcohol abuse should also be noted.
   b. Physical assessment: Nurses need to assess the patient's mobility status, ability to communicate, level of awareness or orientation, and sensory perception.
   c. Accident-prone behavior: Some people seem to be more likely than others to have accidents.
   d. The environment: The nurse must assess every setting in which the patient is at risk for injury, including the home, community, and health care facility.
4. Sample answers:
   a. Age older than 65 years
   b. Documented history of falls
   c. Slowed reaction time
   d. Disorientation or confusion
5. Sample answers: The mother should be informed about safety for toddlers, and a plan should be devised to help her childproof her home. The plan should include the installation of cabinet locks; electrical outlet covers; moving medications, cleaners, poisonous plants, etc. to higher levels; and keeping small or sharp objects out of reach.
6. Sample answers:
   a. Do your children's toys have small or loose parts?
   b. Have you ever left your infant in the bathtub to answer the phone?
   c. Do you have soft pillows or thick blankets in your infant's crib?
7. a. Risk for Injury related to refusal to use child safety seat
   b. Risk for Poisoning related to reduced vision
   c. Risk for Aspiration or Trauma (burns) related to child left unattended in bathtub
   d. Risk for Trauma related to history of previous falls
   e. Impaired Home Maintenance related to insufficient finances
8. a. Screening programs for vision and hearing
   b. Fire prevention programs
   c. Drug and alcohol prevention programs

9. Sample answers:
   a. Impaired circulation
   b. Pressure injuries and diminished bone mass
   c. Fractures
   d. Altered nutrition and hydration
   e. Incontinence
10. Documentation should include alternative strategies that were ineffective, the reason for restraining the patient, the type of restraint and time it was applied, pertinent nursing assessments, and regular intervals when restraints were removed.
11. The nurse completes the safety event report immediately after an accident and is responsible for recording the occurrence of the accident and its effect on the patient in the medical record. The report should objectively describe the circumstances of the accident and provide details concerning the patient's response and the examination and treatment of the patient after the event.
12. Have the patient sit in a straight-backed chair. Observe his posture while seated. Instruct the patient to stand. Assess if he can stand in one fluid motion or needs the use of his hands to push up to a standing position. Does he need multiple attempts to stand? Once standing, ask the patient to keep his eyes open and stand as still as possible. Then ask him to close his eyes and observe his stability with eyes closed. Ask him to open his eyes and walk 10 ft (3 m), and then turn around and walk back to the chair. Using a timed Get Up and Go test: 9 seconds or less indicates full mobility and 10 to 19 seconds means person is almost completely independent. Higher times can indicate impaired mobility.

## APPLYING YOUR KNOWLEDGE

### REFLECTIVE PRACTICE: CULTIVATING QSEN COMPETENCIES

#### Sample Answers

1. What safety interventions might the nurse implement for this patient?
   Mrs. Washington should be advised to have clutter removed from the home, remove throw rugs and fire hazards, and have smoke detectors installed. She should be advised to wear shoes with rubber soles when walking in her home. Mrs. Washington might also benefit from a home alert system in case she falls and needs help.
2. What would be a successful outcome for Mrs. Washington?
   By end of visit, Mrs. Washington points out three safety issues in her home and formulates a plan to correct them.
   By next visit, Mrs. Washington demonstrates walking freely through a clutter-free home with fire alarms installed.
3. What intellectual, technical, interpersonal, and/or ethical/legal competencies are most likely to bring about the desired outcome?
   Intellectual: knowledge of the safety and security needs of older adults and related nursing responsibilities and care
   Interpersonal: ability to establish a therapeutic relationship with an older adult in order to communicate the need for safety interventions in the home
   Ethical/Legal: commitment to patient safety and quality care, including ability to report problem situations immediately
4. What resources might be helpful for Mrs. Washington?
   Home health care services, housekeeping services, smoke detectors, home alert system

## PRACTICING FOR NCLEX

### MULTIPLE CHOICE QUESTIONS

1. b 2. c 3. d 4. b 5. a
6. b 7. a

### ALTERNATE-FORMAT QUESTIONS

#### Multiple Response Questions

1. b, c, e
2. a, b, e
3. a, b, d
4. a, c, f

#### Prioritization Questions

1. 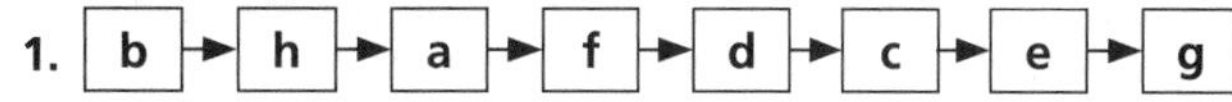


# CHAPTER 28

## ASSESSING YOUR UNDERSTANDING

### FILL IN THE BLANKS

1. Yin-yang
2. Holism
3. Acupuncture
4. guided imagery
5. nutritional supplements
6. aromatherapy

### MATCHING EXERCISES

1. d 2. f 3. b 4. e 5. a
6. c

### SHORT ANSWER

1. a. Allopathy: Generally used to describe "traditional medicine." Has spear-headed remarkable advances in biotechnology, surgical interventions, pharmaceutical approaches, and diagnostic tools
   b. Holism: A theory and philosophy that focuses on connections and interactions between parts of the whole; focuses on reductionism

   **c.** Integrative care: Uses some combination of allopathic and CHA; coordinates best possible treatment plan for patient

**2.** **a.** Ayurveda: The aim of Ayurvedic medicine is to integrate and balance the body, mind, and spirit. Key concepts include universal interconnectedness among people, their health, and the universe as well as the body's constitution and life forces. Nursing considerations: May include dietary needs, time set aside for self-care such as meditation, and desire to continue a herbal/supplement regimen.

   **b.** Yoga: A set of exercises that consist of various physical postures practiced to promote strength and flexibility, increase endurance, or promote relaxation. Nursing considerations: Encourage patients to find a type of yoga that is compatible with their physical condition and goals. Some positions are contraindicated in patients with certain physical conditions.

   **c.** Traditional Chinese medicine: The human body is regarded as an organic entity in which the various organs, tissues, and other parts have distinct functions but are all interdependent; health and disease relate to balance of the functions. Nursing considerations: Teaching about acupuncture, diet, herbs, massage, and energy exercises.

   **d.** Qi gong: System of posture, exercise, breathing techniques, and visualization regulating *qi*. Nursing considerations: Can be learned from videos/DVDs or in a class; encourage students to explore background of instructor.

**3.** **a.** Relaxation techniques: Ultimate goal is to increase the parasympathetic system influence in the body–mind and reduce the effect of stress and stress-related illness

   **b.** Meditation: Seeks to change one's physiology to a more relaxed state and alter one's perception to an increased acceptance of reality

   **c.** Imagery: Involves using all five senses to imagine an event or body process unfolding according to a plan

**4.** **a.** All the life sciences agree that physically a human being is an open energy system.

   **b.** Anatomically, a human being is bilaterally symmetric.

   **c.** Illness is an imbalance in a person's energy field.

   **d.** Human beings have natural abilities to transform and transcend their conditions of living.

**5.** Sample answers:

   **a.** Shamanism: Treatment would consist of first restoring the patient's power and then treating symptoms. Healing techniques may include native plants and herbs, animals, ritual, ceremony, and purification techniques.

   **b.** Relaxation response: Treatment is an alert, hypokinetic process of decreased sympathetic nervous system arousal that may be achieved in many ways, including through breathing exercises, relaxation and imagery exercises, biofeedback, and prayer. A degree of discipline is required to evoke this response, which includes mental and physical well-being.

**6.** Sample answers:

   **a.** Nutritional therapy: It is believed that people have individual needs and preferences with respect to foods.

   **b.** Aromatherapy: It is believed that the fragrance of oils can evoke powerful memories in a split second and change people's perceptions and behaviors.

   **c.** Music: It is believed that music is effective in reducing pain, decreasing anxiety, and promoting relaxation, thereby distracting persons from unpleasant sensations.

   **d.** Humor: It is believed that a good "belly laugh" can help treat acute and debilitating illness.

**7.** **a.** Biology-based practices: Using herbs and special diets

   **b.** Mind–body medicine: Using meditation or yoga

   **c.** Energy medicine: Using energy fields or magnetic fields

   **d.** Manipulative and body-based practices: Manipulating body parts

## APPLYING YOUR KNOWLEDGE

### REFLECTIVE PRACTICE: CULTIVATING QSEN COMPETENCIES

#### Sample Answers

**1.** What type of CHA might the nurse suggest to promote relaxation for Ms. Puentes?
The nurse could teach Ms. Puentes mind–body techniques such as meditation, guided imagery, biofeedback, and relaxation to reduce stressful emotions. Energy healing techniques would also be helpful for pain that lingers after an injury heals, as well as pain complicated by trauma, anxiety, or depression. These CHAs include acupuncture, acupressure, qi gong, and Reiki. Movement-based therapies are also appropriate for postoperative pain. These include physical therapy, yoga, Pilates, and tai chi.

**2.** What would be a successful outcome for Ms. Puentes?
On her next visit, Ms. Puentes lists two CHA measures that promote relaxation and demonstrates the proper use of them.

**3.** What intellectual, technical, interpersonal, and/or ethical/legal competencies are most likely to bring about the desired outcome?
Intellectual: knowledge of available and appropriate complementary and alternative modalities
Technical: ability to properly perform CHA and integrate these measures into patient care
Interpersonal: ability to work collaboratively with other members of the health care team to promote culturally competent care that includes the use of CHA

**4.** What resources might be helpful for Ms. Puentes?
Other health care professionals using CHA, printed and AV materials on CHA, referral to special programs delivering CHA

## PRACTICING FOR NCLEX

### MULTIPLE CHOICE QUESTIONS

**1.** a **2.** c **3.** b **4.** c **5.** a
**6.** d

### ALTERNATE-FORMAT QUESTIONS

### Multiple Response Questions

**1.** a, b, e, f
**2.** a, b, c, f
**3.** a, b, c, d
**4.** c, d, e
**5.** b, d, f
**6.** a, c, d

# CHAPTER 29

## ASSESSING YOUR UNDERSTANDING

### FILL IN THE BLANKS

**1.** 1.5 mL
**2.** 0.5 tab (½ tab)
**3.** 3 tabs
**4.** 0.5 tab (½ tab)
**5.** 3 tabs
**6.** 0.5 tab (½ tab)
**7.** 0.5 tab (½ tab)
**8.** 2 tabs
**9.** 4 mL

### MATCHING EXERCISES

| | | | | |
|---|---|---|---|---|
| **1.** f | **2.** a | **3.** c | **4.** k | **5.** b |
| **6.** j | **7.** d | **8.** g | **9.** i | **10.** h |
| **11.** l | **12.** m | **13.** c | **14.** i | **15.** b |
| **16.** e | **17.** f | **18.** d | **19.** g | **20.** a |

### SHORT ANSWER

**1.** Drugs may be classified by:
   **a.** Pharmaceutical: refers to the mechanism of action (MOA), physiologic effect (PE), and chemical structure (CS) of the drug
   **b.** Therapeutic: refers to the clinical indication for the drug or therapeutic action (e.g., analgesic, antibiotic, or antihypertensive)

**2.** **a.** Drug–receptor interactions: The drug interacts with one or more cellular structures to alter cell function.
   **b.** Drug–enzyme interactions: The drug combines with enzymes to achieve the desired effect.

**3.** Sample answers:
   **a.** Developmental stage of patient: A child's dose of medication is smaller than an adult's dose.
   **b.** Weight: Drug doses for children should be calculated on weight or body surface area. Doses for adults are based on a reference adult (i.e., a healthy adult of 18 to 65 years weighing 150 lb).
   **c.** Sex: Hormonal fluctuations can affect drug action.
   **d.** Genetic factors: Asian patients may require smaller doses of a drug because they metabolize it at a slower rate.
   Cultural: Herbal remedies may interfere with or counteract the action of the prescribed medication.
   **e.** Psychological factors: Patients may attain the same effect with a placebo as with an active drug.
   **f.** Pathology: Liver disease may affect drug action by slowing the metabolism of drugs.
   **g.** Environment: The lower oxygen concentration of air at high altitudes may increase sensitivity to some drugs.
   **h.** Time of administration: The presence of food in the stomach generally delays the absorption of oral medications.

**4.** Sample answers:
   **a.** The nurse knows that the patient is allergic to the drug.
   **b.** The nurse has difficulty reading the order.
   **c.** The nurse knows the drug will be harmful to the patient.

**5.** **a.** Stock supply system (computerized automated dispensing cabinets [ADCs]): A large cabinet containing stock medications for the unit is used. The nurse accesses the system with a user name and password, calling up a medication list for a specific patient or a list of available medications. In many systems, only medications entered for a specific patient are available for withdrawal at any one time.
   **b.** Unit dose dispensing system: In the unit dose system, the pharmacist simplifies medication preparation by packaging and labeling each dosage for a 24-hour period. Unit dose dispensing on a patient-specific basis is now the standard of practice for most hospitals. Pharmaceutical manufacturers should also provide all medications in health systems in unit dose packages. Computerized automated dispensing cabinets are a technology based on stock supply of unit dose medications. A large cabinet containing stock medications for the unit is used. The nurse accesses the system with a user name and password, calling up a medication list for a specific patient or a list of available medications.
   **c.** Medication cart: The standard cart contains individual drawers into which the medications for each patient are placed. The drawer is labeled with the patient's name. If computers are not standard in every patient room and an EHR is used, there may also be a computer attached to the cart that allows for ready access to the eMAR by the administering nurse. The nurse moves the cart from room to room when dispensing medications.
   **d.** Bar code-enabled medication administration (BCMA): When using a computerized bar-coded administration system, each patient and each

nurse wear identification with a unique bar code to identify the person. Each drug is packaged with a bar code that includes its unique National Drug Code number to identify the form and dosage. The nurse scans his or her own ID, the patient's ID, and each package of medication to be administered. The system confirms the nurse's dispensing authority and the patient's ID, matching the patient with his or her medication profile. If any of the information is incorrect or does not match, an alert message will appear on the screen notifying the nurse of the discrepancy. The system also records the medication administration and stores the information.

6. a. Three checks: The medication label should be read (1) when the nurse reaches for the unit dose package or container; (2) after retrieval from the drawer and compared with the eMAR/MAR, or compared with the eMAR/MAR immediately before pouring from a multidose container; and (3) before giving the unit dose medication to the patient, or when replacing the multidose container in the drawer or shelf.
   b. Eleven rights: Ensure that the (1) **right medication** is given to the (2) **right patient** in the (3) **right dosage** (in the right form) through the (4) **right route** at the (5) **right time** for the (6) **right reason** based on the (7) **right (appropriate) assessment data** using the (8) **right documentation** and monitoring for the (9) **right response** by the patient. Additional rights have been suggested to include (10) the **right to education**, ensuring that patients receive accurate and thorough information about the medication, and (11) the **right to refuse**, acknowledging that patients can and do refuse to take a medication.
7. Sample answers:
   a. Crush the medication (if appropriate for the type of medication) and add it to food or a drink so that the patient can swallow it.
   b. Allow the patient to suck on a piece of ice to numb the taste buds.
   c. Give the medication with generous amounts of water.
8. Sample answers:
   a. Route of administration: A longer needle is needed for an intramuscular injection than for an intradermal or subcutaneous injection.
   b. Viscosity of the solution: Some medications are more viscous than others and require a large-lumen needle to be injected.
   c. Quantity to be administered: The larger the amount of medication to be injected, the greater the capacity of the syringe.
   d. Body size: An obese person requires a longer needle to reach muscle tissue than a thin person.
   e. Type of medication: There are special syringes for certain uses.
9. a. Check the patient's condition immediately when the error is noted. Observe for adverse effects.
   b. Notify the nurse manager and the primary care provider to discuss possible courses of action based on the patient's condition.
   c. Report the incident using whatever method is appropriate for your institution. These may include an incident report, a quality assurance report, a risk assessment/root cause analysis report, or a variance report. These forms—generally called *special event, event,* or *unusual occurrence reports*—require an objective, complete account of the medication error. Include the steps taken after the error was recognized. For legal reasons, describe the error fully and accurately.
   d. Medication errors are a common allegation in nursing liability cases. Do not document in the patient's record the fact that an incident report was filed. Your institution is bound by state and national mandates to report certain incidents. Some of this reporting is voluntary and some is required. For example, reporting *near-miss* medication errors, in which an error almost occurred, is voluntary in some instances, but *sentinel events*, in which serious patient harm or death results from the error, require reporting (Wolf & Hughes, 2008; The Joint Commission, 2017b).
10. a. Ampules: An ampule is a glass flask that contains a single dose of medication for parenteral administration. Medication is removed from an ampule after its thin neck is broken.
   b. Vials: A vial is a glass bottle with a self-sealing stopper through which medication is removed. The nurse can remove several doses from the same container.
   c. Prefilled cartridges: These provide a single dose of medication. The nurse inserts the cartridge into a reusable holder and clears the cartridge of excess air.

**11.** See Medical Administration Record below.

## Medical Administration Record

| Ord date | PRN MEDS. | | |
|---|---|---|---|
| 2/24/20 | Dalmane 30 mg | Date | |
| | PO hs prn | Time | |
| | | Init/Site | |
| 2/24/20 | Tylenol with codeine #2 | Date | 2/24/20 |
| | PO q4h prn | Time | 1000 |
| | | Init/Site | CL/PO |

| | SINGLE ORDERS–PREOPERATIVES | | |
|---|---|---|---|
| **Ord date** | **Medication–Dosage–Route of Admin** | **Date/Time** | **Site/Initials** |
| 2/24/20 | Regular Insulin U-100 | 2/24/20 | ® thigh/CL |
| | 10U SQ STAT | | |

| | | | INJECTION SITES MUST BE CHARTED | | | | | | |
|---|---|---|---|---|---|---|---|---|---|
| **Ord date** | **ROUTINE MEDICATIONS** | | **Date/Time** | | | | | | |
| 2/24/20 | **Medication–Dosage–Route of Admin** | **Hr** | 2/25 | 2/26 | 2/27 | 2/28 | 3/1 | 3/2 | 3/3 |
| | Tenormin 50 mg PO od | 1000 | CL | | | | | | |
| 2/24/20 | | | | | | | | | |
| | Hydrodiuril 50 mg PO od | 1000 | CL | | | | | | |
| 2/24/20 | | | 130/90 | | | | | | |
| | NPH Insulin U-100 45U | 7:30AM | CL | | | | | | |
| | SQ daily in AM | | Ⓛ arm | | | | | | |
| 2/24/20 | | | | | | | | | |
| | Cipro 500 mg PO q12h | 1000 | CL | | | | | | |
| | | 10PM | | | | | | | |
| 2/24/20 | | | | | | | | | |
| | Timoptic 0.25% † gtt | 1000 | CL | | | | | | |
| | OD bid | 6PM | | | | | | | |
| 2/24/20 | | | | | | | | | |
| | Nitropaste 1/2" q8h | 8AM | CL $\frac{130}{90}$ | | | | | | |
| | to chest wall | 4PM | | | | | | | |
| | | 12PM | | | | | | | |
| 2/24/20 | | | | | | | | | |
| | Colace 100 mg PO od | 1000 | CL | | | | | | |
| | | | | | | | | | |
| | | | | | | | | | |
| | | | | | | | | | |

*CL: Claire Long, RN*

**12.** See medication chart below.

| Method | Alprazolam | Ranitidine | Ciprofloxacin |
|---|---|---|---|
| Dosage range | 0.25–0.5 mg | 150–300 mg | 250–750 mg |
| Possible route of administration | PO | PO | PO |
| Frequency/schedule | TID | BID | BID |
| Desired effects | Relief of anxiety | Cure/relief of peptic ulcer | Cure/treat infection |
| Possible adverse effects | Drowsiness, lightheadedness, dry mouth, constipation | Malaise, rash, GI upset | GI upset, nausea, diarrhea |
| Signs and symptoms of toxic drug effects | Diminished reflexes, somnolence, confusion | Tachycardia, GI upset | CNS stimulation |
| Special instructions | No alcohol | None | No antacids |
| Nursing/collaborative management of adverse effects | Gastric lavage | None | None |

## APPLYING YOUR KNOWLEDGE

### REFLECTIVE PRACTICE: CULTIVATING QSEN COMPETENCIES

#### Sample Answers

**1.** How might the nurse use blended nursing skills to respond to this medication error?
The nurse would use five rights of medication administration ([1] Give the right medication [2] to the right patient [3] in the right dosage [4] through the right route [5] at the right time) to determine that the medication was labeled incorrectly. The nurse could then call the pharmacy and have new medication delivered with the right patient name.

**2.** What would be a successful outcome for this patient?
Mr. Baptiste receives the prescribed medication with his name on the label.

**3.** What intellectual, technical, interpersonal, and/or ethical/legal competencies are most likely to bring about the desired outcome?
Intellectual: knowledge of intravenous antibiotic therapy, including correct dosages for IV medications
Technical: ability to safely administer IV antibiotics to a patient
Ethical/Legal: ability to provide patient safety via accurate patient identification to ensure medications are delivered in the right dosage to the right patient

## PRACTICING FOR NCLEX

### MULTIPLE CHOICE QUESTIONS

| | | | | |
|---|---|---|---|---|
| **1.** d | **2.** a | **3.** c | **4.** d | **5.** b |
| **6.** a | **7.** b | **8.** d | **9.** b | **10.** a |
| **11.** b | **12.** d | **13.** b | **14.** c | **15.** b |
| **16.** a | **17.** d | | | |

### ALTERNATE-FORMAT QUESTIONS

#### Multiple Response Questions

**1.** a, c, d, e
**2.** b, e, f
**3.** a, b, c
**4.** b, d, e
**5.** a, c, d
**6.** b, e, f
**7.** c, d, f
**8.** a, b, d

# CHAPTER 30

## ASSESSING YOUR UNDERSTANDING

### FILL IN THE BLANKS

**1.** perioperative
**2.** urgency
**3.** elective
**4.** degree of risk
**5.** nerve block
**6.** maintenance
**7.** Conscious (moderate or procedural)
**8.** Informed consent
**9.** Advance directives
**10.** time-out

### MATCHING EXERCISES

| | | | | |
|---|---|---|---|---|
| **1.** a | **2.** c | **3.** d | **4.** b | **5.** d |
| **6.** b | | | | |

### SHORT ANSWER

**1. a.** Preoperative phase: begins with the decision that surgical intervention is necessary and lasts until the patient is transferred to the operating room table

b. Intraoperative phase: extends from admission to the surgical department to transfer to postanesthesia care unit (PACU)
c. Postoperative phase: lasts from admission to the PACU to the complete recovery from surgery and the first health care provider follow-up visit

2. a. Based on urgency: may be classified as elective surgery (preplanned; patient choice), urgent surgery (necessary for patient's health; not emergency), or emergency surgery (preserves patient's life, body part, or body function)
b. Based on degree of risk: may be classified as minor: performed in health care provider's office, an outpatient clinic, or a same-day, outpatient surgery setting (also referred to as ambulatory surgery), or major: requires hospitalization, is prolonged and has higher degree of risk, involves major body organs
c. Based on purpose: descriptors include diagnostic, ablative, palliative, reconstructive, transplant, and constructive.

3. a. Induction: begins with administration of the anesthetic agent and continues until patient is ready for incision
b. Maintenance: continues from point of incision until near completion of procedure
c. Emergence: starts as patient begins to emerge from the anesthesia and usually ends when patient is ready to leave the operating room

4. a. Description of the procedure or treatment
b. The underlying disease process and its natural course
c. Name and qualifications of the person performing the procedure or treatment
d. Explanation of the common risks involved, including potential for damage, disfigurement, or death
e. Patient's right to refuse treatment and withdraw consent
f. Explanation of expected (not guaranteed) outcome, recovery, and rehabilitation plan and course of medication if prescribed

5. a. Cardiovascular disease: increased potential for hemorrhage and hypovolemic shock, hypotension, venous stasis, thrombophlebitis, and overhydration with IV fluids
b. Pulmonary disorders: increased possibility of respiratory depression from anesthesia, postoperative pneumonia, atelectasis, and alterations in acid–base balance
c. Kidney and liver function disorders: influence the patient's response to anesthesia, affect fluid and electrolyte as well as acid–base balance, alter metabolism and excretion of drugs, and impair wound healing
d. Endocrine disorders: endocrine diseases, especially diabetes mellitus, increase the risk for hypoglycemia or acidosis, slow wound healing, and present an increased risk for postoperative cardiovascular complications.

6. a. Fear of the unknown: Encourage the patient to identify and verbalize fears; identify and correct incorrect knowledge; identify patient strengths.
b. Fear of pain and death: Support the patient's spiritual needs through acceptance, participation in prayer, or referral to clergy or chaplain.
c. Fear of changes in body image and self-concept: Identify the need for support systems during initial interview; arrange a preoperative visit from a person who has had the same operation and adapted successfully.

7. The nurse is responsible for ensuring that the tests are ordered and performed, that the results are recorded in the patient's record before surgery, and that abnormal findings are reported.

8. a. Surgical events and sensations: Tell the patient and family when surgery is scheduled; how long it will last; what will be done before, during, and after surgery; and what sensations the patient will be experiencing during the perioperative period.
b. Pain management: The patient should be informed that pain reported by the patient is the determining factor of pain control, pain will be assessed as often as every 2 hours after major surgery, there is little danger of addiction to pain medications, and nonpharmacologic methods of pain control (relaxation techniques, TENS, and PCA) are available.

9. a. Hygiene and skin preparation: Clean the skin with antibacterial soap to remove bacteria (preoperative showers or baths are taken before the scheduled surgery using chlorhexidine gluconate [CHG] soap; children and adult inpatients may be cleansed preoperatively with microfiber cloths impregnated with CHG antimicrobial skin antiseptic, which eliminates skin microorganisms and leaves an antimicrobial film on their skin). Shampoo the hair and clean the fingernails to help to reduce the number of organisms present on the body. Leave hair at the surgical site in place if possible or remove only the hair that will interfere with the procedure with hair clippers.
b. Elimination: Emptying the bowel of feces is no longer a routine procedure, but the nurse should use preoperative assessments to determine the need for an order for bowel elimination. If indwelling catheter is not in place, the patient should void immediately before receiving preoperative medications.
c. Nutrition and fluids: Diet depends on the type of surgery; patients need to be well nourished and hydrated before surgery to counterbalance fluid, blood, and electrolyte loss during surgery. Light meals such as tea and toast may be consumed up to 6 hours before surgery; fatty meals should be consumed up to 8 hours before surgery.

   - **d.** Rest and sleep: The nurse can facilitate rest and sleep in the immediate preoperative period by meeting psychological needs, carrying out teaching, providing a quiet environment, and administering prescribed bedtime sedative medication.

**10.**
   - **a.** Maintain intact skin surfaces
   - **b.** Remain free of neuromuscular damage
   - **c.** Have symmetric breathing patterns

**11.**
   - **a.** Unconsciousness
   - **b.** Response to touch and sounds
   - **c.** Drowsiness
   - **d.** Awake but not oriented
   - **e.** Awake and oriented

**12.** Sample answer:
The person who will be changing the patient's dressing at home should demonstrate proper techniques in wound care and dressing change. Teaching should include the following information: (1) where to buy dressing materials and medical supplies, (2) signs and symptoms of infection, (3) need to eat well-balanced meals and drink fluids, (4) how to modify activities of daily living (as needed), (5) need to wear disposable gloves when changing the dressing and wash hands before and after donning gloves, and (6) how to dispose of old dressings.

**13.** Sample answers:
   - **a.** Developmental considerations: Infants and older adults are at a greater risk from surgery than are children and young or middle-aged adults.
   - **b.** Medical history: Pathologic changes associated with past and current illnesses increase surgical risk.
   - **c.** Medications: Use of anticoagulants before surgery may precipitate hemorrhage.
   - **d.** Previous surgery: Previous heart or lung surgery may necessitate adaptations in the anesthesia used and in positioning during surgery.
   - **e.** Perceptions and knowledge of surgery: The patient's questions or statements are important for meeting his or her psychological needs and those of the family when preparing the patient for surgery.
   - **f.** Lifestyle: Cultural and ethnic background of the patient may affect surgical risk.
   - **g.** Nutrition: Malnutrition and obesity increase surgical risk.
   - **h.** Use of alcohol, illicit drugs, nicotine: Patients with a large habitual intake of alcohol require larger doses of anesthetic agents and postoperative analgesics, increasing the risk for drug-related complications.
   - **i.** Activities of daily living: Exercise, rest, and sleep habits are important for preventing postoperative complications and facilitating recovery.
   - **j.** Occupation: Surgical procedures may require a delay in returning to work.
   - **k.** Coping patterns: The patient needs information and emotional support to recover from surgery.
   - **l.** Support systems: Family members should be encouraged to provide support before and after surgery.
   - **m.** Sociocultural needs: The patient's cultural background may require that nursing interventions be individualized to meet needs in such areas as language, food preferences, family interaction and participation, personal space, and health beliefs and practices.

**14.**
   - **a.** Vital signs: Assess temperature, blood pressure, and pulse and respiratory rates; note deviations from preoperative and PACU data, as well as symptoms of complications.
   - **b.** Color and temperature of skin: Assess for warmth, pallor, cyanosis, and diaphoresis.
   - **c.** Level of consciousness: Assess for orientation to time, place, and person, as well as reaction to stimuli and ability to move extremities.
   - **d.** Intravenous fluids: Assess type and amount of solution, flow rate, securement and patency of tubing, and infusion site.
   - **e.** Surgical site: Assess dressing and dependent areas for drainage. Assess drains and tubes and be sure they are intact, patent, and properly connected to drainage systems.
   - **f.** Other tubes: Assess indwelling urinary catheter, gastrointestinal suction, etc. for drainage, patency, and amount of output.
   - **g.** Pain management: Assess for pain and determine whether analgesics were given in the PACU. Assess for nausea and vomiting.
   - **h.** Position and safety: Place patient in the ordered position; if the patient is not fully conscious, place him or her in the side-lying position. Elevate side rails and place bed in low position.
   - **i.** Comfort: Cover the patient with a blanket, reorient him or her to the room as necessary, and allow family members to remain with the patient after the initial assessment is completed.

**15.** Sample answers:
   - **a.** Nausea and vomiting: Provide oral hygiene as needed; avoid strong-smelling foods.
   - **b.** Thirst: Offer ice chips; maintain oral hygiene.
   - **c.** Hiccups: Rebreathe into paper bag; eat a teaspoon of granulated sugar.
   - **d.** Surgical pain: Assess pain frequently; offer nonpharmacologic measures to supplement medications.

## APPLYING YOUR KNOWLEDGE

### REFLECTIVE PRACTICE: CULTIVATING QSEN COMPETENCIES

#### Sample Answers

1. How might the nurse use blended nursing skills to implement the perioperative care plan in a manner that respects Ms. Greenbaum's human dignity and

addresses her fears and concerns about the surgical experience?
The nurse should assess the patient's psychological, sociocultural, and spiritual dimension since surgery is a major psychological stressor that causes anxiety and fear. The nurse can use cues obtained in a health history to plan nursing interventions to provide information and emotional support for a successful recovery.

2. What would be a successful outcome for this patient?
Following the nursing history, Ms. Greenbaum verbalizes her fears regarding the surgery and lists three coping methods to reduce stress.
3. What intellectual, technical, interpersonal, and/or ethical/legal competencies are most likely to bring about the desired outcome?
Intellectual: ability to identify the common psychological patient responses before and after surgery
Interpersonal: ability to communicate to the patient concerns about the patient and his or her well-being
Ethical/legal skills: ability to participate in care as a trusted and effective advocate, including advocating for a patient who is fearful
4. What resources might be helpful for Ms. Greenbaum?
Printed or AV materials of hysterectomies, counseling, support groups

## PRACTICING FOR NCLEX

### MULTIPLE CHOICE QUESTIONS

| | | | | |
|---|---|---|---|---|
| **1.** a | **2.** c | **3.** b | **4.** d | **5.** b |
| **6.** a | **7.** c | **8.** c | **9.** a | **10.** c |
| **11.** b | **12.** d | **13.** b | **14.** a | **15.** c |
| **16.** a | | | | |

### ALTERNATE-FORMAT QUESTIONS

#### Multiple Response Questions

1. a, d, e, f
2. b, c, d, f
3. b, e, f
4. a, c, d
5. a, b, d, e
6. b, c, e
7. c, d, f
8. a, b, e
9. c, e, f

#### Prioritization Questions

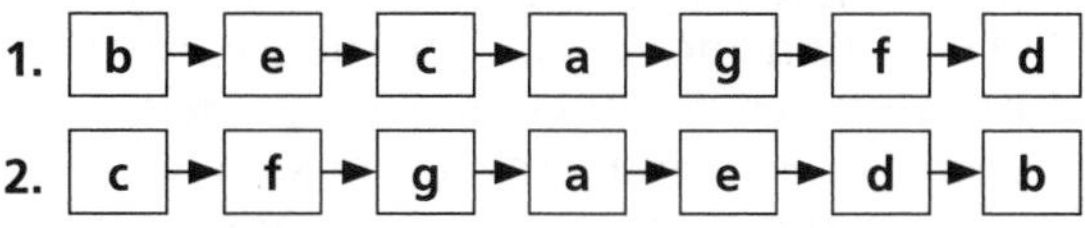

1. b → e → c → a → g → f → d
2. c → f → g → a → e → d → b

# CHAPTER 31

## ASSESSING YOUR UNDERSTANDING

### FILL IN THE BLANKS

1. gingivitis
2. alopecia
3. pediculosis
4. hour of sleep (HS care)
5. disposable bath

### MATCHING EXERCISES

| | | | | |
|---|---|---|---|---|
| **1.** d | **2.** c | **3.** h | **4.** j | **5.** a |
| **6.** i | **7.** f | **8.** b | **9.** e | **10.** g |
| **11.** k | | | | |

### CORRECT THE FALSE STATEMENTS

1. False—ceruminal glands
2. True
3. False—yellowish
4. True
5. False—lowest
6. True
7. False—Oily
8. False—lack of blood circulation
9. True
10. True
11. False—Pediculus humanis corpus
12. False—podiatrist
13. False—morning care (AM care)

### SHORT ANSWER

1. a. Culture: Many people in North America place a high value on personal cleanliness, shower frequently, and use many products to mask odors. Culture may also dictate whether bathing is private or communal.
   b. Socioeconomic class: Financial resources often define the hygiene options available to people. The availability of running water and finances for soap, shampoo, etc. affects hygiene.
   c. Spiritual practices: Religion may dictate ceremonial washing and purification, which may be a prelude to prayer or eating.
   d. Developmental level: Children learn different hygiene practices while growing up. Family practices may dictate morning or evening baths, frequency of shampooing, feelings about nudity, frequency of clothing changes, etc.
   e. Health state: Disease or injury may hinder a person's ability to perform hygiene measures or motivation to follow usual hygiene habits.
   f. Personal preference: People have personal preferences with regard to shower versus tub baths, bar soap versus liquid soap, etc.
2. a. Feeding
   b. Bathing and hygiene
   c. Dressing and grooming
   d. Toileting

3. Bathing/Hygiene Deficit related to mother's lack of knowledge about bathing infants. The mother must be educated on the proper method of bathing her infant. She should be made aware of the need for good hygiene for her baby, and a bath should be demonstrated with a return demonstration. Investigate whether the mother has the financial means to buy the materials necessary for her baby's hygiene (shampoo, oil, powder, diaper rash ointment, etc.).
4. **a.** Early morning care: The patient should be assisted with toileting and provided comfort measures designed to refresh the patient and prepare him or her for breakfast. The face and hands should be washed and mouth care provided.
   **b.** Morning care (AM care): After breakfast, the nurse offers assistance with toileting, oral care, bathing, back massage, special skin care measures, hair care, cosmetics, dressing, and positioning. Bed linens are refreshed or changed.
   **c.** Afternoon care (PM care): The nurse should ensure the patient's comfort after lunch and offer assistance with toileting, handwashing, and oral care to nonambulatory patients.
   **d.** Hour of sleep care (HS care): The nurse again offers assistance with toileting, washing of face and hands, and oral care. A back massage helps the patient relax and fall asleep. Soiled bed linens or clothing should be changed and the patient positioned comfortably.
   **e.** As-needed care (PRN care): The nurse offers individual hygiene measures as needed. Some patients require oral care every 2 hours. Patients who are diaphoretic may need their clothing or linens changed several times a shift.
5. Answers may include: Bathing cleanses the skin, acts as a conditioner, relaxes a restless person, promotes circulation, serves as musculoskeletal exercise, stimulates the rate and depth of respirations, promotes comfort, provides sensory input, improves self-esteem, and strengthens the nurse–patient relationship.
6. Provide the patient with articles for bathing and a basin of water that is at a comfortable temperature; place these items conveniently for the patient. Provide privacy for the patient; remove top linens on patient's bed and replace with a bath blanket. Place cosmetics in a convenient place with a mirror and light, and supply hot water and a razor for a patient who wishes to shave. Assist patients who cannot bathe themselves completely.
7. **a.** A towel bath can be accomplished with little fatigue to the patient.
   **b.** The towel remains warm during the short procedure.
   **c.** Patients state that they feel clean and refreshed.
   **d.** The oil in the bathing solution eliminates dry, itchy skin.
8. **a.** A back rub acts as a body conditioner.
   **b.** Giving a back rub provides an opportunity for the nurse to observe the skin for signs of breakdown.
   **c.** A back rub improves circulation and provides a means of communication with the patient through the use of touch.
9. **a.** Ventilation: It is wise to air the room when the patient is away for a diagnostic or therapeutic procedure to remove pathogens and unpleasant odors associated with body secretions and excretions.
   **b.** Odors: Odors can be controlled by promptly emptying bedpans, urinals, and emesis basins and by being careful not to dispose of soiled dressings or anything with a strong odor in the waste receptacle in the patient's room. Deodorizers may be needed.
   **c.** Room temperature: Whenever possible, patient preference should be followed regarding room temperature. In general, the temperature should be 20° to 23°C.
   **d.** Lighting and noise: The nurse should reduce harsh lighting and noises whenever possible. Conversations should not be carried on immediately outside the patient's room.
10. Sample answers:
   **a.** Rinse off soaps or detergents well when they are used for cleaning the skin.
   **b.** Add moisture to the air through a humidifier.
   **c.** Increase fluid intake.
   **d.** Use an emollient after cleansing the skin.
11. **a.** Lips: color, moisture, lumps, ulcers, lesions, and edema
   **b.** Buccal mucosa: color, moisture, lesions, nodules, and bleeding
   **c.** Gums: lesions, bleeding, edema, and exudate; loose or missing teeth
   **d.** Tongue: color, symmetry, movement, texture, and lesions
   **e.** Hard and soft palates: intactness, color, patches, lesions, and petechiae
   **f.** Eye: position, alignment, and general appearance; presence of lesions, nodules, redness, swelling, crusting, flaking, excessive tearing, or discharge; color of conjunctivae; blink reflex; and visual acuity
   **g.** Ear: position, alignment, and general appearance; buildup of wax; dryness, crusting, discharge, or foreign body; and hearing acuity
   **h.** Nose: position and general appearance; patency of nostrils; presence of tenderness, dryness, edema, bleeding, and discharge or secretions
12. **a.** Eye: Clean the eye from the inner canthus to the outer canthus using a wet, warm washcloth; cotton ball; or compress to soften crusted secretions. Avoid cross-contamination.
   **b.** Ear: Clean the ear with a washcloth-covered finger, instructing patient never to insert objects into the ear for cleaning purposes.

c. Nose: Clean the nose by instructing patient to blow nose while both nares are patent (nasal suctioning may be indicated), remove crusted secretions around the nose, and apply petroleum jelly to tissue.

13. a. Contact lenses: Wash hands before touching eye surfaces or lenses. To allow the cornea to receive a maximal supply of oxygen, contact lenses should be worn and removed according to the type and manufacturer's recommendations. Excessive tearing, pain, and redness signal the need to remove lenses. Lenses should be cleaned and stored as prescribed. Different types of lenses require special care and certain types of products. Sleeping without removing any contact lens is not recommended as the incidence of serious eye infections is greatly increased. Guidelines for Nursing 31-3 demonstrates removal techniques for contact lenses.

b. Artificial eye: Assemble a small basin, soap and water, and solution for rinsing the prosthesis. Ask the patient how he or she cleans the eye area (usually flushed with normal saline before replacing the eye). When the nurse is performing the care, the patient should be lying down so that the prosthesis does not accidentally fall to the floor.

c. Hearing aids: Batteries should be checked routinely and earpieces cleaned daily with mild soap and water.

d. Dentures: Dentures should be cleaned daily to reduce plaque and potentially harmful microorganisms. Daily cleaning includes soaking in and brushing with a nonabrasive denture cleanser. When cleaning dentures, put on gloves and hold the dentures over a basin of water or a sink lined with a washcloth or soft towel so that if they slip from your grasp, they will not fall onto a hard surface and break. If necessary, grasp the dentures with a 4″ × 4″ piece of gauze to help prevent them from slipping out of your gloved hands. Use cool or lukewarm water to cleanse them. Hot water may warp the plastic material of which most dentures are made. Use a soft toothbrush and dental cleanser. Do not use toothpaste as it can be too harsh for denture surfaces. Rinse dentures thoroughly after soaking and brushing, prior to reinsertion into the mouth. Give the patient the opportunity to brush the gums and tongue and rinse the mouth before the dentures are replaced. Assist the patient with care as necessary.

14. Answers may include: deficient self-care abilities, vascular disease, arthritis, diabetes mellitus, history of biting nails or trimming them improperly, frequent or prolonged exposure to chemicals or water, trauma, ill-fitting shoes, or obesity

## APPLYING YOUR KNOWLEDGE

### REFLECTIVE PRACTICE: CULTIVATING QSEN COMPETENCIES

#### Sample Answers

1. What patient teaching should be implemented to help meet the hygienic needs of Ms. Delamordo?
   The nurse should investigate Ms. Delamordo's feelings about being cared for by her daughter since hygiene is such a personal matter. The nurse should encourage her to take care of as many hygienic practices as possible using her left side. Teaching should include how to adapt a bathroom to the needs of a disabled person, for example, by placing a chair in the shower and using hand-held shower heads, checking water temperature, ensuring privacy, helping the patient get in and out of the shower, keeping the bathroom door unlocked, and helping to wash and dry areas that Ms. Delamordo can't reach (such as the back). Ms. Delamordo's daughter should be taught the proper techniques for caring for her mother's hair, dentures, and hearing aids.
2. What would be a successful outcome for this patient?
   By next visit, Ms. Delamordo demonstrates washing areas of her body that she can reach. By next visit, Ms. Delamordo's daughter states that she is comfortable with the care plan for hygienic measures instituted for her mother.
3. What intellectual, technical, interpersonal, and/or ethical/legal competencies are most likely to bring about the desired outcome?
   Intellectual: having basic knowledge about hygiene, hygiene measures, and the products and equipment that facilitate care
   Technical: ability to adapt hygiene care measures to meet the needs of an older adult with right-sided paralysis
   Interpersonal: ability to encourage patients and their caregivers, as appropriate, in learning new self-care measures related to hygiene
4. What resources might be helpful for Ms. Delamordo and her daughter?
   Home health care services, information on adaptive devices for people with paralysis

### PATIENT CARE STUDY

1. Objective data are underlined; subjective data are in boldface.
   Dominic Gianmarco, a <u>78-year-old retired man with a history of Parkinson's disease, lives alone</u> in a small home. He was recently <u>hospitalized for problems with cardiac rhythm, and a pacemaker was installed</u>. The home health care nurse visits 1 week after he was discharged to monitor his recovery and compliance with his medication regimen. The nurse observes that <u>his appearance is disheveled and there are multiple stains on his clothing</u>. Several food

items are in various stages of preparation on the kitchen counter, and some appear to have spoiled. Mr. Gianmarco has several days' growth of beard and a body odor is apparent. He is pleasant and oriented to place and person but cannot identify the time or day of the week. **"I lose track of what day it is. Time is not important when you are my age. The most important thing to me right now is to be able to take care of myself and stay in this house near my friends."** There is a walker visible in a corner of the living room, but Mr. Gianmarco ambulates slowly around the house with a minimum of difficulty and does not use the walker. He comments that he keeps busy **"reading, watching old movies, and going to senior citizen activities with friends who stop by for me."** His daughter, who lives several hours away, visits him every weekend and prepares his medications for the week in a plastic container that is easy for him to open. The nurse observes that all medications appeared to have been taken to date: **"I don't mess around with my medicines. One helps my ticker and the others keep me from shaking so much."**

2. Nursing Process Worksheet
*Health Problem:* Self-care deficit: bathing/hygiene, dressing/grooming
*Etiology:* Neuromuscular impairment secondary to Parkinson's disease, effects of aging
*Signs and Symptoms:* Inability to bathe and groom self independently (disheveled appearance, stains on clothing, unshaven, presence of body odor)
*Expected Outcome:* Within 2 weeks, patient will be able to perform self-care grooming activities with assistance of home health care aide.
*Nursing Interventions:*
   a. Assess patient's ability to care for self in home setting.
   b. Explore availability of home health care aide to visit patient and assist with personal hygiene activities on a regular basis.
   c. Maintain safe environment.
   d. Encourage patient's independent activities.
   e. Investigate need for any adaptive equipment.
*Evaluative Statement:* 3/28/20: Expected outcome partially met. Home health care aide assisting patient for several hours, 3 mornings/wk. Continue to evaluate patient's ability to manage treatment regimen and need for any adaptive equipment.
— *M. Gomez, RN*
3. Patient strengths: has previously been able to care for self, motivated to maintain independence, caring family member able to visit on a regular basis
Personal strengths: commitment to caring, experienced home health care nurse, strong interpersonal skills, good knowledge of gerontologic nursing
4. 3/28/20: Revisited patient 2 weeks after initial visit. Patient alert and oriented. Neat personal appearance—clean shaven, absence of body odor, hair shampooed and combed, wearing clean clothes. Stated, "my girlfriends love me now." Conforming to medication schedule and participating in social activities. Continue periodic observations.
— *M. Gomez, RN*

## PRACTICING FOR NCLEX

### MULTIPLE CHOICE QUESTIONS

**1.** c **2.** a **3.** c **4.** b **5.** b
**6.** d

### ALTERNATE-FORMAT QUESTIONS

#### Multiple Response Questions

1. a, b, d, e
2. d, e, f
3. a, c, e
4. b, d, f
5. a, c, e

# CHAPTER 32

## ASSESSING YOUR UNDERSTANDING

### FILL IN THE BLANKS

1. intentional
2. exudate
3. leukocytes, macrophages
4. granulation
5. fistula
6. sodium chloride solution
7. circular turn
8. pressure injury

### MATCHING EXERCISES

| | | | | |
|---|---|---|---|---|
| **1.** a | **2.** f | **3.** g | **4.** j | **5.** e |
| **6.** n | **7.** k | **8.** p | **9.** i | **10.** m |
| **11.** o | **12.** c | **13.** d | **14.** h | **15.** l |
| **16.** f | **17.** a | **18.** g | **19.** a | **20.** b |
| **21.** d | **22.** c | **23.** e | **24.** g | **25.** e |

### SHORT ANSWER

1. a. Protect the body; immunologic function
   b. Regulate body temperature
   c. Sense stimuli from the environment and transmit these sensations
   d. Absorption and elimination
   e. Help maintain water and electrolyte balance
   f. Produce and absorb vitamin D
2. a. External pressure: compresses blood vessels and causes friction
   b. Friction and shearing forces: tear and injure blood vessels
3. a. Nutrition: Poorly nourished cells are easily damaged (e.g., vitamin C deficiency causes capillaries to become fragile, and poor circulation to the area results when they break).
   b. Hydration: Dehydration can interfere with circulation and subsequent cell nourishment.

c. Moisture on the skin: Moisture associated with urinary incontinence increases the risk for skin damage more than chemical irritation from the ammonia in urine.
d. Mental status: The more alert a patient is, the more likely it is that he or she will relieve pressure periodically and manage adequate skin hygiene.
e. Age: Older people are good candidates for pressure injuries because their skin is susceptible to injury.
f. Immobility: Causes prolonged pressure on body areas

4. Sample answer: Provide the caregivers with a simple, easy-to-understand list of instructions about caring for the pressure injury; address the causative factor for the pressure injury before proceeding with the care plan; consult frequently with the health care provider about the progress of wound healing and products being used; use clean dressings; teach caregivers good handwashing technique; review signs of infection with caregivers and encourage them to contact a health care provider or home health nurse about any problems.
5. a. Hemostasis: Hemostasis occurs immediately after the initial injury. Involved blood vessels constrict and blood clotting begins through platelet activation and clustering. After only a brief period of constriction, these same blood vessels dilate and capillary permeability increases, allowing plasma and blood components to leak out into the area that is injured, forming a liquid called exudate.
   b. Inflammatory phase: The inflammatory phase follows hemostasis and lasts about 2 to 3 days. White blood cells, predominantly leukocytes and macrophages, move to the wound. About 24 hours after the injury, macrophages enter the wound area and remain for an extended period. Macrophages are essential to the healing process. They not only ingest debris, but also release growth factors that are necessary for the growth of epithelial cells and new blood vessels. These growth factors also attract fibroblasts that help to fill in the wound, which is necessary for the next stage of healing. Acute inflammation is characterized by pain, heat, redness, and swelling at the site of the injury.
   c. Proliferative phase: Begins about day 2 or 3 up to 2 to 3 weeks. New tissue is built to fill the wound space (action of fibroblasts). Capillaries grow across the wound, fibroblasts form fibrin that stretches through the clot, a thin layer of epithelial cells forms across the wound, and blood flow is reinstituted. Granulation tissue forms the foundation for scar tissue.
   d. Maturation phase: Begins about 3 weeks after injury, possibly continuing for months or years if wound is large. Collagen is remodeled, new collagen is deposited, and avascular collagen tissue becomes a flat, thin white line.
6. Sample answers:
   a. The patient will participate in the prescribed treatment regimen to promote wound healing.
   b. The patient will remain free of infection at the site of the pressure injury.
   c. The patient will demonstrate self-care measures necessary to prevent the development of a pressure injury.
7. Sample answers:
   a. Overall appearance of skin: Are there any areas on your body where your skin feels paper thin? How does your skin feel in relation to moisture—dry, clammy, oily?
   b. Recent changes in skin condition: Have you noticed any sores anywhere on your body? Do you ever notice any redness over a bony area when you stay in one position for a while?
   c. Activity/mobility: Do you need assistance to walk to the bathroom? Can you change your position freely and painlessly?
   d. Nutrition: Have you lost weight lately? Do you eat well-balanced meals?
   e. Pain: Do you have any painful sores on your body? Do you take any medications for pain?
   f. Elimination: Do you have any problems with incontinence? Have you ever used any briefs or pads for incontinence problems?
8. a. Appearance: Assess for the approximation of wound edges, color of the wound and surrounding areas, drains or tubes, sutures, and signs of dehiscence or evisceration.
   b. Wound drainage: Assess the amount, color, odor, and consistency of wound drainage. Drainage can be assessed on the wound, the dressings, in drainage bottles or reservoirs, or under the patient.
   c. Pain: Assess whether the pain has increased or is constant; pain may indicate delayed healing or an infection.
   d. Sutures and staples: Assess the type of suture and whether enough tensile strength has developed to hold the wound edges together during healing.
9. Provide physical, psychological, and aesthetic comfort; debride (remove necrotic tissue) if appropriate; prevent, eliminate, or control infection; absorb drainage; maintain a moist wound environment; protect the wound from further injury; and protect the skin surrounding the wound.
10. a. R = red = protect: Red wounds are in the proliferative stage of healing and are the color of normal granulation. They need protection by gentle cleansing, using moist dressings, applying a transparent or hydrocolloid dressing, and changing the dressing only when necessary.
    b. Y = yellow = cleanse: Yellow wounds are characterized by oozing from the tissue covering the wound, often accompanied by purulent

drainage. They need to be cleansed using irrigation; wet-to-moist dressings; using nonadherent, hydrogel, or other absorptive dressings; and topical antimicrobial medication.

c. B = black = debride: Black wounds are covered with thick eschar, which is usually black but may also be brown, gray, or tan. The eschar must be debrided before the wound can heal by using sharp, mechanical, chemical, or autolytic debridement.

11. a. Hot water bags or bottles: Relatively inexpensive and easy to use; may leak, burn, or make the patient uncomfortable from their weight.
    b. Electric heating pad: Can be used to apply dry heat locally; it is easy to apply and relatively safe and provides constant and even heat. Improper use can result in injury.
    c. Aquathermia pad: Commonly used in health care agencies for various problems including back pain, muscle spasms, thrombophlebitis, and mild inflammation. Safer than a heating pad but still must be checked carefully.
    d. Chemical heat packs: Commercial hot packs provide a specified amount of dry heat for a specific period.
    e. Warm moist compresses: Used to promote circulation and reduce edema. Must be changed frequently and covered with a heating agent.
    f. Sitz baths: Patient is placed in a tub filled with sufficient water to reach the umbilicus; the legs and feet remain out of the water.
    g. Warm soaks: The immersion of a body area into warm water or a medicated solution to increase blood supply to a locally infected area; to aid in cleaning large sloughing wounds, such as burns; to improve circulation; and to apply medication to a locally infected area. Makes manipulation of a painful area much easier because of the buoyancy.

## APPLYING YOUR KNOWLEDGE

### REFLECTIVE PRACTICE: CULTIVATING QSEN COMPETENCIES

#### Sample Answers

1. What nursing intervention would be appropriate to prevent skin irritation and the development of pressure injuries for Mr. Bentz?
   The nurse should review the patient chart to determine the cause and extent of previous wounds and institute measures to minimize these risks in the future. The nurse should be aware that larger than normal amounts of subcutaneous and tissue fat (which has fewer blood vessels) in people who are obese may slow wound healing because fatty tissue is more difficult to suture, is more prone to infection, and takes longer to heal.
   To protect Mr. Bentz, the nurse should implement turning and positioning schedules, as well as the use of appropriate support surfaces (tissue load management surfaces) and reposition him at least every 2 hours.
   In the event of a recurrence of pressure injuries, nursing interventions should focus on preventing infection, promoting wound healing, preventing further injury or alteration in skin integrity, promoting physical and emotional comfort, and facilitating coping.
2. What would be a successful outcome for this patient?
   Following discharge instructions, Mrs. Bentz will vocalize proper measures to assist her husband with hygiene, diet, positioning, and turning in bed. At follow-up appointment, Mr. Bentz will manifest intact skin free of skin irritations, infections, and wounds.
3. What intellectual, technical, interpersonal, and/or ethical/legal competencies are most likely to bring about the desired outcome?
   Intellectual: knowledge of the phases of wound healing and factors that affect wound healing
   Technical: ability to correctly use the products, protocols, and equipment necessary to prevent and treat pressure injuries and other skin alterations
   Interpersonal: ability to establish trusting professional relationships that enlist patients and their caregivers in a plan to prevent or treat pressure injuries and other skin alterations
4. What resources might be helpful for Mr. Bentz and his wife?
   Home health care visits, printed and/or AV materials on prevention of pressure injuries

### PATIENT CARE STUDY

1. Objective data are underlined; subjective data are in boldface.
   Mrs. Chijioke, an 88-year-old woman who lived alone for years, was brought to the hospital after neighbors found her lying at the bottom of her cellar steps. She had broken her hip and underwent hip repair surgery 3 days ago. The nurse assigned to care for Mrs. Chijioke noticed during the patient's bath that the skin of her coccyx, heels, and elbows was reddened. The skin returned to a normal color when pressure was relieved in these areas. There was no edema, nor was there induration or blistering. Although Mrs. Chijioke can be lifted out of bed into a chair, she spends most of the day in bed, lying on her back with an abductor pillow between her legs. At 5 ft tall and 89 lb, Mrs. Chijioke looks lost in the big hospital bed. Her eyes are bright, and she usually attempts a warm smile, but she has little physical strength and lies seemingly motionless for hours. Her skin is wrinkled and paper thin, and her arms are already bruised from unsuccessful attempts

at intravenous therapy. She was dehydrated on admission since she had **spent almost 48 hours crumpled at the bottom of her steps before being found by her neighbors,** and she was clearly in need of nutritional, fluid, and electrolyte support. A long-time diabetic, Mrs. Chijioke is now spiking a fever (39.0°C or 102.2°F), which concerns her nurse.

2. Nursing Process Worksheet
*Health Problem:* Risk for impaired skin integrity
*Etiology:* Immobility; effects of aging, dehydration, and illness
*Signs and Symptoms:* Skin of her coccyx, heels, and elbows is reddened—returns to normal color when pressure is relieved; lies motionless on her back when unattended; skin is wrinkled and thin; elevated temperature (39°C).
*Expected Outcome:* Whenever observed, the patient's skin will appear clean and intact (no redness, blistering, indurations).
*Nursing Interventions:*
   - **a.** Reposition patient in correct alignment at least every 1 to 2 hours and ensure protection of pressure points where possible; examine skin for signs of breakdown with each position change.
   - **b.** Massage pressure points and keep skin clean and dry.
   - **c.** Keep bed linens dry and free of wrinkles.
   - **d.** Monitor high-risk factors: dehydration, effects of illness.
     Evaluative Statement: 10/6/20: Goal met—patient's skin is clean and intact and shows no signs of breakdown. Continue prevention program
     *— M. Wong, RN*
3. Patient strengths: concerned neighbors; until now has been able to care for herself and keep herself in good health
Personal strengths: ability to recognize patients at high risk for problems such as impaired skin integrity; strong commitment to meeting the needs of geriatric patients; experienced clinician
4. 10/6/20: Patient remains on an every-2-hour positioning regimen. The protective heel and elbow pads have resulted in intact skin in these areas—no redness. The skin on her coccyx appears reddened after she lies on her back, but the redness disappears when the pressure is relieved. No constant redness, edema, or induration. Skin remains dry; lotion applied with each position change.
*— M. Wong, RN*

## PRACTICING FOR NCLEX

### MULTIPLE CHOICE QUESTIONS

| | | | | |
|---|---|---|---|---|
| **1.** b | **2.** d | **3.** a | **4.** c | **5.** d |
| **6.** c | **7.** b | **8.** d | **9.** d | **10.** a |
| **11.** a | | | | |

### ALTERNATE-FORMAT QUESTIONS

#### Multiple Response Questions

1. a, b, c, e
2. b, c, f
3. a, d, e
4. c, d, e
5. a, b, c
6. b, c, d
7. a, e, f
8. c, d, e
9. a, d, e
10. b, c, f

#### Prioritization Question

1.
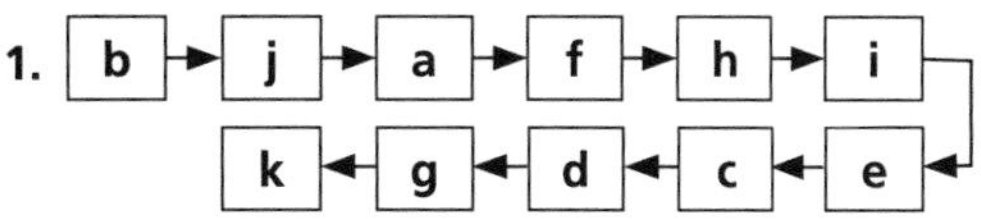


# CHAPTER 33

## ASSESSING YOUR UNDERSTANDING

### IDENTIFICATION

1. **a.** Fowler's position
   **b.** Supine position
   **c.** Side-lying or lateral position
   **d.** Sims' position
   **e.** Prone position

### MATCHING EXERCISES

| | | | | |
|---|---|---|---|---|
| **1.** e | **2.** c | **3.** f | **4.** b | **5.** a |
| **6.** l | **7.** a | **8.** g | **9.** o | **10.** d |
| **11.** k | **12.** b | **13.** n | **14.** c | **15.** m |
| **16.** j | **17.** h | **18.** e | **19.** i | **20.** b |
| **21.** e | **22.** f | **23.** a | **24.** i | **25.** c |
| **26.** d | **27.** g | | | |

### CORRECT THE FALSE STATEMENTS

1. False—irregular bones
2. True
3. True
4. True
5. False—Body mechanics
6. True
7. False—wider
8. False—proprioceptor or kinesthetic
9. False—basal ganglia
10. True
11. True
12. True
13. False—facing
14. True
15. False—slide, roll, push, or pull

## SHORT ANSWER

1. See table below.

| Body System | Effects of Exercise | Effects of Immobility |
|---|---|---|
| Cardiovascular | ↑ Efficiency of heart<br>↓ Resting heart rate and blood pressure<br>↑ Blood flow and oxygenation of all body parts | ↑ Cardiac workload<br>↑ Risk for orthostatic hypotension<br>↑ Risk for venous thrombosis |
| Respiratory | ↑ Depth of respiration<br>↑ Respiratory rate<br>↑ Gas exchange at alveolar level<br>↑ Rate of carbon dioxide excretion | ↓ Depth of respiration<br>↓ Rate of respiration<br>Pooling of secretions<br>Impaired gas exchange |
| Gastrointestinal | ↑ Appetite<br>↑ Intestinal tone | Disturbance in appetite<br>Altered protein metabolism<br>Altered digestion and utilization of nutrients |
| Urinary | ↑ Blood flow to kidneys<br>↑ Efficiency in maintaining fluid and acid–base balance<br>↑ Efficiency in excreting body wastes | ↑ Urinary stasis<br>↑ Risk for renal calculi<br>↓ Bladder muscle tone |
| Musculoskeletal | ↑ Muscle efficiency<br>↑ Coordination<br>↑ Efficiency of nerve impulse transmission | ↓ Muscle size, tone, and strength<br>↓ Joint mobility, flexibility<br>Bone demineralization<br>↓ Endurance, stability<br>↑ Risk for contracture formation |
| Metabolic | ↑ Efficiency of metabolic system<br>↑ Efficiency of body temperature regulation | ↑ Risk for electrolyte imbalance<br>Altered exchange of nutrients and gases |
| Integumentary | Improved tone, color, and turgor, resulting from improved circulation | ↑ Risk for skin breakdown and formation of decubitus ulcers |
| Psychological Well-Being | Energy, vitality, general well-being<br>Improved sleep<br>Improved appearance<br>Improved self-concept<br>Positive health behaviors | ↑ Sense of powerlessness<br>↓ Self-concept<br>↓ Social interaction<br>↓ Sensory stimulation<br>Altered sleep–wake pattern<br>↑ Risk for depression |

2. a. Motion
   b. Maintenance of posture
   c. Heat production
3. a. Point of origin: attachment of a muscle to the more stationary bone
   b. Point of insertion: attachment of a muscle to the more movable bone
4. a. The afferent nervous system conveys information from receptors in the periphery of the body to the central nervous system.
   b. Nerve cells called neurons are responsible for conducting impulses from one part of the body to another.
   c. This information is processed by the central nervous system, and a response is decided on.
   d. The efferent system conveys the desired response from the CNS to skeletal muscles by way of the somatic nervous system.
5. a. Body alignment or posture: The alignment of body parts that permits optimal musculoskeletal balance and operation and promotes healthy physiologic functioning
   b. Balance: A body in correct alignment is balanced; its center of gravity is close to the base of support, the line of gravity goes through the base of support, and the object has a wide base of support.
   c. Coordinated body movement: Using major muscle groups rather than weaker ones and taking advantage of the body's natural levers and fulcrums.
6. Sample answers:
   a. Develop a habit of maintaining erect posture and begin activities by broadening the base of support and lowering the center of gravity.

b. Use the weight of the body as a force for pulling or pushing by rocking on the feet or leaning forward or backward.
c. Slide, roll, push, or pull an object rather than lifting it to reduce the energy needed to move the weight against the pull of gravity.
d. Use the weight of the body to push an object by falling or rocking forward, and to pull an object by falling or rocking backward.

7. a. Aerobic exercises (running, swimming, tennis): Sustained muscle movements that increase blood flow, heart rate, and metabolic demand for oxygen over time, thereby promoting cardiovascular conditioning.
b. Stretching exercises (warm-up and cool-down exercises): Movements that allow muscles and joints to be stretched gently through their full range of motion; increase flexibility.
c. Strength and endurance exercises (weight training): Weight training, calisthenics, and specific isometric exercises can build both strength and endurance, increase the power of the musculoskeletal system, and improve the body.
d. Activities of daily living (shopping, cleaning): All activities of daily living have an effect on health and provide increased fitness that does not require a gym.

8. Sample answers:
a. Increased energy, vitality, and general well-being
b. Improved sleep
c. Improved self-concept
d. Increased positive health behaviors

9. a. Pillows: Pillows are used primarily to provide support or to elevate a part. Pillows of different sizes are useful for different body parts.
b. Mattresses: A mattress should be firm but should have sufficient "give" to permit good body alignment to be comfortable and supportive. A well-made and well-supported foam-rubber mattress retains a uniform firmness.
c. Adjustable bed: The head of an adjustable bed can be elevated to the desired degree, and the distance from the floor can be altered to allow the patient to get in and out of bed more easily or to allow health care workers to give care without back strain.
d. Bed side rails: They help to remind patients that they are not in their usual environment and keep them from falling out of bed.
e. Trapeze bar: This handgrip suspended from a frame near the head of the bed makes moving and turning considerably easier for many patients and facilitates transfers into and out of bed.
f. Cradle: A metal frame that keeps the top bedding off the patient's lower extremities while providing privacy and warmth.
g. Sandbags: Sandbags immobilize an extremity and support body alignment. They are not hard or firmly packed but should be placed so they do not create pressure on bony prominences.
h. Trochanter rolls: Used to support the hips and legs so that the femurs do not rotate outward.
i. Hand/wrist splints or rolls: A commercial plastic or aluminum splint is used to hold the thumb in place no matter what position the hand is in.

10. a. Quadriceps drills: Have the patient contract the muscles on the front of the thighs by pulling kneecaps toward hips; hold the position to the count of four; relax muscles for count of four. Frequency: two or three times each hour, four to six times a day.
b. Pushups: Sitting in bed: Instruct patient to lift hips off the bed by pushing down with hands on mattress. Lying on abdomen: Instruct patient to place hands near the outstretched body at shoulder level with palms down on the mattress and elbows bent sharply; then have patient straighten elbows while lifting head and shoulders off bed. Wheelchair: Instruct patient to place hands on arms of chair and raise body three or four times a day and increase frequency as upper body strength is increased.
c. Dangling: Instruct the patient to sit on the edge of the bed with legs and feet dangling over the side. Rest the patient's feet on the floor or footstool. Have patient assume a marching position. (Remain with patient in case he or she feels faint.)

11. a. Physical assessment: The nurse would assess the following:
General ease of movement: Are body parts moving fluidly and is voluntary movement controlled and coordinated?
Gait: Is head erect? Are the vertebrae straight, knees and feet forward, and arms swinging freely in alternation with leg swings?
Alignment—in standing position: Can a straight line be drawn from the ear through the shoulder and hip?
Joint structure and function: Are there any joint deformities or limitations in full range of motion?
Muscle mass tone and strength: Are they adequate to accomplish movement and work?
Endurance: Is patient able to turn in bed, maintain correct alignment when sitting and standing, ambulate, and perform self-care activities?
b. Diagnosis: Activity intolerance related to decreased muscle mass, tone, and strength.
c. Exercise program: Do range-of-motion exercises twice a day to build up muscles and joint capabilities. Use quadriceps drills two or three times an hour, four to six times a day. Do settings twice a day and pushups three or four times a day.

12. Sample answers:
   a. General ease of movement: Normal: Body movements are voluntarily controlled, fluid, and coordinated.
   Abnormal: Involuntary movements, tremors, tics, chorea, etc.
   b. Gait and posture: Normal: Head erect, vertebrae straight.
   Abnormal: Spastic hemiparesis, scissors gait.
   c. Alignment: Normal: In the standing and sitting position, a straight line can be drawn from the ear through the shoulder and hip; in bed, the head, shoulders, and hips are aligned.
   Abnormal: Abnormal spinal curvatures, inability to maintain correct alignment independently.
   d. Joint structure and function: Normal: Absence of joint deformities, full range of motion.
   Abnormal: Limitations in the normal range of motion, increased joint mobility.
   e. Muscle mass, tone, and strength: Normal: Adequate muscle mass and tone. Abnormal: Atrophy, hypotonicity.
   f. Endurance: Normal: Ability to turn in bed, maintain correct alignment.
   Abnormal: Weakness, pallor.

---

## APPLYING YOUR KNOWLEDGE

### REFLECTIVE PRACTICE: CULTIVATING QSEN COMPETENCIES

#### Sample Answers

1. What patient teaching might the nurse incorporate into the care plan to help Kelsi's parents minimize the complications of immobility for their daughter?
   The nurse should review the nursing history to assess Kelsi's activity level prior to the accident and develop a teaching plan that maximizes her level of functioning. The nurse should communicate with Kelsi and her parents and explain what is happening to her and the reasoning behind the positioning and turning schedules and range-of-motion exercises. The parents could also be taught to assist with these interventions.
2. What would be a successful outcome for this patient?
   By next visit, Kelsi's parents will demonstrate range-of-motion exercises to help restore mobility to their daughter. By next visit, Kelsi will manifest appropriate muscle strength and freedom from skin alterations.
3. What intellectual, technical, interpersonal, and/or ethical/legal competencies are most likely to bring about the desired outcome?
   Intellectual: knowledge of common problems associated with mobility and inactivity
   Technical: ability to use correctly the protocols, products, and equipment necessary to promote body alignment and to prevent or treat complications related to immobility
   Interpersonal: ability to demonstrate respect for a patient's human dignity and autonomy and to encourage patients and their caregivers to maximize their mobility and functional status
   Ethical/Legal: ability to act as a patient advocate to promote the maximum level of patient functioning
4. What resources might be helpful for the Lester family?
   Home health care services, physical rehabilitation services, printed or AV materials on range-of-motion exercises

### PATIENT CARE STUDY

1. Objective data are underlined; subjective data are in boldface.
   Robert Witherspoon, a <u>42-year-old university professor</u>, presents for a checkup shortly after his father's death. His father died of complications of coronary artery disease. Mr. Witherspoon is <u>5 ft 9 in, weighs 235 lb</u>, has a decided "paunch," and **reports that until now he has made no time for exercise because he preferred to use his free time reading or listening to classical music. He enjoys French cuisine, including rich desserts**, and <u>has a total cholesterol level of 310 mg/dL (optimal is under 200 mg/dL)</u>. **He admits being frightened by his father's death and is appropriately concerned about his elevated cholesterol level. "I guess I've never given much thought to my health before, but my Dad's death changed all that,"** he tells you. **"I know coronary artery disease runs in families, and I can tell you that I'm not ready to pack it all in yet. Tell me what I have to do to fight this thing."** He admits that he used to tease a colleague—who lowered his own cholesterol from 290 to 200 mg/dL by diet and exercise alone—by accusing him of being a fitness freak. **"Now, I'm recognizing the wisdom of his health behaviors and wondering if diet and exercise won't do the trick for me. Can you help me design an exercise program that will work?"**
2. Nursing Process Worksheet
   *Health Problem:* Altered health maintenance; lack of exercise program
   *Etiology:* Low value placed on fitness and self-care behaviors in the past
   *Signs and Symptoms:* 5 ft 9 in tall; 235 lb; until now "no time" for exercise; "I've never given much thought to my health before," "Tell me what I have to do to fight this thing," "Can you help me design an exercise program that will work?"
   *Expected Outcome:* At next visit, 10/27/20, patient will report adherence to the exercise program developed 9/30/20 (additional goals will describe desired changes in weight and cholesterol level).
   *Nursing Interventions:*
   a. Explore the patient's fitness goals, interest, skills, exercise opportunities, and exercise capacity.
   b. Assist the patient in obtaining medical clearance for exercise.

c. Explore feasible exercise activities with the patient, considering health benefits sought, time involved, need for special equipment, precautions, and risk.
d. Develop an exercise program that specifies warm-up and cool-down activities and three or four major exercise activities from which the patient can choose. Specify frequency, duration, and intensity.
e. Encourage the patient to complement the exercise program with everyday activities that require exercise.
f. Try to identify with the patient potential threats to the exercise program's successful implementation. Plan support strategies.

*Evaluative Statement:* 10/27/20: Goal partially met—patient reports that the second week into his program his "jogging buddy" got sick and that without the support of his friend he stopped exercising regularly; wants to resume. Revision: Explore new strategies to strengthen resolve/adherence.
— *J. McKeough, RN*

3. Patient strengths: Patient is highly motivated to develop new self-care behaviors as a result of his father's death—asking for help.
Personal strengths: Good understanding of the relationship between self-care behaviors (exercise, nutrition) and health; experienced in designing exercise programs; knowledge of benefits/risks associated with exercise; strong interpersonal/counseling skills
4. 10/27/20: Whereas the patient left the last session "enthusiastic" about beginning an exercise program, he reported today that he "feels like a failure" since he wasn't faithful to the goals he set for himself. After losing his exercise buddy, he found it easy to "skip runs," and he hasn't found another racquetball partner. We identified and reinforced the progress he has made and developed new expected outcomes that are less dependent on external support. — *J. McKeough, RN*

## PRACTICING FOR NCLEX

### MULTIPLE CHOICE QUESTIONS

| | | | | |
|---|---|---|---|---|
| **1.** b | **2.** a | **3.** c | **4.** d | **5.** a |
| **6.** c | **7.** b | **8.** c | **9.** d | **10.** c |
| **11.** a | **12.** a | **13.** b | **14.** d | **15.** d |

### ALTERNATE-FORMAT QUESTIONS

#### Multiple Response Questions

1. c, d, f
2. a, c, e
3. b, c, d
4. a, e, f
5. b, d, e
6. c, e, f
7. a, b, c
8. b, c, e

# CHAPTER 34

## ASSESSING YOUR UNDERSTANDING

### FILL IN THE BLANKS

1. reticular activating system (RAS) and bulbar synchronizing region
2. delta sleep
3. parasomnias
4. insomnia
5. hypersomnia
6. narcolepsy

### MATCHING EXERCISES

| | | | | |
|---|---|---|---|---|
| **1.** g | **2.** a | **3.** b | **4.** c | **5.** d |
| **6.** h | **7.** i | **8.** f | **9.** e | **10.** c |
| **11.** a | **12.** a | **13.** d | **14.** b | **15.** c, d |
| **16.** b | **17.** d | **18.** a | | |

### CORRECT THE FALSE STATEMENTS

1. True
2. True
3. False—at stage I, NREM sleep
4. False—4 or 5
5. False—12 to 15
6. True
7. False—protein and carbohydrate
8. False—hinders
9. True
10. True
11. False—sleep apnea

### SHORT ANSWER

1. **a.** Restores physical well-being
   **b.** Relieves stress and anxiety
   **c.** Restores the ability to cope and to concentrate on activities of daily living
2. **a.** Infants: 12 to 15 hrs/day
   **b.** Growing children: 9 to 11 hrs/day
   **c.** Adults: 7 to 9 hrs/day
   **d.** Older adults: May require a longer time to go to sleep and wake earlier and more frequently during the night
3. **a.** Physical activity: Activity increases fatigue and promotes relaxation that is followed by sleep. It also increases both REM and NREM sleep.
   **b.** Psychological stress: The person experiencing stress tends to find it difficult to obtain the amount of sleep he or she needs, and REM sleep decreases.
   **c.** Motivation: A desire to be wakeful and alert helps overcome sleepiness and sleep; when there is minimal motivation to be awake, sleep generally follows.
   **d.** Culture: Bedtime rituals, sleeping place, and pattern of sleep may vary according to culture.
   **e.** Diet: Carbohydrates appear to have an effect on brain serotonin levels and promote feelings of calmness and relaxation; protein may actually increase brain energy alertness and concentration.

f. Alcohol and caffeine: Alcohol in moderation seems to help induce sleep in some people, but large quantities limit REM and delta sleep. Caffeine is a CNS stimulant and may interfere with the ability to fall asleep.
g. Smoking: Nicotine has a stimulating effect, and smokers usually have a more difficult time falling asleep.
h. Environmental factors: Most people sleep best in their usual home environments.
i. Lifestyle: Sleep disorders are the major problem associated with shift work, and developing a sleep pattern is especially difficult if the shift changes periodically. Sleep can be affected by watching some types of television shows, participating in stimulating activity, and level of activity or exercise.
j. Exercise: Moderate exercise is a healthy way to promote sleep, but exercise that occurs within 2 hours before normal bedtime can hinder sleep.
k. Illness: Illness is a physiologic and psychological stressor and, therefore, influences sleep.
l. Medications: Sleep quality is influenced by certain drugs that may decrease REM sleep.

4. The cause of the sleep disturbance, the related signs and symptoms, when it first began and how often it occurs, how it affects everyday living, the severity of the problem and whether it can be treated independently by nursing, how the patient is coping with the problem, and the success of any treatments attempted
5. a. Energy level
   b. Facial characteristics
   c. Behavioral characteristics
   d. Data suggestive of potential sleep problems
6. Make sure the patient has a comfortable bed, with bottom linens tight and clean. The upper linens should allow freedom of movement and not exert pressure. A quiet, darkened room with privacy, with proper ventilation and a comfortable temperature, should be provided.
7. Sample answers:
   a. Disturbed sleep pattern: difficulty remaining asleep related to noise of hospital environment and need for periodic treatments
   b. Disturbed sleep pattern: excessive daytime sleeping related to effects of biologic aging
   c. Disturbed sleep pattern: altered sleep–wake patterns related to frequent rotations of shift
   d. Disturbed sleep pattern: premature wakening related to alcohol dependency
   e. Disturbed sleep pattern: difficulty falling asleep related to worries about family
8. a. Eyes: Dart back and forth quickly
   b. Muscles: Small muscle twitching, large muscle immobility
   c. Respirations: Irregular; sometimes interspersed with apnea
   d. Pulse: Rapid or irregular
   e. Blood pressure: Increases or fluctuates
   f. Gastric secretions: Increase
   g. Metabolism: Increases; body temperature increases
   h. Sleep cycle: REM sleep enters from stage II of NREM sleep and reenters NREM sleep at stage II; arousal from sleep difficult
9. Sample answers:
   a. Prepare a restful environment.
   b. Offer appropriate bedtime snacks and beverages.
   c. Promote comfort and relaxation.
10. Sample answers:
    a. Usual sleeping and waking times: Do you usually go to bed and wake up around the same time?
    b. Number of hours of undisturbed sleep: Do you have any difficulty falling asleep? Do you wake up during the night?
    c. Quality of sleep: Do you feel rested after the amount of sleep you get?
    d. Number and duration of naps: Do you find yourself falling asleep during the day?
    e. Energy level: Do you feel refreshed after a night's sleep?
    f. Means of relaxing before bedtime: Do you watch television or read before bedtime?
    g. Bedtime rituals: What do you do before going to bed?
    h. Sleep environment: What is your bedroom environment like?
    i. Pharmacologic aids: Do you ever take medications to help you fall asleep?
    j. Nature of sleep disturbance: What do you think is causing your sleep problem?
    k. Onset of a disturbance: When did you first notice that you had trouble falling asleep?
    l. Causes of a disturbance: Are you doing anything different before bedtime?
    m. Severity of a disturbance: Do you have breathing problems during the night?
    n. Symptoms of a disturbance: Do you grind your teeth at night?
    o. Interventions attempted and results: What measures have you taken to promote a comfortable sleep environment? Have these measures been successful?

## APPLYING YOUR KNOWLEDGE

### REFLECTIVE PRACTICE: CULTIVATING QSEN COMPETENCIES

**Sample Answers**

1. What nursing interventions might the nurse employ to help alleviate Mr. Bitner's sleep disturbances?

Nursing strategies for promoting rest and sleep in older adults include encouraging physical activity, discouraging napping, arranging an assessment for depression and treatment, reviewing medications, assessing for any side effects of sleep pattern disturbance, and decreasing fluids in the evening.

2. What would be a successful outcome for this patient?
At next visit, Mr. Bitner lists three strategies to follow to help alleviate his sleep disturbance.
In 3 weeks, Mr. Bitner reports obtaining 6 undisturbed hours of sleep at night.
3. What intellectual, technical, interpersonal, and/or ethical/legal competencies are most likely to bring about the desired outcome?
Intellectual: knowledge of the factors that affect rest and sleep, including developmental variables
Interpersonal: ability to assist older adults to develop methods to promote adequate sleep and cope with disturbed sleep patterns
Ethical/Legal: ability to practice in an ethically and legally defensible manner when providing care to patients experiencing disturbed sleep pattern
4. What resources might be helpful for Mr. Bitner?
Printed materials on sleep enhancement strategies, relaxation therapy, consultation with a sleep therapist

## PATIENT CARE STUDY

1. Objective data are underlined; subjective data are in boldface.
Gina Cioffi, a 23-year-old graduate nurse, has been in her new position as a critical care staff nurse in a large tertiary care medical center for 3 months. **"I was so excited about working three 12-hour shifts a week when I started this job, thinking I'd have lots of time for other things I want to do, but I'm not sure anymore," she says. "I've been doing extra shifts when we're short-staffed because the money is so good, and right now it seems I'm always tired and all I think about all day long is how soon I can get back to bed. Worst of all, when I do finally get into bed, I often can't fall asleep, especially if things have been busy at work and someone 'went bad.'** Does everyone else feel like me?" Looking at Gina, you notice dark circles under her eyes and are suddenly struck by the change in her appearance from when she first started working. At that time, she "bounced into work" looking fresh each morning, and her features were always animated. Now, her skin is pale, her hair and clothes look rumpled, and the "brightness" that was so characteristic of her earlier is strikingly absent. With some gentle questioning, you discover that **she frequently goes out with new friends she has made at the hospital when her shift is over, and sometimes goes for 48 hours without sleep. "I know I've gotten myself into a rut. How do I get out of it? I used to think my sleep habits were bad at school, but this is a hundred times worse because there never seems to be time to crash. I just have to keep on going."**
2. Nursing Process Worksheet
*Health Problem:* Sleep pattern disturbance: altered sleep–wake patterns.
*Etiology:* Twelve-hour shift work and stress of new job.
*Signs and Symptoms:* Works three 12-hour shifts plus two or three extra shifts per week; "right now it seems like I am always tired and all I think about all day long is how soon I can get back to bed; when I do finally get into bed I often can't fall asleep." Dark circles under eyes; pale skin; sometimes goes 48 hours without sleep; reports being less animated.
*Expected Outcome:* By this time next month (7/22/20), patient will report she is sleeping soundly for a minimum of 6 hours per night at least 6 days a week, as evidenced by her feeling less fatigued and more in control of sleep situation.
*Nursing Interventions:*
   a. Instruct patient to keep a sleep diary for 7 days and analyze its contents at the end of the week.
   b. Counsel patient about the need to reevaluate priorities (e.g., working extra shifts).
   c. Develop stress management strategies, including relaxation exercises.
   d. Identify and reduce (where possible) factors interfering with sleep.

*Evaluative Statement:* 10/6/20 Expected outcome met: Sleeping 7 to 8 hours per night and generally feels refreshed upon awakening. — *N. McLoughlin, RN*
3. Patient strengths: Strongly motivated to address this problem
Personal strengths: Comprehensive knowledge of the physiology of sleep and sleep requirements and patterns; familiarity with the stresses of clinical nursing, especially for the graduate nurse; strong interpersonal skills; creative problem solver
4. 10/6/20: Patient "bounced into the office" with the vigor and enthusiasm she displayed when she first started working. Her skin had regained its usual coloring and glow, and her face was animated. She expressed gratitude for "helping me recover my old self" and reported that she is sleeping 7 to 8 hours per night and usually wakes up refreshed and ready to tackle the new day. On questioning, she expressed an appreciation for the need to balance rest and activity and appears to have developed a workable plan for ensuring adequate rest.
— *N. McLoughlin, RN*

## PRACTICING FOR NCLEX

### MULTIPLE CHOICE QUESTIONS

| | | | | |
|---|---|---|---|---|
| **1.** b | **2.** a | **3.** d | **4.** b | **5.** a |
| **6.** d | **7.** c | **8.** d | **9.** b | **10.** c |
| **11.** b | **12.** b | | | |

## ALTERNATE-FORMAT QUESTIONS

### Multiple Response Questions

1. a, c, e
2. b, d, e
3. a, d, f
4. a, b, c
5. b, c, e
6. a, b, d, e

### Prioritization Question

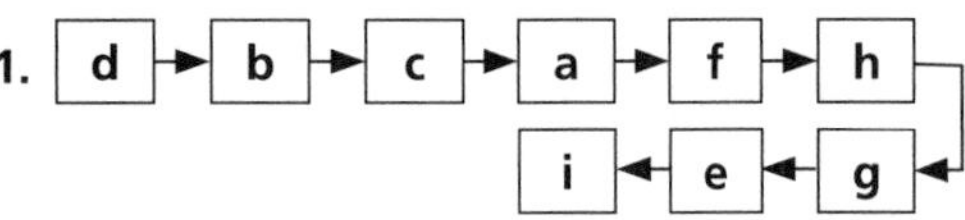


# CHAPTER 35

## ASSESSING YOUR UNDERSTANDING

### FILL IN THE BLANKS

1. nociceptive
2. cutaneous
3. visceral
4. allodynia
5. referred

### MATCHING EXERCISES

| | | | | |
|---|---|---|---|---|
| 1. e | 2. k | 3. f | 4. j | 5. a |
| 6. c | 7. g | 8. b | 9. d | 10. h |
| 11. c | 12. d | 13. b | 14. a | 15. c |
| 16. a | 17. b | 18. c | 19. j | 20. b |
| 21. d | 22. k | 23. a | 24. i | 25. c |
| 26. f | 27. h | 28. g | | |

### SHORT ANSWER

1. See Box 35-1 on page 227. Sample answers:
   Situation A: Pain, acute migraine, related to unrelieved stress as manifested by furrowed brows, nausea, and anxiety
   Situation B: Pain related to animal scratch and fear, as manifested by pulling back from cat, swelling and redness around scratch, and exaggerated weeping
   Situation C: Pain, acute postoperative, related to cesarean section as manifested by refusal to move, muscle tension, and rigidity and helplessness
   Situation D: Chronic pain related to degenerative joint disease as manifested by grimacing, refusal to walk, increased blood pressure, and exaggerated restlessness
2. The injured tissue releases chemicals that excite nerve endings. A damaged cell releases histamine, which excites nerve endings. Lactic acid accumulates in tissues injured by lack of blood supply and is believed to excite nerve endings and cause pain or lower the threshold of nerve endings to other stimuli. Bradykinin, prostaglandins, and substance P are also released.
3. Referred pain can be transmitted to a cutaneous site different from where it originated because afferent neurons enter the spinal cord at the same level as the cutaneous site to which the pain has been referred.
4. The theory states that small nerve fibers conduct excitatory pain stimuli toward the brain, exaggerating the effect of the arriving impulses through a positive feedback mechanism. Large nerve fibers appear to inhibit the transmission of pain impulses from the spinal cord to the brain through a negative feedback system (Melzack & Wall, 1965). There is a transmission mechanism that is believed by some to be located in substantia gelatinosa cells in the dorsal horn of the spinal cord. This serves as the gate. Only a limited amount of sensory information can be processed by the nervous system at any given moment. When too much information is sent through, certain cells in the spinal column interrupt the signal as if closing a gate (Pasero & McCaffery, 2011).
5. **a.** Acute pain: Generally rapid in onset, varying in intensity from mild to severe, and lasting from a brief period up to 6 months (e.g., surgery pain)
   **b.** Chronic pain: May be limited, intermittent, or persistent, but lasts for 6 months or longer and interferes with normal functioning (e.g., arthritis pain)
   **c.** Intractable pain: Pain that is resistant to therapy and persists despite a variety of interventions
6. Sample answers:
   **a.** Culture/ethnicity: In one culture, it may be acceptable to express pain vocally, whereas in another culture, such vocal expressions of pain are unacceptable.
   **b.** Family, biologic sex, or age: Spouses may reinforce pain behavior in their partners.
   **c.** Religious beliefs: In some religions, pain is viewed as suffering and as a means of purification to make up for individual or community sin.
   **d.** Environment and support people: Caring support people can help a patient cope with the strangeness of the health care environment.

| Situation | Behavioral | Physiological | Affective |
|---|---|---|---|
| A | Furrowed brows | Nausea | Anxiety |
| B | Crying | Swelling and redness on scratched area | Fear |
| C | Refusal to move | Muscle tension, rigidity | Helplessness |
| D | Grimacing, refusal to walk | Increased blood pressure | Exaggerated restlessness |

e. Anxiety and other stressors: Fear of the unknown may compound anxiety and aggravate pain.
f. Past pain experience: A child may have no fear of pain because he has never experienced pain.

7. Answers will vary with student experiences.
8. Sample answers:
   a. "You are the authority on your pain experience, and you must let your nurse know when you are in pain or when the medication isn't working anymore."
   b. "Physical addiction may occur with chronic opioid use, but this is not the same as the psychological dependence of addiction. Studies suggest that only half of 1% of all people with cancer pain and other severe types of pain will become addicted to opioids."
   c. "It is a myth that pain in the older adult is part of the normal aging process. Opioid drugs can be used to manage your pain safely as long as we take the appropriate precautions and conscientiously assess any side effects."
9. Sample answers:
   a. Duration of pain: "For how long have you been experiencing this pain?"
   b. Quantity and intensity of pain: "How frequently do you get these attacks? On a scale of 1 to 10, how would you rate the intensity of this pain?"
   c. Quality of pain: "How would you describe the pain (sharp, intense, dull, throbbing, etc.)?"
   d. Physiologic indicators of pain: "Have you noticed any physical changes since you've been experiencing this pain?"
10. Answers will vary with student experiences and may include the following: If a patient suspects a plot to trick him or her into feeling better, the patient is unlikely to respect or appreciate the good intentions of the health care providers and nurses involved.
11 a. A patient with a cognitive impairment: Many cognitively impaired patients cannot verbally report their pain or express concepts; therefore, nurses must rely on their own careful assessments, their empathetic qualities, and the expectation that this patient will experience pain if a verbal patient usually reports this event as painful.
   b. A 5-year-old patient: Children cannot always express their pain; the nurse must observe facial expressions, body positions, crying, and physiologic responses. Communication with parents or guardians is vital for accurate pain assessment.
   c. An older adult: Nurses should be aware that older adults fear that admitting pain may limit their independence; boredom, loneliness, and depression may affect an older adult's perception of pain and willingness to report it. Also, their choice of terms in describing pain may be deceptive.

## APPLYING YOUR KNOWLEDGE

### REFLECTIVE PRACTICE: CULTIVATING QSEN COMPETENCIES

#### Sample Answers

1. What nursing interventions might the nurse use to help minimize the effects of premenstrual syndrome on Ms. Potter?
   The nurse should investigate Ms. Potter's symptoms and pain history to determine what pharmaceutical or CAM measures might help relieve the pain and anxiety she is experiencing.
   The nurse should also keep in mind that stress and fatigue intensify the effects of pain.
2. What would be a successful outcome for this patient?
   By next visit, Ms. Potter vocalizes pain relief related to learned relaxation measures.
3. What intellectual, technical, interpersonal, and/or ethical/legal competencies are most likely to bring about the desired outcome?
   Intellectual: knowledge of the pain experience, pain process, and factors influencing the pain experience, such as stress and fatigue
   Interpersonal: ability to communicate and interact effectively with patients experiencing pain
4. What resources might be helpful for Ms. Potter?
   Consultation with an experienced CAM practitioner, printed materials on PMS, and relief measures

### PATIENT CARE STUDY

1. Objective data are underlined; subjective data are in boldface.
   Tabitha Wilson is a <u>24-month-old infant with AIDS who is hospitalized with infectious diarrhea</u>. She is well known to the pediatric staff, and there is real concern that she might not pull through this admission. She has suffered many of the complications of AIDS and is no stranger to pain. At the present time, <u>the skin on her buttocks is raw and excoriated, and tears stream down her face whenever she is moved. Her blood pressure also shoots up when she is touched</u>. The severity of her illness has left her <u>extremely weak and listless,</u> and **her foster mother reports that she no longer recognizes her child.** When alone in her crib, <u>she seldom moves, and she moans softly</u>. Several nurses have expressed great frustration caring for Tabitha because they find it hard to perform even simple nursing measures like turning, diapering, and weighing her when they see how much pain these procedures cause.
2. Nursing Process Worksheet
   *Health Problem:* Pain
   *Etiology:* Excoriated skin on buttocks and debilitating effects of illness
   *Signs and Symptoms:* Tears stream down face when moved and blood pressure shoots up; moans; skin on buttocks is raw and excoriated

*Expected Outcome:* By 2/15/20, patient's behaviors will indicate that pain is sufficiently relieved for patient to rest comfortably—even during clinical procedures

*Nursing Interventions:*

**a.** Report pain assessment to MD and collaborate on designing effective pain management program.

**b.** Ensure that the analgesia administration schedule produces consistent comfort.

**c.** Collaborate with wound care specialist in implementing program for healing of lesions on buttocks.

*Evaluative Statement:* 2/15/20: Expected outcome partially met—patient's behavior (absence of tears, decreased moaning, decreased BP) indicates some pain relief, but procedures that involve moving the patient still result in great discomfort. Revision: consult with health care provider again.
— *E. Daniel, RN*

3. Patient strengths: Patient and her foster parents are greatly liked by the staff; parents show great willingness to be involved in care.
Personal strengths: Knowledge of pain experience; experience in designing and monitoring pain management regimens; experience with pain management in infants and children; good rapport with wound and skin care specialist; strong interpersonal skills
4. Tabitha's response to procedures is markedly improved since the new analgesic regimen was implemented. However, although she no longer "tears up" when touched, and her blood pressure is more stable during procedures, she continues to cry during her bath and during procedures that involve more movement. Will speak with MD about modifying analgesic regimen.
— *E. Daniel, RN*

## PRACTICING FOR NCLEX

### MULTIPLE CHOICE QUESTIONS

| | | | | |
|---|---|---|---|---|
| **1.** c | **2.** d | **3.** a | **4.** d | **5.** a |
| **6.** c | **7.** b | **8.** d | **9.** a | **10.** c |
| **11.** d | **12.** b | **13.** c | **14.** b | **15.** c |

### ALTERNATE-FORMAT QUESTIONS

#### Multiple Response Questions

1. a, c, d
2. c, e, f
3. b, d, e
4. b, c, d, f
5. c, d, e

# CHAPTER 36

## ASSESSING YOUR UNDERSTANDING

### FILL IN THE BLANKS

1. 27.5
2. 2,178
3. 45% to 65%
4. 10% to 35%
5. 50% to 60%
6. aspiration
7. Basal metabolism

### MATCHING EXERCISES

| | | | | |
|---|---|---|---|---|
| **1.** a | **2.** c | **3.** b | **4.** a | **5.** b |
| **6.** c | **7.** a | **8.** c | **9.** b | **10.** b |

11. d, milk, eggs, nuts
12. a, dairy products
13. g, salt
14. i, seafood
15. e, salt and processed foods
16. k, liver
17. m, fish and tea
18. f, wheat
19. o, liver and whole grains
20. b, milk products and soft drinks
21. h, liver
22. j, oysters
23. l, beans and fruit
24. n, whole grains

| | | | | |
|---|---|---|---|---|
| **25.** e | **26.** a | **27.** g | **28.** b | **29.** i |
| **30.** c | **31.** f | | | |

32. d

### SHORT ANSWER

1. Nitrogen balance is a comparison between catabolism and anabolism and can be measured by comparing nitrogen intake and nitrogen excretion. When catabolism and anabolism are occurring at the same rate, as in healthy adults, the body is in a state of neutral nitrogen balance.
2. **a.** Saturated fatty acids: Cannot bind additional hydrogen atoms (i.e., their carbon bonds are all saturated). Example: animal fats. Saturated fats raise cholesterol.
**b.** Unsaturated fatty acids: Have one or more double bonds between carbon atoms. When double bonds are broken, carbons can bind with additional hydrogen atoms. Example: vegetable fats. Unsaturated fats lower serum cholesterol levels.
3. **a.** Certain age groups: infants, adolescents, pregnant and lactating women, and older adults

b. Smoking, alcohol abuse, and long-term use of certain medications
c. Chronic illnesses
d. Poor appetite

4. a. Infancy: The period from birth to 1 year of age is the most rapid period of growth. Nutritional needs per unit of body weight are greater than at any other time in the life cycle.
b. Toddlers and preschoolers. During this stage, the growth rate slows. Mobility, autonomy, and coordination increase, as do muscle mass and bone density. This age group develops an attitude toward food. Appetite decreases and becomes erratic.
c. School-aged children: Nutritional implications focus on health promotion. Increasing energy requirements should be balanced with foods of high nutritional value. The appetite improves but may still be irregular.
d. Adolescents: Nutrient needs increase to support growth. Weight consciousness becomes compulsive in 1 of 100 teenage girls and results in an eating disorder.
e. Adults: Growth ceases, and nutritional needs level off.
f. Pregnant women: Nutrient needs increase to support growth and maintain maternal homeostasis, particularly during the second and third trimesters. Caloric needs are higher for lactation than for pregnancy.
g. Older adults: Because of the decreases in BMR and physical activity and loss of lean body mass, energy expenditure decreases. The calorie needs of the body decrease.

5. See table below.

6. Sample answers:
a. Eat a variety of high-fiber foods daily.
b. Drink water: 2,200 to 3,000 mL/day for adults.
c. Substitute high-fiber foods for lower-fiber foods.
d. Add bran to diet slowly to decrease likelihood of flatus and distention.

7. a. Anorexia nervosa: Characterized by denial of appetite and bizarre eating patterns; may result in extremely dangerous amount of weight loss; can be fatal. Typical person is adolescent girl from middle or upper socioeconomic class; competitive; obsessive; distorted body image.
b. Bulimia: Characterized by gorging followed by purging with self-induced vomiting, diuretics, and laxative use. Typical person is college student who fears gaining weight but is overwhelmed by periods of intense hunger.

8. a. Biologic sex: Men have higher caloric and protein requirements than women because of their larger muscle mass.
b. State of health: The alteration in nutrient requirements that results from illness and trauma varies with the intensity and duration of stress.
c. Alcohol abuse: Alcohol can alter the body's use of nutrients and thereby its nutrient requirements by numerous mechanisms.
d. Medications: Nutrient absorption may be altered by drugs that change the pH of the gastrointestinal tract, increase gastrointestinal motility, damage the intestinal mucosa, or bind with nutrients, rendering them unavailable to the body.
e. Megadoses of nutrient supplements: An excess of one nutrient can lead to a deficiency of another.

| Nutrient | Function | Recommended % |
|---|---|---|
| **a.** Carbohydrates | Supply energy (4 cal/g); also spares protein, helps burn fat efficiently, and prevents ketosis | 45–65% |
| **b.** Proteins | Maintain body tissues; support new tissue growth; component of body framework | 10–35% |
| **c.** Fats | Important component of cell membranes; synthesis of bile acids; precursor of steroid hormones and vitamin D; most concentrated source of energy (9 cal/g); aids in absorption of fat-soluble vitamins; provides insulation, structure, and body temperature control | Saturated <10%<br>Unsaturated <35% |
| **d.** Vitamins | Metabolism of carbohydrates, protein, and fat; support vital functions and prevent deficiency diseases | |
| **e.** Minerals | Key components of body structures; regulation of body processes | |
| **f.** Water | Essential for all biochemical reactions; participates in many biochemical reactions; helps regulate body temperature, helps lubricate body joints; needed for adequate mucous secretions; supports blood volume and blood pressure | 2,200–3,000 mL/day |

**f.** Religion: Nurses need to be aware of dietary restrictions associated with religions that might affect a patient's nutritional requirements.
**g.** Economics: A person's food budget affects dietary choices and patterns.

**9. a.** Food diaries: The patient records all food and beverages consumed in a specified time period (3 to 7 days).
**b.** Diet history: This is a 24-hour recall, food frequency record, plus interview designed to determine past and present food intake and habits.
**c.** Food frequency record: Food frequency records give a general picture of nutritional consumption. The nurse would ask patients questions to elicit an average number of times certain foods or food groups are consumed in a given period of time: per day, per week, or per month.

**10.** Sample answer:
The nurse should explain the diet order to the patient, screen patients at home who are at nutritional risk, observe intake and appetite, evaluate patient's tolerance for specific types of foods, assist the patient with eating, address potential for harmful drug–nutrient interactions, and teach nutrition.

**11.** Sample answers:
**a.** Provide simple verbal instructions; include family members when appropriate.
**b.** Advise the patient to eliminate any foods that are not tolerated.
**c.** Offer support and encouragement.

**12. a.** Clear liquid diet: Only foods that are clear liquids at room temperature, such as gelatins, fat-free bouillon, ice pops, clear juices, etc.; inadequate in calories, proteins, and most nutrients
**b.** Full liquid diet: All liquids that can be poured at room temperature, such as clear liquids plus milk, plain frozen desserts, pasteurized eggs, cereal gruels; high-calorie, high-protein supplements are recommended if used for more than 3 days

**13. a.** Nasogastric feeding tube: Inserted through nose and into stomach. Advantage: Allows stomach to be used as natural reservoir, regulating amount of food that enters intestine. Disadvantage: Introduces risk for aspiration of tube feeding solution into lungs.
**b.** Nasointestinal feeding tube: Passed through the nose into the upper portion of the small intestine. Advantage: Minimal risk for aspiration. Disadvantage: Dumping syndrome may develop.

**14. a.** Patient's progress toward meeting nutritional goals
**b.** Patient's tolerance of and adherence to the diet when appropriate
**c.** Patient's level of understanding of the diet and need for further diet instruction
**d.** Findings should be communicated to other health care team members.
**e.** Plan should be revised or terminated as needed.

## APPLYING YOUR KNOWLEDGE

### REFLECTIVE PRACTICE: CULTIVATING QSEN COMPETENCIES

#### Sample Answers

**1.** What patient teaching might the nurse provide to help Mr. Johnston meet his nutritional and exercise needs?
The nurse should assess Mr. Johnston's eating habits by conducting a diet history. A diet plan could then be devised that would contain foods low in fat and cholesterol, enabling him to lose 1 to 2 lb/wk. The nurse should also set up an exercise program for Mr. Johnston that he could adapt to his busy lifestyle. For the greatest chance of success, the nurse should tailor diet instructions individually to Mr. Johnston's lifestyle, culture, intellectual ability, and level of motivation.

**2.** What would be a successful outcome for this patient?
By the end of the visit, Mr. Johnston lists recommended allowances of grains, vegetables, fruits, milk, and meat and beans as seen in the MyPlate Food Guide
By next visit, Mr. Johnston manifests a weight loss of 2 lb and has lower blood pressure and cholesterol levels.

**3.** What intellectual, technical, interpersonal, and/or ethical/legal competencies are most likely to bring about the desired outcome?
Intellectual: knowledge of nutrients and nutritional requirements for patients across the life span; knowledge of hypertension and high cholesterol and strategies for managing these conditions through dietary restrictions
Interpersonal: special interpersonal competencies to help the executive see the value in making lifestyle changes necessary to improve his nutritional status
Ethical/Legal: ability to act as a trusted and effective patient advocate

**4.** What resources might be helpful for Mr. Johnston?
Consultation with a nutritionist, printed materials on hypertension and high cholesterol, exercise programs

### PATIENT CARE STUDY

**1.** Objective data are underlined; subjective data are in boldface.
Mr. Church, a <u>74-year-old White man</u>, is being admitted to the geriatric unit of the hospital for a diagnostic workup. He was <u>diagnosed with Alzheimer's disease 4 years ago</u>, and <u>1 year ago, he was admitted to a long-term care facility</u>. His wife of 49 years is extremely devoted and informs the nurse taking the admission history that she instigated his admission to the hospital because she **was alarmed by the amount of weight he was losing**. Assessment reveals a <u>6-ft, 1-in tall, emaciated man who weighs 149 lb. His wife reports he has lost 20 lb in the past 2 months</u>. The staff at the long-term care facility report that <u>he was eating his meals, and his wife validated that this was the case.</u> No one seems sure, however, of the caloric content of his diet. **Mrs. Church nods her head vigorously when asked if her husband had**

**seemed more agitated and hyperactive recently.** Mr. Church has dull, sparse hair; pale, dry skin; and dry mucous membranes.

2. Nursing Process Worksheet
   *Health Problem:* Altered nutrition: less than body requirements
   *Etiology:* Imbalance between energy expenditure and caloric intake
   *Signs and Symptoms:* 6 ft tall, 149 lb; appears "emaciated"; 20-lb weight loss over 2 months; is eating meals; more hyperactive and agitated than usual; dull, sparse hair; pale, dry skin; dry mucous membranes
   *Expected Outcome:* In 1 month (1/20/20), patient will demonstrate signs of ingesting enough calories to meet energy needs, as evidenced by a 5- to 10-lb weight gain.
   *Nursing Interventions:*
   a. Do a 72-hour diet history to determine the average number of calories he ingests daily.
   b. Provide whatever assistance he needs with feeding. Add high-calorie snacks to his diet, increasing calories progressively until the pattern of weight loss is replaced by weight gain.
   c. Until the desired weight is regained and maintained, weigh the patient daily and keep an accurate fluid I&O and calorie intake record.
   d. Explore nursing strategies to reduce agitation and hyperactivity, such as music, balance between solitude and social interaction, rest periods, etc.

   *Evaluative Statement:* 1/20/20: Expected outcome met—patient gained 8 lb over past month and seems to enjoy high-calorie snacks. — *M. Bendyma, RN*
3. Patient strengths: Patient has a very supportive wife. Personal strengths: Sound knowledge of nutrition and Alzheimer's disease; experienced in working with persons with Alzheimer's disease and their families; experienced gerontologic nurse.
4. Over the past month, the patient's intake has increased by 2,000 cal/day. He enjoys high-calorie snacks of peanut butter and jelly sandwiches, milkshakes, dried fruit and nuts, pasta salads, and an occasional Snickers bar. He has regained 8 of the 20 lb he lost, and his wife is delighted. He remains hyperactive, but scheduled walks have decreased some of his agitation. Will continue to monitor his nutritional needs. — *M. Bendyma, RN*

## PRACTICING FOR NCLEX

### MULTIPLE CHOICE QUESTIONS

| | | | | |
|---|---|---|---|---|
| **1.** a | **2.** b | **3.** c | **4.** c | **5.** b |
| **6.** a | **7.** c | **8.** b | **9.** c | |

### ALTERNATE-FORMAT QUESTIONS

#### Multiple Response Questions

1. c, d, f
2. a, d, e
3. a, d, e
4. a, c, d
5. c, d, e, f
6. c, d, e
7. a, c, d

# CHAPTER 37

## ASSESSING YOUR UNDERSTANDING

### MATCHING EXERCISES

| | | | | |
|---|---|---|---|---|
| **1.** f | **2.** h | **3.** k | **4.** a | **5.** d |
| **6.** c | **7.** j | **8.** l | **9.** e | **10.** g |
| **11.** i | **12.** d | **13.** a | **14.** c | **15.** c |
| **16.** b | **17.** e | **18.** d | | |

### SHORT ANSWER

1. a. Developmental considerations: Infants are born with no urinary control. Most children develop urinary control between the ages of 2 and 5 years. Physiologic changes that accompany normal aging may affect urination in the older adult.
   b. Food and fluid: The kidneys should preserve a careful balance of fluid intake and output. Caffeine-containing beverages have a diuretic effect and increase urine production. Alcohol produces the same effect by inhibiting the release of antidiuretic hormone. Foods high in water may increase urine production. High-sodium foods and beverages cause sodium and water reabsorption and retention.
   c. Psychological variables: People experiencing stress often find themselves voiding smaller amounts of urine at more frequent intervals. Stress can also interfere with the ability to relax perineal muscles and the external urethral sphincter.
   d. Activity and muscle tone: Exercise increases metabolism and optimal urine production and elimination. With prolonged periods of immobility, decreased bladder and sphincter tone can result in poor urinary control and urinary stasis.
   e. Pathologic conditions: Certain renal or urologic problems can affect both the quantity and quality of urine produced.
   f. Medications: Medications have numerous effects on urine production and elimination. Nephrotoxic drugs are a serious concern. Abuse of analgesics can result in nephrotoxicity. Certain drugs cause urine to change color.
2. a. The child should be able to hold urine for 2 hours.
   b. The child should recognize bladder fullness.
   c. The child should be able to express the need to void and control urination until reaching the toilet.
3. a. Infants and young children: It is important to assess whether the child has achieved bladder control and whether a toileting schedule has been established for the child. It is also important to identify the words the child uses to indicate the need to void.
   b. Older adults: Decreased bladder tone may be a problem. The nursing history should note how the person handles these problems and the adequacy of the solution.

   c. Patients with limited or no bladder control or urinary diversions: The procedures and equipment used should be assessed to make sure they follow accepted guidelines and are not predisposing the person to infection or other risk.
4. a. Kidneys: Palpation of the kidneys is usually performed as part of a more detailed assessment. This technique requires deep palpation and is generally assessed by an advanced health care professional, such as an advanced practice nurse or health care provider.
   b. Bladder: The bladder cannot be assessed by the nurse when it is empty. When it is distended, the nurse observes the lower abdominal wall, noting any swelling, and palpates the area for tenderness, noting the smoothness and roundness of the bladder.
   c. Urethral orifice: This is inspected for any signs of inflammation or discharge. Foul odors should be noted.
   d. Skin integrity and hydration: The skin should be carefully assessed for color, texture, turgor. The integrity of the skin in the perineal area should also be assessed.
   e. Urine: Each time a patient's urine is handled, it should be assessed for color, odor, clarity, and the presence of sediment. Abnormalities should be noted.
5. Sample answers:
   a. The patient will produce urine output about equal to fluid intake.
   b. The patient will maintain fluid and electrolyte balance.
   c. The patient will report ease of voiding.
   d. The patient will maintain skin integrity.
6. a. Schedule: Some patients report voiding on demand in no apparent pattern; others have inflexible patterns that have developed over the years and become anxious if these are interrupted.
   b. Privacy: Many adults and children cannot void in the presence of another person; privacy should be offered in the health care and home settings.
   c. Position: Helping patients assume normal voiding positions may be all that is necessary to resolve an inability to void.
   d. Hygiene: Patients confined to bed will find it difficult to perform their usual genital hygiene. The nurse should place these patients on a bedpan and pour warm soapy water over the perineal area, followed by clear water.
7. Sample answers:
   a. To relieve urinary retention
   b. To obtain a sterile specimen from a woman
   c. To empty the bladder before, during, and after surgery
8. Sample answers:
   a. The patient will explain the cause for the urinary diversion and the rationale for treatment.
   b. The patient will demonstrate self-care behaviors and manage the diversion effectively.

## APPLYING YOUR KNOWLEDGE

### REFLECTIVE PRACTICE: CULTIVATING QSEN COMPETENCIES

1. How might the nurse respond to Mrs. Morita's remarks regarding her husband's home care?
   Mr. Morita has the right to a urinary assessment to determine if there are any underlying causes, either physical or psychological, for the incontinence. The nurse should speak to the couple to assess their feelings regarding the incidents. Nursing strategies could be implemented to promote urinary continence prior to inserting a urinary catheter. If these measures fail, the nurse might suggest using a condom catheter for Mr. Morita as a possible alternative, rather than an indwelling catheter, which would increase his risk for infection. The nurse could also look into home health care personnel for the couple to assist with toileting and/or light housekeeping.
2. What would be a successful outcome for this patient?
   By next visit, Mr. Morita states two methods to promote urinary continence.
   By next visit, Mrs. Morita expresses satisfaction with urinary strategies to promote continence and receives outside help in the home.
3. What intellectual, technical, interpersonal, and/or ethical/legal competencies are most likely to bring about the desired outcome?
   Intellectual: knowledge of the anatomy and physiology of the urinary systems and developmental variables that influence urination
   Technical: ability to use the equipment and protocols necessary to diagnose and treat urinary problems
   Ethical/Legal: strong sense of accountability for the health and well-being of patients experiencing urinary problems
4. What resources might be helpful for the Morita family?
   Home health care services, printed information on urinary incontinence, and care of urinary catheters

### PATIENT CARE STUDY

1. Objective data are underlined; subjective data are in boldface.
   Mr. Eisenberg, <u>age 84</u>, was admitted to a long-term care facility when his wife of 62 years died. He has <u>two adult children</u>, neither of whom feels prepared to care for him the way his wife did. **"We don't know how Mom did it year after year,"** his son says. **"After he retired from his law practice, he was terribly demanding, and it just seemed nothing she did for him pleased him. His Parkinson's disease does make it a bit difficult for him to get around, but he's able to do a whole lot more than he is letting on. He's always been this way."** The aides have reported to you that Mr. Eisenberg is <u>frequently incontinent of both urine and stool during the day as well as during the night.</u> He is <u>alert and appears capable of recognizing the need</u>

to void or defecate and signaling for any assistance. His son and daughter report that this was never a problem at home and that he was able to go into the bathroom with assistance. He has been depressed about his admission to the home and seldom speaks, even when directly approached. He has refused to participate in any of the floor social events since his arrival.

2. Nursing Process Worksheet
   *Health Problem:* Toileting self-care deficit
   *Etiology:* Depression on entering a long-term care facility and decreased will to live
   *Signs and Symptoms:* Incontinent of both urine and stool during the day and night (need to determine the frequency); alert and capable of recognizing and signaling the need to void/defecate; able to walk to bathroom with assistance
   *Expected Outcome:* Within 2 weeks (6/17/20), patient will communicate the need to void/defecate appropriately, as evidenced by reduction in incontinent episodes to one "accident" daily.
   *Nursing Interventions:*
   a. Initiate a regular toileting schedule with the patient in which he is assisted to the bathroom; use these interactions to reinforce the importance of his maintaining his independence.
   b. Refrain from using adult incontinent pads or in any way communicating that incontinence is "OK."
   c. Call an interdisciplinary conference to develop a strategy to ease his transition to the home.

   *Evaluative Statement:* 6/17/20: Expected outcome partially met—when assisted to the bathroom, the patient voids/defecates; but if the staff neglects to offer assistance, the patient will not use his call light to request it, and incontinent episodes recur (more than one a day on some days). Revision: Continue to counsel regarding transition to the home and importance of independence. — *P. Wu, RN*
3. Patient strengths: Patient is alert and capable of expressing his needs for assistance. Mobile with assistance.
   Personal strengths: Good knowledge of gerontologic nursing and experience in caring for older adults; experienced counselor and teacher of appropriate self-care measures.
4. 6/15/20: A review of the patient's record reveals three incontinent episodes in the past 24 hours (two urine, one stool). When asked why he did not ask for assistance to get to the bathroom, the patient refused to answer. Generally, he cooperates with the toileting regimen, and when taken to the bathroom voids/defecates as needed. Will continue to counsel regarding the importance of his independently managing his toileting needs. Will reevaluate his ability to recognize the need to void/defecate and ask for assistance. — *P. Wu, RN*

## PRACTICING FOR NCLEX

### MULTIPLE CHOICE QUESTIONS

**1.** a **2.** b **3.** d **4.** a **5.** c
**6.** d **7.** c **8.** d **9.** a **10.** d
**11.** d

### ALTERNATE-FORMAT QUESTIONS

#### Multiple Response Questions

1. b, c, e, f
2. a, d, f
3. b, e, f
4. a, c, e, f
5. a, b, d, e
6. b, c, d
7. a, c, e

#### Hot Spot Questions

Refer to figures.

1. Urethra positions.

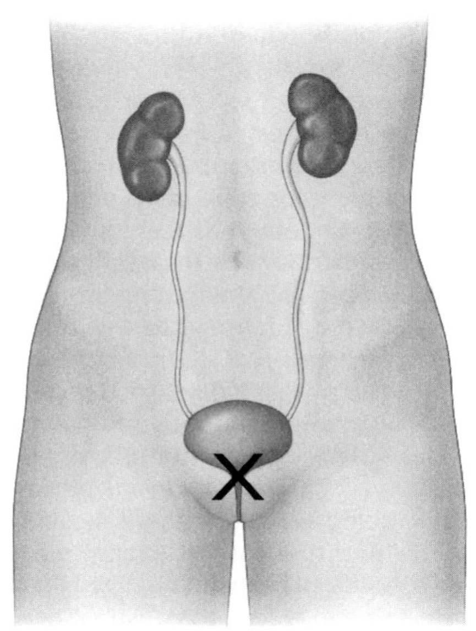


A

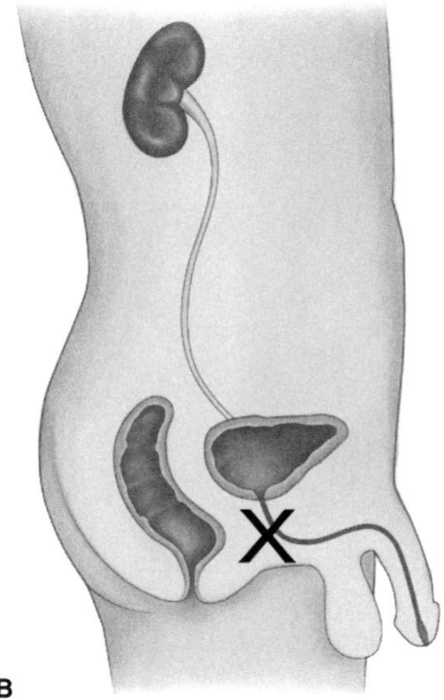


B

**2.** External sphincter location.

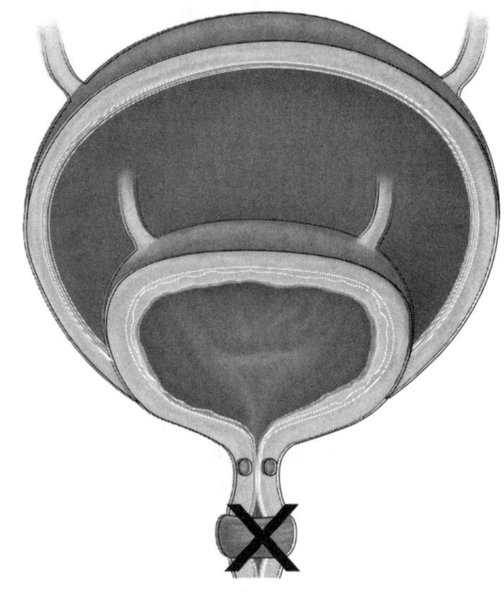


**3.** Bladder location and size (male).

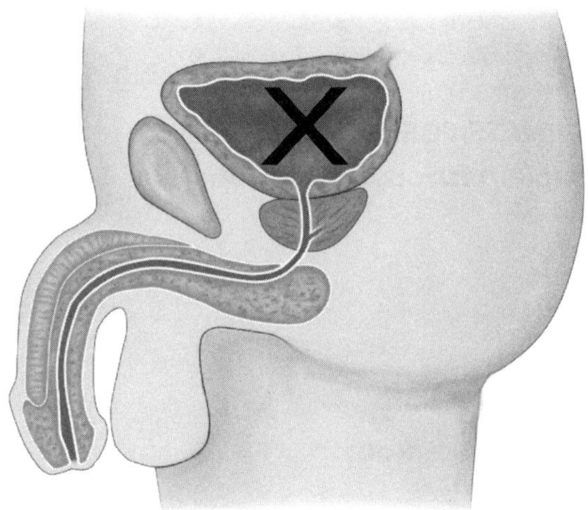


**4.** Suprapubic catheter position.

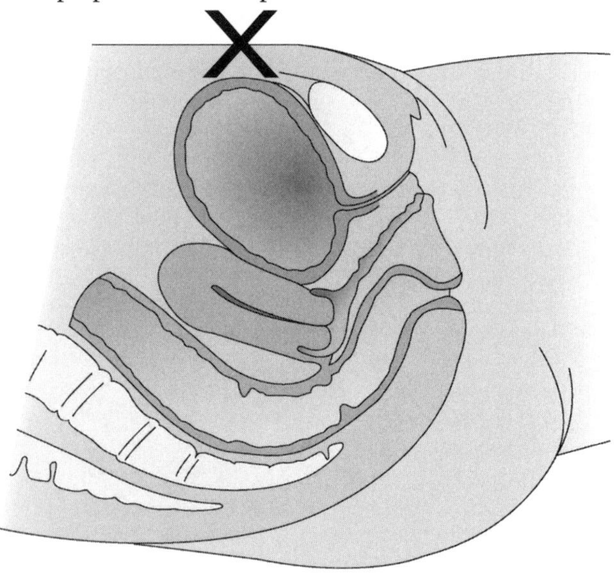


# CHAPTER 38

## ASSESSING YOUR UNDERSTANDING

### IDENTIFICATION

**1. a.** Rectum
**b.** Internal anal sphincter
**c.** External anal sphincter
**d.** Anal valve
**e.** Anal canal

**2. a.** Sigmoid colostomy—formed
**b.** Descending colostomy—formed
**c.** Transverse (single B) colostomy—soft
**d.** Ascending colostomy—soft to liquid
**e.** Ileostomy—liquid

### MATCHING EXERCISES

| | | | | |
|---|---|---|---|---|
| **1.** h | **2.** a | **3.** d | **4.** f | **5.** c |
| **6.** e | **7.** b | **8.** g | **9.** j | **10.** a |
| **11.** d | **12.** c | **13.** b | **14.** g | **15.** a |
| **16.** h | **17.** b | **18.** d | **19.** i | **20.** c |
| **21.** e | **22.** k | **23.** g | **24.** f | **25.** a |
| **26.** m | **27.** h | **28.** b | **29.** n | **30.** c |
| **31.** i | **32.** q | **33.** o | **34.** r | **35.** d |
| **36.** l | **37.** p | **38.** e | **39.** k | **40.** j |

### SHORT ANSWER

**1. a.** Completion of absorption
**b.** Manufacture of certain vitamins
**c.** Formation of feces
**d.** Expulsion of feces from the body

**2. a.** One is situated in the medulla.
**b.** A subsidiary center is situated in the spinal cord.

**3. a.** Direct manipulation of the bowel during surgery inhibits peristalsis, causing a condition termed paralytic ileus. This temporary stoppage lasts 24 to 48 hours.
**b.** Inhalation of anesthetic agents inhibits peristalsis by blocking parasympathetic impulses to the intestinal musculature.

**4. a.** Inspection: The nurse observes the contour of the abdomen, noting any masses or areas of distention.
**b.** Auscultation: The nurse uses a warmed stethoscope to listen for bowel sounds in a systematic, clockwise manner in all abdominal quadrants.
**c.** Percussion: The nurse percusses all quadrants of the abdomen in a systematic, clockwise manner to identify any masses, fluid, or air.
**d.** Palpation: The nurse performs light palpation in each quadrant while watching the patient's face for nonverbal signs of pain during palpation. The nurse palpates each quadrant in a systematic manner, noting muscular resistance, tenderness, enlargement of the organs, or masses.

**5. a.** Developmental considerations: The stool characteristics of an infant depend on whether the infant is being fed breast milk or formula.
**b.** Daily patterns: A change in a person's daily routine may lead to constipation.

c. Food and fluids: Both the type and the amount of foods eaten affect elimination.
d. Activity and muscle tone: Regular exercise improves gastrointestinal motility.
e. Lifestyle: A person's daily schedule, occupation, and leisure activities may contribute to a habit of defecating at regular times or to an irregular pattern.
f. Psychological variables: In some people, anxiety may have a direct effect on gastrointestinal motility, and diarrhea accompanies periods of high anxiety.
g. Medications: Medications may influence the appearance of the stool—for instance, iron salts result in a black stool from the oxidation of iron.
h. Diagnostic studies: Patients may need to fast for tests, which may alter elimination patterns.

6. Sample answer:
When you were first diagnosed with diverticular disease? How long have you had the pain? Have you ever had this pain before? How often do you move your bowels? What do your stools look like? Have you noticed any changes in stool lately? What is your regular diet like? Are there any foods you avoid? Are there any foods that help relieve the pain?
7. a. Daily fluid intake of 2,000 to 3,000 mL
b. Increased intake of high-fiber foods
c. Regular exercise
d. Acceptance of bowel elimination as a normal process of life
8. a. Constipating: Processed cheese, lean meat, eggs, pasta
b. Laxative: Certain fruits and vegetables, bran, chocolate
c. Gas producing: Onions, cabbage, beans, cauliflower
9. a. The patient will have a soft, formed bowel movement every 1 to 3 days without discomfort.
b. The patient will explain the relationship between bowel elimination and dietary fiber, fluid intake, and exercise.
c. The patient will relate the importance of timing, positioning, and privacy to healthy bowel elimination.
10. a. Constipation: Increase intake of high-fiber foods and fluid.
b. Diarrhea: Prepare and store food properly, avoid highly spiced foods or laxative-type foods, increase intake of low-fiber foods, and replace lost fluids.
c. Flatulence: Avoid gas-producing foods such as beans, cabbage, onions, cauliflower, and beer.
d. Ostomies: A low-fiber diet is usually recommended, although patients may experiment with their diet to determine how much fiber they can tolerate.
11. a. Abdominal settings: Lying in a supine position, tighten and hold the abdominal muscles for 6 seconds and then relax them. Repeat several times every waking hour.
b. Thigh strengthening: Flex and contract the thigh muscles by slowly bringing the knees up to the chest—one at a time—and then lowering them to the bed. Perform several times for each knee, each waking hour.
12. a. To relieve constipation or fecal compaction
b. To prevent involuntary escape of fecal material during surgical procedures
c. To promote visualization of the intestinal tract by radiographic or instrument examination
d. To help establish regular bowel function during a bowel training program
13. a. Ileostomy: allows liquid fecal content from the ileum of the small intestine to be eliminated through the stoma
b. Colostomy: permits formed feces from the colon to exit through the stoma
14. a. Timing: Patients should be allowed to heed the natural urge to defecate.
b. Positioning: The squatting position best facilitates defecation.
c. Privacy: Most patients consider elimination of a private act, and nurses should provide privacy for their patients.
d. Nutrition: Patients with elimination problems may need a dietary analysis to determine which foods and fluids are contributing to their problem.
e. Exercise: Regular exercise improves gastrointestinal motility and aids in defecation.

## APPLYING YOUR KNOWLEDGE

### REFLECTIVE PRACTICE: CULTIVATING QSEN COMPETENCIES

#### Sample Answers

1. What nursing interventions might the nurse implement for this patient?
The nurse should address methods to counteract the constipating effects of the medication on Mr. Cobbs' gastrointestinal system. The nurse could then prepare a teaching plan for Mr. Cobbs that lists the foods that he should eat to stimulate peristalsis. Nursing interventions to remove the fecal impaction in a competent manner should also be initiated.
2. What would be a successful outcome for Mr. Cobbs?
By next visit, Mr. Cobbs lists three foods to include in his diet to prevent constipation.
By next visit, Mr. Cobbs verbalizes having regular, pain-free bowel movements.
3. What intellectual, technical, interpersonal, and/or ethical/legal competencies are most likely to bring about the desired outcome?

Intellectual: knowledge of the anatomy and physiology of bowel elimination and variables, such as medications, that influence bowel elimination
Technical: ability to perform digital extraction of fecal matter in a safe and competent manner
Interpersonal: ability to interact in a nonjudgmental and professional manner when interacting in situations involving bowel elimination, a typically private matter
Ethical/Legal: adherence to safety and quality when performing nursing interventions to promote bowel elimination

4. What resources might be helpful for Mr. Cobbs? Consultation with a dietitian, printed or AV materials discussing the effect of medications on the gastrointestinal system, and appropriate interventions

## PATIENT CARE STUDY

1. Objective data are underlined; subjective data are in boldface.
   Ms. Elgaresta, <u>age 54, a single Hispanic woman,</u> is being followed by a cardiologist who monitors her arrhythmia. <u>Last month, she started taking a new heart medication</u>. At this visit, she says to the nurse practitioner who works with the cardiologist: **"Right after I started taking that medication, I got terribly constipated, and nothing seems to help. I'm desperate and about ready to try dynamite unless you can think of something else!" She reports a change in her bowel movements from one soft stool daily to one or two hard stools weekly, stools that cause much straining.** The nurse practitioner realizes that regulating Ms. Elgersma's heart is difficult and that her best cardiac response to date has been with the medication that is now causing constipation. Reluctant to suggest substituting another medication too quickly, she asks more questions, and Ms. Elgaresta responds, **"I've never been much of a drinker, two cups of coffee in the morning and maybe a glass of wine at night. Water? Almost never. And I don't drink juices or soft drinks."** Analysis of her diet reveals a <u>diet low in fiber</u>: **"I never was one much for vegetables, and they can just keep all this bran stuff that's out on the market! Coffee and a cigarette. That's for me!"** Ms. Elgaresta is a workaholic computer programmer and spends what little spare time she has watching TV. She reports **tiring after walking one flight of stairs and says she avoids all forms of vigorous exercise.**
2. Nursing Process Worksheet
   *Health Problem:* Constipation
   *Etiology:* New medication, deficient fiber and fluid intake, and insufficient exercise
   *Signs and Symptoms:* Change in bowel habits from one soft, formed stool daily to one or two hard stools per week and straining
   *Expected Outcome:* One month after new regimen begins (5/4/20), patient reports one soft, formed stool every 1 to 2 days
   *Nursing Interventions:*
   a. Counsel patient about the relationship between diet (fiber intake and fluids) and bowel elimination, and exercise and bowel elimination.
   b. Assess patient's willingness and motivation to make lifestyle changes and develop a workable plan.
   c. Reinforce importance of continuing medication.
   *Evaluative Statement:* Expected outcome met—patient now passing a soft, formed stool almost every day.
   *— B. Shevorkis, RN*
3. Patient strengths: Patient is highly motivated to learn new self-care behaviors.
   Personal strengths: Knowledge of the physiology of elimination; experienced patient educator and counselor; excellent role model of healthy self-care behaviors.
4. 5/4/20: Patient in for 1-month follow-up. Expressed delight with effects of new self-care behaviors: (1) decreased fat consumption and increased fiber in diet, (2) increased fluid intake—especially water, (3) increased exercise—four 30-minute periods of aerobic exercise per week. Constipation problem is resolved—passes soft stool almost every day—and reports having much more energy for work. Progress reinforced.
   *— B. Shevorkis, RN*

## PRACTICING FOR NCLEX

### MULTIPLE CHOICE QUESTIONS

**1.** d **2.** c **3.** b **4.** a **5.** d
**6.** b **7.** c

### ALTERNATE-FORMAT QUESTIONS

#### Multiple Response Questions

1. c, d, f
2. b, c, f
3. c, d, f
4. b, e, f
5. a, c, d, e
6. b, d, e
7. c, d, e
8. a, c
9. b, d, f

#### Prioritization Question

1. 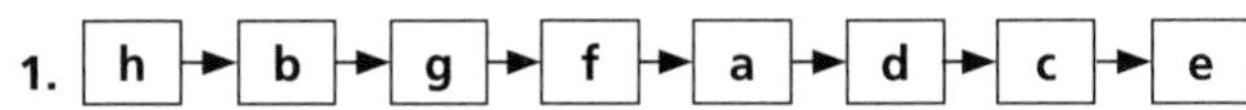


# CHAPTER 39

## ASSESSING YOUR UNDERSTANDING

### IDENTIFICATION

1. a. Frontal sinus
   b. Nasal cavity
   c. Epiglottis

d. Right lung
e. Right bronchus
f. Terminal bronchiole
g. Diaphragm
h. Left lung
i. Mediastinum
j. Trachea
k. Esophagus
l. Larynx and vocal cords
m. Laryngeal pharynx
n. Oropharynx
o. Nasopharynx
p. Sphenoidal sinus

2. Cuffed tracheostomy set

## MATCHING EXERCISES

| | | | | |
|---|---|---|---|---|
| **1.** b | **2.** f | **3.** i | **4.** k | **5.** a |
| **6.** e | **7.** d | **8.** g | **9.** h | **10.** j |
| **11.** c | **12.** e | **13.** f | **14.** a | **15.** h |
| **16.** d | | | | |

## SHORT ANSWER

1. a. The integrity of the airway system to transport air to and from the lungs
   b. A properly functioning alveolar system in the lungs to oxygenate venous blood and remove carbon dioxide from the blood
   c. A properly functioning cardiovascular system to carry nutrients and wastes to and from body cells
2. a. Upper airway: The upper airway comprises the nose, pharynx, larynx, and epiglottis. Its main function is to warm, filter, and humidify inspired air.
   b. Lower airway: The lower airway comprises the trachea, right and left mainstem bronchus, segmental bronchi, and terminal bronchioles. The major functions are conduction of air, mucociliary clearance, and production of pulmonary surfactant.
3. a. Any change in the surface area available for diffusion will have a negative effect on diffusion.
   b. Incomplete lung expansion or lung collapse (atelectasis) prevents pressure changes and exchange of gases by diffusion in the lungs.
   c. Any disease or condition that results in thickening of the alveolar–capillary membrane makes diffusion more difficult.
   d. The partial pressure, or pressure resulting from any gas in a mixture depending on its concentration, can also affect diffusion.
4. a. It is dissolved in plasma.
   b. Most oxygen (97%) is carried in the body by red blood cells in the form of oxyhemoglobin.
5. a. Infant: Respiratory activity is abdominal. The chest wall is so thin that the ribs, sternum, and xiphoid process are easily identified.
   b. Preschool and school-aged child: Some subcutaneous fat is deposited on the chest wall, so landmarks are less prominent than in an infant; preschool child's eustachian tubes, bronchi, and bronchioles are elongated and less angular than in an infant, so the number of routine colds and infections decreases until the child enters school.
   c. Older adult: Bony landmarks are more prominent; kyphosis contributes to appearance of leaning forward and can limit respiratory ventilation; barrel chest deformity may result; senile emphysema may be present; power of respiratory and abdominal muscles is reduced.
6. Before: Collect baseline data; prepare the patient physically and emotionally, instruct patient to remain still; administer analgesics as ordered.
   During: Observe patient for reactions; report any deviation from normal color, pulse, and respiratory rates to health care provider; ensure that specimens, if obtained, are taken to the laboratory immediately.
   After: Observe patient for changes in vital signs, particularly respirations; chest radiograph.
7. The inhalation of cigarette smoke increases airway resistance, reduces ciliary action, increases mucus production, causes thickening of the alveolar-capillary membrane, and causes bronchial walls to thicken and lose their elasticity.
8. a. Deep breathing: The nurse instructs the patient to make each breath deep enough to move the bottom ribs. The patient should start slowly, inspiring deeply through the nose and expiring slowly through the mouth.
   b. Incentive spirometry: The patient takes a deep breath and observes the results of his or her efforts as they register on the spirometer as the patient sustains maximal inspiration.
   c. Pursed lip breathing: While sitting upright, the patient inhales through the nose while counting to three and then exhales slowly and evenly against pursed lips while tightening the abdominal muscles. During exhalation, the patient counts to seven. To purse the lips, the patient should position the lips as though he or she was sucking through a straw or whistling. When walking and using pursed lip breathing, the patient should inhale while taking two steps and then exhale through pursed lips while taking the next four steps, and then repeat the cycle.
   d. Diaphragmatic breathing: The patient places one hand on the stomach and the other on the middle of the chest. He or she breathes in slowly through the nose, letting the abdomen protrude as far as it will go. Then the patient breathes out through pursed lips while contracting the abdominal muscles, with one hand pressing inward and upward on the abdomen. He or she repeats these steps for 1 minute, followed by a rest for 2 minutes several times during the day.
   e. Voluntary coughing: The nurse encourages the patient to cough voluntarily; coughing is more effective when combined with deep breathing.

9. a. Avoid open flames in the patient's room.
   b. Place "No Smoking" signs in conspicuous places in the patient's room.
   c. Check to see that electric equipment is in good working order.
   d. Avoid wearing and using synthetic fabrics, which build up static electricity.
   e. Avoid using oils in the area.
10. a. Oropharyngeal/nasopharyngeal airway: Semicircular tube of plastic or rubber inserted into the back of the pharynx through the mouth or nose in a spontaneously breathing patient; used to keep the tongue clear of the airway and to permit suctioning of secretions; often used for postoperative patients until they regain consciousness
   b. Endotracheal tube: Polyvinylchloride tube that is inserted through the nose or mouth into the trachea using a laryngoscope as guide; used to administer oxygen by mechanical ventilator, to suction secretions easily, or to bypass upper airway obstructions
   c. Tracheostomy tube: An artificial opening made into the trachea. The curved tracheostomy tube is inserted into this opening to replace an endotracheal tube, provide a method to mechanically ventilate the patient, bypass an upper airway obstruction, or remove tracheobronchial secretions.
11. Nursing responsibilities include assisting with insertion and removal of a chest tube. Once the tube is in place, monitor the patient's respiratory status and vital signs, check the dressing, and maintain the patency and integrity of the drainage system.
12. a. Help the patient assume a position that allows free movement of the diaphragm and expansion of the chest wall to promote ease of respiration.
   b. Keep the patient's secretions thin by asking the patient to drink 2 to 3 quarts of clear fluids daily.
   c. Provide humidified air.
   d. Perform chest physiotherapy on the patient's lungs to loosen pulmonary secretions.
   e. Use vibration to help loosen respiratory secretions.
   f. Provide postural drainage.
   g. Help patient maintain good nutrition.
13. The nurse is responsible for replacing a disposable inner cannula or cleaning a nondisposable one and regularly changing dressings and ties.
14. a. Chest Compression: Check the pulse for no more than 10 seconds. If the victim has no pulse, initiate chest compressions to provide artificial circulation.
   b. Airway: Tilt the head and lift the chin; check for breathing. The respiratory tract must be opened so that air can enter.
   c. Breathing: If the victim does not start to breathe spontaneously after the airway is opened, give two breaths lasting 1 second each.
   d. Defibrillation: Apply the AED as soon as it is available.

## APPLYING YOUR KNOWLEDGE

### REFLECTIVE PRACTICE: CULTIVATING QSEN COMPETENCIES

#### Sample Answers

1. How might the nurse respond to Ms. McIntyre's request for a DNR order while taking into consideration the wishes of her daughter?
   The nurse could check Ms. McIntyre's chart for advance directives or a living will and if one is not executed, the nurse could help Ms. McIntyre fill one out. The nurse should consult with the daughter and inform her of her mother's wishes for a DNR order. A counselor could be called in to facilitate the process. When planning patient care, the nurse should take into consideration age-related changes that may be increasing Ms. McIntyre's symptoms and that may respond to appropriate treatment and therapy.
2. What would be a successful outcome for this patient?
   By next visit, Ms. McIntyre vocalizes understanding of, and signs, an advance directive to direct her future care and protect her rights as a patient.
3. What intellectual, technical, interpersonal, and/or ethical/legal competencies are most likely to bring about the desired outcome?
   Intellectual: knowledge of developmental variables affecting respiratory function
   Technical: ability to use the equipment and protocols necessary to diagnose and treat respiratory problems
   Ethical/Legal: knowledge of patients' and families' rights related to refusal of care
4. What resources might be helpful for Ms. McIntyre?
Legal counseling, family counseling, advance directives, and living wills

### PATIENT CARE STUDY

1. Objective data are underlined; subjective data are in boldface.
   Toni is a <u>14-year-old</u> girl who is in the adolescent mental health unit following a suicide attempt. Her chart reveals that on several occasions when her mother was visiting, she began <u>hyperventilating (respiratory rate of 42 and increased depth).</u> Gasping for breath on these occasions, she nevertheless pushed away all who approached her to assist. Her mother confided that she and her husband are in the midst of a divorce and that it hasn't been easy for Toni at home: **"I know she's been having a rough time at school, and I guess I've been too**

**caught up in my own troubles to be there for her."** When you attempt to discuss this with Toni and mention her mother's concern, she begins hyperventilating again.

2. Nursing Process Worksheet
*Health Problem:* Ineffective breathing patterns
*Etiology:* Anxiety
*Signs and Symptoms:* Periods of hyperventilation (increased RR [42] and increased depth) associated with stressful situations (visits by mother)
*Expected Outcome:* By her second week in the unit (3/22/20), Toni will demonstrate an effective respiratory rate and rhythm (not to exceed 24) during her mother's visits.
*Nursing Interventions:*
   a. Use interview questions directed to Toni and her mother to determine the nature of the problem, its probable cause, and its effect on her lifestyle.
   b. Demonstrate consciously controlled breathing and encourage her to use it during periods of anxiety or activity.
   c. Maintain an emotionally "safe" environment. The same nurses should always work with this patient and maintain eye contact during conversations with her.
   d. If fear is the cause of her anxiety, encourage her to express concerns. Reduce cause of fear, if feasible.
   e. If there is a strong emotional component, discuss with the patient the possibility of developing effective coping skills with professional counseling.

*Evaluative Statement:* 3/22/20: Expected outcome partially met—on two occasions, Toni remained in control of her breathing during her mother's visits. On at least one occasion, she hyperventilated.
— *K. O'Leary, RN*

3. Patient strengths: The patient's strengths still need to be identified; mother seems to be gaining an appreciation of her needs.
Personal strengths: Good understanding of the effects of stress and experienced in helping patients replace maladaptive coping strategies with adaptive strategies.
4. 3/22/20: This morning, Toni began talking about the difficult situation at home. When asked about her relationship with her mother, she began gulping for air but "caught herself" and quickly reestablished control of her breathing, consciously decreasing her rate and depth. Whereas she has shown no signs of hyperventilation on two of her mother's last visits, she had one episode in which she hyperventilated and totally "lost control" and needed sedation. She stated that she feels like she is making progress but still has a long way to go before she will feel comfortable at home and in control of simple, everyday things like breathing.
— *K. O'Leary, RN*

## PRACTICING FOR NCLEX

### MULTIPLE CHOICE QUESTIONS

| | | | | |
|---|---|---|---|---|
| **1.** d | **2.** a | **3.** b | **4.** d | **5.** b |
| **6.** c | **7.** c | **8.** a | **9.** d | **10.** b |
| **11.** b | **12.** d | **13.** a | **14.** d | **15.** d |

### ALTERNATE-FORMAT QUESTIONS

#### Multiple Response Questions

1. a, b, e
2. b, c, e
3. a, d, e
4. b, c, d, e,
5. a, b, e
6. b, e, f
7. a, d, e

#### Prioritization Questions

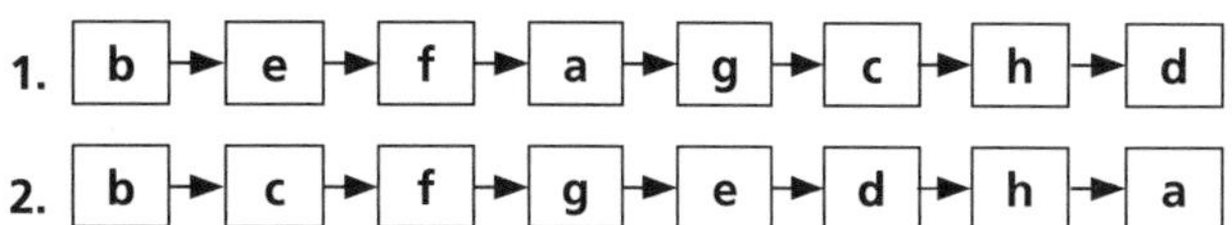
1. b → e → f → a → g → c → h → d
2. b → c → f → g → e → d → h → a

# CHAPTER 40

## ASSESSING YOUR UNDERSTANDING

### MATCHING EXERCISES

| | | | | |
|---|---|---|---|---|
| **1.** b | **2.** c | **3.** a | **4.** a | **5.** d |
| **6.** c | **7.** b | **8.** d | **9.** a | **10.** c |
| **11.** a | **12.** b | **13.** c | **14.** a | **15.** c |
| **16.** b | **17.** a | **18.** d | **19.** c | **20.** c |
| **21.** f | **22.** p | **23.** b | **24.** o | **25.** l |
| **26.** h | **27.** a | **28.** d | **29.** e | **30.** j |
| **31.** m | **32.** n | **33.** g | **34.** k | |

### CORRECT THE FALSE STATEMENTS

1. True
2. False—electrolytes
3. False—hypotonic solution
4. True
5. False—hydrogen
6. False—alkali
7. False—alkaline
8. False—lungs
9. True
10. False—hypernatremia
11. False—disproportionate
12. True

### SHORT ANSWER

1. a. Osmosis: The solvent water passes from an area of lesser solute concentration to an area of greater solute concentration until an equilibrium is established.
   b. Diffusion: The tendency of solutes to move freely throughout a solvent. The solute moves from an area of higher concentration to an area

of lower concentration until an equilibrium is established.

c. Active transport: A process that requires energy for the movement of substances through a cell membrane from an area of lesser concentration to an area of higher concentration.

2. a. Ingested liquids: Fluid intake is regulated by the thirst mechanism and is stimulated by intracellular dehydration and decreased blood volume.
   b. Food: The amount of water depends on the food (e.g., melons have a higher water content than bread).
   c. Metabolic oxidation: Water is an end product of oxidation that occurs during the metabolism of food.
3. Water is lost:
   a. through the kidneys as urine
   b. through the skin as perspiration
   c. through insensible water loss
4. a. Kidneys: Approximately 170 L of plasma is filtered daily in the adult, while only 1.5 L of urine is excreted. They selectively retain electrolytes and water and excrete wastes.
   b. Cardiovascular system: The heart and blood vessels are responsible for pumping and carrying nutrients and water throughout the body.
   c. Lungs: The lungs regulate oxygen and carbon dioxide levels of the blood.
   d. Thyroid: Thyroxine, released by the thyroid gland, increases blood flow in the body. This in turn increases renal circulation, which results in increased glomerular filtration and urinary output.
   e. Parathyroid glands: The parathyroid glands secrete parathyroid hormone, which regulates the level of calcium in ECF.
   f. Gastrointestinal tract: The GI tract absorbs water and nutrients that enter the body through this route.
   g. Nervous system: The nervous system acts as a switchboard and inhibits and stimulates mechanisms that influence fluid balance.
5. a. Acidosis: Characterized by a high concentration of hydrogen ions in ECF, which causes the pH to fall below 7.35
   b. Alkalosis: Characterized by a low concentration of hydrogen ions in ECF, which causes the pH to exceed 7.45
6. a. Respiratory acidosis: An excess of carbonic acid in ECF caused by decreased alveolar ventilation and resulting in the retention of carbon dioxide. The lungs cannot compensate for the rise in carbonic acid levels. As the carbonic acid concentration increases, the kidneys retain more bicarbonate and increase their excretion of hydrogen.
   b. Respiratory alkalosis: A deficit of carbonic acid in ECF caused by increased alveolar ventilation and resulting in a decrease in carbon dioxide. Respiratory rate and depth increase because carbon dioxide is being excreted faster than normal; depression or cessation of respirations can occur. The kidneys attempt to alleviate this imbalance by increasing bicarbonate excretion and hydrogen retention.
   c. Metabolic acidosis: A deficit of bicarbonate in ECF resulting from an increase in acidic components or an excessive loss of bicarbonate. The lungs attempt to increase the rate of carbon dioxide excretion by increasing the rate and depth of respirations; the kidneys attempt to compensate by retaining bicarbonate and excreting more hydrogen. May result in loss of consciousness and death.
   d. Metabolic alkalosis: An excess of bicarbonate in ECF resulting from loss of acid or ingestion or retention of base. The body attempts to compensate by retaining carbon dioxide. Respirations become slow and shallow, and periods of apnea may occur. The kidneys excrete potassium and sodium along with excess bicarbonate and retain hydrogen within carbonic acid.
7. a. Increased hematocrit: severe dehydration and shock (when hemoconcentration rises considerably)
   b. Decreased hematocrit: acute, massive blood loss; hemolytic reaction following transfusion of incompatible blood
   c. Increased hemoglobin: hemoconcentration of the blood
   d. Decreased hemoglobin: anemia, severe hemorrhage, and following a hemolytic reaction
8. a. Urine pH and specific gravity: Specific gravity is a measure of the kidney's ability to concentrate urine. Normal range: 1.005 to 1.030. Both may be obtained by dipstick measurement on a fresh voided specimen or through lab analysis.
   b. Serum electrolytes: Indicates plasma levels of select electrolytes
   c. Arterial blood gases: Indicate the adequacy of oxygenation and ventilation and acid–base status
9. a. Note the patient's fluid and food intake and learn what the patient's previous eating and drinking patterns have been.
   b. Note whether thirst is excessive or whether patient experiences little or no thirst.
   c. Note excessive losses of fluid from the body and attempt to prevent losses when possible.
   d. Physiologic changes that accompany the aging process may affect the patient's ability to maintain fluid balance.
10. Handling all equipment, performing dressing changes, assessing patient for evidence of infection or other complications, and maintaining the supplies necessary to continue home infusion.

## APPLYING YOUR KNOWLEDGE

### REFLECTIVE PRACTICE: CULTIVATING QSEN COMPETENCIES

#### Sample Answers

1. Based on the data in this scenario, what body systems are involved in Mr. Park's fluid volume excess? What interventions would be appropriate?
   Fluid has accumulated in Mr. Park's heart and lungs as manifested by his bounding pulse, distended neck veins, and abnormal lung sounds. The nurse should make careful assessments of Mr. Park's IV infusion to ensure the proper flow rate. The nurse should also be aware that fluid restriction may be ordered and prepare the patient by explaining the reason for the restriction and what foods to avoid (dry, salty, or sweet foods or fluids). The nurse could then work with the patient to develop short-term outcomes for accomplishing the overall task and discuss with the patient the time intervals at which fluids will be served. Fluids could be served in small cups to make the cup appear to contain more liquid and ice chips could be offered at intervals. The nurse should provide oral hygiene at regular intervals so that the patient's mouth remains clean and moist, and the nurse should lubricate the lips and mucous membranes as indicated.
2. What would be a successful outcome for Mr. Park?
   By end of shift, Mr. Park lists the reasons for fluid restrictions and states that he is breathing more easily following implementation of treatment regimen.
3. What intellectual, technical, interpersonal, and/or ethical/legal competencies are most likely to bring about the desired outcome?
   Intellectual: knowledge of how to promote and maintain fluid, electrolyte, and acid–base balance
   Technical: ability to use the equipment and protocols necessary to maintain and restore fluid, electrolyte, and acid–base balance
   Ethical/Legal: strong sense of accountability for the health and well-being of patients and willingness to hold colleagues accountable for safe quality practice
4. What resources might be helpful for Mr. Park?
   Patient teaching plan, printed materials on overhydration

### PATIENT CARE STUDY

1. Objective data are underlined; subjective data are in boldface.
   Rebecca is a <u>college freshman</u> who had her wisdom teeth removed yesterday morning. She had a sore throat several days before the extraction but did not mention this to the oral surgeon. **Because of her sore throat, she had greatly decreased both her food and fluid intake.** The night of the surgery, she had an <u>oral temperature of 39.5°C (103.1°F)</u>. Friends gave her some Tylenol, which brought her temperature down, and encouraged her to drink more fluids. When they checked on her this morning, <u>her temperature was elevated again</u>, and she said **she had felt too weak during the night to drink.** They took her to the student health service, where the admitting nurse noticed her <u>dry mucous membranes, decreased skin turgor, and rapid pulse. At 5 ft 2 in and 98 lb</u>, **Rebecca had lost 4 lb in the past week.**
2. Nursing Process Worksheet
   *Health Problem:* Fluid volume deficit
   *Etiology:* Decreased fluid intake (sore throat and weakness) and loss of water and electrolytes in fever
   *Signs and Symptoms:* Elevated temperature (39.5°C), 4-lb weight loss in 1 week, dry mucous membranes, decreased skin turgor, and rapid pulse
   *Expected Outcome:* By 3/19/20, patient will demonstrate corrected fluid volume deficit by (1) balanced fluid intake and output, averaging 2,500 mL fluid/day; (2) urine specific gravity within normal range (1.010 to 1.025); (3) moist mucous membranes and adequate skin turgor; and (4) pulse returned to baseline.
   *Nursing Interventions:*
   a. Assess for worsening of fluid volume deficit.
   b. Give oral fluids that are nonirritating, as tolerated.
   c. If oral fluids are not tolerated, confer with MD regarding IV replacement therapy.
   d. Monitor response to fluid therapy: vital signs, urine volume and specific gravity, increased skin turgor, moist mucous membranes, increased body weight.

   *Evaluative Statement:* 3/19/20: Goals met—patient has corrected fluid volume deficit; fluid intake and output average 2,700 mL fluid/day; pulse returned to baseline; skin turgor improved; mucous membranes are moist. — *J. Barclay, RN*
3. Patient strengths: Previously healthy; concerned friends; highly motivated to correct deficit
   Personal strengths: Strong knowledge of fluid, electrolyte, and acid–base balance; good interpersonal skills
4. 3/19/20: Patient tolerating oral replacement fluids and understands importance of increasing fluids until the deficit is corrected. Friends remind her to drink at frequent intervals. Pulse returned to baseline. Yesterday's fluid intake was 2,900-mL fluid, output 2,500 mL. Improved skin turgor and moist mucous membranes. Gained 2 lb. — *J. Barclay, RN*

## PRACTICING FOR NCLEX

### MULTIPLE CHOICE QUESTIONS

| | | | | |
|---|---|---|---|---|
| **1.** c | **2.** a | **3.** b | **4.** b | **5.** d |
| **6.** c | **7.** a | **8.** d | **9.** b | **10.** b |
| **11.** a | **12.** b | **13.** b | | |

### ALTERNATE-FORMAT QUESTIONS

#### Multiple Response Questions

1. c, d, f
2. a, b, d, f
3. b, d, f

**4.** d, e, f
**5.** a, b, c
**6.** b, d, f
**7.** a, b, e
**8.** c, d, e
**9.** b, c, e

## Chart/Exhibit Questions

**1.** c
**2.** a
**3.** d
**4.** a
**5.** b
**6.** See table below.

| | | | | Comp. Present? | | If Yes | | If Yes | |
|---|---|---|---|---|---|---|---|---|---|
| **pH** | **$PaCO_2$** | **$HCO_3^-$** | **Nature of Disturbance** | **Yes** | **No** | **Renal** | **Respiratory** | **Partial** | **Complete** |
| 7.28 | 63 | 25 | respiratory acidosis | | × | | | | |
| 7.20 | 40 | 14 | metabolic acidosis | | × | | | | |
| 7.52 | 40 | 35 | metabolic alkalosis | | × | | | | |
| 7.16 | 82 | 30 | respiratory acidosis | × | | × | | × | |
| 7.36 | 68 | 35 | respiratory acidosis | × | | × | | | × |
| 7.56 | 23 | 26 | respiratory alkalosis | | × | | | | |
| 7.40 | 40 | 26 | None | | | | | | |
| 7.56 | 23 | 26 | respiratory alkalosis | | × | | | | |
| 7.26 | 70 | 25 | respiratory acidosis | | × | | | | |
| 7.52 | 44 | 38 | metabolic alkalosis | | × | | | | |
| 7.32 | 30 | 18 | metabolic acidosis | × | | | × | × | |
| 7.49 | 34 | 26 | respiratory alkalosis | | × | | | | |

## Hot Spot Questions

**1.** See figure below for PICC placement.

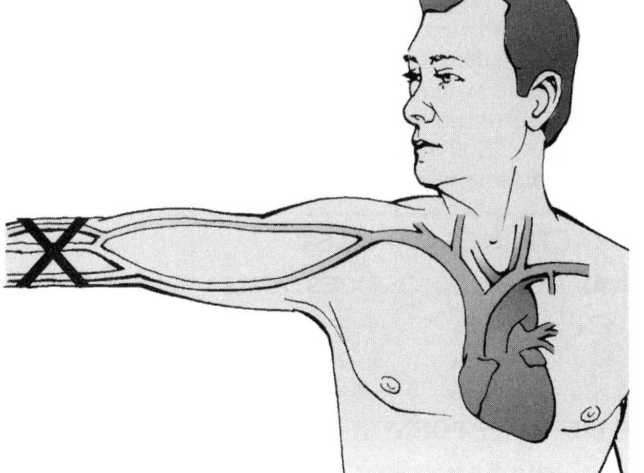

**2.** See figure below for triple-lumen nontunneled percutaneous central venous catheter placement.

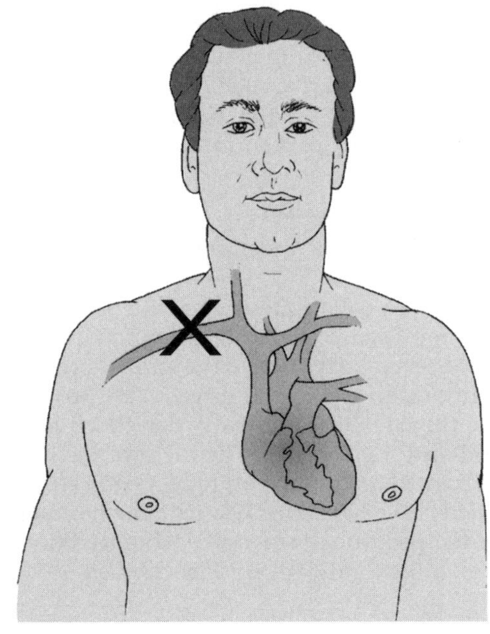

# CHAPTER 41

## ASSESSING YOUR UNDERSTANDING

### FILL IN THE BLANKS

1. self-actualization
2. self-concept
3. global self
4. ideal self
5. false self
6. Personal identity

### MATCHING EXERCISES

| | | | | |
|---|---|---|---|---|
| **1.** a | **2.** d | **3.** h | **4.** e | **5.** f |
| **6.** c | **7.** g | **8.** d | **9.** b | **10.** c |
| **11.** a | **12.** d | **13.** b | **14.** c | **15.** d |
| **16.** a | | | | |

### SHORT ANSWER

1. Sample answer:
   Nurses interacting with older adults need to take simple measures such as addressing older adults respectfully, communicating that you take their concerns seriously, noticing and affirming their personal strengths, and interacting with them as people.
2. Answers will vary with student experiences.
3. Sample answers:
   a. Significance: Do you feel loved and appreciated by the key people in your life?
   b. Competence: Does anything interfere with your ability to do your life work?
   c. Virtue: How would you describe your ability to follow your moral code?
   d. Power: Do you feel you are in control of your life?
4. Sample answers:
   a. Developmental considerations: A teenager needs to be trusted and guided to make good choices that affect his or her life.
   b. Culture: As a child internalizes the values of parents and peers, culture begins to influence his or her sense of self.
   c. Internal and external resources: The amount of money a person earns may influence his or her self-concept.
   d. History of success or failure: A child who repeatedly fails in school may have difficulty succeeding in life.
   e. Stressors: Self-concept determines the way a person perceives stressors in his or her life and reacts to them.
   f. Aging, illness, or trauma: A paralyzing injury will most likely affect self-concept.
5. Sample answers:
   a. Dispel the myth that it is necessary to know all there is to know about nursing to be a good nurse: Nurses must accept the fact that they must constantly learn new theories and procedures to keep up with medicine.
   b. Realistically evaluate strengths and weaknesses: A periodic review of a nurse's skills, strengths, and weaknesses should be built into the practice.
   c. Accentuate the positive: Nurses should not dwell on one mistake they may have made but should recall what they did right and learn from their mistakes.
   d. Develop a conscious plan for changing weaknesses into strengths: If a nurse has weak technical skills in one area, he or she should focus on this area and strengthen his or her knowledge and competency through research, study, and practice.
   e. Work to develop team self-esteem: Congratulate colleagues and celebrate when the nursing team is successful.
   f. Actively demonstrate your commitment to nursing and concern about the nursing profession's public image: Nurses should be aware of their impact on society, and the image they project should be positive.
6. Answers will vary with student experiences.
7. Sample answers:
   a. Personal identity: How would you describe yourself to others?
   b. Patient strengths: What special talents and abilities do you have?
   c. Body image: What are your positive physical attributes?
   d. Self-esteem: What do you like most about yourself?
   e. Role performance: What major roles describe you?
8. Sample answers:
   a. Diagnosis: Anxiety related to unwelcome change in body image (mastectomy).
   Patient goal: Patient will express satisfaction with ability to live with altered body image.
   b. Diagnosis: Anxiety related to inability to accept or manage new role.
   Patient goal: Patient reports feeling less anxious about being pregnant.
   c. Diagnosis: Ineffective health maintenance related to low self-esteem and inability to cope with grief.
   Patient goal: Patient will acknowledge his own self-worth and express a desire to take care of himself despite his grief.
   d. Diagnosis: Deficient knowledge: How to help child develop self-esteem, related to lack of experience with parenting.
   Patient goal: Patient will describe methods of developing self-esteem in children.
   e. Diagnosis: Risk for physical trauma, domestic abuse, related to low self-esteem and sense of hopelessness.
   Patient goal: Patient will verbalize that she is liked and deserves to live without fear of abuse.

f. Diagnosis: Ineffective sexuality pattern related to changed body image, disturbance in self-concept. Patient goal: Patient will describe self realistically, identifying strengths that make her desirable to husband.

9. a. Encourage patients to identify their strengths.
   b. Notice and reinforce patient strengths.
   c. Encourage patients to will for themselves the strengths they desire and to try them on.

10. a. Using looks, touch, and speech to communicate worth
    b. Speaking respectfully to the patient and addressing the patient by preferred name
    c. Moving the patient's body respectfully if the patient cannot move on his or her own

11. Sample answers:
    a. Help her find meaning in the experience, regain mastery to the extent that this is possible, and realistically evaluate the adequacy of her coping strategy. Teach her to develop a "game plan" for confronting anxiety-producing situations. Identify and secure interventions for treatable depression. Remedy treatable causes of self-identity disturbances, such as pain or substance abuse.
    b. Notice and affirm positive physiologic characteristics of the patient. Teach preventive self-care measures that reduce uncomfortable signs of aging. Explore new activities (which may include old hobbies) that are within the changing physical abilities of the patient.
    c. Help patient identify and use personal strengths. Let him know that you value him simply for who he is. Use the name he prefers. Ask him questions about his life, interests, and values. Engage him in activities in which he can be successful. Empower him to meet his needs. Provide necessary knowledge, teach new behaviors, and instill in him the belief that he can change.
    d. Explore with patient the many roles she has fulfilled throughout her lifetime. Encourage her to reminisce. Facilitate grieving over valued roles that she can no longer perform.

## APPLYING YOUR KNOWLEDGE

### REFLECTIVE PRACTICE: CULTIVATING QSEN COMPETENCIES

1. What interventions might the nurse employ to try to resolve Mr. Santorini's self-image disturbance?
   The nurse would need to assess Mr. Santorini's self-knowledge, self-expectations, and self-evaluation for each component of self-concept to determine if he will still be able to fulfill his role expectation to function as a complete, intact man. The nurse should keep in mind that major stressors place anyone at relative risk for maladaptive responses, such as withdrawal, isolation, depression, extreme anxiety, substance abuse, or exacerbation of physical illness. How Mr. Santorini perceives the amputation and his ability to mobilize personal strengths and other resources are determined largely by his self-concept, which, in turn, is influenced by the response he chooses. Following a complete history and assessment, the nurse could work with Mr. Santorini and assist with adapting to the loss of his leg. Patient teaching involving the use of a prosthesis may be helpful as he begins to adapt to his body change.
2. What would be a successful outcome for Mr. Santorini?
   By next visit, Mr. Santorini lists three positive aspects of his self-image.
   By next visit, Mr. Santorini reports acceptance of his amputation and successful use of his new prosthesis.
3. What intellectual, technical, interpersonal, and/or ethical/legal competencies are most likely to bring about the desired outcome?
   Intellectual: knowledge of measures to modify a negative self-concept for a middle-aged man with a new amputation
   Interpersonal: strong interpersonal skills to establish a trusting relationship with a middle-aged man with an amputation
   Ethical/Legal: commitment to patient advocacy, including getting Mr. Santorini the help needed to achieve his health goals
4. What resources might be helpful for Mr. Santorini?
   Counseling services, printed or AV materials on the use of prostheses

### PATIENT CARE STUDY

1. Objective data are underlined; subjective data are in boldface.
   An English teacher asks you, the school nurse, to see one of her students, Julie, whose <u>grades have recently dropped</u> and who <u>no longer seems to be interested in school</u> or anything else. "She was one of my best students, and I can't figure out what's going on," the teacher says. "She seems reluctant to talk about this change." When Julie, a <u>16-year-old junior</u>, walks into your office, you are immediately struck by her <u>stooped posture, unstyled hair, and sloppy appearance</u>. Julie is <u>attractive, but at 5 ft 3 in and 150 lb, she is overweight</u>. Julie is initially reluctant to talk, but she breaks down at one point and confides that for the first time in her life she feels **"absolutely awful"** about herself. **"I've always concentrated on getting good grades and achieved this easily. But now, this doesn't seem so important. I don't have any friends.** All I hear the girls talking about is boys, and <u>I was never even asked out by a boy</u>, which I guess isn't surprising. Look at me." After a few questions, it becomes clear that Julie has new expectations for herself based on what she observes in her peers, and she finds herself falling far short of her new, ideal self. Julie admits **that in the past, once she set a goal for herself, she was always able to achieve it because she is strongly self-motivated.**

Although she has withdrawn from her parents and teachers, she admits that she does know adults she can trust who have been a big support to her in the past. She says, "If only I could become the kind of teenager other kids like and have lots of friends!"

2. Nursing Process Worksheet
*Health Problem:* Situational low self-esteem
*Etiology:* Perceived inability to meet newly accepted peer standards regarding socialization/dating
*Signs and Symptoms:* Feels "absolutely awful" about herself; 5 ft 3 in, 150 lb; "I don't have any friends"; never dated; grades have dropped recently; new lack of interest/vitality; stooped posture; unstyled hair; sloppy appearance
*Expected Outcome:* In 1 month, by 10/10/20, patient will report that she feels better about herself, based on new socialization experiences with peers and improved body image
*Nursing Interventions:*
   a. Help patient develop workable self-care strategies to lose weight and enhance physical appearance.
   b. Explore patient's interest in activities that will serve two goals: (1) enable patient to develop friendships and (2) improve her body image (e.g., sports, dancing, hiking clubs).
   c. Counsel patient about peer relationships, sexuality, and dating.

*Evaluative Statement:* 10/10/20: Goal partially met—patient states that she feels "great" about losing weight (150 lb, down to 145 lb) and likes her "new look" but still feels shy with peers and is not dating. Revision: Celebrate new self-care behaviors and reevaluate efforts to enhance peer relationships.
— *M. Stenulis, RN*
3. Patient strengths: physically attractive; past history of achieving personal goals; strongly self-motivated; has trusting relationships with adults (parents and teachers)
Personal strengths: ability to establish trusting nurse–patient relationships with high school students; knowledge of teen social "norms"; successful history of motivating teens to develop and take pride in health self-care behaviors
4. 10/10/20: Met with patient 1 month after initial meeting. In that time, she lost 5 lb, which she attributes to decreased snacking and increased activity (joined field hockey team). She walked into the office with erect posture and exhibited more interest/vitality than at last meeting. She reports still feeling very shy with her peers and is uncomfortable with boys. She is very interested, however, in participating in group activities in which she can overcome her shyness and hopes to make new friends. — *M. Stenulis, RN*

## PRACTICING FOR NCLEX

### MULTIPLE CHOICE QUESTIONS

| | | | | |
|---|---|---|---|---|
| **1.** b | **2.** a | **3.** b | **4.** c | **5.** d |
| **6.** c | **7.** c | **8.** a | **9.** a | |

### ALTERNATE-FORMAT QUESTIONS

#### Multiple Response Questions

1. b, c, f
2. a, d, e, f
3. a, b, d

# CHAPTER 42

## ASSESSING YOUR UNDERSTANDING

### FILL IN THE BLANKS

1. psychosocial
2. local adaptation
3. inflammatory
4. fight-or-flight
5. psychosomatic
6. anxiety
7. coping mechanisms
8. caregiver burden

### MATCHING EXERCISES

| | | | | |
|---|---|---|---|---|
| **1.** c | **2.** i | **3.** l | **4.** f | **5.** b |
| **6.** e | **7.** a | **8.** d | **9.** g | **10.** h |
| **11.** j | **12.** m | **13.** c | **14.** i | **15.** b |
| **16.** h | **17.** a | **18.** e | **19.** f | **20.** g |

### SHORT ANSWER

1. a. Mind–body interaction: Humans react to threats of danger as if they were real. The person perceives the threat on an emotional level, and the body prepares itself either to resist it or turn away and avoid the danger. For example: An executive has an important presentation to make in the morning and is restless the night before, cannot eat breakfast, and feels apprehensive and has a rapid heartbeat before the presentation.
   b. Local adaptation syndrome: A localized response of the body to stress. It does not involve the entire body, only a body part. LAS is an adaptive response, primarily homeostatic and short term. For example: reflex pain response and inflammatory response.
   c. General adaptation syndrome: A biochemical model of stress developed by Hans Selye that describes the body's general response to stress and serves as part of the knowledge base essential to all areas of nursing care. For example: Alarm reaction—various defense mechanisms are activated; resistance—body attempts to adapt to the stressor; exhaustion—the body either rests and mobilizes its defenses to return to normal or reaches total exhaustion and dies.

2. a. The inflammatory response is a local response to injury or infection. It serves to localize and prevent the spread of infection and promote wound healing. When you cut your finger, for example, you often develop the symptoms of the inflammatory response: pain, swelling, heat, redness, and changes in function.
3. a. Severity and duration of the stressor
   b. Previous health of the person
   c. Immediacy and effectiveness of health care interventions
4. a. Mild anxiety: Present in day-to-day living; increases alertness and perceptual fields and motivates learning and growth
   b. Moderate anxiety: Narrows a person's perceptual fields so that the focus is on immediate concerns, with inattention to other details
   c. Severe anxiety: Creates a very narrow focus on specific detail; causes all behavior to be geared toward relief
   d. Panic: Causes the person to lose control and experience dread and terror; characterized by increased physical activity, distorted perceptions and relations, and loss of rational thought
5. Answers will vary with student experiences.
6. Sample answers:
   a. Stressors in health facilitate normal growth and development.
   b. Fear of developing cardiovascular disease can motivate a person to exercise regularly.
   c. Fear of failure in business can motivate a person to attend classes.
7. Sample answers:
   a. Developmental stress: An infant learns that his hunger will be taken care of in a timely manner; a school-aged child learns the rewards of studying; an older adult man accepts the limitations of age on his social life.
   b. Situational stress: A child contracts a life-threatening illness; a spouse loses her job; a spouse asks for a divorce.
8. Sample answers:
   a. "It must have been frightening being in an automobile accident."
   b. "I notice that you seem distracted; would you care to talk about it?"
9. Sample answers:
   Confront the mother in an understanding manner and question her about her daily schedule and ability to do all the things necessary to take care of her family. Refer the mother to outside agencies (e.g., daycare programs), supportive friends and family members, or resources for hired help to give her a break from her responsibilities. Help the mother arrange her daily care to schedule some time for herself, if possible.
10. a. Exercise: The benefits of exercise include an improved musculoskeletal system, more effective cardiovascular function, weight control, and relaxation. It improves one's sense of well-being, relieves tension, and enables one to cope with life better.
    b. Rest and sleep: Allows the body to maintain homeostasis and restore energy levels; provides insulation against stress.
    c. Nutrition: Plays an active role in maintaining the body's homeostatic mechanisms and in increasing resistance to stress.
11. a. Identify the problem.
    b. List alternatives.
    c. Choose from among the alternatives.
    d. Implement a plan.
    e. Evaluate the outcome.
12. a. Age affects the ability to adapt.
    b. Nutrition affects stress levels.
    c. Sleep affects stress levels.
    d. Social factors and life events affect stress level.
13. a. Provide social support.
    b. Provide emotional and physical support.
    c. Help with problem-solving and teaching–learning activities.

## APPLYING YOUR KNOWLEDGE

### REFLECTIVE PRACTICE: CULTIVATING QSEN COMPETENCIES

#### Sample Answers

1. What might be the cause of the flare-up of Ms. Rogerrios's inflammatory bowel disease? What nursing interventions would be beneficial for this patient?
   The stress of having to return to work for financial reasons following a 15-year absence may have exacerbated Ms. Rogerrio's inflammatory bowel disease. The nurse could teach Ms. Rogerrio coping mechanisms to minimize this effect of stress. Examples of interventions appropriate for this patient include patient teaching regarding meditation and/or relaxation techniques and maintaining a proper diet and exercise program.
2. What would be a successful outcome for this patient?
   By next visit, Ms. Rogerrio lists three benefits of using stress reduction strategies and their effect on relieving diarrhea related to her inflammatory bowel disease.
3. What intellectual, technical, interpersonal, and/or ethical/legal competencies are most likely to bring about the desired outcome?
   Intellectual: knowledge about the physiologic and psychological responses to stress
   Interpersonal: strong interpersonal skills to establish a trusting relationship with a woman returning to the workforce; ability to assist patients to develop positive coping mechanisms to deal with stress

Ethical/Legal: familiarity with facility policy and role responsibilities related to stress management

4. What resources might be helpful for Ms. Rogerrio? Exercise classes, printed or AV materials on stress reduction techniques

**PATIENT CARE STUDY**

1. a. On a scale of 1 to 10, with 10 being most able to control this situation, how would you rate yourself at this time? What does that number mean to you?
   b. Who do you talk to when you feel sad or nervous?
   c. What has helped you handle stressful situations in the past? (Also, see samples of questions in text.)
2. Heart palpitations, dry mouth, difficulty breathing, increased perspiration, nausea, tremors, increased pulse rate, increased blood pressure, crying, sleep disturbances, eating disturbances.
3. a. Anxiety related to multiple stressors occurring in relatively short period of time
   b. Altered Thought Processes related to severe anxiety
   c. Risk for Altered Nutrition: Less Than Body Requirements related to decreased food intake
   d. Risk for Social Isolation related to perceived need to be family caregiver
4. a. Verbalize a decrease in anxiety with increased feelings of comfort.
   b. Develop effective coping skills through problem-solving and anxiety-reducing techniques.
   c. Maintain or slightly increase body weight.
   d. Actively participate in at least one social activity outside the home each week.
5. A crisis occurs when previous coping and defense mechanisms are no longer effective. This failure causes high levels of anxiety, disorganized behavior, and an inability to function adequately.
6. Identify the problem, list alternatives, choose from among alternatives, implement a plan, and evaluate the outcome.
7. Exercise: Exercise helps maintain physical and emotional health; it also improves ability to cope with stressors. Recommend an exercise program of 30 to 45 minutes of enjoyable exercise three or four times a week.
   Rest and sleep: Rest and sleep restore energy levels and provide insulation against stress. Relaxation techniques are often helpful in inducing sleep.
   Nutrition: Nutrition plays an active role in increasing resistance to stress. Follow recommended guidelines for amounts and types of foods to eat. (See Chapter 36 for more information about nutrition.)
8. Mrs. Brent will meet expected outcomes if she verbalizes the causes of stress and anxiety, identifies and uses sources of support, uses problem-solving techniques to reduce the number of stressors, practices healthy lifestyle habits, and verbalizes a decrease in anxiety and an increase in comfort.

## PRACTICING FOR NCLEX

### MULTIPLE CHOICE QUESTIONS

| | | | | |
|---|---|---|---|---|
| **1.** a | **2.** c | **3.** b | **4.** b | **5.** a |
| **6.** d | **7.** c | **8.** c | **9.** a | **10.** a |
| **11.** d | **12.** a | **13.** b | | |

### ALTERNATE-FORMAT QUESTIONS

#### Multiple Response Questions

1. b, d, f
2. d, e
3. c, e, f
4. c, d, f
5. a, e, f

#### Prioritization Question

1. 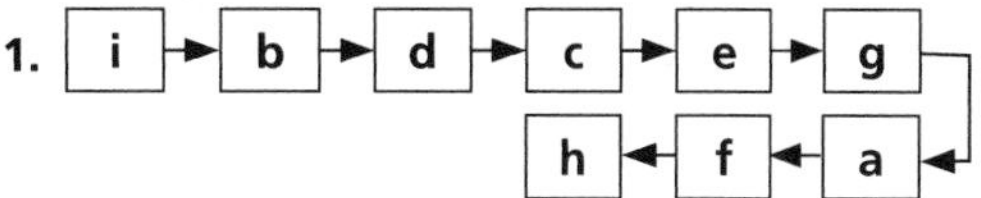


# CHAPTER 43

## ASSESSING YOUR UNDERSTANDING

### FILL IN THE BLANKS

1. perceived
2. Bereavement
3. outcome
4. dysfunctional
5. irreversible cessation of all functions of the entire brain, including the brainstem
6. palliative

### MATCHING EXERCISES

| | | | | |
|---|---|---|---|---|
| **1.** h | **2.** e | **3.** a | **4.** g | **5.** b |
| **6.** d | **7.** c | **8.** d | **9.** a | **10.** e |
| **11.** b | **12.** c | **13.** f | | |

### CORRECT THE FALSE STATEMENTS

1. False—unresolved grief
2. False—anger
3. True
4. False—durable power of attorney for health care
5. True
6. False—no-code or do-not-resuscitate
7. True
8. False—mortician
9. False—nurse

### SHORT ANSWER

1. a. Care of the body: Place body in normal anatomic position; remove soiled dressings and tubes (unless an autopsy is being performed); place ID tags on shroud, ankle, and prostheses.
   b. Care of the family: Be an attentive listener; attend funeral (if family permits); make follow-up call to assess family's well-being.
   c. Discharging legal responsibilities: The mortician assumes responsibility for handling and filing the death certificate with proper authorities. A

clinician's signature is required on the certificate (check your state law to see if nurses can sign death certificates), as well as that of the pathologist, the coroner, and others in special cases. The nurse is responsible to ensure that the death certificate is signed.

**2. a.** Denial and isolation: The patient denies that he or she will die, may repress what is discussed, and may isolate self from reality.
   **b.** Anger: The patient expresses rage and hostility and adopts a "why me?" attitude.
   **c.** Bargaining: The patient tries to barter for more time.
   **d.** Depression: The patient goes through a period of grief before death.
   **e.** Acceptance: The patient feels tranquil; he or she has accepted death and is prepared to die.

**3.** As soon as possible, the patient should be told her diagnosis and prognosis, how the disease is likely to progress, and what this will mean for her.

**4.** Answers will vary with student experiences.

**5.** Nursing's role is to participate in the decision-making process by offering helpful information about the benefits and burdens of continued ventilation and description of what to expect if it is initiated. Supporting the patient's family and managing sedation and analgesia are critical nursing responsibilities.

**6.** Sample answers:
   **a.** Communicate openly with patients about their losses and invite discussion of the adequacy of their coping mechanisms.
   **b.** Respond genuinely to the concerns and feelings of dying patients and their families; do not be afraid to cry with the patient and to allow feelings to show.
   **c.** Value time spent with patients and family members in which supportive presence is the primary intervention.

**7.** Sample answers:
   **a.** The patient shall make health care decisions reflecting his values and goals.
   **b.** The patient shall experience a comfortable and dignified death.
   **c.** The patient and family shall accept need for help as appropriate and use available resources.

**8.** Sample answers:
   **a.** In favor of: It is a beneficent and compassionate act. It takes the matter outside the reach of "medical power" and scrupulosity. It respects autonomy by preserving the patient's control of the manner, method, and timing of death.
   **b.** Against: It undermines the value of, and respect for, all human life. A focus on euthanasia will divert attention from other valuable palliative techniques. If legalized, it is predicted patients will feel a subtle pressure to conform in order to relieve the economic and emotional burdens they impose on family and friends.

**9. a.** No-code: If a health care provider has written DNR on the chart of a patient, the patient or surrogate has expressed a wish that there be no attempts made to resuscitate the patient in the event of a cardiopulmonary emergency. The nurse must clarify the patient's code status.
   **b.** Comfort measures only: Nurses should be familiar with the forms used to indicate patient preferences about end-of-life care. The goal of a comfort measures only order is to indicate that the goal of treatment is a comfortable, dignified death and that further life-sustaining measures are no longer indicated.
   **c.** Do-not-hospitalize orders: These orders are used by patients in long-term care facilities and other residential settings who have elected not to be hospitalized for further aggressive treatment. The nursing responsibilities would be the same as for comfort measures only.
   **d.** Terminal weaning: The nurse's role is to participate in the decision-making process by offering helpful information about the benefits and burdens of continued ventilation and a description of what to expect if terminal weaning is initiated.

**10. a.** Durable power of attorney: Nurses must facilitate dialog about this advance directive, which appoints an agent the person trusts to make decisions in the event of the appointing person's subsequent incapacity.
   **b.** Living will: Nurses must also facilitate dialog about this advance directive, which provides specific instructions about the kinds of health care that should be provided or avoided in particular situations.

## APPLYING YOUR KNOWLEDGE

### REFLECTIVE PRACTICE: CULTIVATING QSEN COMPETENCIES

#### Sample Answers

1. How might the nurse react to Ms. Malic in a manner that respects her right to privacy while at the same time helping her through the grief process? The nurse should realize that Ms. Malic is experiencing anticipatory loss and use this knowledge to help her cope with the potential loss of her baby. To develop meaningful communication, the nurse must develop a trusting relationship with the patient. The nurse needs to use open-ended questions to elicit information and listen to Ms. Malic, recognizing both her verbal and nonverbal cues. The nurse should also be encouraging without giving false reassurances. If she agrees to participate, Ms. Malic would benefit from grief counseling.
2. What would be a successful outcome for this patient?

By next visit, Ms. Malic vocalizes her fears for her baby and herself and lists the benefits of grief counseling.

3. What intellectual, technical, interpersonal, and/or ethical/legal competencies are most likely to bring about the desired outcome?
   Intellectual: ability to identify the impact that loss, grief, and death and dying have on the patient and his or her family members
   Interpersonal: ability to establish trusting relationships, even in times of great crisis related to anticipatory loss
   Ethical/Legal: commitment to safety and quality, strong sense of responsibility and accountability, and strong advocacy skills
4. What resources might be helpful for Ms. Malic?
   Grief counseling, information on premature babies

## PATIENT CARE STUDY

1. Objective data are underlined; subjective data are in boldface.
   LeRoy is a <u>40-year-old architect</u> whose life partner, Michael, is dying of AIDS. Although both LeRoy and Michael "did the bathhouse scene" in the early 1980s and had multiple unprotected sexual encounters, they have been in a monogamous relationship for the past 14 years. Michael has been in and out of the hospital during the past 3 years and is now dying of end-stage AIDS at home. He is enrolled in a hospice program. LeRoy has been very supportive of Michael throughout the different phases of his illness but at present **seems to be "losing it."** Michael noticed that LeRoy is <u>sleeping at odd times and seems to be losing weight</u>. **He suspects that LeRoy may be drinking more than usual and using recreational drugs.** He also says that **he is "acting strangely"; he seems emotionally withdrawn and unusually uncommunicative. "I don't think he's able to deal with the fact that I am dying,"** Michael tells you. "He won't let me talk about it at all." The hospice nurse notes that <u>LeRoy is now rarely home when he comes to visit</u>. When the hospice nurse calls to arrange a meeting with LeRoy, LeRoy informs him that he is **"managing quite well, thank you,"** and that **he has no concerns or problems to discuss.**
2. Nursing Process Worksheet
   *Health Problem:* Anticipatory grieving
   *Etiology:* Inability to allow himself to think about what his life will be like without his life partner; history of using denial as a coping mechanism
   *Signs and Symptoms:* Partner reports that LeRoy is sleeping at odd times and seems to be losing weight. He suspects that LeRoy is drinking more than usual and using recreational drugs. He also says that he is "acting strangely" and that he seems emotionally withdrawn and unusually uncommunicative. LeRoy is now rarely home when the hospice nurse visits. When the nurse called to arrange a meeting with him, LeRoy informed him that he was "managing quite well, thank you" and that he had no concerns or problems to discuss.
   *Expected Outcome:* LeRoy will openly express his grief over Michael's impending death and participate in decision making for the future.
   *Nursing Interventions:*
   a. Determine what is making this anticipated loss so "unthinkable."
   b. Encourage patient to share concerns. Normalize the experience of grieving by sharing experiences of other gay partners who have successfully grieved over the death of their friends and loved ones. Respect patient's use of denial to make time to work things through. Let him know you are available to help at a later date, if necessary.
   c. Help the patient explore his usual strategies for adjusting to loss (i.e., denial) and determine how they are serving him now. If he feels they are inadequate, help him develop new strategies.
   d. Promote grief work through each phase of the grieving process: denial, isolation, depression, anger, guilt, fear, rejection. Help Michael understand LeRoy's grief and need to move in and out of each stage at his own pace.
   e. Refer patient to community-based support groups.

   *Evaluative Statement:* 5/1/20: Goal not met. LeRoy is still denying that he is experiencing any difficulty dealing with Michael's impending death; appears fearful of even discussing this subject. Revision: Reiterated stages of grieving and importance of grief work; offered a listening ear should he decide he wishes to talk about this later.
   *— C. Taylor, RN*
3. Patient strengths: LeRoy's long-standing relationship with Michael and desire to be present and supportive is a powerful motivator for getting him to address his inability to consciously work through his grief. LeRoy is intelligent and trusts health care professionals, with whom he has had good experiences in the past.
   Personal strengths: Knowledge about stages of grief and grief work; strong interpersonal skills; teaching and counseling skills.
4. 5/13/20: LeRoy, the patient's life partner and significant other, called today to arrange a time to meet. He noted that he finally had a long talk with Michael and can see that he hasn't been able to deal with his dying in a conscious manner at all: "I guess I just kept hoping that if I didn't think about it, it wouldn't happen." He says he realizes that if he continues in this manner, he won't be able to provide Michael the support he needs. He also admits feeling "totally overwhelmed." Brief discussion of stages of grieving and grief work, and appointment made for follow-up.
   *— C. Taylor, RN*

## PRACTICING FOR NCLEX

### MULTIPLE CHOICE QUESTIONS

| | | | | |
|---|---|---|---|---|
| **1.** c | **2.** d | **3.** b | **4.** a | **5.** b |
| **6.** d | **7.** d | **8.** b | | |

### ALTERNATE-FORMAT QUESTIONS

#### Multiple Response Questions

1. a, c, f
2. b, d, e
3. d, e, f
4. a, c, d
5. a, d, e, f
6. b, d, e, f

# CHAPTER 44

## ASSESSING YOUR UNDERSTANDING

### FILL IN THE BLANKS

1. Sensory reception
2. Kinesthesia
3. Stereognosis
4. impaired memory
5. sensory deficit

### MATCHING EXERCISES

| | | | | |
|---|---|---|---|---|
| **1.** h | **2.** d | **3.** a | **4.** c | **5.** b |
| **6.** f | **7.** e | **8.** a | **9.** c | **10.** d |
| **11.** b | **12.** c | **13.** d | **14.** b | **15.** a |

### SHORT ANSWER

1. **a.** A stimulus, an agent, act, or other influence capable of initiating a response by the nervous system.
   **b.** A receptor or sense organ must receive the stimulus and convert it into a nerve impulse.
   **c.** The nerve impulse must be conducted along a nervous pathway from the receptor or sense organ to the brain.
   **d.** A particular area in the brain must receive and translate the impulse into a sensation.
2. Sample answers:
   **a.** Environment: A patient with AIDS in isolation is at high risk for sensory deprivation.
   **b.** Impaired ability to receive environmental stimuli: A patient who is visually impaired is at high risk for sensory deprivation.
   **c.** Inability to process environmental stimuli: A patient who is confused cannot process environmental stimuli.
3. **a.** Perceptual responses: inaccurate perception of sights, sounds, tastes, smells, and body position; poor coordination and equilibrium; mild to gross distortions in perception, ranging from daydreams to hallucinations
   **b.** Cognitive responses: inability to control the direction of thought content; decreased attention span and ability to concentrate; difficulty with memory, problem solving, and task performance
   **c.** Emotional responses: inappropriate emotional responses: apathy, anxiety, fear, anger, belligerence, panic, depression; rapid mood changes
4. Sample answers:
   **a.** A patient is disoriented by the strange sights, odors, and sounds in a CCU.
   **b.** A burn victim is in constant pain and cannot concentrate on his environment.
   **c.** A confused patient panics at the sight of doctors and nurses probing his body.
5. Cultural care deprivation is a lack of culturally assistive, supportive, or facilitative acts (e.g., touching is viewed as a natural and welcome custom in certain cultures, while in other cultures it is taboo).
6. Sample answers:
   **a.** Infant: soothing sounds, rocking, holding and changing position, changing patterns of light and shade, developing appropriate play
   **b.** Adult: use of music, poetry, drama to alleviate boredom
   **c.** Older adult: use of art classes or organizing a book club in a long-term care facility
7. Sample answers:
   **a.** Patient will report feeling safe and in control of his or her environment.
   **b.** Patient will verbalize acceptance of the sensory deficit.
8. Sample answer:
   This patient is suffering from sensory deprivation. Measures should be taken to stimulate as many senses as possible. The curtains could be opened to allow light into the room; soft music could be played to stimulate auditory functioning; flavorful meals could be prepared to stimulate taste; flowers, cards, and pictures could be displayed to stimulate visual functioning.
9. **a.** Avoid damage from UV rays.
   **b.** Use caution with aerosol sprays.
   **c.** Have regular eye examinations and tests for glaucoma.
   **d.** Know the danger signals that indicate serious eye problems.
10. Sample answers:
    **a.** Visual: Read different types of books to the child; limit television watching; plan various outings.
    **b.** Auditory: Teach the child songs; play records; join a storytelling group.
    **c.** Olfactory: Have child identify different odors; prepare enticing meals and savor the aromas.
    **d.** Gustatory: Encourage the child to experiment with different foods with varying colors, tastes, shapes, and textures; introduce finger foods into diet.
    **e.** Tactile: Use games and sports to increase body contact with child; demonstrate affection by hugging, holding child in lap, etc.

11. Sample answers:
    a. Developmental considerations: The adult may experience the need to compensate for the loss of one type of stimulation by increasing other sources of sensory stimuli.
    b. Culture and lifestyle: A person's culture may dictate how much sensory stimulation is considered normal.
    c. Personality: Different personality types demand different levels of stimulation.
    d. Stress: Increased sensory stimulation may be sought during periods of high stress.
    e. Illness and medication: Illness can affect the reception of sensory stimuli; medications that alert or depress the central nervous system may interfere with the perception of sensory stimuli.
12. Sample answers:
    a. Stimulation: Assess for recent changes in sensory stimulation if the type of stimulation present is developmentally appropriate.
    b. Reception: Assess for anything that may interfere with sensory reception and prescribe any corrective devices the patient may use to overcome sensory impairment.
    c. Transmission–perception–reaction: High-risk patients include confused patients and patients with nervous system impairments. Assess the patient's abilities to transmit, perceive, and react to stimuli during everyday interactions.
13. Sample answers:
    a. Visually impaired patients: Acknowledge your presence in the patient's room, identify yourself by name, and speak in a normal tone of voice.
    b. Hearing-impaired patients: Avoid excessive noise, avoid excessive cleaning of ears, and know the symptoms of hearing loss.
    c. Unconscious patients: Be careful of what is said in the patient's presence; assume the person can hear you, and speak to the person before touching him.

## APPLYING YOUR KNOWLEDGE

### REFLECTIVE PRACTICE: CULTIVATING QSEN COMPETENCIES

#### Sample Answers

1. What nursing interventions might be appropriate for Mr. Pirolla?
   Sensory deprivation can lead to perceptual, cognitive, and emotional disturbances. Therefore, the nursing care plan should include sensory stimulation for Mr. and Mrs. Pirolla. The nurse should also investigate if hearing aids would help Mr. Pirolla with his hearing loss. The nurse should assess both Mr. Pirolla and his wife to see how they are coping with the changes in their social environment. Safety in the home and community is also an issue that needs to be addressed. The nurse should incorporate knowledge of the guidelines for communicating both with persons with reduced vision and hearing when developing a teaching plan to assist Mrs. Pirolla in dealing with her husband's condition.
2. What would be a successful outcome for this patient?
   By next visit, Mr. Pirolla states that he is adapting to his condition and receiving new sensory stimulation from his environment.
3. What intellectual, technical, interpersonal, and/or ethical/legal competencies are most likely to bring about the desired outcome?
   Intellectual: Knowledge of the arousal mechanism and how the body responds, including sensoristasis and adaptation; ability to integrate knowledge of sensory alterations, including factors contributing to disturbed sensory perceptions.
   Interpersonal: Demonstration of the ability to empathize and communicate with patients with sensory deficits and interact effectively with patients and their caregivers.
4. What resources might be helpful for Mr. Pirolla?
   Social services, printed materials on sensory deficits, community services

### PATIENT CARE STUDY

1. Objective data are underlined; subjective data are in boldface.
   George Gibson, an <u>81-year-old, married, African-American man</u>, reluctantly reports, after much prodding from his wife, that he is not hearing as well as he used to be. **"I don't know what the trouble is," he tells you. "I'm in perfect health, always have been. More and more, people just seem to be mumbling instead of talking."** You notice <u>he is seated on the edge of his chair and bends toward you when you speak to him. His wife reports that he has stopped going out and pretty much stays in his room whenever people come to visit</u> because **he is embarrassed** by his inability to hear. "This is really a shame, because <u>George was always the life of the party,</u>" she says. You ask Mr. Gibson if he has ever had his hearing evaluated, and he tells you no, until now, he's been trying **to convince himself that nothing's wrong with his hearing.**
2. Nursing Process Worksheet
   *Health Problem:* Sensory/perceptual alteration: auditory.
   *Etiology:* Reluctance to accept that he has an auditory problem and to seek help.
   *Signs and Symptoms:* Leans forward to hear speaker; attempts to deny hearing loss and attributes problem to others who are "mumbling"; has greatly reduced opportunities for conversation; has not sought help until now.
   *Expected Outcome:* After medical evaluation of hearing loss and treatment, patient demonstrates

better coping skills by increasing amount of time he spends socializing.
*Nursing Interventions:*
**a.** Explain that hearing loss often accompanies aging and that a medical evaluation is important to provide proper treatment.
**b.** Help patient make an appointment for evaluation.
**c.** Explore strategies for improving his communication skills and preventing social isolation.
*Evaluative Statement:* 12/5/20: Goal partially met—hearing aid has enabled patient to comprehend most one-to-one conversations, but ability to hear well in groups is still impaired. Is willing to investigate possibility of learning to lip-read. No longer avoids company, especially if it is only one or two people. *— D. Mason, RN*

**3.** Patient strengths: healthy until now; wife is supportive; previous history of strong interactional skills
Personal strengths: recognize significance of sensory/perceptual alterations; able to distinguish changes in perceptual abilities normally related to aging from those indicating treatable medical problems; able to establish trusting relationship with older adults

**4.** 12/5/20: Patient presents after auditory examination revealed a partial sensorineural loss that was distorting his perception of certain frequencies; partially correctable with amplification. Patient still leans close to speaker, but in a one-to-one conversation, his responses demonstrate his ability to correctly interpret most of what the speaker is saying. He reports that he still has great difficulty listening in groups. His wife notes with delight that he seems "more like his old self" when one or two friends come to visit. He expresses an interest in learning to lip-read. *— D. Mason, RN*

## PRACTICING FOR NCLEX

### MULTIPLE CHOICE QUESTIONS

**1.** c **2.** d **3.** b **4.** a **5.** b
**6.** d **7.** b

### ALTERNATE-FORMAT QUESTIONS

#### Multiple Response Questions

**1.** b, c, e, f
**2.** c, d, e
**3.** a, c, e
**4.** d, e, f
**5.** a, d, f
**6.** b, d, f
**7.** c, e, f

# CHAPTER 45

## ASSESSING YOUR UNDERSTANDING

### FILL IN THE BLANKS

**1.** Sexuality
**2.** Gender identity
**3.** Sexual orientation
**4.** premenstrual syndrome (PMS)
**5.** erogenous zones
**6.** Norplant
**7.** transdermal contraceptive

### MATCHING EXERCISES

**1.** d **2.** a **3.** h **4.** b **5.** g
**6.** e **7.** c **8.** f

### SHORT ANSWER

**1.** Sample answers:
**a.** Chronic pain: Teach altered or modified positions for coitus.
**b.** Diabetes: Some men may be candidates for a penile prosthesis; pharmacologic management of erectile dysfunction may be indicated.
**c.** Cardiovascular disease: Teach gradual resumption of sexual activity, comfortable position for affected partner.
**d.** Loss of body part: Teach acceptance of body image.
**e.** Spinal cord injury: Promote stimulation of other erogenous zones.
**f.** Mental illness: Provide counseling for depression.
**g.** Sexually transmitted infections: Educate the public about the prevention and treatment of STIs.

**2. a.** Follicular phase: Days 4 to 14; a number of follicles mature, but only one produces a mature ovum; at the same time, in the uterus the endometrium is becoming thick and velvety in preparation for the fertilized egg.
**b.** Proliferation phase: Ovulation occurs on day 14; the mature ovum ruptures from the follicle and is swept into the fallopian tube. If sperm are present, the ovum is fertilized at this time.
**c.** Luteal phase: Days 15 to 28; the empty follicle fills with a yellow pigment and is then called the corpus luteum, which produces hormones that encourage a fertilized egg to grow. If fertilization does not occur, the corpus luteum disintegrates.
**d.** Secretory phase: The endometrial lining becomes thick; in the absence of fertilized egg, the corpus luteum dies, and the endometrial lining disintegrates; menses begins on day 28 as a result of the uterus shedding the endometrial lining.

**3. a.** Excitement phase:
Female: The breasts of the woman swell and nipples become erect; vaginal lubricant seeps out of body; upper two thirds of vagina expand; clitoris enlarges and emerges slightly from clitoral hood; labia enlarge and turn deep rosy red.

Male: Erection of the penis caused by increased congestion with blood; scrotum noticeably elevates, thickens, and enlarges. The skin of the penis and scrotum turns deep reddish-purple; male nipples may harden and become erect.

**b.** Plateau:
Female: The clitoris retracts and disappears under clitoral hood; intensity is greater than that of excitement phase but not enough to begin orgasm.
Male: Secretions from Cowper's glands may appear at the glans of the penis during this phase.

**c.** Orgasm:
Female: The orgasm phase begins with a heightened feeling of physical pleasure followed by overwhelming release and involuntary contractions of the genitals. Loss of muscular control can cause spastic contractions.
Male: Involuntary spasmodic contractions of the genitals occur in the penis, epididymis, vas deferens, and rectum; most often accompanied by ejaculation.

**d.** Resolution:
Female: Return to normal body functioning; feelings of relaxation, fatigue, and fulfillment; the woman is physiologically capable of immediate response to sexual stimulation and may achieve multiple orgasms.
Male: Return to normal body functioning accompanied by same feelings as above; men experience a refractory period during which they are incapable of sexual response.

**4. a.** Any inpatient or outpatient who is receiving care for pregnancy, an STI, infertility, or conception
**b.** Any patient who is currently experiencing a sexual dysfunction or problem
**c.** Any patient whose illness will affect sexual functioning and behavior in any way

**5.** Sample answers:
**a.** "How would you describe this problem?"
**b.** "What do you think caused the problem, or what was happening when you first noticed it?"
**c.** "What have you tried in the past to correct the problem?"

**6. a.** A change in knowledge
**b.** A change in patient attitude
**c.** A change in behavior

**7.** See table below.

| Method | Advantages | Disadvantages |
|---|---|---|
| **a.** Behavioral | Methods can be effective in avoiding pregnancy if mutual understanding, support, and motivation exist between the woman and her partner. There are no side effects (as in hormonal methods) and no messy devices to insert. Periodic abstinence and fertility awareness methods are two methods of contraception that involve charting a woman's fertility pattern. The best approach to monitoring fertility is a combination of temperature methods, cervical mucus method, and calendar method, called the symptothermal method. | Requires abstinence during ovulation and complete understanding of the signs and symptoms of ovulation. Continuous abstinence involves not having any sex with a partner at all. It is 100% effective in preventing pregnancy and STIs. However, people may find it difficult to abstain for long periods of time. |
| **b.** Barrier methods | Condoms help to prevent STIs; appropriate for women with sensitivity to the pill; effective when used correctly; relatively inexpensive methods. | Devices must be applied before intercourse; not all women can wear them; threat of toxic shock syndrome with vaginal sponge. |
| **c.** Intrauterine devices | High rate of effectiveness; little care or motivation on part of patient is necessary; excellent method for women who have completed their families but are not ready for sterilization. | Serious side effects and complications. |
| **d.** Hormonal methods | Many beneficial noncontraceptive effects, for example, protecting women against development of breast, ovarian, and endometrial cancer; almost 100% effective when taken as directed. | Cost may be prohibitive to some; compliance is necessary; some women should not take the pill due to physiologic disorders or diseases. |
| **e.** Sterilization | After initial surgery and recheck, no further compliance is necessary; almost 100% effective. | Should be considered permanent and irreversible. |

## APPLYING YOUR KNOWLEDGE

### REFLECTIVE PRACTICE: CULTIVATING QSEN COMPETENCIES

#### Sample Answers

1. What issues might the nurse address in the care plan for Mr. Smith? What patient teaching should be incorporated into the care plan?
   The nurse should review the effects of Mr. Smith's conditions on sexual function and assess his current status, as well as the effect of the medications he is taking to see if they are a contributing factor. The nurse could consult with the primary health care provider to see if an adjustment in the medications might alleviate the problem. The nurse should also explore the emotional and psychological effects of the dysfunction on Mr. Smith and his wife and consult with other members of the health care team to develop an effective care plan. Patient teaching could include information about medications to treat impotence and the possibility of having a penile implant.
2. What would be a successful outcome for this patient?
   Following an adjustment to his medications, Mr. Smith vocalizes an improvement in his sexual functioning.
3. What intellectual, technical, interpersonal, and/or ethical/legal competencies are most likely to bring about the desired outcome?
   Intellectual: Ability to integrate knowledge about sexual health into nursing care, including the ability to identify areas of sexual dysfunction for the patient with a history of diabetes and hypertension experiencing impotence.
   Interpersonal: Strong interpersonal skills to establish trusting relationships and build rapport with a patient experiencing impotence.
4. What resources might be helpful for Mr. Smith?
   Counseling, printed materials on impotence and corrective measures, information on the effect of medications on sexual functioning

### PATIENT CARE STUDY

1. Objective data are underlined; subjective data are in boldface.
   Anthony Piscatelli, <u>a 6-ft-tall, muscular, healthy 19-year-old college freshman in the School of Nursing,</u> confides to his nursing advisor that "**everything is great**" about college life, with one exception: "**All of a sudden, I find myself questioning the values I learned at home about sex and marriage.** My Mom was really insistent that each of her sons should respect women and that intercourse was something you saved until you were ready to get married. If she told us once, she told us a hundred times, that we'd save ourselves, the girls in our lives, and her and Dad a lot of heartache if we could just learn to control ourselves sexually. Problem is that no one here seems to subscribe to this philosophy. **I feel like I'm abnormal in some way to even think like this.** There's a lot of sexual activity in the dorms, and no one even thinks you're serious if you talk about virginity positively. What do you think? Did my Mom sell me a bill of goods? Is it true that if you take the proper precautions, no one gets hurt and everyone has a good time?" Tony reports that **he is a virgin and that he really misses his close family back home: "I do get lonely at times and would love to just cuddle with someone or even give and get a big hug, but no one seems to understand this."**
2. Nursing Process Worksheet
   *Health Problem:* High risk for altered sexuality patterns
   *Etiology:* Discrepancy between his family's values about sex and marriage and those he is discovering in peer group
   *Signs and Symptoms:* "All of a sudden, I find myself questioning the values I learned at home about sex and marriage"; feels like he is "abnormal" in some way to value virginity; lonely—wants intimacy; "Is it true that if you take the proper precautions, no one gets hurt and everyone has a good time?"
   *Expected Outcome:* By next meeting, 11/17/20, patient will report personal satisfaction with the results of his reevaluation of his beliefs/values concerning sex and marriage.
   *Nursing Interventions:*
   a. Assess patient's knowledge of sexual development and need for intimacy and belonging, and correct any misinformation.
   b. Explore with the patient the source of the beliefs/values he learned at home and assist in determining the role he wants these beliefs/values to play in his life.
   c. Compare the options of abstinence and becoming sexually active and perform related sexual teaching.
   d. Refer to appropriate on-campus sexuality classes, counseling center, or seminars, as indicated.

   *Evaluative Statement:* 11/17/20: Goal not met. Patient reports that his confusion has only deepened and he now feels like "my head is warring with my body." Reports sleeping with his girlfriend but feeling very guilty afterward—now ignores this girl. Revision: See if he's willing to talk with a peer or professional counselor regarding sexual concerns.
   *— R. LeBon, RN*
3. Patient strengths: healthy; caring family; ability to voice his concerns; very "likable" person
   Personal strengths: sound knowledge of sexuality; respect for and appreciation of sexuality; understanding of developmental challenges of young adults and self-identity and intimacy needs; ability to create trusting relationships with young adults
4. 11/17/20: Patient states he is "more confused now" than when we last met. He yielded to peer pressure and slept with girlfriend; used condom. While he "enjoyed this experience," he has been "wracked

with guilt" ever since. He cannot reconcile this behavior with what he learned at home and continues to feel "unsure" of who he wants to be. He definitely wants some resolution of this conflict and is interested in speaking with a professional sexuality counselor. Referral made. — *R. LeBon, RN*

## PRACTICING FOR NCLEX

### MULTIPLE CHOICE QUESTIONS

**1.** a **2.** c **3.** c **4.** b **5.** d
**6.** c **7.** b **8.** b **9.** c

### ALTERNATE-FORMAT QUESTIONS

#### Multiple Response Questions

1. a, b, c, e
2. b, c, f
3. b, c, d
4. d, e, f
5. b, d, e
6. c, d, e, f
7. a, b, e

#### Prioritization Questions

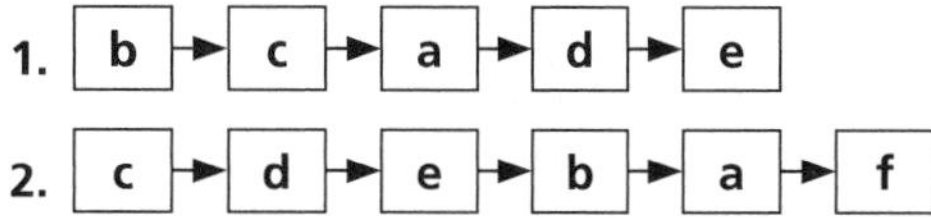


# CHAPTER 46

## ASSESSING YOUR UNDERSTANDING

### FILL IN THE BLANKS

1. alienation
2. Spiritual distress
3. forgiveness
4. spiritual guilt
5. Christian scientist

### MATCHING EXERCISES

**1.** d **2.** a **3.** e **4.** b **5.** g
**6.** c **7.** a **8.** d **9.** c **10.** b
**11.** a **12.** d **13.** c

### SHORT ANSWER

1. a. Need for meaning and purpose
   b. Need for love and relatedness
   c. Need for forgiveness
2. Sample answers:
   a. Offering a compassionate presence
   b. Assisting in the struggle to find meaning and purpose in the face of suffering, illness, and death
   c. Fostering relationships with God/humans that nurture the spirit
   d. Facilitating the patient's expression of religious or spiritual beliefs and practices
3. a. Life-affirming influences: enhance life, give meaning and purpose to existence, strengthen feeling of self-worth, encourage self-actualization, and are health giving and life-sustaining
   b. Life-denying influences: restrict or enclose life patterns, limit experiences and associations, place burdens of guilt on people, encourage feelings of unworthiness, and are generally health denying and life inhibiting
4. Sample answers:
   a. Many religions prescribe dietary requirements and restrictions.
   b. Some religious faiths restrict birth control practices.
5. Sample answers:
   a. As a guide to daily living: Religions may specify dietary requirements or birth control measures.
   b. As a source of support: It is common for people to seek support from religious faith in times of stress; this support is often vital to the acceptance of an illness. Prayer, devotional reading, and other religious practices often do for the person spiritually what protective exercises do for the body physically.
   c. As a source of strength and healing: People have been known to endure extreme physical distress because of strong faith; patients' families have taken on almost unbelievable rehabilitative tasks because they had faith in the eventual positive results of their effort.
   d. As a source of conflict: There are times when religious beliefs conflict with prevalent health care practices; for example, the doctrine of Jehovah's Witnesses prohibits blood transfusions. For some, illness is viewed as punishment for sin and is inevitable.
6. a. Developmental considerations: As a child matures, life experiences usually influence and mature his or her spiritual beliefs. With advancing years, the tendency to think about life after death prompts some people to reexamine and reaffirm their spiritual beliefs.
   b. Family: A child's parents play a key role in the development of the child's spirituality.
   c. Ethnic background: Religious traditions differ among ethnic groups. There are clear distinctions between Eastern and Western spiritual traditions, as well as among those of individual ethnic groups, such as Native Americans.
   d. Formal religion: Each of the major religions has several characteristics in common.
   e. Life events: Both positive and negative life experiences can influence spirituality and in turn are influenced by the meaning a person's spiritual beliefs attribute to them.
7. Answers will vary with student experiences.
8. a. Basis of authority or source of power
   b. Scripture or sacred word
   c. An ethical code that defines right and wrong
   d. A psychology and identity that allow its adherents to fit into a group and the world to be defined by the religion
   e. Aspirations or expectations
   f. Some ideas about what follows death

9. Sample answers:
   a. Spiritual pain: "This seems to be a source of deep pain for you."
   b. Spiritual alienation: "Does it seem like God is far away from your life?"
   c. Spiritual anxiety: "Are you afraid that God might not be there for you when you need Him?"
   d. Spiritual anger: "I sense a great deal of anger in your statements about God taking away your daughter. Can you share more about this?"
   e. Spiritual loss: "Tell me more about how your inability to get to the synagogue is affecting you."
   f. Spiritual despair: "So you are saying that no matter how hard you try, you'll never be able to be close to God?"
10. Diagnosis: Hopelessness related to belief that God doesn't care
    Nursing care plan: The nurse should offer a supportive presence, facilitate the patient's practice of religion, counsel the patient spiritually, or contact a spiritual counselor.
11. Answers will vary with student experiences.
    a. The room should be orderly and free of clutter.
    b. There should be a seat for the counselor at the bedside or near the patient.
    c. The top of the bedside table should be free of items and covered with a clean, white cover if a sacrament is to be administered.
    d. The bed curtains should be drawn to provide privacy, or the patient should be moved to a private setting.
13. Sample answers:
    a. Deficit: Meaning and purpose: Explore with the patient what has given his or her life meaning and purpose to the present, sources of meaning for other people, and possible meaning of illness. Refer the patient to a spiritual advisor and appropriate support groups.
    b. Deficit: Love and relatedness: Treat the patient at all times with respect, empathy, and genuine caring.
    c. Deficit: Forgiveness: Offer a supportive presence to the patient that demonstrates your acceptance of him or her. Explore the patient's self-expectations and assist the patient in determining how realistic they are. Explore the importance of learning to accept oneself and others.

## APPLYING YOUR KNOWLEDGE

### REFLECTIVE PRACTICE: CULTIVATING QSEN COMPETENCIES

#### Sample Answers

1. How might the nurse use blended nursing skills to provide holistic, competent nursing care for Ms. Zeuner?
   Ms. Zeuner is in need of assistance at home to help her care for her husband. The nurse could check with social services or look into community services that would allow her to attend her church services and other community support groups.
2. What would be a successful outcome for this patient?
   By next visit, Ms. Zeuner vocalizes a connectedness with her church and community stimulated by receiving help at home with her husband.
3. What intellectual, technical, interpersonal, and/or ethical/legal competencies are most likely to bring about the desired outcome?
   Intellectual: ability to identify spirituality as a source of patient support, strength, or conflict, incorporating this information into the patient's care plan
   Interpersonal: ability to establish trusting relationships, even in times of distress, crisis, and conflict. Ability to demonstrate respect, empathy, and caring for the patient
4. What resources might be helpful to Ms. Zeuner?
   Respite care, meals-on-wheels, parish nursing, community support groups

### PATIENT CARE STUDY

1. Objective data are underlined; subjective data are in boldface.
   Jeffrey Stein, a 31-year-old attorney, is in a step-down unit following his transfer from the cardiac care unit, where he was treated for a massive heart attack. **"Bad hearts run in my family, but I never thought it would happen to me," he says. "I jog several times a week and work out at the gym, eat a low-fat diet, and I don't smoke."** Jeffrey is **5 ft 7 in tall, weighs about 150 lb, and is well built**. During his second night in the step-down unit, he is unable to sleep and tells the nurse, **"I've really got a lot on my mind tonight. I can't stop thinking about how close I was to death.** If I wasn't with someone who knew how to do CPR when I keeled over, I probably wouldn't be here today." Gentle questioning reveals that Mr. Stein is worried about what would have happened had he died. **"I don't think I've ever thought seriously about my mortality, and I sure don't think much about God.** My parents were semiobservant Jews, but I don't go to synagogue myself. I celebrate the holidays, but that's about all. **If there is a God, I wonder what he thinks about me."** He asks if there is a rabbi or anyone he can talk with in the morning who could answer some questions for him and perhaps help him get himself back on track. **"For the last couple of years, all I've been concerned about is paying off my school debts and making money.** I guess there's a whole lot more to life, and maybe this was my invitation to sort out my priorities."
2. Nursing Process Worksheet
   *Health Problem:* Spiritual distress: spiritual anxiety.
   *Etiology:* Challenged belief and value system.
   *Signs and Symptoms:* Recent massive heart attack; unable to sleep; raised in semiobservant Jewish

family but, "for the last couple of years all I've been concerned about is paying off my school debts and making money"; questions about afterlife.
*Expected Outcome:* After meeting with Rabbi White 2/12/20, patient reported feeling "less anxious" about his religious belief system and reevaluated sense of priorities.
*Nursing Interventions:*
**a.** Encourage patient to continue to share concerns about his religious beliefs and value system.
**b.** Arrange for patient to talk with the hospital's Jewish chaplain in the morning.
**c.** Normalize this experience by sharing with the patient that serious illness often prompts a life review.
**d.** Recommend that the patient begin to list the things in life that are most important to him.
*Evaluative Statement:* Patient slept past two nights after meeting with Rabbi White and reports being "less anxious" about "religion." He says there are some things he wants to change about his life, and that this is a good time to start.
— *T. Michael Gray, RN*

**3.** Patient strengths: Healthy; practices healthy self-care behaviors; strongly motivated to attain life goals. Knows himself well enough to "name his problems" and cares enough about himself to seek the assistance he needs.
Personal strengths: Belief that meeting spiritual needs is an important component of good nursing; excellent rapport with the hospital's pastoral care department; history of establishing therapeutic relationships with patients.

**4.** 0200, 2/14/20: Before patient fell asleep, he thanked me for arranging for him to meet with Rabbi White. "I guess I did what a lot of people do—forget all about God while they try to make a living." He appears less anxious about his religious beliefs and feels that his "recent bout with death" was a timely reminder to evaluate his priorities in life and make some needed changes. Sleeping peacefully at present.
— *T. Michael Gray, RN*

## PRACTICING FOR NCLEX

### MULTIPLE CHOICE QUESTIONS

**1.** b **2.** d **3.** c **4.** a **5.** b
**6.** d **7.** b **8.** a

### ALTERNATE-FORMAT QUESTIONS

### Multiple Response Questions

**1.** a, b, e
**2.** a, b, d
**3.** d, e
**4.** b, d, e
**5.** c, d